Conduct disorders in childhood and adolescence

Condu... ... ... cal
referra ... ... urs
in you ... ... ult
proble ...

   This ... ith
contrib ... ity
and pr ... o-
psychol ... n-
ces. Infl ... re
reviewe ... n-
siderati ... ok
develop ...

   Integ ... ve
survey ... th
practiti ... d
behavio ...

Jonatha ... ol
and Ald ... r,
Menning ...
with Der ...
ment in ...
Barbara ...
Developi ...
published ...
Fifteen Th

Cambridge Child and Adolescent Psychiatry

Child and adolescent psychiatry is an important and growing area of clinical psychiatry. The last decade has seen a rapid expansion of scientific knowledge in this field and has provided a new understanding of the underlying pathology of mental disorders in these age groups. This series is aimed at practitioners and researchers both in child and adolescent mental health services and developmental and clinical neuroscience. Focusing on psychopathology, it highlights those topics where the growth of knowledge has had the greatest impact on clinical practice and on the treatment and understanding of mental illness. Individual volumes benefit both from the international expertise of their contributors and a coherence generated through a uniform style and structure for the series. Each volume provides firstly an historical overview and a clear descriptive account of the psychopathology of a specific disorder or group of related disorders. These features then form the basis for a thorough critical review of the etiology, natural history, management, prevention and impact on later adult adjustment. Whilst each volume is therefore complete in its own right, volumes also relate to each other to create a flexible and collectable series that should appeal to students as well as experienced scientists and practitioners.

Editorial board

Already published in this series:

Conduct disorders in childhood and adolescence

Edited by

Jonathan Hill

and

Barbara Maughan

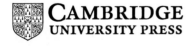 CAMBRIDGE
UNIVERSITY PRESS

CAMBRIDGE UNIVERSITY PRESS
Cambridge, New York, Melbourne, Madrid, Cape Town, Singapore, São Paulo

Cambridge University Press
The Edinburgh Building, Cambridge CB2 2RU, UK

Published in the United States of America by Cambridge University Press, New York

www.cambridge.org
Information on this title: www.cambridge.org/9780521786393

First published 2001

A catalogue record for this publication is available from the British Library

Library of Congress Cataloguing in Publication data

Conduct disorders in childhood and adolescence / edited by Jonathan Hill and Barbara Maughan.
    p.   cm. – (Cambridge child and adolescent psychiatry)
Includes index.
ISBN 0 521 78639 8 (pb)
1. Conduct disorders in children. 2. Conduct disorders in adolescence. I. Hill,
Jonathan, Prof. II. Maughan, Barbara, 1946– . III. Cambridge child and adolescent
psychiatry series
[DNLM: 1. Conduct Disorder – Adolescence. 2. Conduct Disorder – Child. WS 350.6
C7468 2000]
RJ499.C615 2000
618.92′89 – dc21   99-057084

ISBN-13 978-0-521-78639-3 paperback
ISBN-10 0-521-78639-8 paperback

Transferred to digital printing 2006

Every effort has been made in preparing this publication to provide accurate and up-to-date information which is in accord with accepted standards and practice at the time of publication. Nevertheless, the authors, editors and publisher can make no warranties that the information contained herein is totally free from error, not least because clinical standards are constantly changing through research and regulation. The authors, editors and publisher therefore disclaim all liability for direct or consequential damages resulting from the use of material contained in this publication. Readers are strongly advised to pay careful attention to information provided by the manufacturer of any drugs or equipment that they plan to use.

Contents

Contributors

Adrian Angold
Developmental Epidemiology Program
Box 3454, Duke University Medical Center
Durham NC 27710, USA

William M. Bukowski
Department of Psychology
Concordia University
PY 170
7141 Sherbrooke Way
Montreal, Quebec
Canada H4B 1R6

John Coie
Department of Psychology
Social and Health Sciences
Duke University
Durham NC 22710, USA

E. Jane Costello
Developmental Epidemiology Program
Box 3454, Duke University Medical Center
Durham NC 27710, USA

Michelle DeKlyen
Children's Hospital and Regional Medical
Center
4800 Sand Point Way
PO Box 5371, Seattle
Washington 98105–0371, USA

Thomas J. Dishion
Oregon Social Learning Center
207 East 5th Avenue
Suite 202, Eugene
Oregon 97401, USA

Judy Dunn
Social, Genetic and Developmental
Psychiatry Research Centre
Institute of Psychiatry
111 Denmark Hill
London SE5 8AF, UK

Bill Henry
Department of Psychology
Colby College
Waterville ME 04901, USA

Joe Herbert
Department of Anatomy
University of Cambridge
Downing Street
Cambridge CB2 3DY, UK

Jonathan Hill
University Child Mental Health Unit
Mulberry House
Royal Liverpool Children's Hospital
Alder Hey, Eaton Road,
Liverpool L12 2AP, UK

Robert A. Hinde
St John's College
Cambridge CB2 1TP, UK

Alan E. Kazdin
Department of Psychology
Yale University
PO Box 208205
New Haven
Connecticut
06520–8205, USA

Jeff Kiesner
Dipartimento di Psicologia dello
Sviluppo e della Socializzazione
Università degli Studi di Padova
via Venezias
35131 Padova
Italy

Martin Knapp
Centre for the Economics of Mental Health
Institute of Psychiatry
7 Windsor Walk
Denmark Hill
London SE5 8BB, UK

David LeMarquand
Rehabilitation and Forensic Programs
North Bay Psychiatric Hospital
4700 Highway 11 North
PO Box 3010
North Bay, ON
P1B 8L1, Canada

Rolf Loeber
Life History Studies
Western Psychiatric Institute and Clinic
3811 O'Hara Street
Pittsburgh PA 15213, USA

Donald R. Lynam
Department of Psychology
College of Arts and Sciences
University of Kentucky
115 Kastle Hall, Lexington
Kentucky 40506–0044, USA

Manuela Martinez
Area of Psychobiology
Faculty of Psychology
University of Valencia, Spain

Barbara Maughan
Social, Genetic and Developmental
Psychiatry Research Centre
Institute of Psychiatry
111 Denmark Hill
London SE5 8AF, UK

Jacquelyn Mize
Human Development and Family Studies
School of Human Sciences
Auburn University
AL 36849, USA

Gregory S. Pettit
Human Development and Family Studies
School of Human Sciences
Auburn University
AL 36849, USA

Jodi A. Polaha
Department of Psychology
Auburn University
AL 36849, USA

François Poulin
Départment de Psychologie
Université de Québec à Montréal
Case postale Centre-ville
Montréal
Québec H3C 3P8
Canada

Michael Rutter
Social, Genetic and Developmental
Psychiatry Research Centre
Institute of Psychiatry
111 Denmark Hill
London SE5 8AF, UK

Emily Simonoff
Department of Child and Adolescent
Psychiatry and Psychology
Bloomfield Clinic, Guy's Hospital
St Thomas Street
London SE1 9RT, UK

Matthew L. Speltz
Children's Hospital and Medical Center
4800 Sand Point Way
PO Box C5371, Seattle
Washington 98105, USA

Richard E. Tremblay
Research Unit on Children's Psychosocial
Maladjustment
3050 Edouard-Montpetit Blvd
CP6128, Succ. Centre-Ville
Montreal, Quebec, H3C 3J7
Canada

Frank Vitaro
Research Unit on Children's Psychosocial
Maladjustment
3050 Edouard-Montpetit Blvd
CP6128, Succ. Centre-Ville
Montreal, Quebec, H3C 3J7
Canada

Preface

Conduct disorder is a complex and puzzling topic. Viewed from one perspective, it might seem that oppositionality and aggression, lying and stealing are problems of social deviance, with little place in the research and clinical practice of mental health professionals. But closer investigation suggests a different view. Overlaps with social disadvantage are strong, but by no means complete; in addition, the long-term legacy of childhood conduct problems lies not only in continuing antisocial behaviours but in problems with interpersonal functioning and increased psychiatric risk. Conduct disorders are defined both socially and individually, and are influenced by both individual and social risks. Only a multifaceted approach will do them justice. That is the aim of this book.

Specifically, the volume aims both to inform and to equip the reader. The task of informing is in many ways straightforward. The chapters that follow – all written by leading experts in their fields – cover a wide spectrum of conceptual and empirical approaches, and synthesize and review current literature in their fields. The opening contributions set current debates in context, providing an historical perspective on changing societal responses to 'bad behaviour' in childhood, setting out links between normal and abnormal social development, and detailing current understandings of the neural and biosocial bases of aggression and antisocial behaviour. An overview of epidemiological findings then forms the backdrop to a series of chapters examining the broad spectrum of causal factors implicated in the genesis of childhood conduct problems: genetic and environmental, psychological and neuropsychological, social and interactional. The final chapters turn to broader issues: mechanisms for the persistence of antisocial behaviours in childhood; the personal and social burdens they presage for adult functioning; new approaches to applying health economic costings to conduct disorders; and the crucial issues of prevention and treatment. To conclude, Michael Rutter highlights some of the key challenges facing clinicians and researchers in the field of childhood conduct problems today.

The chapters bear witness to the range and depth of current research on childhood antisocial behaviour, and to the important advances made in our understanding of conduct problems over recent years. But as they also underline, many fundamental questions remain to be addressed. As a result, we need to approach emerging evidence both critically and creatively. The second main aim of the volume is to equip the reader for that task by addressing a series of more general themes.

The first concerns the nature of the phenomena we are attempting to explain. As currently conceptualized, conduct disorders are almost certainly heterogeneous. The ICD and DSM diagnostic criteria encompass a wide range of behaviours, arising at different ages, and showing varying patterns of correlated problems and comorbidity. Quite different mechanisms may underlie different subgroups in the conduct-disordered population; the key challenge lies in 'parsing' that heterogeneity in ways that can provide for real advances in both clinical practice and etiological understanding. Individual chapters illustrate a wide spectrum of approaches here. Perhaps, for example, we should focus on subtypes of aggression, elucidating their differing motivations (Hinde, chapter 2) and underlying neural systems (Herbert & Martinez, chapter 4). Alternately, the key distinction may be between covert and overt acts (Loeber & Coie, chapter 14), or problems that arise at different developmental periods, or show differing patterns of comorbidity (Angold & Costello, chapter 6). But there may also be arguments for casting our net more widely. The long-term outcomes of childhood conduct problems lie not only in antisocial behaviours but in a broader constellation of difficulties – in problems in relationship functioning, risks of psychiatric disorder, and difficulties in performing social roles (Maughan & Rutter, chapter 18). Perhaps we need a similarly broad characterization of antisocial problems in childhood? Difficulties in peer relationships, for example, are frequently associated with childhood conduct problems; although the nature of that association is complex (Vitaro et al., chapter 13), the combination of conduct problems and difficulties in social relationships may constitute an early indication of the group of problems characterized as antisocial personality disorder in adult life. Clarifying how these and other features contribute to the identification of clinically meaningful subtypes constitutes one major agenda for future research.

A second key issue concerns the interface between biological, psychological and social influences on childhood conduct problems. Most individual chapters focus on individual domains of risk, highlighting likely causal mechanisms in specific spheres. But our ambition has been that there should be no mystery about the ways in which they interact. Although we still do not have the detail in many areas, the general principles are clear. Crucially, the contributions bring out that the brain is a social organ, so that there is no useful division between the 'bio' and the 'social'. From birth onwards infants seek out social stimuli, and aggression forms part of the repertoire of social behaviours shown by all children. As Herbert and Martinez (chapter 4) outline, the neural underpinnings of aggression differ depending on the social function it performs. Furthermore, neural systems, psychological processes and social stimuli are in constant interaction. The development of the brain comes about through an interplay of genetically timed events and social experiences, each of which can have short and long-term consequences (Hill, chapter 5). Testosterone may influence aggression, and equally is influenced by patterns of social dominance. Early stressors can impact on neuroendocrine systems and on social cognitive and attachment processes. In a similar way, genetically informative studies are highlighting not only heritable contributions to conduct problems (Simonoff, chapter 8) but also the complex interplay between genetic and environmental effects (Maughan, chapter 7).

Many of the most fruitful recent lines of research have elucidated particular mechanisms in the social generation of antisocial problems in children. As Dunn (chapter 3) outlines, learning to cope with conflict is an important developmental task for all children, and goes hand in hand with increasing social understanding. How do these developments go awry in children with conduct problems? At the individual level, neuropsychological deficits – especially impairments in verbal skills and in planning and self-control – seem likely to constitute key vulnerability factors (Lynam & Henry, chapter 9). In terms of social processes, current research highlights the role of social reinforcement (Kiesner et al., chapter 10), social cognitive processes (Pettit et al., chapter 11) and attachment processes (DeKlyen & Speltz, chapter 12). Each is capable of illuminating the other. The elegant studies of micro processes in the reinforcement of deviant behaviours described by Kiesner and colleagues are further illuminated by the social cognitive processes described by Pettit. Studies of reinforcement have shown that the negative behaviours of peers, siblings or parents can increase the likelihood of a child behaving aggressively. The child's aggressive behaviours in turn increase the likelihood of further negative behaviour from others, giving rise to 'coercive cycles'. And aggressive children, perhaps especially those who have been harshly treated, are more likely to perceive threat in the actions of others. Social and individual risks are in continuing interaction, and contribute, as Loeber and Coie (chapter 14) discuss, to risks not only for the early genesis but also for the persistence of childhood conduct problems over time.

In this as in all areas that concern normal and deviant development, we need to be equipped to interpret research findings. Although it is beyond the scope of a book of this breadth and size to consider detailed methodological issues, the authors have all indicated strengths and limitations in relation to key studies they discuss. Representativeness of samples, sample size, possible biases, methods of measurement, strengths of associations and effects of multiple analyses are all referred to where they are important to the interpretation of data, and are all seen as critical to scientific advance. To tackle complex personal problems, appropriately sophisticated methodologies are crucial; key methodological concerns are thus highlighted throughout the volume.

The interplay between research and practice constitutes a fourth central theme. For those who treat conduct-disordered children in their day to day practice, or who aim to intervene to prevent their difficulties, the acid test of theoretical advances must lie in their capacity to inform and improve our responses to conduct-disordered children and their families. In the past, conduct disorders were often regarded as among the most recalcitrant of childhood difficulties, that little in the clinician's armamentarium could effectively reach. As Kazdin (chapter 15) discusses in relation to treatment, and LeMarquand and colleagues (chapter 16) in relation to prevention, that situation is gradually changing. We can now identify promising treatment modalities, and careful re-analysis of the prevention literature, alongside major new large-scale trials, are also highlighting effective strategies in that domain. Importantly, as these authors underline, the tasks of evaluating interventions and developing theory interact, each casting light on the other. As we enter the new millennium, we are at major growing-points in both our understanding of childhood conduct disorders, and in our approaches to treatment; the chapters in this volume mark important steps in that advance.

Jonathan Hill and Barbara Maughan

Bad behaviour: an historical perspective on disorders of conduct

E. Jane Costello and Adrian Angold

Introduction

Conduct disorder is by many centuries the oldest of the diagnostic categories used in contemporary child psychiatry. Long before psychiatry and psychology were born, people agonized over what to do with out-of-control children. We are still agonizing. Furthermore, we are still agonizing about the same questions.

The questions that have troubled people over the centuries about out-of-control children fall into three overlapping groups:

Questions of the relationship between family and state in the control of children

Can the state control how parents treat children?

Can the state hold parents responsible for children's behaviour?

What are the state's responsibilities in the raising of children, including children whose families cannot control them?

Questions of the development of personal responsibility

What makes an action reprehensible? Is it the act itself, or the intention behind the act?

At what age or developmental stage should individuals be held accountable for their reprehensible actions? Is responsibility an all-or-nothing phenomenon, or is it graduated? Does personal responsibility vary with the nature of the act?

Is the same set of behaviours sanctionable at all ages, or are there 'status offences' that should only be punishable if committed by children?

Questions about the appropriate regulatory agencies for out-of-control children

In what circumstances are out-of-control children the responsibility of the family, the legal system, the religious system, the educational system, the social services system or the medical system?

What should be the relative roles of prevention, restitution, deterrence, and reform in the response of these agencies to out-of-control children?

In the first section of this chapter we take a rapid historical tour of how different societies have grappled with these questions. Over 3000 years and countless attempts to regulate human social behaviour, one can see five overlapping approaches to dealing with deviant children: the religious (deviance as sin), the legal (deviance as crime), the medical (deviance as sickness), the social (deviance as response to environment) and the educational (deviance as ignorance). Given limited space, we concentrate here on the first three of these approaches. We discuss how each has been used in attempts to answer the kinds of question listed above. Finally, we suggest another approach within which to consider conduct disorder: that of evolutionary psychology, which looks at the two major components of conduct disorder, deceit and aggression, in the light of the selection pressures operating on our species over the past few million years.

A note about terminology

In the words of August Aichhorn, the first person to apply psychoanalytic concepts and methods to out-of-control children: 'A strict definition or delimitation of these groups is difficult because they tend to merge into each other, but you are familiar with these cases from everyday observation, in social work, in the child guidance clinic, in the Juvenile Court, and in similar contacts' (Aichhorn, 1935, p. 4). In this chapter we have used a wide variety of terms to describe bad children – out-of-control, incorrigible, delinquent, deviant, vagrant, wayward, dissocial – depending on the historical period and context. A history specific to 'conduct disorder' would have to be confined to the past few decades, when this term has been adopted by the ICD and DSM taxonomies to cover a subset of out-of-control behaviours.

Relationship between family and state in the control of children

Early written records

Some of the earliest evidence about the control of undesirable behaviour, adult or child, presents a picture of the individual or family unit as the sole responsible agency, with little or no outside interference available or sought. For example, in the *Iliad*, written around 800 BC, when Agamemnon took Achilles's favourite slave girl, Briseis, it was Achilles's job to take action (by withdrawing from the battle against the Trojans) and to force Agamemnon to return her; although the elders tried to persuade Agamemnon to return the booty he took, they did not use force or invoke the law – there was no law governing such behaviour, and no agency to enforce punishment (Mackenzie, 1981). Even when public authority, vested in the ruler and, later, the state, took over responsibility for defining crime and punishing it, as we see happening under the legal codes of Draco and Solon in the seventh and sixth centuries BC, the family, in the person of the father, retained absolute power and responsibility in the raising of children.

However, leaving parents with power of life and death in bringing up their children does not mean that society did not have an interest in the results of that upbringing. From as far back as we have records, humans have been clear that parents who bring their children up badly are putting society at risk. For example, in the sixth century BC in India the Buddha described meeting a group of young men who were 'quick tempered, rough, greedy'. He commented that their families and friends had given them sweetmeats and always petted them, with the result that they went about 'plundering and eating; they slapped the women and girls of the clan on the back' (*Anguttara-Nikaya*, III: 63). It is clear that the Buddha held parents responsible for training their children in right behaviour.

They should restrain a child from vice, train him to a profession, contract a suitable marriage for him, and in due time hand over his inheritance. In return the child is conscious of maintaining the family tradition and thus not becoming a participant in committing crimes which will bring a bad name not only to him but to the entire family. *Sacred Books of the Buddhists*, IV, 181 (quoted in Ratnapala & Ward, 1993)

Within the Hebrew tradition, while the story of Abraham and Isaac reflects absolute parental power of life and death over a child, the book of *Deuteronomy*, written down around the seventh century BC, shows parents turning to the state for help in dealing with a child-rearing problem:

18. If a man have a stubborn and rebellious son, which will not obey the voice of his father, or the voice of his mother, and that, when they have chastened him, will not hearken unto them:
19. Then shall his father and his mother lay hold on him, and bring him out unto the elders of his city, and unto the gate of his place;
20. And they shall say unto the elders of his city, This our son is stubborn and rebellious, he will not obey our voice; he is a glutton, and a drunkard.
21. And all the men of his city shall stone him with stones, that he die: so shalt thou put evil away from you; and all Israel shall hear, and fear. (*Deuteronomy 21*, 18-21)

These texts from several continents, written down over 2000 years ago and probably reflecting much older traditions, exemplify three themes that reappear constantly over following centuries: that families have considerable (even absolute) power over their children, but at the same time have responsibilities to them; that the rest of the population has expectations of how families should raise their children; and that the state will intervene to punish children if the parents fail in their child-rearing task.

The Anglo–American tradition

A tradition of joint responsibility of a 'kinship' for a crime committed by one person underpinned early English law. For example, a law from a seventh century AD codex states:

If any one steal, so that his wife and his children know it not, let him pay LX shillings as his wite (punishment). But if he steal with the knowledge of all his household, let them all go into slavery. A boy of X years may be privy to a theft. (Thorpe, 1840, p. 103)

Here the child of 10 is treated as an adult in sharing in the family's responsibility for the crime, even when the actual offence was committed by an adult. However, the attitude to the culpability of children appears to have shifted during the latter half of the first millennium AD. The tenth century AD laws of King Aethelstan state that a thief shall be released to his kinsmen so long as they pay *bohr* (security) for him, but that a child under 12 years of age shall not be taken up for theft, and 'no younger person should be slain than XV years, except he should make resistance or flee, and would not surrender himself', when he should be put in prison until redeemed by his kinsmen (Thorpe, 1840).

As the state began to impose punishments directly on the culprit, rather than relying on the kinship system to control behaviour, it was forced to deal with delinquent children directly.

Not all of the legislation applied to conduct disorder or delinquency as we think of it today. For example, a great deal of medieval legislation affecting children's behaviour aimed at enforcing a master's control over his apprentices; most of these cases seem to have been dealt with by arbitration rather than formal court proceedings. We also find reports of children accused of heresy and witchcraft, and in these cases youth appears to have been no defence: for example, as late as 1716 an 11-year-old girl, Elizabeth Hicks, was executed for witchcraft. But many young people were arraigned for out-of-control behaviour as we think of it today, and the courts had to decide how to deal with them. In the process, they had to deal with the problem of whom to hold responsible for a crime.

The development of personal responsibility

Plato, responsibility and culpability

The Platonic tradition that forms one of the threads of western attitudes to morality offers one of the earliest, and still one of the most sophisticated, analyses of the relationship between harmful actions and the development of criminal responsibility. Where English law defines criminal responsibility in terms of culpable intention (*mens rea*), Plato makes a crucial distinction between responsibility and culpability. No-one does wrong willingly (*Laws, Book 9*); nevertheless, we are responsible for our own actions (*Gorgias 467*). Individuals, even small children, are responsible for any harm they do, and restitution is owed to the victim, even if the damage was unintentional or the perpetrator an infant. Culpability, however, is a different matter, and is a matter of disposition. In essence, Plato views the distinction between a good man and a criminal as one of disposition rather than of action. He identifies three sources of criminal disposition: crime as ignorance (e.g. *Republic*); crime as psychic disorder or disorganization (*Laws*), and crime as disease (*Timaeus*). However, he does not imply that the criminal intends or wants to do wrong; rather, the criminal acts in ignorance of his own best interests and therefore against his true desires (Mackenzie, 1981). Rather than demanding retribution, the law's response should therefore have as its focus (1) establishing appropriate restitution for the harm done and (2) changing the criminal's disposition through education and conditioning (*Laws*).

Plato's view of delinquent behaviour is reflected in the history of attempts to deal with childhood conduct disorder, which shows repeated efforts to move away from punishment toward responding to childhood deviance as the manifestation of a faulty disposition that needs to be taught, guided or treated. Attempts to deal with the problem of childhood deviance as 'ignorance' to be ameliorated through education can be found from at least the sixteenth century on. Plato's suggestion that crime is caused by psychic disorder is reflected in attempts through the centuries to use moral codes, especially religious ones, to direct children toward good behaviour. His analogy between disease and deviance is also a theme that runs through the history of conduct disorder, particularly in the past century, as medicine and psychology have tried their hand at treating it. It is interesting that just as Plato leaves unanswered the question of which model or metaphor for deviance he finds most compelling, so we still vacillate among religious, legal, educational and psychiatric models of the origins and treatment of childhood misconduct.

The law and criminal responsibility

Plato's distinction between responsibility and culpability has not taken firm hold in the Anglo-American legal tradition, which still wrestles, as it has for centuries, with the question: At what age or developmental stage are people to be held responsible for their behaviour? We can see people struggling with this problem in a contemporary account of the court of Henry VIII:

This year, the 29th of January (1537/8) was arraigned at Westminster in the afternoon a boy of Mr. Culpepers, Gentleman of the Kings Privie Chamber, which had stolen his masters purse and £11 of money, with a jewel of the Kings which was in the same purse, and there condemned to death; but the morrow after when he was brought to the place of execution . . . and that the hangman was taking the ladder from the gallowes, the Kinge sent his pardon for the sayde boy, and so he was saved from death, to the great comfort of all the people there present. (*Charles Wriothesley*, Hamilton, 1894, p. 73)

The interesting point here is that, while no-one protested the justice of punishing the boy, and there is no evidence that he was not held responsible for the theft, yet his pardon was 'to the great comfort of all the people there present'. As we saw, tenth century law exempted children younger than 12 from punishment for theft, and those under 15 from capital punishment, even when it was clear that they had committed an illegal act, so long as they did not compound the crime. Over the centuries we can see a struggle in legal thought to justify this tendency toward mercy for young criminals. It is a struggle that forced writers to grapple with basic philosophical principles of the law as it deals with the nature of human responsibility.

Sir Edward Coke, the attorney general at the end of the sixteenth century, was of the view that until the age of 14 a child should not be punished as an adult, on the grounds that *actus non fecit reum, nisi mens sit rea*: the deed did not make the person culpable, unless the intention were culpable, and a child was *non compos mentis*, and therefore not culpable (Thomas, 1826). In the same period a guide for Justices of the Peace stated that anyone aged 8 or above who committed homicide should be hanged for it 'if it may appeare (by hyding of the person slaine, by excusing it, or by any other act) that he had knowledge of good and eville, and of the perill and danger of that offence . . . But an infant of such tender years, as that he hath no discretion or intelligence, if he kill a man, this is no felony in him' (Brydall, 1635). If, on the other hand, a young person murdered someone to whom they owed 'faith, duties, and obedience', such as a parent or a master or mistress, this crime of 'Petie Treason' was more culpable than ordinary murder 'in respect of the duties of nature violated', and was punishable by being drawn and hanged (boys) or burned alive (girls)

(Brydall, 1635). This theme, that the law treats children sometimes less severely, sometime more severely than adults, will appear again in our review. In general, though, Justices were advised to class children under 14 with 'natural fools, . . . an Ideot, Lunaticke, dumbe and deafe person . . .' in being *non compos mentis* unless shown otherwise (Brydall, 1635) Another widely cited reason why children should not be punished like adults was that the purpose of punishment was to deter others from similar offences. But, it was argued, madmen, or children below the age of discretion, cannot be deterred by example, and so such punishments are futile (Brydall, 1635).

Thinking about juvenile responsibility had not changed much by the middle of the nineteenth century, when Sir William Blackstone, in his *Commentaries on the Laws of England*, wrote:

Infants, under the age of discretion, ought not to be punished by any criminal prosecution whatever. What the age of discretion is, in various nations, is a matter of some variety . . . by the law (of England), as it now stands, and has stood ever since the time of Edward the Third, the capacity of doing ill, or contracting guilt, is not so much measured by years and days, as by the strength of the delinquent's understanding and judgment. For one lad of eleven years old may have as much cunning as another of fourteen; and in these cases our maxim is, that '*malitia supplet aetatem*' (*malice adds years*). Under seven years of age, indeed, an infant cannot be guilty of felony, for then a felonious discretion is almost an impossibility in nature; . . . under fourteen, although an infant shall be *prima facie* adjudged to be *doli incapax* (*incapable of doing harm*), yet if it appear to the court and jury that he was *doli capax*, and could discern between good and evil, he may be convicted and suffer death . . . But in all such cases, the evidence of that malice which is to supply age, ought to be strong and clear beyond all doubt and contradiction. (Blackstone, 1857, Vol IV, p. 19)

How to establish 'a felonious discretion' was the problem. It is a complex concept, involving public consensus on what constitutes a felonious act, knowledge of the developmental stages of moral understanding, and a decision in the individual case about the stage of moral understanding reached by the child in question. Blackstone was clear that rough-and-ready guidelines about age as the standard of 'felonious discretion' must be adjusted to the individual case.

In summary, in response to the problem of personal responsibility, legal codes through the centuries have tried to lay down a satisfactory basis for what appears to be a universal tendency to want to treat children more leniently than adults committing the same action. Indeed, a revisionist explanation for why juvenile courts and reformatories were set up is the increasing use of the judicial power of 'nullification': judges were persistently refusing to pass sentence on clearly delinquent children because they shrank from committing them to the adult penal system. A juvenile system was the only way to enforce consistent punishment (Parsloe, 1978).

The concept of culpable intent (*mens rea*) has been invoked to provide a decision rule, in conjunction with the developmental argument that children below a certain age or stage are not capable of acting with culpable intent. However, the problem of how to tell whether a child is acting culpably has not been solved satisfactorily. Rules of thumb, such as age, are widely applied. That this approach is unsatisfactory is shown every time children commit particularly heinous acts, and arouse a public demand that they be tried 'as adults'. The somewhat contradictory implication is that, while children may not be 'responsible' for committing minor offences, they must be held personally responsible for committing truly horrendous acts. The logic of this very human response is far from clear. Plato ruthlessly cut through the problem by removing intention from the field, and separating responsibility from culpability. We are all responsible for our actions, and should make restitution for harm done to others. However, culpability is a different issue, redefined in terms of ignorance, psychic disorder or disease, and treated through education, training or treatment. Before we address some of these approaches to conduct disorder in the third section of this chapter, we turn to another aspect of personal responsibility that has caused endless problems over the centuries: what to do about children who have not done anything that would bring them under the aegis of the law if they were adults, but who nevertheless create an offence to public order.

Vagrancy and status offences

Alongside legislation to deal with children who commit crimes, we find complaints about, and attempts to deal with, another group of out-of-control children: those who offend adults by their mere existence.

Public attitudes to child vagrants is conveyed in this account, typical of (if more poetic than) many official reports, written in 1849 for the Mayor of New York by the city's Chief of Police:

I deem it to be my duty to call the attention of your Honor to a deplorable and growing evil which exists amid this community . . . for which the laws and ordinances afford no adequate remedy.

I allude to the constantly increasing numbers of vagrant, idle, and vicious children of both sexes, who infest our public thoroughfares, hotels, docks, etc. Children who are growing up in profligacy, only destined to a life of misery, shame, and crime, and ultimately to a felon's doom . . . to those whose business and habits do not permit them a searching scrutiny, the degrading and disgusting practices of these almost infants in the schools of vice, prostitution, and rowdyism, would certainly be beyond belief. The offspring of always careless, generally intemperate, and oftentimes immoral and dishonest parents, . . . a large proportion of these juvenile vagrants are in the daily practice of pilfering wherever opportunity offers, and begging where they cannot steal. In addition to which, the female portion of the youngest class, those who have only seen some eight to twelve summers, are addicted to immoralities of the most loathsome description . . . from this corrupt and festering fountain flows on a ceaseless stream to our lowest brothels – to the Penitentiary and the State Prison. (Matsell, 1850, p. 14)

The first administrative response to this group of children was to get them off the streets; the second, to dispatch them back to their own parish or to whomever the authorities could persuade to accept responsibility for them. The remainder of the children had then to be dealt with somehow, and created a problem to be struggled with by public and private agencies. The general consensus of the hundreds of plans, proposals and recommendations for dealing with these children published during this period was to treat them as criminals in the making: the literature of the period is full of proposals for reformatories, asylums, refuges, institutional training, penitentiaries, agricultural workhouses, compulsory emigration to the colonies, or transportation for life. In the words of one treatise, published in 1829:

The difficulty of dealing with the destitute children of the Metropolis consists not so much in providing a suitable punishment for the actually delinquent as in disposing of the multitudes against whom no offence can be proved. However much their waywardness and wretchedness may be deplored, and however strongly their incipient guilt may be suspected, still having committed no offence known to the law, they are not within cognizance of the civil power. Now it appears to us that it would be real humanity toward these unfortunate creatures to subject them to compulsory and perpetual exile from England. (Wade, 1829, p. 164)

The conflict between protecting children, and protecting the adult community from children, can be seen in hundreds of legal, sociological, and religious publications over the past 1000 years; the extent of progress that we have made toward resolving the conflict can be measured in the recent debate over Newt Gingrich's suggestion that more orphanages would be one solution to America's current crisis.

Regulatory agencies for out-of-control children: the last two centuries

As the nineteenth century progressed, we see a gradual movement toward making distinctions among the mad and the bad, and developing different institutions to house them: asylums for the profoundly retarded, orphanages for the parentless, workhouses for the destitute, reformatories for the delinquent. As a part of this process, the question of who could or should take responsibility for the subgroup of delinquent or conduct disordered youth was the subject of intense debate. Accompanying the debate has come a plethora of professional bodies with an interest in explaining and treating childhood deviance from their own point of view. Until the middle of the nineteenth century almost no-one made a living out of delinquent youth; 150 years later they provide a livelihood for thousands of professionals. Different groups position themselves to 'own' different types of delinquents – girls, boys, substance abusing, violent, comorbid, sexually abusive, sexually abused – and to pass other varieties on to someone else. There is not space in this chapter to consider the different ideas of all the educators, social workers, psychologists, physicians, lawyers, clergy and other professionals who have their own views about the causes and treatment of deviance. Here we concentrate on two traditions that currently hold powerful sway over the way we dispose of out-of-control children: the law and psychiatry.

Conduct disorder as crime: the role of the law

The law affects the lives of deviant children in two ways: in a personal way, when the child is accused of contravening specific laws and faces the consequences, and in a general way, as legislation is passed that affects the treatment of children as a group, or more specifically the treatment of deviant youth.

As the agency of last resort, the law continues to play a central role in the definition and disposition of deviant children. While the current (DSM–IV) definition of conduct disorder refers to 'violations of social norms' or 'rules', in fact all the symptoms listed are or under some circumstances can be violations of law, when perpetrated by children (Table 1.1). Thus, stealing with or without confrontation, forced sex, use of a weapon, breaking in, vandalism, fire setting and cruelty to animals are all illegal for both children and adults, while cruelty to people, fighting and lying may be, depending on severity and circumstances. Running away and truancy fall into the category of status offences: behaviours that are not illegal for adults but can in many parts of the United States be grounds for arrest and court proceedings. In some States, girls can come to the attention of the law by behaviour deemed sexually promiscuous (not counted toward DSM Conduct Disorder), while there is a range of behaviours that are legal for adults but not for children, notably alcohol and tobacco use, and driving motor vehicles. Thus, the law defines as deviant not only children who break the laws set for adults, but also those who break any of a separate set of rules for the behaviour of children.

In the past two centuries the courts have moved backward and forward between treating children like adults and treating them differently, in the

Table 1.1. Behaviours included in DSM–IV Conduct Disorder

Aggression to people and animals	*Deceitfulness or theft*
Bullies, threatens, intimidates	Breaking in
Initiates physical fights	Conning
Use of a weapon	Stealing without confrontation
Physically cruel to people	
Physically cruel to animals	*Serious violation of rules*
Stealing with confrontation	Staying out at night
Forced sexual activity	Running away from home
	Truancy from school
Destruction of property	
Deliberate fire-setting	
Deliberate destruction of property	

attempt to prevent them from becoming 'career criminals'. The law has been concerned with two main aspects of the treatment of deviant youth: how to treat them at the trial stage, and how to deal with those found guilty. Around the turn of the century, there were major efforts around the English-speaking world to get children out of the regular courts and into courts run specifically to deal with minors. A separate juvenile court was set up in Adelaide, Australia, in 1890, and at about the same time in England (in Birmingham). A juvenile court system was formally mandated in England and Wales through an Act of Parliament passed in 1908. In the United States, Massachusetts required separate hearings for children's cases in the 1870s, but the court in other respects resembled the adult court system. Illinois opened a juvenile court in 1899, and by 1925 every State but Maine and Wyoming had juvenile courts, and every State except Wyoming had a system for juvenile probation (Schlossman, 1977).

More important than the creation of separate physical and organizational entities was the decision to implement a different system of legal proceedings in many of these courts; a system that was more sensitive to children's developmental stage, and more focused on prevention and rehabilitation than on punishment. All of the American States except for New York adopted this 'socialized' model; juvenile courts dealt with youth under the civil rather than the criminal code. England and Wales dealt with juveniles at special sittings of magistrates' courts, with both criminal and civil (but not chancery) jurisdiction. These courts dealt with all offences committed by 7–16-year-olds except murder. In criminal cases either the child or the court could opt for trial by jury, when the case would move to the regular criminal court. The magistrates' courts also dealt with destitute and neglected, out-of-control children.

The differences between the juvenile courts and the adult model are interesting for the light they throw on the legal system's view of young deviants. In some ways children are less protected than adults: rules of search and seizure are less stringent; children may not have the right to trial by jury; rules of evidence are often more casual, and sentencing can be out of proportion to the sentence for the same offence committed by an adult, as in the case of 15-year-old Gerald Gault of Arizona, who in the 1960s was sentenced to six years in a State reformatory for making an obscene telephone call. On the other hand, children's identities are more stringently protected, and in most jurisdictions the record is sealed when the age of majority is reached. Children do not need to find bail, but can be released into the custody of their parents. Probation officers or other court officials play a big role in juvenile cases, devoting considerable efforts to diverting or adjudicating a case so that it never comes to trial.

Parens patriae
The treatment of out-of-control children in England and the United States has been heavily influenced by the common law concept of *parens patriae*, the interest that the state has in the welfare of the individual. *Parens patriae* is a doctrine with its origins in civil law dealing with issues of equity, and is, in the words of the historian Steven Schlossman, 'a doctrine of nebulous origin and meaning . . . (which) sanctioned the right of the Crown to intervene or supplant natural family relations whenever the child's welfare was threatened. Applied at first only where the property of well-to-do minors was at issue, a broader construction of the doctrine gradually became common. During the nineteenth century every American state affirmed its right to stand as guardian or superparent of all minors as part of its legal inheritance from Great Britain' (Schlossman, 1983, p. 962). Under this principle the State has a responsibility both to individual children, who must be protected even, if necessary, from their own parents, and to the community, which must be protected from the damage caused by individuals. An important corollary of this history is that the juvenile courts opened in the United States took their inspiration from civil, rather than criminal law; in Schlossman's words 'The juvenile court, as described by its founders, was to be as much a school as a court – a new branch of public education for errant children and negligent parents' (Schlossman, 1983, p. 962).

Critics throughout the history of the juvenile court movement, in both Britain and the United States, have argued about the 'social' versus 'legal' approach to delinquent youth. One side rejects the notion that juvenile offenders should be treated differently from others who have committed a similar offence: it is the offence that should be punished, not the person. The other side objects to the role of the state, under *parens patriae*, as an intermediary between the child and the family. They see it as a threat to parental rights, while often doubting the competence of the state either to judge when it should intervene or to provide an effective alternative to family management of childhood problems. A more extreme group sees the exercise of *parens patriae* as a plot to impose social control over all the nation's children (*New American*, 1996, Does the State own your child? American Opinion Publishing, Incorporated).

Many critics of the legal system's response to deviant children would argue that the similarities between its treatment of adults and children are still much too great, while the differences are the wrong ones. Thus, they find fault with extending the adversarial approach typical of Anglo-American law to cases involving children (King & Piper, 1995), arguing that a different style of proceedings, modelled more on the European fact-finding than the English adversarial approach, makes more sense for children. Others argue that the battle over *parens patriae* is being fought over the wrong issue; the critical issue is not whether the parents or the State have the greater right to control the child's behaviour, but rather the relative weight of the two purposes of *parens patriae*: help for the individual child versus social defence for the public. Historically, the second has taken precedence (Faust & Brantingham, 1974). However, in the past 30 years efforts have been made to enforce the supremacy of the first, under the general principle of there being a legal right to treatment. Pressure to enforce the right to treatment principle implicit in *parens patriae* is increasingly bringing the legal and medical approaches to child deviance into contact, and in the process raising questions about the validity and legal status of both the 'treatment' model and current legal practice. For example, if imprisonment is shown to increase the likelihood of recidivism, does the State have a responsibility to force sentencing reforms that run counter to the prevailing code of law, on the grounds that they would be better for children? On the other hand, does a court have the right to require a course of treatment for which there is no scientifically established benefit? (King & Piper, 1995).

Rehabilitation versus punishment

As the nineteenth century progressed, juvenile law reformers were influenced not only by rudimentary research on the later careers of convicted children, but also by the contagion theories that were having such a dramatic effect upon public health (Gerry, 1892). One response was to segregate children from adults, both before and after conviction. In the first decades of the century, when convicted criminals often spent months or years in the 'hulks' (old warships used as floating prisons) awaiting transportation, a separate hulk, the *Euryalus*, was set aside for boys. This 'simply created a floating gaol even more verminous and vice-ridden than its adult counterparts' (Harris & Webb, 1987, p. 11). In 1837 a separate 'training prison' for boys aged 9 to 19 was opened at Parkhurst, on the Isle of Wight; the aim was not to provide a substitute for imprisonment but to 'train' boys before transporting them to the colonies. The experiment ended 26 years later amid a public outcry against its brutality and corruption. England passed the Reformatory School Act in 1854, which encouraged (but did not require) the establishment of separate institutions for criminal children, but the Act mandated a 10–21 day prison sentence in a regular prison before removal to a Reformatory School, and a 2–6 year committal. It was not until 1899 that a child could be sent straight to a Reformatory School. Here again, we find children treated in some ways more generously than adults, with requirements for their education and health care carefully specified, while in other ways they forfeited some basic rights of the adult criminal, such as the right to a fixed term of sentencing or clear-cut rights of probation and appeal. In some cases, as in the provisions made in New York and other large cities to apprentice criminal children to farmers in the mid-West, a child could be 'sentenced' until the age of 18 (girls) or 21 (boys). Schemes that sent English delinquents to the colonies could be seen as a form of life sentence.

Conduct disorder as sickness: the role of medicine and psychiatry

At the same time that legal and social reformers were arguing over whether deviant children needed punishment or treatment, the medical professions were developing distinctions among children with different kinds of behavioural problems. The first distinction that emerged was between 'imbeciles' and 'lunatics'; between children showing developmental delays and those whose cognitive development was normal but who showed serious emotional or behavioural problems. James Prichard (1786–1848), a physician, wrote that 'idiotism and imbecility are observed in childhood, but insanity, properly so termed, is rare before the age of puberty' (Prichard, 1837, p. 127). Following Pinel, the French psychiatrist who had first described 'madness without delirium', Prichard distinguished moral insanity from, on the one hand, 'mania, or raving madness . . . in which the mind is totally deranged' (p. 16), and which he attributed to physical causes such as convulsions, and, on the other hand, imbecility or mental retardation. Pritchard used the word 'moral' in its eighteenth-century sense of pertaining to personality or character. Henry Maudsley, writing 30 years later, used the term in its nineteenth-century sense, referring to ethics and norms. He distinguished between instinctive insanity, which was 'an aberration and exaggeration of instincts and passions', moral insanity, which was a defect of the moral qualities along a dimension of 'viciousness to those extreme manifestations which pass far beyond what anyone would call wickedness' (p. 289), and moral imbecility, diagnosed by the 'total defect of moral faculties from birth and always associated with violent, mischievous and criminal acts' (von Gontard, 1988). Drawing on the new knowledge about evolution, Maudsley argued that the moral qualities are the most vulnerable to disease of all human mental capabilities, because they are located in the cerebral cortex, evolutionarily the most recently developed part of the brain; 'the finest flowers of evolution, the finest function of mind to be affected at the beginning of mental derangement of the individual' (Maudsley, 1883, p. 244).

The dominant causal theory of psychopathology in the second half of the nineteenth century was genetic: heredity and degeneration caused disease, which started with scarcely perceptible signs in early childhood, but took a progressive and irreversible course and would probably be transmitted to future generations if the affected individual were permitted to breed. Even when the proximal cause of insanity was a moral one, '. . . the different forms of insanity that occur in young children . . . are almost always traceable to nervous disease in the preceding generation' (Maudsley, 1879, p. 68).

Typical of the views held by the medical profession in the mid-nineteenth century is a volume entitled *The Hereditary Nature of Crime*, published in 1870 by the Resident Surgeon of the General Prison for Scotland, J. B. Thomson (Thomson, 1870). His conclusion was that crime is so nearly allied to insanity as to be chiefly a psychological study, and that its hereditary and intractable nature offered little hope for curing young criminals, even with extensive early treatment; transportation was probably the best remedy, for the sake of society (the contagion model again).

This extremely gloomy view of the prospects for delinquent children set medicine and psychiatry apart from religion (except, perhaps, for the extremes of Calvinism), education, social work and the law, which had in common an incurable optimism about the possibilities of reform, by one means or another. This gap began to shrink toward the end of the century, with a new view introduced, paradoxically, by that most gloomy of psychiatric models: psychoanalysis.

Psychoanalysis and conduct disorder
Although Sigmund Freud himself accepted that individuals had innate or constitutional characteristics, he developed what his daughter, Anna Freud,

described as an 'etiological formula of a sliding scale of internal and external influences: that there are people whose sexual constitution would not have led them into a neurosis if they had not had certain experiences, and these experiences would not have had a traumatic effect on them if their libido had been otherwise disposed' (S. Freud, 1916–17, p. 347, in A. Freud, 1965, p. 520). 'Hereditary factors depend for their pathogenic impact on the accidental influences with which they interact' (A. Freud, 1965, p. 138). Children whose libido 'disposed' them to pathology could be saved by the right environment, or therapy, or both. Thus, although even mild symptoms could be ominous, the course was not inevitable. In the words of Anna Freud:

> This endeavor (psychoanalysis) also disposes effectively of the conception of dissociality as a nosological entity which is based on one specific cause, whether this is thought to be internal (such as 'mental deficiency' or 'moral insanity') or external (such as broken homes, parental discord, parental neglect, separations, etc.). As we abandon thinking in terms of specific causes of dissociality, we become able to think increasingly in terms of successful or unsuccessful transformations of the self-indulgent and asocial trends and attitudes which normally are part of the original nature of the child. This helps to construct developmental lines which lead to pathological results, although these are more complex, less well defined, and contain a wider range of possibilities than the lines of normal development. (A. Freud, 1965, pp. 166–167)

The application of psychoanalytic developmental principles to children with primarily behavioural problems can be seen in its clearest form in the work of August Aichhorn, a student of Sigmund Freud's and the author of 'Wayward Youth' (Aichhorn, 1935), a book based on a series of case histories of delinquent children collected in the first two decades of this century. Aichhorn, the son of a banker turned baker, grew up in Austria surrounded by his father's apprentices, and became first a teacher, then the director of an institution for delinquent youth, adviser to Vienna's Child Welfare Department, and then director of a child guidance clinic. The psychoanalytic view of delinquency held that, in Aichhorn's words, 'Every child is at first an asocial being in that he demands direct primitive instinctual satisfaction without regard for the world around him. This behaviour, normal for the young child, is considered asocial or dissocial in the adult' (Aichhorn, 1935, p. 4). Children were seen as inherently 'dissocial' and in need of training to help them to adjust to the demands of society. Training is only complete when 'suppression of instinctual wishes is transformed into an actual renunciation of these wishes' (Aichhorn, 1935, p. 5).

Thus in the psychoanalytic approach to deviant children that dominated the child guidance clinics of the Unites States for several decades, we see an integration of educational, religious and medical approaches to delinquency.

Aichhorn referred to the therapist's role as one of a 'remedial educator', taking over when standard educational methods have failed, working together with educators on the task of making the child 'fit for his place in society'. 'When symptoms of delinquency are not predominantly neurotically determined, pedagogical skill is important because of the necessity to regulate the child's environment . . . (but) in every case, the educator should consult a psychoanalytically trained physician so that disease will not be overlooked' (Aichhorn, 1935, p. 9). Neuroses demanding psychoanalytic therapy were present in some, but not all, cases, and where present needed treatment as part of what would nowadays be called 'multi-system therapy'.

Modern medicine and conduct disorder
In this section we discuss modern medicine's taxonomy, rather than its treatment of conduct disorder, which is dealt with elsewhere in this volume. Medicine has only recently included 'conduct disorder' as a disease category. The International Classification of Diseases first included disorders of the nervous system and sense organs in its fifth revision, published in 1938, and then only under a single three-digit code with four categories. The sixth revision (1948) was the first to contain a section on mental disorders, and the eighth revision, adopted in 1965, was the first to contain any categories referring specifically to disorders of conduct (see Table 1.2). ICD–9, published in both research (1977) and clinical (1978) formats (World Health Organization, 1978), greatly expanded the ICD–8 format for conduct disorder to include ten categories and one V-code (Table 1.2). ICD–10 (World Health Organization, 1992) reorganized the classification to bring it into closer alignment with the American Diagnostic and Statistical Manual (American Psychiatric Association, 1994), although it bears more relation to the 1987 edition (DSM–III–R) (American Psychiatric Association, 1987) than to the current, 1994, version (DSM–IV), which has many fewer categories.

In the United States, the first version of the Diagnostic and Statistical Manual to mention conduct disorder was the second edition (American Psychiatric Association, 1968), which created four categories. The next edition (American Psychiatric Association, 1980) split antisocial behaviour under two diagnostic labels: Oppositional and Conduct Disorders. Oppositional Disorder was re-labelled Oppositional Defiant Disorder in DSM–III–R and DSM–IV, and adopted by ICD–10. The main justification for doing this was evidence that age distinguished youth who had different clusters of symptoms. The symptoms that define Oppositional Defiant Disorder are those of 'negative, hostile, or defiant behaviour', while the symptoms specified for Conduct Disorder

Table 1.2. Diagnoses of behavioural disorders in DSM and ICD

DSM–II (1968)	307.1, 307.2 Transient situational disturbance of childhood or adolescence
	308.4 Unsocialized aggressive reaction of childhood (or adolescence)
	308.5 Group delinquent reaction of childhood (or adolescence)
	316.3 Dyssocial behaviour
DSM–III (1980)	309.30 Adjustment reactions of childhood or adolescence with disturbance of conduct
	309.40 Adjustment reactions of childhood or adolescence with disturbance of emotions and conduct
	312.00 Conduct disorder, undersocialized, aggressive
	312.10 Conduct disorder, undersocialized, nonaggressive
	312.21 Conduct disorder, socialized, nonaggressive
	312.23 Conduct disorder, socialized, aggressive
	313.81 Oppositional disorder
	V71.02 Childhood or adolescent antisocial behaviour
DSM–III–R (1987)	309.30 Adjustment disorder with disturbance of conduct
	309.40 Adjustment disorder with mixed disturbance of emotions and conduct
	312 Conduct disorder:
	312.00 Conduct disorder, solitary aggressive type
	312.20 Conduct disorder, group type
	312.90 Conduct disorder, undifferentiated type
	313.81 Oppositional defiant disorder
	V71.02 Child or adolescent antisocial behaviour
DSM–IV (1994)	309.3 Adjustment disorder with disturbance of conduct
	309.4 Adjustment disorder with mixed disturbance of emotions and conduct
	312.8 Conduct disorder, childhood- or adolescent-onset type
	313.81 Oppositional defiant disorder
	312.9 Disruptive behaviour disorder NOS
	V71.02 Child or adolescent antisocial behaviour
ICD–8 (1969)	308 Behaviour disorders of childhood
ICD–9 (1977)	301.3 Aggressive personality reaction
	301.7 Amoral personality, asocial personality, antisocial personality
	309.3 Adjustment reaction with predominant disturbance of conduct
	309.4 Adjustment reaction with mixed disturbance of emotions and conduct

Table 1.2. (*cont.*)

	312 Disturbance of conduct without specifiable personality disorder, Disturbance of conduct NOS
	312.0 Unsocialized disturbance of conduct
	312.1 Socialized disturbance of conduct
	312.2 Compulsive conduct disorder
	312.3 Mixed disturbance of conduct and emotions, neurotic delinquency
	314.2 Hyperkinetic conduct disorder
	V71.0 Dyssocial behaviour without manifest psychiatric disorder
ICD–10 (1992)	F90.1 Hyperkinetic conduct disorder
	F91 Conduct disorders:
	F91.0 Conduct disorder confined to the family context
	F91.9 Unsocialized conduct disorder
	F91.2 Socialized conduct disorder
	F91.3 Oppositional defiant disorder
	F91.8 Other conduct disorders
	F91.1 Conduct disorder, unspecified
	F92 Mixed disorders of conduct and emotion:
	F92.0 Depressive conduct disorder
	F92.8 Other mixed disorders of conduct and emotion
	F92.9 Mixed disorder of conduct and emotions, unspecified

concentrate on behaviours that violate 'the basic rights of others or major age-appropriate societal norms or rules'.

Over the past 20 years the power and impact of this medical taxonomy has grown enormously, helped by, among other things, the availability of glossaries and volumes of casebooks, quick reference books, and other clinical aids, which have helped to standardize the use of descriptive terms; a multiaxial classification system collecting information on intellectual functioning and etiological factors; separate versions for clinical and research use; and in the United States by the growing influence of managed care, which increasingly limits those whom clinicians can treat to subcategories defined by the currently accepted taxonomy. In another chapter in this volume we discuss the effects of the current taxonomy on which children and adolescents are defined as conduct disordered. Here we would simply draw attention to one or two effects. First, by concentrating on rule-breaking as the defining characteristic of conduct disorder, the current taxonomy effectively excludes from consideration many girls who would have been identified as status offenders, vagrants, wayward youth, morally diseased or any of the earlier classifications discussed here. Second, the definition concentrates on behaviours rather than the mental state or motivation driving the behaviour. Thus, the DSM–IV symptom list (Table 1.1) is divided into four classes of behaviour: aggression to people and animals, (deliberate) destruction of property, deceitfulness or theft, and serious violations of rules. The definitions and examples provided play down the problem of *mens rea*, or culpable intent, the concept that, in the early English legal system, was the criterion for punishing a child who had done something that would be punishable in an adult. Even more interestingly, the section on 'associated features' of DSM–IV Conduct Disorder contains the following:

Individuals with Conduct Disorder may have little empathy and little concern for the feelings, wishes, and well-being of others . . . They may be callous and lack appropriate feelings of guilt or remorse. It can be difficult to evaluate whether displayed remorse is genuine because the individuals learn that expressing guilt may reduce or prevent punishment. (American Psychiatric Association, 1994, p. 87)

Thus, in DSM–IV terminology a conduct-disordered child may be both guilty in the sense of having *mens rea*, culpable intent (as in, e.g. 'deliberate destruction of others' property') and pathologically guiltless, in the sense of lacking remorse. In general, however, the current taxonomy comes down on the side of the law in defining the act as the focus of concern, rather than on the side of religion and psychoanalysis, which have focused on the state of mind in which the act was performed more than on the act itself. This is not to say that psychiatry is not concerned to change children's attitudes and beliefs: clearly many forms of therapy are directed at this. We simply make the point that a newly arrived Martian reading DSM–IV on conduct disorder could be forgiven for wondering whether it was a codex for doctors or for lawyers.

Another approach looks at the distribution of human characteristics from a statistical or actuarial viewpoint. Relatively few aspects of biology, particularly of personality characteristics or traits, are categorical, and some people have to be at the extremes of any distribution. Extremes of aggression and cooperation, trust and deceit are likely to place individuals at higher risk of not fitting into social organizations in which most people can more easily select their behaviour from either end of the distribution. Even more risky is being at an extreme on more than one distribution: aggressive and deceitful (or unrealistically trusting and cooperative). However, such combinations are going to occur in the population with a certain probability, and there may not be much that society can do about it. The empirical question is whether these characteristics co-occur at a higher level than expected by chance, in which case one could make the case for a 'syndrome' or disease process (or, to pursue the other line of argument, for an evolutionarily advantageous trait). For example, our data on 1400 youth studied annually for four years showed that young people who admitted to being frequent liars, i.e. deceitful, were six times more likely than the rest to confess to frequent fighting. This suggests a syndromal rather than a purely statistical association between deceit and aggression. It cannot, however, tell us anything about the distribution of the individual behaviours or traits. A lot more work needs to be done on this topic.

Evolutionary psychology and conduct disorder

In this section we bring this brief history of conduct disorder up to the present with some thoughts on what evolutionary psychology has to say about conduct disorder. Evolutionary psychology is a fairly new branch of psychology, practiced by a multidisciplinary band of anthropologists, philosophers, and economists as well as by psychologists. What brings them together is an interest in applying what we know about evolution to understanding more about human behaviour, in the belief that 'there is . . . a general theory of behaviour and that the theory is evolution, to just the same extent and in almost exactly the same ways that evolution is the general theory of morphology' (Roe & Simpson, 1958).

The problem of conduct disorder is central to the concerns of evolutionary psychology, because a disorder defined in terms of 'violations of social norms' raises important evolutionary questions. It is abundantly clear that humans evolved in the past and survive in the present through their ability to live in social groups. How is it, then, that individuals who persistently violate social norms appear in generation after generation, as this review of the historical literature suggests?

One explanation put forward is that what is disadvantageous in some circumstances conveys an advantage in other circumstances. A physiological example is heavily pigmented skin, which protects against skin cancer in sunny climates, but increases the risk of vitamin D deficiency in less sunny regions. So, just for a moment, let us look at childhood deviance not from the point of view of what is wrong with these children, but rather from the point of view of adaptation and survival.

Ever since mathematicians worked out that under many circumstances the 'selfish gene' triumphs in apparently paradoxical ways, 'calculating' its chances for survival across multiple generations as much as in a specific individual (Dawkins, 1976; Hamilton, 1964; Paradis & Williams, 1989), attention has been directed toward the inter-relationships between individual development and survival within a group. Recently evolutionary psychology has focused on behavioural predispositions that appear to have been 'hard-wired' into organisms, particularly complex organisms like humans, that live in social groups. Two areas of behaviour that have attracted attention have considerable importance for conduct disorder: trust/deceit and cooperation/aggression. Deceitful behaviour includes lying, cheating, conning and defaulting on agreements; the range of 'covert' (Loeber & Schmaling, 1985) antisocial behaviours listed among the criteria for conduct disorder (Table 1.2). Aggressive behaviour includes the 'overt' aspects of conduct disorder: fighting, rape, stealing with confrontation, etc. Here we consider the evolutionary aspects of these behaviours separately, although of course they may coexist in behavioural complexes (e.g. terrorism).

Trust and deceit

Trust is 'as vital a form of social capital as money is a form of actual capital' (Ridley, 1996, p. 250). A social organization without trust is unthinkable, and, as Ridley demonstrates, low-trust societies do markedly worse economically and socially than those that have developed strong norms encouraging trust and cooperation. Yet taking advantage of another's trust by stealing her property or reneging on a promise very often brings rewards to the perpetrator. From the viewpoint of evolution, then, how should we view deceit, a form of behaviour that has clear survival advantage for the individual, but is harmful to the group? Conversely, we can see clearly enough that societies in which no-one trusted anyone else would quickly fall apart (even if the others were in fact trustworthy), so why have humans not evolved to be completely trusting and trustworthy? If trust is critical to social life, why do we all cheat sometimes, and why do some seriously deceitful people survive and flourish?

Research on this theme has used as its paradigm the 'prisoner's dilemma', a problem in game theory first formalized by Albert Tucker in 1950. The basic structure of the problem is shown in Fig. 1.1. Two individuals accused of a serious crime (which they did in fact commit) are interrogated separately. They know that if neither confesses, the evidence is only enough to convict them of a minor offence, with a short sentence. If both confess, both will be punished for the serious crime. If one talks, he will go free, while the other will be punished very severely, for the serious crime and for refusing to confess. What should each one do? Trust his partner in crime, and stay silent, or talk on the assumption that this is what his partner will do? Even if the criminals knew the rules and agreed before they were arrested that they would stay silent, does it

		Prisoner Y	
		Confess	Remain silent
Prisoner X	Confess	5 years for each	0 years for X 20 years for Y
	Remain silent	20 years for X 0 years for Y	1 year for each

Fig. 1.1. Format of the 'Prisoner's dilemma'.

still make sense to do so, or does the advantage lie with the criminal who defects first? When first posed, the problem for trust seemed acute, because studies showed unequivocally that, if played as a single game, trust was disadvantageous and defection always the winning strategy. However, intensive computer simulation research, using more realistic assumptions in which individuals are likely to meet similar situations repeatedly, have shown that over the long haul the strategy that works best on one occasion does not continue to work best if the players have time to get to know one another and to get to know who cheats and who doesn't. Over the long haul, the most beneficial strategy for either party has been called 'Win-stay/Lose-shift' or 'Pavlov' (Nowak et al., 1995). This strategy requires the individual to behave well in the first rounds of the game (i.e. not cheat), and thereafter, while forgiving occasional defections, to do to his colleague whatever that person did to him. The only time that persistent betrayal of your colleague pays off is if he persistently and naively refuses to cheat, whatever you do to him. In this case, it clearly makes sense to cheat every time, since there are no harmful consequences for doing so. Simulation studies have shown that the 'Pavlov' strategy, a combination of decent behaviour, forgiveness of the odd error, firm reciprocity in the face of persistent defection, and a willingness to beat a genuine 'sucker', brings greater benefits over time than a strategy of unmitigated deceit or one of high-minded refusal to betray one's colleague. That is, when simulated societies operating by different rules are pitted against one another, over multiple 'generations' those that play 'Pavlov' survive (Nowak et al., 1995).

The question of why selection pressures have not wiped out cheating is answered by appeal to the basic evolutionary idea of random mutation combined with frequency-dependent fitness. In a world of good guys, a single, randomly appearing, cheater would win every time, because the costs to the good guys of maintaining the cognitive capacities needed to detect and defeat cheaters would previously have had no evolutionary advantage and would either not have developed or would have disappeared, so that society would have no defences against deception. A society of good guys would thus be taken over by cheaters, who would however be unable to maintain the social structure necessary for survival because they could not trust or be trusted. Simulation studies suggest that social groups need a certain ratio of good guys to cheaters, in order to maintain a reasonably stable equilibrium (Frank, 1988).

How could social organisms like humans develop the capacity to live in groups that contain both trustworthy and deceitful people, and even people who are sometimes trustworthy and sometimes deceitful? The system can only work if people are usually able to detect deceit when cheating occurs, and are inclined to punish or withhold support from cheaters. This suggests that humans would need to have developed certain sets of mental capacities: memory for different individuals, the ability to signal and respond to honesty and deceit, and a reward system that makes trustworthy behaviour worthwhile even when behaving honestly loses a particular, short-term, reward.

Evolutionary psychologists argue that these capacities are among the major distinguishing characteristics of the human brain (Barkow et al., 1992; Frank et al., 1993). Developmental psychology has demonstrated that human infants recognize human faces and distinguish them from other, equally complex, stimuli when only a few days old (Bower, 1974; Cole, 1998; Kagan, 1984). By seven or eight months, they not only distinguish among individuals but also show distress when separated from caregivers and handed over to someone less well-known, indicating that memory for individual humans, and an associated feeling of trust, develops very early (Kagan, 1984). Comparative studies of other animals suggests that ability to distinguish among large numbers of individuals of the species is strongly correlated with the development of the neocortical brain areas (Ridley, 1996). It has been argued (Cosmides & Tooby, 1992) that the extraordinary development of the human neocortex may have been driven to a significant degree by the need to recognize and characterize large numbers of people.

Not only can we distinguish among individuals, we also learn quickly to know a lot about their emotional state. Some of the earliest work in evolutionary biology was Darwin's studies of facial expression and their links to emotion (Darwin, 1872). He suggested that facial expressions have the same meaning (fear, anger, surprise) in every society, and noted that many of the muscle groups that create them are very difficult to control deliberately, so that our facial expressions often express our feelings more clearly than we might wish. It is, as Darwin points out, hard to understand why humans should have so many facial muscles and such clear links between their use and emotional states if there were no evolutionary advantage to so costly a system.

The economist Robert Frank (Frank, 1988) has developed an argument that links these observations together, proposing that emotions provide the reward and punishment system that carries us across the short-term losses associated with being cheated because we were honest, or being honest when no-one could detect us if we cheated. Emotions tell us very rapidly how we would feel about ourselves if we were to do something that we haven't yet done, using a store of accumulated knowledge of how we did feel when we did something similar. Emotions enable us to deal with the 'discounting' factor that makes a distant reward less appealing than a smaller one close at hand (Rogers, 1994). They also tell us how someone else would feel if we cheated or played straight. This empathy leads to the development of the emotions of guilt and shame, which can be triggered even by behaviour that leads to clear material reward – behaviour that in other respects makes all sorts of rational sense. Frank argues that

Emotion is often an important motive for irrational behaviour. Abundant evidence suggests that emotional forces lie behind our failure to maximize (i.e., to behave 'rationally' in terms of currently available rewards and risks). Developmental psychologists tell us that moral behaviour emerges hand-in-hand with the maturation of specific emotional competencies. The psychopath fails not because of an inability to calculate self-interest, but because of an inability to empathize, a fundamental lack of emotional conditionability. (Frank, 1988, p. 255)

This chain of argument leads to the conclusion that, given the premise that deviance in the form of deceitful behaviour will sometimes arise by chance, stable societies will remain stable precisely because they contain a certain proportion of exceptionally untrustworthy people. The behaviour of these individuals will be shaped by their failure to develop the cognitive and emotional links that enable most people to maintain trustworthy behaviour over time with no immediate reward. This may be because they 'discount' distant reward more steeply than the rest of us, or because they fail to develop empathy, and thus develop no commitment beyond the immediate set of payoffs. Whatever the process, the interesting point for this chapter is the argument that a certain degree of 'covert' evil keeps society alert and reasonably honest; too much and too little are both destabilizing.

Aggression

It is perfectly clear that aggressive behaviour in males, and the physical qualities that support it, have been rewarded for as long as we have records. However, aggression in all species that have been studied is highly controlled by developmental and social stimuli (Cairns et al., 1989, 1993). The same is true of humans. Many of the behaviours listed under DSM–IV's criteria for conduct disorder can be seen as pathological or acceptable depending on the circumstances in which they are performed. Several (fighting, using a weapon, threatening, being physically cruel) are sanctioned, if not demanded, in times of war; killing animals and birds not needed for food is a popular hobby; 'deliberate destruction of property' is a skilled profession. Problems occur when children fail to learn, or to apply, rules about the appropriate circumstances for employing the underlying capacities for aggression that these behaviours demand. All the signs are that we are driving aggressive behaviour into more and more highly formalized settings, such as professional games, and out of everyday life. The level of schoolboy fighting one reads about in Victorian novels is simply not tolerated today, nor are physical assaults on spouses or children. The fact that we are so concerned about 'street violence' probably has more to do with the lethality of the weapons that modern aggressors have than with their number relative to the past. The interesting question for current urban societies dealing with conduct disorder is whether the level and distribution of aggression in social groups that supported survival when our species evolved is consistent with the stability of our present social structures, and if not, what level or type of aggressive behaviour are we willing to tolerate.

Anthropological studies of the last remaining hunter-gatherer societies, which probably approximate the kind of social organizations within which humans developed, show that aggression and deceit are far from being routinely disapproved of or socially disadvantageous (Chagnon, 1988; Hill & Hurtado, 1953; Knauft, 1991). For example, among the Yanomamo of Amazonia, men who engaged in revenge killings, either within or outside the immediate kinship group, have more wives and more children than men who do not (Chagnon, 1988). A recent study of young men growing up in inner-city Pittsburgh found that those who became fathers by age 18 (12% of the sample) were significantly more likely than the rest of the sample to rate themselves, or be rated by parents or teachers, as untrustworthy, cruel to people, drug-abusing, and/or delinquent (Stouthamer-Loeber & Wei, 1998). Furthermore, these young fathers were four times as likely as the other youth to report serious delinquency in the year after they became fathers; parenthood did not change them. It has been suggested that in some environments, specifically those in which childhood is stressful and early mortality is high, it 'makes more sense' to breed early and often, putting more effort into the aspects of reproduction concerned with 'mating' (number of offspring) rather than 'parenting' (nurturing of offspring) (Chisholm, 1993). As discussed elsewhere in this volume, conduct disorder is highly associated with correlates of environmental stress and risk: poverty, disrupted family life, poor schools and neighbourhoods. Following this line of argument, we could construe what Robert Hinde (chapter 2, this volume) calls 'distrustful aggression' as highly adaptive in such circumstance, assuming a reproductive strategy of early procreation. There is anthropological evidence (Rogers, 1994) that increasing environmental risk is associated with increasingly steep time-discounting, as well as higher tolerance of aggression.

In summary, evolutionary psychology challenges us to turn our ideas about conduct disorder on their head and ask why a pattern of behaviour that adults find so objectionable has nevertheless persisted for at least as long as we have written records.

Conclusions

It is unlikely that a modern textbook on, for example, rheumatoid arthritis would include an entire chapter on the history of the diagnosis. The fact that such a chapter is included in this volume is an indication that the problems of definition and ownership are far from being solved. The history of society's definition of, and response to, deviant children is more confused and contradictory than even this most difficult group of individuals should have to put up with. We still have not made up our minds how to respond to the basic issues of responsibility and culpability laid out by Plato 2500 years ago. Is it surprising that treatment has been so varied and, on the whole, so ineffective, given that we do not appear to have decided whose problem we are treating: the child's? the parents'? society's?

Some progress has been made. Mainly, as in other areas of medicine, this has been done by creating categories that (1) better reflect differences among subgroups, and (2) better reflect what society wants to do with subgroups. Thus, out of the amorphous mass of what Mary Carpenter called 'the perishing and dangerous classes' (Carpenter, 1851) we now distinguish children from adults, the abused and neglected from the criminal, the mentally retarded from the behaviourally deviant, those with attention deficit hyperactivity disorder from those with conduct disorder. We have a tremendous array of different institutions for the care and control of these different groups. None of this was true 150 years ago. However, unlike many other branches of medicine that were equally primitive 150 years ago, we have made painfully little progress toward an etiology that carries strong implications for prevention, treatment and control. This failure is reflected in our institutional responses to conduct disorder, which are heavily weighted toward isolation and control – the contagion model of public health that we associate with diseases that we don't understand very well and have not learnt to prevent or cure. We no longer treat leprosy this way, but conduct disordered youth are still more likely to be isolated in a reformatory than to receive effective treatment.

In this chapter we have presented examples of public responses to conduct disordered children over the centuries, concentrating on religious, philosophical, legal and psychiatric writings. The viewpoints of education and social work have been neglected here not because they have not been important, but because of lack of space to do them justice. Returning to the set of questions with which we began, we show that remarkably little progress has been made in reaching consensus on the first two issues: the relative roles of parents and state, and appropriate norms for the development of personal responsibility. On the first of these issues, it is possible to trace a process of increasing state regulation of parental control of children – for example, states increasingly regulate parents' rights to punish their children physically, and in many societies schools take responsibility for moral as well as factual education. There is a marked shortage of evidence, however, about the effects of this takeover on rates of conduct disorder in society. It is interesting to see that some evolutionary psychologists are coming out against large-scale units of social organization, including publicly funded and organized schooling, arguing that they foster aggression and deceit rather than trust and cooperation (Ridley, 1996). Voices from the political right ('family values') and the left ('it takes a village to raise a child') are being heard in favour of greater support for families in their child-rearing tasks, as a way of combating conduct disorder.

Questions about norms for the development of personal responsibility should be more amenable to empirical answers than issues of parent–state relationships. There is a burgeoning literature on children's moral development, showing that some very basic constructs, like empathy, shame and fairness, develop extraordinarily early (Kagan, 1984; Wilson, 1993). However, we are a long way from applying this knowledge in the form of criteria for culpability that use anything more subtle than the old age-based norms described in this chapter.

The third set of questions, about who should be responsible for defining and dealing with the behaviours that we do not wish to tolerate, can only be answered satisfactorily when we have a clearer set of responses to the first two issues. It is, of course, being answered practically, but the answers are unsatisfactory by any standard that one would want to apply. As in medieval London we have vagrant children roaming the streets of our cities, whom we treat as criminals; as in nineteenth-century Philadelphia the organizations we set up to 'reform' these children only perpetuate their problems; like August Aichhorn we know that these children need multi-system treatment services, and we have a multitude of agencies offering services – but no service system. In sum, it is hard to imagine a topic that provides less encouragement about human ability to solve a social problem than does conduct disorder.

REFERENCES

Aichhorn, A. (1935). *Wayward Youth.* New York: The Viking Press.

American Psychiatric Association (1968). *Diagnostic and Statistical Manual of Mental Disorders* (2nd edn) (DSM–II). Washington, DC: American Psychiatric Press.

American Psychiatric Association (1980). *Diagnostic and Statistical Manual of Mental Disorders* (3rd edn) (DSM–III). Washington, DC: American Psychiatric Press.

American Psychiatric Association (1987). *Diagnostic and Statistical Manual of Mental Disorders* (3rd edn revised) (DSM–III–R). Washington, DC: American Psychiatric Press.

American Psychiatric Association (1994). *Diagnostic and Statistical Manual of Mental Disorders* (4th edn) (DSM–IV). Washington, DC: American Psychiatric Press.

Barkow, J., Cosmides, L. & Tooby, J. (1992). *The Adapted Mind.* Oxford: Oxford University Press.

Blackstone, W. (1857). *Commentaries on the Laws of England.* London: Murray.

Bower, T.G.R. (1974). *Development in Infancy.* San Francisco: W.H. Freeman and Company.

Brydall, J. (1635). *A Compendious Collection of the Laws of England.* London: John Bellinger and Tho. Dring.

Cairns, R.B., Cairns, B.D., Neckerman, H.J., Ferguson, L.L. & Gariépy, J.L. (1989). Growth and aggression: 1. Childhood to early adolescence. *Developmental Psychopathology, 25,* 320–30.

Cairns, R.B., McGuire, A.M. & Gariépy, J.L. (1993). Developmental behavior genetics: fusion, correlated constraints, and timing. In D.F. Hay & A. Angold (Eds.), *Precursors and Causes in Development and Psychopathology* (pp. 87–122). Chichester: John Wiley & Sons.

Carpenter, M. (1851). *Reformatory Schools for the Children of the Perishing and Dangerous Classes, and for Juvenile Offenders.* London: C. Gilpin.

Chagnon, N. (1988). Life histories, blood revenge, and warfare in a tribal population. *Science, 239,* 985–92.

Chisholm, J. (1993). Death, hope, and sex: life-history theory and the development of reproductive strategies. *Current Anthropology, 34,* 1–24.

Cole, J. (1998). *About Face.* Cambridge: MIT Press.

Cosmides, L. & Tooby, J. (1992). Cognitive adaptations for social exchange. In J.H. Barkow, L. Cosmides & J. Tooby (Eds.), *The Adapted Mind* (pp. 163–228). New York: Oxford University Press.

Darwin, C. (1872). *The Expression of Emotions in Man and Animals.* Chicago: University of Chicago Press.

Dawkins, R. (1976). *The Selfish Gene.* Oxford: Oxford University Press.

Faust, F. & Brantingham, P. (1974). *Juvenile Justice Philosophy*. St. Paul, Minnesota: West Publishing Company.

Frank, R.H. (1988). *Passions Within Reason: The Strategic Role of The Emotions*. New York: W.W. Norton and Company.

Frank, R.H., Gilovich, T. & Regan, D.T. (1993). The evolution of one-shot cooperation. *Ethology and Sociobiology, 14*, 247–56.

Freud, A. (1965). *Normality and Pathology in Childhood*. New York: International Universities Press.

Gerry, E.T. (1892). Cause of juvenile delinquency. *The Independent* (March 3, 1892), p. 294.

Hamilton, D. (1964). The genetical evolution of social behavior. *Journal of Theoretical Biology, 7*, 1–52.

Hamilton, W. D. (1894). *A Chronicle of England During the Reigns of the Tudors*. London: Camden Society.

Harris, R. & Webb, D. (1987). *Welfare, Power, and Juvenile Justice*. London: Tavistock Publications Ltd.

Hill, K. & Hurtado, M. (1953). *Ache Life History*. New York: Aldine De Gruyter.

Kagan, J. (1984). *The Nature of the Child*. New York: Basic Books, Inc.

King, M. & Piper, C. (1995). *How the Law Thinks About Children*. Vermont: Arena Ashgate Publishing Ltd.

Knauft, B.M. (1991). Violence and sociality in human evolution. *Current Anthropology, 32*, 391–428.

Loeber, R. & Schmaling, K.B. (1985). Empirical evidence for overt and covert patterns of antisocial conduct problems: a metaanalysis. *Journal of Abnormal Child Psychology, 13*, 337–52.

Mackenzie, M. (1981). *Plato on Punishment*. Berkeley and Los Angeles, California: University of California Press.

Matsell, G.W. (1850). Report of the chief of police concerning destitution and crime among children in the city. In T.L. Harris (Ed.), *Juvenile Depravity and Crime in Our City. A Sermon* (pp. 14–15). New York: Norton.

Maudsley, H. (1879). *The Pathology of Mind*. London: Macmillan.

Maudsley, H. (1883). Body and will, an essay concerning will in its metaphysical and pathological aspects. *Journal of Child Psychology and Psychiatry and Allied Disciplines, 29*, 244.

Nowak, M.A., May, R.M. & Sigmund, K. (1995). The arithmetics of mutual help. *Scientific American, 272*, 50–5.

Paradis, J. & Williams, G.C. (1989). *Evolution and Ethics: T.H. Huxley's Evolution and Ethics with New Essays on its Victorian and Sociobiological Context*. Princeton: Princeton University Press.

Parsloe, P. (1978). *Juvenile Justice in Britain and the United States: The Balance of Needs and Rights*. London: Routledge & Kegan Paul Ltd.

Prichard, J.C. (1837). *A Treatise on Insanity and Other Disorders Affecting the Mind*. Philadelphia: Haswell, Barrington & Haswell.

Ratnapala, N. & Ward, R.H. (1993). *Crime and Punishment in the Buddhist Tradition*. New Delhi, India: Mittal Publications.

Ridley, M. (1996). *The Origins of Virtue*. New York, NY: Penguin Books.

Roe, A. & Simpson, G. (1958). *Behavior and Evolution*. New Haven: Yale University Press.

Rogers, A.R. (1994). Evolution of time preference by natural section. *American Economic Review*, 84, 460–81.

Schlossman, S. (1977). *Love and the American Delinquent*. Chicago: Univeristy of Chicago Press.

Schlossman, S.L. (1983). *Studies in the History of Early 20th Century Delinquency Prevention*. Santa Monica: Rand Corp.

Stouthamer-Loeber, M. & Wei, E.H. (1998). The precursors of young fatherhood and its effect on delinquency of teenage males. *Journal of Adolescent Health*, 22, 56–65.

Thomas, J.H. (1826). *The Reports of Sir Edward Coke*. London: J. Butterworth and Son.

Thomson, J.B. (1870). *The Hereditary Nature of Crime*. London: Howard League Lib.

Thorpe, B. (1840). *Ancient Laws and Institutes of England*. London: G.E. Eyre and A. Spottiswoode.

von Gontard, A. (1988). The development of child psychiatry in 19th century Britain. *Journal of Child Psychology and Psychiatry*, 29, 569–88.

Wade, J. (1829). *A Treatise on the Police and Crimes of the Metropolis; Especially Juvenile Delinquency, Female Prostitution, Mendacity, Gaming*. London: British Museum.

Wilson, J.Q. (1993). *The Moral Sense*. New York: The Free Press.

World Health Organization (1978). *Manual of the International Classification of Diseases, Injuries, and Causes of Death*. Geneva: WHO.

World Health Organization (1992). *The Tenth Revision of the International Classification of Diseases and Related Health Problems* (ICD–10). Geneva: WHO.

2

Can the study of 'normal' behaviour contribute to an understanding of conduct disorder?

Robert A. Hinde

Introduction

Conduct disorder embraces a wide spectrum of antisocial behaviours, only a proportion of which is necessary for diagnosis (Earls, 1994). That, and the fact that it is often associated with other conditions such as hyperactivity and cognitive impairment, suggest that it is far from being a clear-cut category. The variability in definitions of conduct disorder is highlighted by Angold & Costello (chapter 6, this volume), and the complexity of possible causal factors is illustrated by the range of chapters in this volume. It can be presumed that the causal factors interact in development: for instance, those antisocial children with an early onset of behavioural problems may have subtle neuro-psychological problems which affect functions including language, memory and self-control (Moffitt et al., 1996; Lynam & Henry, chapter 9, this volume). These contribute to 'difficult temperament', and that in turn to an increased likelihood of exposure to negative environmental influences which exacerbate the condition (Kiesner et al., chapter 10, this volume).

An apparently complex symptomatology and etiology raises a number of questions, one being the extent to which it is reasonable to expect each individual symptom to depend on a relatively simple causal basis. To exemplify this issue, the initial discussion here centres on aggressive behaviour, though there is no implication that aggressiveness per se is central to conduct disorder or basic to its many symptoms.

Another set of questions concerns the extent to which the several symptoms have distinct causal bases, whether they can be divided up into distinct groups differing in their etiology, and whether some common factor can be found. It will be suggested that the symptoms listed, for instance, in the Child Behavior Problem Checklist or the Rutter scales, could be related to a number of aspects of cognitive and behavioural functioning. This chapter will cover some topics which have not received much attention with respect to aggressive children, yet may be important for understanding this symptomatic and etiological heterogeneity. The extent of the motivational complexity will be reviewed and three possible inter-related possibilities considered: perception of inequity in relationships, a feeling of reactive autonomy coupled with a perception of being constrained by others, and disruption of the self-system.

Aggressive behaviour

Definitions

Aggressive behaviour can be defined as behaviour directed towards causing harm to others. Physical injury caused deliberately is thus unequivocally aggressive, but accidental injury is not. Inflicting psychological harm may or may not be included. Behaviour that is simply assertive is not included, so what the lay-person calls 'aggressive salesmanship' falls outside the definition. Assertiveness with neglect of the possibility that injury to others may result, as in reckless driving, may or may not be seen as aggressive.

Categorization of aggressive and prosocial behaviour

Aggressive behaviour is phenomenologically diverse, and can be divided into a number of categories. Numerous classificatory systems have been proposed, and two may be cited as examples.

Aggression in nursery school children has been divided (e.g. by Feshbach, 1964; Manning et al., 1978) into:

(a)   Instrumental aggression (manipulative aggression, specific hostility) – concerned with obtaining or retaining particular objects or situations or access to desirable activities.

(b)   Harassment (teasing aggression) – directed primarily towards annoying or injuring another individual, without regard to any object or situation.

(c)   Defensive aggression – hostility provoked by the actions of others.

(d)   Games aggression – aggression escalating out of the rough-and-tumble play often shown by children of this age.

Violence shown by adolescents and adults has been classified by Tinklenberg & Ochberg (1981) into:

(a)   Instrumental – motivated by a conscious desire to injure or eliminate the victim. Not committed in anger. (It will be apparent that this does not correspond with 'Instrumental' in the nursery school system.)

(b)   Emotional – hot-blooded, angry, or performed in extreme fear. Impulsive. Usually involves intimates.

(c)   Felonious – committed in the course of another crime.

(d)   Bizarre – severely psychopathic.

(e)   Dyssocial – violent acts that gain approbation from the reference group and are regarded by them as correct responses to the situation. Usually associated with group membership.

Although such categorizations may have heuristic value, it will be apparent that the categories are not clear-cut. For instance harassment is not always easily distinguished from instrumental aggression in children, for it may be related to long-term goals concerned with access to desirable situations; and in adults felonious aggression may have a strong fear component, and thus overlap with emotional violence, which in turn may overlap with bizarre violence. Some reasons for this are discussed in the next section.

Motivational complexity

The diversity of aggressive behaviour must be seen as a consequence of its motivational heterogeneity – using the concept of motivation here in a rather loose sense. In the first instance, causing harm to another nearly always involves exposing oneself to risk of injury. Thus aggressive behaviour is often seen as a sub-category of 'Agonistic behaviour', which covers a spectrum from attack to flight. In animals ambivalence between the two may result in threat postures or displacement activities (Huntingford, 1991; Tinbergen, 1952), and the boxer's stance, involving a readiness both to hit the opponent and to defend the self, provides a parallel in humans.

But the diversity of aggression depends on more that just attack and flight motivation. Even the relatively simple instrumental aggression of school children may involve also 'Acquisitiveness' (motivation to obtain the object or situation) and 'Assertiveness' (motivation to show off to the rival or to peers). Considering only these three, one can picture the relations between them as in Fig. 2.1, where the three types of motivation are represented three-dimensionally as lying along three orthogonal axes, with aggression occurring only if the motivational state is above the striped area.

Aggressiveness with a low component of acquisitiveness would appear as harassment (see above), though there may be additional motives such as the bolstering of self-esteem or compensating for imagined slights (Hartup, 1974) which appear as assertiveness. Defensive aggression, and emotional aggression in adulthood, may involve strong frustration – either of fleeing motivation or of some other motivation, as in the anticipation of loss in jealousy (Buunk & Bringle, 1987). And dyssocial aggression must depend on the need for social approval from the peer group.

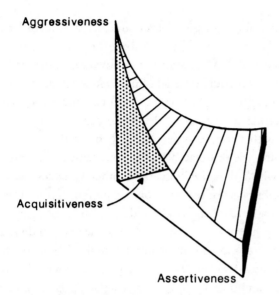

Fig. 2.1. Proposed relationship between acquisitiveness, assertiveness and aggressiveness.

In this context it is salutary to remember that what appears to be the same behaviour may have quite different bases in different individuals. This is strikingly exemplified in Straker's (1992) analysis of the 'Youth' who were involved in violent demonstrations against the apartheid regime in South Africa. Many of them came from deprived backgrounds but refused to accept deprivation as inevitable and preferred to deal with adversity by confrontation. However the groups contained diverse personality types, including the well-balanced, idealistic, dedicated and independently-minded 'leaders'; the 'followers' who were searching for a script as warrior heroes; the 'conduits' who lacked a firm sense of self and were using the group to define it; the 'conformists', motivated by a search for camaraderie in the group rather than by ideals; and the near psychopaths. The basic motivations, or the balance between them, were clearly different in each case. What is especially interesting about Straker's data in the present context is that the violent actions of the 'Youth' can be seen as involving not only aggressive behaviour and (though not in the eyes of the authorities) prosocial behaviour.

Some problems

It will be apparent that 'explaining' the diversity of aggression prosocial behaviour in terms of mixed motivations can be a useful heuristic device, since excessive aggression with a strong element of acquisitiveness calls for measures different from those required for aggression based on fear, jealousy, or lack of self-esteem. However explanations in terms of mixed motivations can pose problems. In the first place, the postulation of motivations must not be associated with the misleading Freudian model of motivation (or libido) being dissipated in action. Second, aggressive behaviour can not be understood solely in terms of processes internal to the actor: the social context (such as the presence of peers), and how that context is perceived by the parties concerned, are essential elements. Third, the postulated motivations can explain only the types of behaviour with which they are concerned: other variables must be postulated to explain other aspects of the syndrome. And fourth, the relation between strength of motivation and the likelihood or strength of aggressive behaviour is influenced by many other issues: for instance two individuals might be similarly motivated (in a loose sense) but differ in the degree to which aggression is inhibited. A central issue in all cases of aggression is a readiness or willingness to harm others, and that implies a deficiency in social inhibitions: poor impulse control is a common characteristic of conduct disorder (Moffitt et al., 1996; Pulkkinen, 1986). Fifth and related to the last, postulated motivations are not to be seen as amorphous driving forces, but as cognitively based and affectively coloured (Pettit et al., chapter 11, this volume). Of relevance here is the finding that highly aggressive children see the world in more aggressive terms, and are less dissatisfied with their own aggressive solutions to problems than are nonaggressive children (Guerra & Slaby, 1989).

Aggressiveness in conduct disorder

Aggressive behaviour is a common characteristic of conduct disorder, and appears not only as straight aggression, but also as disruptive behaviour, annoying others and cruelty, and may be responsible for the dislike of conduct-disordered children often shown by other children. However the preceding discussion indicates that this does not necessarily mean that there is excessive aggressive motivation – the aggressive behaviour could be a consequence of assertiveness. We shall consider later how far that view fits other aspects of conduct disorder. First another background issue must be put in place.

Levels of complexity

The understanding of any aspect of human behaviour requires the recognition of a series of levels of complexity – psychological processes, individual behaviour, short-term interactions between individuals, longer-term relationships, groups and societies (Fig. 2.2). Each of these involves problems not relevant to

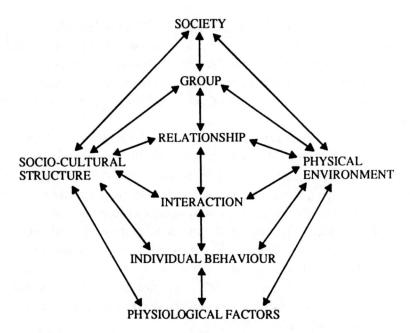

Fig. 2.2. Levels of complexity in psychological processes, behaviours and social relationships.

less complex levels: for instance a relationship may involve one or many types of interaction, but this is a property irrelevant to individual interactions. And at each level we tend to use additional explanatory concepts: thus an aggressive interaction between two siblings might be explained in terms of their both wanting the same toy, but frequent aggression in their relationship might be ascribed to sibling rivalry.

Each of these levels may be influenced by what we may conveniently call the socio-cultural structure – the system of values, beliefs, norms and institutions relevant to the level in question. The symptomatology of conduct disorder clearly indicates that social norms and values, or rather their absence or neglect, are likely to play an important role. It is important to note that these norms and values may be peculiar to the individual, dyad, group or society, though those at each level are likely to be closely related to those at others.

Finally, each of these levels affects, and is affected by, the others as well as by the socio-cultural structure (and also, though not discussed here, by the physical environment). Thus the course of any particular interaction is influenced by the nature of the relationship in which it is embedded, while the nature of the relationship depends on that of the component interactions. Similar dialectic relations occur with the socio-cultural structure: thus norms concerned with marriage both influence and are influenced by the incidence of divorce. In view of these facts, the successive levels of complexity (including the individual) and the socio-cultural structure are to be seen not as entities but as processes undergoing continuous creation, maintenance or disintegration through the agency of the dialectical relations between them (Hinde, 1991, 1997).

Aggressive behaviour between individuals is almost always influenced by these dialectical relations. As we have seen, even the aggressive behaviour of young children may be influenced by the presence of bystanders, and the same is true of defensive aggression. Emotional aggression may be instigated by third parties, as in sexual jealousy; and dyssocial aggression depends on group norms and values. Dyssocial aggression is likely to occur in the context of intergroup conflict, which in turn depends on factors promoting cohesion of the in-group(s). (This is in harmony with the view that behaviour may be simultaneously aggressive and prosocial. We have already noted an example of aggression directed towards outsiders for the good of the group in Straker's analysis of the 'Youth'.)

We have seen that any one instance of aggressive behaviour may depend on several types of motivation, and that the diversity of these types of behaviour can be partially understood in terms of differing combinations of motivational factors. Of course, the facts that different types of aggression may have different causal bases, and that the etiology of any one type may be complex, does not necessarily mean that the aggression seen in the context of conduct disorder is diverse or complexly based. It does, however, indicate a danger in postulating motivation (or a temperamental characteristic) isomorphous with the behaviour it is supposed to 'cause', and raises the possibility that the aggressiveness seen in conduct disorder, although involving few inhibitions about hurting others, may spring not just from aggressiveness per se but from other sources – for instance assertiveness or a need to show off, which could contribute also to the other types of antisocial behaviour shown.

We have also seen how understanding requires us to take into account the total situation, including the level of complexity. Furthermore a motivational approach involves some difficulties and is likely to be incomplete, and must soon involve the use of some cognitive concepts, such as self-esteem, norms and values. The following sections, concerned with the possibility of identifying factors common to many of the symptoms of conduct disorder, explore these issues further.

Cognitive issues

Morality and the issue of what is 'fair'

Many of the symptoms of conduct disorder, including aggressiveness, involve an apparent disregard of others, or a failure to empathize with them. Disruptiveness, selfishness, sulking, boasting, teasing, impatience, and many others, as well as aggressiveness (Quay, 1983), all have such characteristics. Furthermore the antisocial behaviour often appears to be spontaneous and to depend on, for instance, a sudden outburst of anger. While most children use 'moral emotions' to make judgements about the consequences of their actions (Arsenio & Lover, 1995; Dunn, 1988), it seems as though the norms of acceptable behaviour, of what is and is not fair, are simply inoperative for conduct-disordered individuals. The antisocial acts are accompanied by a neglect or down-grading by the actor of social norms and of the other's point of view.

It may be helpful to consider this from another point of view – the issue of fairness in close interpersonal relationships. Considerable evidence shows that individuals assess 'equity', an individual perceiving a relationship to be equitable if the rewards received appear to be commensurate with the costs in comparison with the partner or comparable others. If the relationship is perceived as inequitable, the individual feels anxiety – and there is evidence that feeling over-benefited as well as under-benefited can induce anxiety (Prins et al., 1993; Walster et al., 1976). Anxiety induces attempts to restore equity – either 'actual equity' by the manipulation of rewards or costs, or 'perceived equity' by distortion of the perception of relative outcomes. Thus a harmdoer may either restore actual equity by compensating the victim, or restore his (or her) 'perceived equity' by convincing himself that the victim deserved what he got, or did not really suffer, or that he (the harmdoer) was not really responsible (Walster et al., 1976). In so far as an individual diagnosed as having conduct disorder reflects on such issues, it is not unreasonable to suppose that his or her behaviour is associated with a tendency to perceive psychological equity in his (her) actions when victims or third parties would perceive the situation differently.

In harmony with this view, studies of close relationships indicate that an individual at fault tends to make attributions about the situation and to excuse his behaviour (Kelley, 1979; Weiner et al., 1987). This is not just because actor and other have different information available to them: attributions are coloured by intention and anticipation (Orvis et al., 1976). Again, in close relationships individuals who have dysfunctional or unrealistic beliefs about relationships tend to perceive the behaviour of a partner as due to stable and global characteristics (Fincham & Bradbury, 1989): sufferers from conduct disorder may see the world as having unfavourable stable characteristics. In general, attributions depend on past experience involving both cultural conventions and individual memory (Fletcher & Fitness, 1993), and involve the elaboration of complex causal accounts (Howe, 1987): those made in conduct disorder would seem to depend on and contribute to a complex account of a world seen as hostile and constraining (Pettit et al., chapter 11, this volume).

This also raises the issue of how individuals acquire moral values. There is much evidence that those values depend on experience with parents, peer groups and others (Dunn, 1988; Eisenberg & Mussen, 1989; Grusec & Goodnow, 1994; Kohlberg, 1984; Piaget, 1932). Parents and peer groups are diverse, and it is to be expected that the moral values acquired should vary according to the precise nature of the experience with them, and also indirectly with the socio-cultural structure (Fig. 2.2) (Miller & Bersoff, 1995; Wainryb & Turiel, 1995). In these interactions, an element of conflict with others, at any rate from time to time, is inevitable, and conflict with others involves perception both of the self and of the other in relation to the self. The ways in which conflicts are or are not resolved play a role in the development of the child's understanding of other people and of itself (Dunn & Slomkowski, 1992): they often require the individual to reconcile her own legitimate claims with concern for the other (Killen & Nucci, 1995). For most people a norm that people should help those who help them is acquired early in life: and a norm of responsibility, prescribing that we should help others who need one's help, somewhat later (Eisenberg & Mussen, 1989).

The acquisition of moral values involves individuals as 'active contributors to their own development, interpreting their world and making judgements that determine their actions in it' (Hart & Killen, 1995, p. 7). If a child feels its actions to be condemned unfairly by others – for instance by a parent who fails to understand its behaviour – he or she might well come to abandon any tendency to take the perspective of others, disregard the norms of behaviour, and act solely to further his or her own interests. It has indeed been found that children with insecure attachments to their parents, a condition associated with inadequate sensitive parenting (Ainsworth et al., 1978) are likely to believe that others treat them unfairly. They tend to be less compliant and less cooperative, and are more attention-seeking and disruptive as toddlers or preschool children (Arend et al., 1979; Bates et al., 1985; DeKlyen & Speltz, chapter 12, this volume). However, not all such children are aggressive: the aggressiveness may arise from parental mishandling of the conflicts that arise. The parents may reinforce aggressiveness, escalate conflicts, emphasize the aggressiveness in their children's behaviour, or behave in a hostile manner themselves (Hart et al., 1990; Keane et al., 1990; Patterson, 1982; Perry et al., 1992). Such children would feel their autonomy to be improperly constrained, and see the rights of others in a manner that might seem distorted to those others or to third parties.

Autonomy and inner endorsement of actions

It is important to note here that autonomy is not the same as intentionality, for autonomy involves a feeling of inner endorsement of one's actions. The behaviour of one who is desperately seeking approval or a fair deal or who is avoiding guilt is intentional but not autonomous. A distinction may also be made between 'reactive autonomy', a tendency to prefer to act independently, without being influenced by others, and 'reflective autonomy', the tendency to experience a feeling of choice about one's behaviour. While the latter is associated with open and honest interactions and relationships, reactive autonomy is associated with disagreeableness, poor social adjustment and dependency (Deci & Ryan, 1987). Many of the symptoms of conduct disorder can be seen in these terms – a need to act independently while feeling constrained by others: these include disobedience, uncooperativeness, negativity, impertinence, argumentativeness and quarrelling, refusal to be told what to do, sulking and pouting, bullying and trying to dominate others, picking on others, selfishness and impatience. The aggression could also be seen as a consequence of frustration due to felt constraint or to the assertiveness consequent upon this. That conduct disordered individuals do suffer from frustration is suggested by the frequent occurrence of temper tantrums.

Another issue, concerned with the perception of what is fair, may be important here. Even within any one society, a number of different rules of justice may develop, applicable by each individual in different situations. In some cases, notions of equality prevail – everyone deserves equal outcomes. In others equality is subordinated to equity – each person's outcomes should be related to what he (or she) has put in, in terms of costs incurred in the endeavour in question or investments (skill, social status, etc.). In yet others social justice – the view that each deserves outcomes in proportion to his needs – is recognized: this is most frequent when the actor identifies in some way with the needy other, as in family relationships or when people have been struck by unavoidable disaster. Lerner (1974) has suggested that what is considered as fair depends on the participants' definition of the relation in terms of two dimensions – the extent to which the partners identify with each other, and whether the other person is seen as an individual or as the incumbent of a position in society (Table 2.1). This is in harmony with the view that individuals

Table 2.1. Forms of justice in different types of relationship. Modified from Lerner (1974). (For explanation, see text.)

		Perceived relationship		
		Identity	Unit	Non-unit
Object of relationship	Person	Perception of 0 as self	Perception of similarity with or belonging with 0	Perception of contrasting interests
				Law
		Needs (Marxist)	Parity (Equality)	Darwinian Justice
	Incumbent	Perception of self in 0's circumstances Entitlement	Perception of equivalence with 0	Scarce resources, with equally legitimate claims
		Social obligations	Equity	Justified self-interest

with conduct disorder may fail adequately to identify with or empathize with others and/or to see others as individuals rather than mere incumbents of positions in society. And this again is in harmony with seeking to act independently and feeling constrained from doing so. In Lerner's view, this would result in behaviour based on self-interest.

The ability to make moral judgements influences aggressive behaviour, but does not determine it. A good intention may be over-ridden by acquisitiveness or assertiveness, or an individual may be able to make moral judgements but, perhaps as a consequence of prior experience, be unwilling or unable to trust others (Boon & Holmes, 1991). In both these cases the ontogenetic bases are likely to lie in earlier experiences in relationships.

The self-system

A number of the issues raised in the previous paragraphs are likely to be related to characteristics of the self-system: some recent work on the nature of the self-system, and more specifically on the nature of self-understanding, is relevant here.

Both introspection and objective data (Hinde et al., 1995) show that individuals may behave differently in different contexts, yet we see ourselves as having continuity in time, place and situation. But precisely how we see ourselves changes with age through a series of stage-like reorganizations (Damon & Hart, 1988). Thus the proportion of self-descriptions that involve references to others decreases with age, girls using more social references than boys, and the descriptions become less concrete and more abstract. There are also differences related to the context. Children and adolescents describing themselves tend to emphasize passivity in the family context but activity in relation to school. To illustrate the effect of context, McGuire & McGuire (1988, p. 102) write: 'a woman psychologist in the company of a dozen women who work at other occupations thinks of herself as a psychologist; when with a dozen male psychologists she thinks of herself as a woman'. Damon & Hart (1988), discussing cultural differences in self-understanding, refer to it as 'a cognizing interaction between subject and environment' (p. 172).

Self-understanding is by no means unidimensional. Understanding of the physical, active, social and psychological selves, and senses of continuity, distinctness and agency, have been distinguished by Damon & Hart (1988). These do not necessarily develop in parallel, so that at one age an individual may reason about the several components at different developmental levels. It is important to emphasize here especially the importance of links between how one perceives oneself and how one perceives others. An individual's self-perception is derived from her perceptions of how others behave to her (Higgins, Loeb & Moretti, 1995; Mead, 1934), and the characteristics of others that are most salient tend to be those in which they either most resemble or differ from the self (Andersen & Cole, 1990; Markus et al., 1985). Indeed, the evidence suggests that the self-concept is normally organized around relationships (Aron & Aron, 1996; Fiske et al., 1991; Fletcher & Fitness, 1996; Planalp, 1985). For instance, errors in naming individuals often involve the substitution for the name intended of the name of someone in a similar relationship to the speaker, and close relationships may involve sharing the other's characteristics (identification).

At this point we may summarize the arguments in the preceding paragraphs. We have seen that the appearance of both prosocial and aggressive behaviour may depend on the perception of 'fairness', and that what is considered fair is in part an aspect of the moral values of the group or individual. Judgements about moral values, or the extent to which they influence behaviour, are affected by the attributions that an individual makes, by self-perceptions, and by his or her capacity to identify with others and to see others as individuals. The effectiveness of moral values must depend on the ability to make judgements in or about situations of conflict with others. The self-system is concerned in large part with relationships with others (Hinde, 1997).

This raises a number of possibilities for basic conditions underlying many of the symptoms of conduct disorder, all of which are related to the nature of the self-system. A negative or deficient view of relationships with others could be associated with reactive autonomy and a perception of being constrained by others. Such individuals would then be deficient in their capacity to identify with others or to see others as individuals, and thus have aberrant views about what is fair. They might be prone to act impulsively, without consideration of moral issues, or be impervious to moral judgements, in either case making self-justificatory attributions. They would also be likely to have distorted views of the trustworthiness of others. They may seem to lack self-esteem, with the self-assertiveness or acquisitiveness becoming paramount motivations because they are perceived to raise the individual's image in the eyes of others, but it would be more in harmony with the other symptoms if the assertiveness, showing off, and attention-seeking stemmed from a feeling of being constrained, with no necessary lack of self-esteem. All of these issues point to abnormalities in self-understanding related to their experience in relationships.

A number of other sources of evidence are in harmony with the suggested importance of self-understanding. Thus self-understanding is associated with sustained moral action (Hart et al., 1995). There is some evidence that enhancing a person's capacity to deal with conflict situations is therapeutically effective (Kendall & Braswell, 1985). A tentative proposal might link disruption of the self-system to differences between early and later appearing conduct disorders (Moffitt et al., 1996; Maughan, chapter 7, and Hill, chapter 5, this volume). It has been suggested that some disruption of the self-system in adolescence occurs in normal development (Erikson, 1963). Although this view is controversial, it is consistent also with the finding that conduct problems starting in adolescence are usually self-limiting. By contrast, early appearing aggression is likely to persist and may be associated with more fundamental and persistent deficits in the self-system.

Some further empirical evidence in harmony with the view that the self-system plays a role are available. B. Melcher (cited in Damon & Hart, 1988) tested the hypothesis that the relation between moral judgement and moral behaviour is mediated by self-understanding. Studying groups of conduct-disordered and normal adolescents, she found a significant relation between moral judgement and self-understanding, and a near significant one between self-understanding and conduct. She also found that the conduct-disordered group showed a developmentally immature lack of concern with the future integration of the self into the networks of family, friends and society, and had difficulty in envisioning the future of the self at all. Thus the data suggested that they 'have difficulties in developing a sense of personal identity that allows for future planning to guide current behavior' (Damon & Hart, 1988, p. 155). The developmental delay was most evident in the understanding of the self over time and of agency: the disordered adolescents also had little sense of agency, feeling that the self is shaped by experience. Thus Damon and Hart conclude that the conduct-disordered individual is not concerned with the future self's appeal to others, and thus feels few inhibitions about behaviour that results in social estrangement.

Conclusion

Based on data drawn from studies of normal individuals, two approaches to the bases of conduct disorder have been outlined, and an approach to unravelling the nexus of factors associated with conduct disorder has been discussed. A motivational approach applied to the particular symptom of aggressiveness demonstrates the dangers of a simplistic approach to etiology, but beyond that has only limited usefulness. A cognitive approach is more likely to be relevant to the wide range of symptoms that such individuals show. In particular, it leads to a focus on the self-system, and especially to deficiencies in the understanding of self-in-relation-to-others. The preceding discussion leads to the speculation that a critical issue may be an unsatisfied need to act independently of others whilst feeling constrained from doing so. This could be basic to aggressiveness stemming from assertiveness, to a disregard of group moral values, to a tendency to make self-justificatory attributions, to an ability to identify others as individuals and to see them merely as incumbents of positions in society, and not to trust them. Such issues embrace many, perhaps all, of the generally recognized symptoms of conduct disorder – but it must be emphasized that this is a post hoc explanation, awaiting confirmation.

REFERENCES

Ainsworth, M. D. S., Blehar, M. C., Waters, E. & Wall, L. (1978). *Patterns of Attachment*. Hillsdale, NJ: Lawrence Erlbaum.
Andersen, S.M. & Cole, S.W. (1990). 'Do I know you?': the role of significant others in general social perception. *Journal of Personality and Social Psychology, 59*, 384–99.
Arend, R., Gove, F. & Sroufe, L.A. (1979). Continuity of individual adaptation from infancy to kindergarten. *Child Development, 50*, 950–9.
Aron, A. & Aron, E.N. (1996). Self and self-expansion in relationships. In G.J.O. Fletcher & J.

Fitness (Eds.), *Knowledge Structures and Interaction in Close Relationships* (pp. 325–44). Hillsdale, NJ: Lawrence Erlbaum.

Arsenio, W. & Lover, A. (1995). Children's conceptions of sociomoral affect: happy victimizers, mixed emotions, and other expectancies. In M. Killen & D. Hart (Eds.), *Morality in Everyday Life* (pp. 87–130). Cambridge: Cambridge University Press.

Bates, J.E., Maslin, C.A. & Franklel, K.A. (1985). Attachment security, mother-child interaction, and temperament as predictors of behavior-problem ratings at age three years. In I. Bretherton & E. Waters (Eds.), *Monographs of the Society for Research in Child Development*, 50, No. 209.

Boon, S.D. & Holmes, J.G. (1991). The dynamics of interpersonal trust: resolving uncertainty in the face of risk. In R.A. Hinde & J. Groebel (Eds.), *Cooperation and Prosocial Behaviour* (pp. 190–211). Cambridge: Cambridge University Press.

Buunk, B. & Bringle, R.G. (1987). Jealousy in close relationships. In D. Perlman & S. Duck (Eds.), *Intimate Relationships* (pp. 123–47). Beverley Hills: Sage.

Damon, W. & Hart, D. (1988). *Self-understanding in Childhood and Adolescence*. Cambridge: Cambridge University Press.

Deci, E.L. & Ryan, R.M. (1987). The support of autonomy and the control of behaviour. *Journal of Personality and Social Psychology*, 53, 1024–37.

Dunn, J. (1988). *The Beginnings of Social Understanding*. Cambridge, MA: Harvard University Press.

Dunn, J. & Slomkowski, C. (1992). Conflict and the development of social understanding. In C. Shantz & W.W. Hartup (Eds.), *Conflict in Child and Adolescent Development* (pp. 70–92). Cambridge: Cambridge University Press.

Earls, F. (1994). Oppositional-defiant and conduct disorders. In M. Rutter, E. Taylor & L. Hersov (Eds.), *Child and Adolescent Psychiatry* (pp. 308–29). Oxford: Blackwell.

Eisenberg, N. & Mussen, P.H. (1989). *The Roots of Prosocial Behavior in Children*. Cambridge: Cambridge University Press.

Erikson, E.H. (1963). *Childhood and Society*. New York: Norton.

Farrington, D.P. et al. (1990). Advancing knowledge about the onset of delinquency and crime. In B.B. Lahey & A.E. Kazdin (Eds.), *Advances in Clinical Child Psychology*, 13, 283–342. New York: Plenum Press.

Feshbach, S. (1964). The functions of aggression and the regulation of aggressive drive. *Psychological Review*, 71, 257–62.

Fincham, F.D. & Bradbury, T.N. (1989). Perceived responsibility for marital events: ego-centric or partner-centric bias. *Journal of Marriage & the Family*, 51, 27–35.

Fiske, A.R., Haslam, N. & Fiske, S.T.(1991). Confusing one person with another: what errors reveal about elementary forms of social relations. *Journal of Personality & Social Psychology*, 60, 656–74.

Fletcher, G.J.O. & Fitness, J. (1993). Knowledge structures and explanations in personal relationships. In S. Duck (Ed.), *Individuals in Relationships*, pp. 121–43. Newbury Park, CA: Sage.

Fletcher, G.J.O. & Fitness, J. (1996). *Knowledge Structures and Interaction in Close Relationships*. Hillsdale, NJ: Lawrence Erlbaum.

Grusec, J. & Goodnow, J. (1994). Impact of parental discipline methods on the child's internalisation of values. *Developmental Psychology*, 30, 4–19.

Guerra, N.G. & Slaby, R.G. (1989). Evaluative factors in social problem solving by adolescent boys. *Journal of Abnormal Child Psychology*, 17, 277–89.

Hart, C.H., Ladd, G.W. & Burleson, B.R. (1990). Children's expectations of the outcomes of social strategies: relations with sociometric status and maternal disciplinary style. *Child Development*, 61, 127–37.

Hart, D. & Killen, M. (1995). Introduction: perspectives on morality in everyday life. In M. Killen & D. Hart (Eds.), *Morality in Everyday Life*, pp. 1–22. Cambridge: Cambridge University Press.

Hart, D., Yates, M., Fegley, S. & Wilson, G. (1995). Moral commitment in inner-city adolescents. In M. Killen & D. Hart (Eds.), *Morality in Everyday Life* (pp. 317–41). Cambridge: Cambridge University Press.

Hartup, W.W. (1974). Aggression in childhood: development perspectives. *American Psychologist*, 29, 336–41.

Higgins, E.T., Loeb, I. & Moretti, M. (1995). Self-discrepancies and developmental shifts in vulnerability: Life transitions in the regulatory significance of others. In D. Cicchetti & S.L. Toth (Eds.), *Emotion, Cognition and Representation*, pp. 191–230. Rochester, NY: University of Rochester Press.

Hinde, R.A. (1991). A biologist looks at anthropology. *Man*, 26, 583–608.

Hinde, R.A. (1997). *Relationships: A Dialectical Approach*. Hove: Psychology Press.

Hinde, R.A., Tamplin, A. & Barrett, J. (1995). Consistency within and between relationships. *Cztowiek i spoleczenstwo*, 12, 7–18.

Howe, G.W. (1987). Attributions of complex cause and perception of marital conflict. *Journal of Personality and Social Psychology*, 111, 9–28.

Huntingford, F. (1991). War and peace revisited. In M. Dawkins, T.R. Halliday & R. Dawkins (Eds.), *The Tinbergen Legacy* (pp. 40–59). London: Chapman & Hall.

Keane, S.P., Brown, K.P. & Crenshaw, T.M. (1990). Children's intention-cue detection as a function of maternal social behavior. *Developmental Psychology*, 26, 1004–9.

Kelley, H.H. (1979). *Personal Relationships*. Hillsdale, NJ: Lawrence Erlbaum Associates.

Kendall, P.C. & Braswell, L. (1985). *Cognitive Behavioral Therapy for Impulsive Children*. New York: Guilford. (Cited Earls, 1994.)

Killen, M. & Nucci, L.P. (1995). Morality, autonomy and social conflict. In M. Killen & D. Hart (Eds.), *Morality in Everyday Life* (pp. 52–86). Cambridge: Cambridge University Press.

Kohlberg, L. (1984). *Essays on Moral Development*. New York: Harper & Row.

Lerner, M. (1974). Social psychology of justice and interpersonal attraction. In T.L. Huston (Ed.), *Foundations of Interpersonal Attraction* (pp. 331–55). New York: Academic Press.

Manning, M., Heron, J. & Marshall, T. (1978). Styles of hostility and social interactions at nursery, at school and at home. In L. A. Hersov & D. Shaffer (Eds.), *Aggression and Anti-social Behaviour in Childhood and Adolescence*. Oxford: Pergamon.

Markus, H., Smith, J. & Moreland, R.L. (1985). Role of the self-concept in the perception of others. *Journal of Personality and Social Psychology*, 49, 1494–512.

McGuire, W.J. & McGuire, C.V. (1988). Content and process in the experience of self. *Advances in Experimental Social Psychology*, 21, 97–144.

Mead (1934). *Mind, Self and Society*. Chicago: University of Chicago Press.

Miller, J.G. & Bersoff, D.M. (1995). Development in the context of everyday family relationships: culture, interpersonal morality and adaptation. In M. Killen & D. Hart (Eds.), *Morality in Everyday Life* (pp. 259–82). Cambridge: Cambridge University Press.

Moffitt, T.E., Caspi, A., Dickson, N., Silva, P. & Stanton, W. (1996). Childhood-onset versus adolescent-onset antisocial conduct problems in males: natural history from ages 3 to 18 years. *Development and Psychopathology, 8*, 399–424.

Orvis, B.R., Kelley, H.H. & Butler, D. (1976). Attributional conflict in young couples. In J.H. Harvey, W. Ickes & R.E. Kidd (Eds.), *New Directions in Attribution Research*. Hillsdale, NJ: Lawrence Erlbaum.

Patterson, G.R. (1982). *Coercive Family Processes*. Eugene, OR: Castalia.

Perry, D.G., Perry, L.C. & Kennedy, E. (1992). Conflict and the development of antisocial behavior. In C.U. Shantz & W.W. Hartup (Eds.), *Conflict in Child and Adolescent Development* (pp. 301–29). Cambridge: Cambridge University Press.

Piaget, J. (1932, 1965). *The Moral Judgement of the Child*. New York: Free Press.

Planalp, S. (1985). Relational schemata. *Human Communication Research, 12*, 3–29.

Prins, K.S., Buunk, B.P. & van Yperen, N.W. (1993). Equity, normative disapproval and extra marital relationships. *Journal of Social and Personal Relationships, 10*, 39–53.

Pulkkinen, L. (1986). The role of impulse control in the development of antisocial and prosocial behavior. In D. Olweus, J. Block & M. Radke-Yarrow (Eds.), *Development of Antisocial and Prosocial Behavior* (pp. 149–76). Orlando: Academic Press.

Quay, H.C. (1983). A dimensional approach to children's behavior disorder: the Revised Behavior Problem Checklist. *School Psychology Review, 12*, 244–9. (Cited Earls, 1994.)

Straker, G. (1992). *Faces in the Revolution*. Cape Town: David Philip.

Tinbergen, N. (1952). Derived activities: their causation, biological significance, origin, and emancipation during evolution. *Quarterly Review of Biology, 27*, 1–32.

Tinklenberg, J.R. & Ochberg, F.M. (1981) Patterns of violence: a California sample. In D.A. Hamburg & M.B. Trudeau (Eds.), *Biobehavioral Aspects of Aggression*. New York: Alan Liss.

Wainryb, C. & Turiel, E. (1995). Diversity in social development. In M. Killen & D. Hart (Eds.), *Morality in Everyday Life* (pp. 283–316). Cambridge: Cambridge University Press.

Walster, E., Berscheid, E. & Walster, G.W. (1976). New directions in equity research. *Advances in Experimental Social Psychology, 9*, 1–42.

Weiner, B., Amirkhan, J., Folkes, V.S. & Verette, J.A. (1987). An attributional analysis of excuse-giving. *Journal of Personality and Social Psychology, 52*, 316–24.

3

The development of children's conflict and prosocial behaviour: lessons from research on social understanding and gender

Judy Dunn

Introduction

The goal of this chapter is to consider normal developmental patterns in children's handling of conflict, their prosocial behaviour and moral understanding in early childhood, and in particular, some of the questions and challenges to developmental accounts raised by recent research on children's social understanding. Clearly, conflict management and moral sensibility reflect only two facets of the disparate behaviours grouped under the umbrella of conduct disorder. However, a focus on children's handling and resolution of disputes and their moral reasoning can provide a useful window on the broad developmental themes implicated in patterns of oppositional, antisocial and aggressive behaviour within the normal population. If we consider either normal developmental changes or individual differences in children's conflict behaviour, we are alerted to the major changes in children's regulation of their own emotions, their understanding of social rules, their understanding of and concern for others' feelings, and their moral sensibility during childhood. All of these are implicated in the development of 'ordered' behaviour, and by analogy, potentially important in the growth of 'disordered' conduct.

It is important to note at the outset that conflict (both intrapsychic and interpersonal) is recognized as a major force in individual developmental change in the grand theories of psychological development – those of Freud, Vygotsky, Piaget, Sullivan, Erikson and Lewin, for example (Shantz & Hartup, 1992). Thus while a focus on conflict means attention to what is only one aspect of conduct disorder, it does entail facing some central developmental issues. Conflict between young children and their parents or companions, for example, is seen as a major route through which children begin to take account of and interpret others' perspectives and feelings, to grasp the principles and sanctions of their culture, to reflect on their own actions and beliefs. Its potential for individual development, and for the development of relationships and social organizations is great (Ross & Conant, 1992). Yet common observations tell us that children's conflicts also include uninhibited aggression, loss of emotional control, moral principles overwhelmed. Such conflicts can reflect destructive and damaging relationships between bullies and their victims, and the pain and betrayal of broken friendships. These very different aspects of conflict highlight how important it is that we should gain clarification on the development of conflict behaviour, on the place of conflict in children's relationships, and on the influences on individual differences within the normal range in both the frequency of their conflict experiences and their management of such discord.

We know that a wide range of factors are implicated in individual differences in how children behave in conflict situations, and how frequently they are involved in disputes – both within their families and in the worlds of peers, teachers and other adults. The list of potential influences on these individual differences is long. It includes family relationships – those between parents (Cummings & Davies, 1994; Grych & Fincham, 1990), between parents and children (Herrera & Dunn, 1997), and siblings (Patterson, 1981). It also includes friendships and children's relations with the wider peer group, the broader social context in which children grow up (neighbourhood, school, inner city, ethnic community), the psychosocial risks implicated in such contexts, gender, and children's individual characteristics (personality, adjustment, powers of emotional regulation and social understanding). A summary of the research evidence on such a wide range of factors is well beyond the scope of this chapter. The focus here will be on just two of these sources of potential influence – sources on which there has been considerable recent research – namely social understanding, and gender.

In this chapter, the first section summarizes briefly the key developmental changes that have been described in children's angry and aggressive behaviour, in their behaviour in conflict, their prosocial behaviour and moral sensibility. Patterns of gender differences in these broad normative patterns are noted. The second section considers the relation of individual differences in these aspects of development to children's growing social understanding. Recent longitudinal studies linking individual differences in conflict management to early differences in social understanding are summarized. In the third section a series of questions and challenges to our understanding of conflict behaviour within the normal population are considered. It is argued that an approach which focuses on children's conflict behaviour within particular relationships, rather than on group differences (such as gender), is likely to be most fruitful. Such an approach includes an appreciation of the emotional dynamics of particular relationships and of bidirectional influences within relationships.

Developmental changes in childhood

Anger, aggression and conflict

Descriptions of developmental changes in babies' and children's expression of anger and aggression differ considerably depending on the particular measures chosen; the most recent research is reviewed in detail by Coie & Dodge (1998). In brief, anger is clearly displayed by babies of 4 months of age, and by 12 months, infants respond to situations of frustration and to peer provocation with protest and retaliation. Goodenough's (1931) classic studies describe marked increases in angry outbursts – with for instance stamping and hitting – between 12 and 30 months at home. Conflict with peers, especially over favoured objects, increases in frequency over the second year, while tantrums, and lack of tolerance of frustration both within the family and with peers are very common indeed during this period, but decline during the third and fourth years. The decline in children's angry and distressed behaviour with their siblings is particularly notable during their fourth year: in a longitudinal study of children between 2 and 5 years we found that while at 33 months around 21% of the children's interactions with their siblings involved the expression of intense anger or distress, this proportion had dropped to 9% by the children's fourth birthday (Dunn et al., 1996). The increase in children's opposition to their parents during the second and third years has been seen as related directly to children's increasing awareness of self and other, of autonomy and indepen-dence (Spitz, 1957).

In contrast to the decline in tempers and aggressive response to frustration in the preschool years, verbal aggression sharply increases between 24 and 48 months as children's linguistic and communicative powers increase. It is usually argued that children's growing verbal skills play a key role in the decline of uninhibited angry outbursts.

Gender differences in the early school years?

As they grow up through the primary school years, most children show much less frequent aggression with their peers, though conflict, overt aggression and verbal hostility between siblings remain high in many families (Boer & Dunn, 1990); physical aggression to siblings is commonly shown by both girls and boys. In general, the form of aggressive behaviour changes, too, in the school years. It becomes more clearly directed to individuals, and related to social issues, key elicitors come to include perceived threats, for instance, and manipulation of relationships within the peer group. 'Relational aggression' (in contrast to overt aggression) has been highlighted in recent accounts of school-aged children's conflicts, especially those of girls: this category includes attempts to exclude others from close peer networks, to damage reputations, and gossip in malicious ways (Crick, 1995; Crick & Grotpeter, 1995).

By the later preschool period, gender differences in the rates of aggressive behaviour that children show in group situations are evident in a wide range of cultures and socioeconomic groups. Boys become more frequently involved in conflict than girls do, they play more roughly and assert their views more forcefully, and they are more often physically aggressive (for review see Coie & Dodge, 1998). These gender differences increase as children grow towards adolescence. What underlies these differences between boys and girls? While it is likely that biological differences are implicated in the early stages of gender differences in aggression and conflict – for example in the greater propensity of boy babies to grab impulsively at toys (Hay et al., 1983) – these gender differences are fostered by the gender segregation of groups of peers that develops in early childhood (Maccoby, 1986). Boys, it is thought, develop styles of relating to one another that encourage and maintain assertive, competitive and even aggressive ways of interacting, while girls develop more cooperative styles of group interaction, and make more attempts to resolve conflicts through conciliation. And differences in adults' perceptions of and reactions to aggression and conflict involvement by boys and girls are also very likely to influence the development of gender differences. The distinction between overt and relational aggression is in some respects valuable. It has led, for example, to the inclusion of girls as well as boys in studies of children at risk for conduct problems, and it has highlighted aspects of aggressive behaviour that have been relatively neglected. However three notes of caution should be acknowledged in relation to the gender differences in these forms of aggressive behaviour.

The first is that these forms of behaviour are shown by boys as well as girls; given that girls tend to be more verbally skilled, and more focused on relationships within groups than are boys, it is not surprising that in group contexts the gender differences in relational aggression are found. However the motivation for aggressive and conflicted behaviour clearly crosses the gender divide. The second point is that 'relational' aggression is not a developmental achievement limited to school-aged children, but is evident among preschool children, as any observer in a daycare setting will confirm (Crick et al., 1997). It clearly becomes more frequently used as a weapon in the armoury of conflict strategies as children's interest in and understanding of others in their group become more mature. The third point is that there may well be cultural differences in the expression of these different forms of aggressive behaviour, which are seen as gender-related on the basis of studies chiefly conducted in the US. Thus a recent study of children in central Italy reported that relational aggression was more common among boys than girls (Tomada & Schneider, 1997).

Developmental themes

Two general themes are evident in these normative changes. First, it seems that the same underlying constructs such as aggression are reflected in different aspects of behaviour at different ages. For children at the extremes of opposi-tional behaviour and conduct disorder this has been described for example by Lahey & Loeber (1994), with their account of a developmental trajectory by which aggressive conduct problems begin with temper tantrums, irritable and annoying behaviour. Such behaviour is common among preschool children but usually has largely disappeared by 8 or 9 years (Loeber et al., 1991). Children who are clinically referred for conduct problems during the primary school years have usually failed to outgrow these difficulties. (It is of course possible that these children were different in their social behaviour even as preschoolers from the children who outgrew their toddler and preschool temper tantrums.)

In a parallel way, Farrington (1995) has argued that the same underlying construct of antisocial behaviour is reflected in different measures as children grow up (for instance, fighting frequently at 8 years, vandalism at 12, and so on). Our own study of preschoolers at risk for the development of antisocial behaviour suggests that there are changes even earlier: the 4-year-olds we studied engaged frequently in violent fantasy play with their friends, while as 5–6-year-olds, they had begun to be interested also in sex games. For children within the normal range, the extent of continuities and discontinuities in the developmental trajectories are perhaps less clear. For instance, within the family, siblings continue to irritate and deliberately annoy each other well into middle childhood and early adolescence, although overt physical aggression decreases.

The second general theme evident in the descriptive developmental data on nonclinic populations is that these changes in aggressive and angry behaviour are likely to be linked to broad developmental changes in language and communicative skills, in perspective-taking and understanding of social rules, in emotion regulation and in cognitive strategies for coping with delay of gratification (Mischel, 1974). Such developmental trends are evident, for instance, in the changes in children's management of conflict between the toddler and middle childhood years, the example we consider next.

Conflict strategies

During the toddler and preschool years, children make increasing use of justification, denial of intention, excuses and blaming others when they are in disputes. All these reflect children's growing understanding of what will influence other people's reactions to transgressions, or make them more likely to submit to the children's own goals. Children give increasingly explicit accounts of why they should get their own way, and of why their goals are legitimate.

While these developmental changes are paralleled by a decrease in outright physical aggression in conflict, they by no means ensure an increase in harmony within relationships. In our longitudinal studies of children observed within their families, we distinguished between children's use of reasoning and justification to gain their own way in disputes ('self-oriented' conflict management), and their use of reasoning to resolve the conflict by taking account of the other person's desires or goals ('other-oriented' management). While there was a clear developmental increase in the use of reasoning (as opposed to simple protest or physical hostility) within disputes with mothers and siblings, the increase was in the use of self-oriented management, not in reasoning strategies aimed at resolving conflict in the interests of both antagonists. That is, children were using their new skills of argument to gain their own ends, rather than to resolve conflict, and family harmony did not increase in parallel with the new understanding. Gender differences in these skills of argument were not found at an above-chance level.

Particularly striking changes are evident during middle childhood not only in the breadth of social knowledge that is reflected in children's justifications and excuses, but in their grasp of what will comfort or distress others. As their comprehension of complex social emotions increases between 5 and 9 or 10 years, they use this understanding of others in notable ways. The following examples are quotations from 6–7-year-olds studied at home (Bretherton et al., 1986).

Statements	Context
'And I tried to go up to Jim to play with him again, but he won't come near me. And he's not . . . when a kid isn't really your friend yet, they don't know you didn't mean to do it to them.'	Explaining to mother about an incident at school where he accidentally hit another boy.

'Well that's all right. Sometimes when I hit you and then I want to comfort you, you push me away because you're still angry.'	Explaining to a friend why another child did not respond to friend's efforts to comfort her.
'If you can't remember to kiss me, then you're not thinking about me enough.'	When mother forgot to kiss her goodnight.

During these middle childhood years children also become better able to read social cues of hostility or exclusion (Dodge, 1986). Again, such sophistication certainly does not guarantee kinder behaviour; skills at reading others' intentions can be used either to resolve conflicts, or to exacerbate disputes.

Gender differences in conflict strategies within close relationships

Gender differences have been described in children's conflict strategies in group situations. Girls were reported by Eisenberg and her colleagues, for instance, to use more verbal negotiation during conflicts than boys, and this may have prevented the escalation of their conflicts into major aggression (Eisenberg et al., 1994).

However, it is not clear that such gender differences are evident in children's intimate relationships in childhood.

In two longitudinal studies, in the US and in the UK, our observations of children's management of conflict, and the frequency or duration of conflict with their mothers, siblings at 33 and 47 months, and when alone with a friend at 47 months and 6 years did not reveal an above-chance level of gender differences. The findings suggest that within the intimate world of the family, and the intimate context of dyadic interaction with a friend, the marked individual differences in young children's conflict behaviour in these normal samples of children drawn from the local communities were not explained by gender (Pethick, unpublished data).

Prosocial behaviour

The evidence for developmental changes in prosocial behaviour has been recently reviewed by Eisenberg & Fabes (1998). Signs of empathetic concern for others' distress are shown by babies during the first year, and children's attempts to provide practical help and comfort increase in effectiveness and frequency during the second year, paralleling their growing ability to understand others' perspectives and feelings. Sharing and helping also become increasingly frequent in the second year. The question of how far these prosocial actions change with age over the following years has been a matter of dispute. Some research suggests a decrease over the early childhood years (Hay, 1979, 1994), however a recent comprehensive meta-analysis of the available research suggests overall increases in prosocial behaviour with age (Fabes & Eisenberg, 1996). The picture given by this analysis is that as children get older, they are more likely to act in helpful and empathetic ways – at least during early childhood and primary school years. However the changes are complex, and the design of studies importantly affects the pattern of findings (Eisenberg & Fabes, 1998).

The developmental processes that underlie these changes are not yet well understood. Clearly, children's increasing understanding of emotions and others' perspectives, their developing skills at decoding emotional expression, and at appreciating complex social situations are importantly implicated. So too are developments in attentional and planning processes (Krebs & Van Hesteren, 1994). And there are also developmental changes in children's motivation to help and support others (Eisenberg, 1986). Proposals for stage-changes in motivation to act prosocially have been put forward, as in the model outlined by Bar-Tal and colleagues (Bar-Tal et al., 1980), in which children change from being primarily motivated by material rewards or avoidance of punishment, through compliance with social demands to altruism without self-focused concerns. There is some support for such a model (Eisenberg & Fabes, 1998).

Gender differences in prosocial behaviour?
According to the stereotypic views within our own cultures, females are more sympathetic, empathetic, and more prosocial in their responses to others. Girls are thought – and indeed expected – to be more helpful, responsive and empathetic than boys. Some cross-cultural studies report that support and helpfulness are more frequently shown by girls than by boys across widely differing cultures, at least among children in middle childhood (Whiting & Edwards, 1973). It is usually assumed that sex-role stereotypes and cultural expectations play a key role in fostering such differences, and such assumptions are supported by some experimental studies (Eisenberg & Fabes, 1998). However, as the recent overview by Eisenberg & Fabes (1998) establishes, the empirical evidence for differences in prosocial behaviour is inconsistent and equivocal. The results emerging from a meta-analysis indicate, for instance, that sex differences were evident for aggregated measures reflecting kindness or considerateness (with girls showing more frequent kindness), but much less clear for measures reflecting instrumental help or sharing. The sex differences were also greater for situations when the target was an adult than when the target was another child. Sex differences were also greater when the measure was self-report rather than observational – and this may in part explain the

greater differences in domains such as considerateness (usually measured by self-report) as compared with instrumental help (usually measured by observation).

Eisenberg & Fabes (1998) make a number of important general points in relation to gender and prosocial behaviour, on the basis of their thorough review. They note that although boys and girls apparently do not differ in some measures of prosocial behaviour, girls may be viewed as more prosocial because they are lower in overt aggression. In general, evidence for sex differences in empathy, sympathy and prosocial behaviour all depend on the particular method used to assess the behaviour. Sex differences were clearer in studies in which individuals had control over the responses, as in self-report assessments – and non-existent when physiological indices, for example (over which the respondent had no control) were employed. As to developmental changes in gender differences in empathy or prosocial behaviour, Eisenberg & Fabes conclude that the developmental trajectory of sex differences in both prosocial and empathic behaviour is unclear. Although sex differences become evident with age if univariate measures of prosocial behaviour are used, there was no effect of age in their meta-analysis when the methods of the study (see above) were taken into account.

Gender differences in normal and troubled children?

This evidence on the development of prosocial and conflict behaviour in normal young children has raised some questions, then, about conventional assumptions about the ubiquity of gender differences in early childhood. Yet gender differences are striking among conduct-disordered children. How can we reconcile these different patterns? Three possibilities need to be considered. The first is that the developmental period considered here is chiefly early-to-middle childhood, and generalizations to early adolescence, when gender differences in prosocial behaviour, for instance, are more apparent, may well not be appropriate. More interestingly, the second possibility is that there is a difference between oppositional behaviour and conduct disorder that must be considered. Some large-scale studies report the former to be shown at similar rates by boys and girls, while gender differences in the latter are marked. Much of the conflict behaviour discussed for normal children would fall more appropriately into the former than the latter category.

A third possibility – perhaps the most plausible – is that the pattern of gender differences described for conduct-disordered children represents a real difference between the extreme and the middle range of children. That is, simple extrapolation from the 'normal' range of oppositional behaviour in conflict, or helpful, empathetic actions as regards gender are not appropriate, because the processes implicated in the development and maintenance of these behaviours differ for children at the extreme in key respects. Each of these possibilities merit investigation.

Moral reasoning

The literature on moral reasoning, and children's reactions to transgressions involving other people is clearly relevant to any consideration of children's conflict and prosocial behaviour, both for children within the normal range and for children at risk for conduct disorder, but the issues raised are beyond the scope of this chapter. A recent review of current theoretical and empirical work can be found in Turiel (1998), here I will simply highlight two general points. The first is that as regards general developmental trends, the accounts given by different researchers are set in very different theoretical frameworks, and this means that we are as yet far from having a single – or simple – developmental story. A fundamental distinction in approaches to moral development, for example, is between formulations that are based on moral actions in terms of moral judgements, and those that are based on emotion-social or motivational terms. Examples of the former, such as the accounts of Kohlberg or Piaget, posit stages of moral thinking that are based on underlying cognitive capacities. In contrast, Hoffman's (1991) account proposes a sequence in which developments in empathy drive not only moral actions but moral judgements as well.

In all these accounts, of course, taking the perspective of the other person involved plays a key role. But even within accounts that emphasize the centrality of emotions in moral sensibility (within the tradition of Hume, 1751/1966; Smith, 1759/1956) there are inconsistencies in the developmental findings and their interpretations. For example, these formulations discuss developmental changes in terms of children's growing understanding of mixed or ambivalent emotions. Thus the response of a transgressor to the results of a breach for which he is responsible is seen as centrally related to his appreciation of the feelings of the victim, and also of the possibility that a victimizer may feel both positive emotions (as when he wins a game by cheating) and sadness or guilt given the feelings of the victim. According to some research within this tradition, it is not until around 8 years of age that children appreciate the mixed emotions that a victimizer may feel, and may begin to feel concerned about reparation. However there are inconsistencies in the results of different studies; some show that children continue to be 'happy victimizers' well into middle childhood, with no decrease in children's view that victimizers will feel simply happy at the results of transgressions by the age of 7–10 years (Arsenio &

Kramer, 1992; Arsenio & Lover, 1995). This issue of understanding the complexity of the feelings of victims and victimizers may be of key significance for conduct-disordered children. Arsenio & Fleiss's (1996) recent study showed that behaviourally disruptive children viewed the feelings of those involved in transgressions differently from other children. They minimized the fear associated with being a victim, and explained victimizers' emotions with more references to desirable consequences – both material and psychological. They made fewer references to the loss, harm and unfairness created by the victimizers' acts.

Gender differences in moral development and reasoning?
The second point concerns the issue of gender differences in moral development. This has been a topic of much controversy, highlighted for instance in Gilligan's argument that the morality of females is different in nature from that of males (see Gilligan & Wiggins, 1987). She and others have argued that the 'morality of justice' that focuses on rules, rights and autonomy (on which males score more highly than females in many studies) contrasts with 'the logic underlying an ethic of care [which] is a psychological logic of relationships' (p. 73), an aspect of morality originating in attachment and other relationship experiences, which has special significance for females.

It is a powerful argument. Is there evidence for gender differences in moral reasoning during early childhood – as might be expected within Gilligan's framework? In two longitudinal studies, one in the US and one in the UK, we examined the children's responses to scenarios involving transgressions within close relationships. When the children were 4-year-olds we conducted interviews in which they were asked directly about transgressions in which they were either protagonists or victims, in situations in which the other person was either a sibling or a friend. One and two years later, we assessed the children's moral orientation with the procedures developed by Kochanska (1991) (see Dunn et al., 1995a). Here, the procedures focused on different transgressions in which the child was asked to take the role of the protagonist in the transgression; the child was then asked a series of questions involving the feelings of both victim and victimizer, and what would happen next in the story.

In these studies, gender differences were not found in the 4-year-olds' reasoning about moral breaches within sibling or friend relationships in either the US or the UK samples at an above-chance level. In the later assessments, which differed in that they were not directly focused on family relationships, but were based on scenarios that involved peers, some gender differences were found. The girls showed more mature moral orientation – less concern with external punishment and more with the feelings of the victim. What is not yet clear is whether the lack of gender differences in the 4-year-old interviews reflects an age difference from the later assessments, or whether the focus on real-life sibling and friend relationships was the explanation. That is, boys and girls may not differ from one another in their moral orientation when the focus is upon moral issues involving intimate or family relationships, rather than those involving the world of peers.

Individual differences in social understanding and their links to conflict and prosocial behaviour

The work summarized above clearly implicates changes in social understanding in the general developmental changes in conflict and prosocial behaviour. And studies of children at the extremes of aggressive behaviour implicate problems in social understanding clearly in the development of their adjustment problems (Crick & Dodge, 1994; Dodge, 1986). How far are differences in understanding others' feelings and intentions important in relation to differences within the normal range of children's management of conflict, and their prosocial and moral reasoning? Such individual differences in understanding of mind and emotion are marked in every study of children whether preschoolers or older. And are these differences in social understanding related to gender?

The series of longitudinal studies in the US and the UK we conducted can serve as an illustration of some general principles here. First, the evidence from a study in Pennsylvania showed that early differences in understanding of mind and emotion (assessed when the children were 40 months) were linked to later differences in the children's handling of conflict with their mothers, their siblings, and their close friends (Dunn & Herrera, 1997; Dunn et al., 1995b; Slomkowski & Dunn, 1992; Tesla & Dunn, 1992). The children who had been successful at mindreading and emotion understanding as young 3-year-olds were, several years later, more likely to use reasoning in their disputes – rather than simply protesting, or becoming overtly aggressive.

But an important second point was that the children's use of their understanding in one relationship was not related to their handling of conflict in the other two that we studied. That is, some children used negotiation and reasoning with their mothers, but not with their siblings or friends. Others used reasoning with their friends, but not with their family members, and so on. The lack of correlation of conflict management strategies across children's various relationships makes an important principle clear. This is that the dynamics and quality of particular relationships importantly affect the way that children use their powers of understanding, to resolve or exacerbate conflict. We need to move away from the assumption that children's understanding of mind is a unitary cognitive capacity that is independent of children's emotional state, or the particular setting in which children are assessed (Dunn et al., 1996).

A third point was that, unsurprisingly, there were other important over-time associations with the individual differences in children's conflict management. For instance, the way in which mothers had handled conflict when the children were 2 years old was correlated with the children's management of conflict with their own friends, as 6-year-olds. Individual differences in children's language skills were also implicated (Herrera & Dunn, 1997). Clearly this is a pattern which – if replicated for other samples – carries important implications for understanding the development of conduct-disordered children's behaviour in conflict.

Research on children's moral reasoning about transgressions in standardized assessments provides evidence for the same general points concerning both links with early social understanding, and the importance of particular relationships in how that understanding affects judgements or action. First, in both the US study and our ongoing research in London, children's early understanding of mind and feelings was indeed related over time to their moral reasoning (Dunn et al., 1995a). In the London studies of 4- and 5-year-olds, for instance, individual differences in understanding feelings and understanding of mind made independent contributions to the variance in moral reasoning and these links were not simply a function of IQ or verbal skills. Children who scored highly on assessments of understanding emotions, and mindreading showed more mature moral reasoning concerning transgressions involving friends and siblings than the children who had performed less well on the social understanding tasks, and these associations were not explained by differences in verbal skills (though these were independently related to the moral reasoning scores). Second, the children made different judgements and reasoned differently concerning transgressions, victimization and reparation, depending on whether their antagonist or victim was their best friend, or their sibling.

Conclusions

In this concluding section, some key issues raised by recent developmental research on conflict and prosocial behaviour within normal groups of children, and the relation of such behaviour to social understanding and gender are briefly summarized.

The first issue is the distinction between understanding of other people's feelings, intentions and goals, and the use to which children put that understanding in real-life conflicts or sociomoral dilemmas. This is a distinction that is likely to be as relevant for children at risk for conduct disorder as for children within the normal range. It is clearly of key importance to clarify the extent to which conduct-disordered children's behaviour in conflict reflects underlying problems in understanding others of a very general sort, or whether it is the use to which they put their understanding in particular social settings that differs from that of other children.

The second issue, which directly follows from the first, is that children use their understanding differently within their various close relationships. It appears that whether they use their grasp of others' feelings and intentions in the interests of solving and resolving conflict, or rather to get their own way, or indeed do not use their capacity to reason and negotiate at all depends on other qualities of the children's particular relationship with their antagonists. The emotional dynamics of particular relationships, the history of the relations between the participants, for instance, are likely to be of core importance.

Here again, the implications for understanding how conduct-disordered children behave in disputes, or when faced with someone in distress, are important. Do conduct-disordered children show a general failure to understand others' feelings and intentions, across all their relationships? Or are there differences in their conflict behaviour within different social relationships – as with the children we studied? To clarify the bases for conduct-disordered children's difficulties in social situations we may need to take a broad-based approach to studying their relationships, rather than focusing chiefly on conflict and control issues. An ongoing study of secondary school students at risk for exclusion from school because of conduct problems has highlighted how the relationships that these children have with their various teachers differ notably, and the extent of troublesome behaviour a child shows not only varies across his or her different classes, but is closely linked to the quality of the child's relationship with the teacher of each of these classes (O'Connor, personal communication).

And with prosocial behaviour and moral sensibility as with conflict interactions, it is the particular relationship between child and other that is centrally important in relation to children's propensity to act in an altruistic or helpful way towards another. Again, it appears likely that this will apply to conduct-disordered children too – but we have no systematic information on the matter.

A related point concerns the social context in which children are studied. It seems that sex differences in aggressive or prosocial behaviour are most consistently found in 'public' settings – within classrooms, playgrounds, neighbourhood gangs – rather than within intimate or family relationships. We should be conscious of the different picture that emerges within family relationships – such as the overt aggression shown by girls towards their siblings even within middle childhood. Again, whether these points are echoed for behaviourally disruptive or conduct-disordered children remains unclear.

The third issue is a more general one. There is increasing concern among those studying social development to clarify the nature and role of bidirectional influences in children's relationships. It is now widely recognized that we need to move beyond a general acknowledgement that children play a part in precipitating or eliciting conflict and disputes; we need to tackle the intractable questions of how far, when and which children elicit hostile reactions from others, or create situations that foster disruptive or aggressive behaviour. This issue – important in considering general developmental patterns – is of special significance for children at risk for conduct disorder, and deserves our research attention.

Acknowledgements

The research on social understanding and conflict in the US and UK described here was supported by the Medical Research Council in Great Britain and the National Institutes of Health (HD 23158). We are very grateful to the families who participated in the studies.

REFERENCES

Arsenio, W. & Fleiss, K. (1996). Typical and behaviourally disruptive children's understanding of the emotional consequences of socio-moral events. *British Journal of Developmental Psychology*, 14, 173–186.

Arsenio, W. & Kramer, R. (1992). Victimizers and their victims: Children's conceptions of the mixed emotional consequences of moral transgressions. *Child Development*, 63, 915–27.

Arsenio, W. & Lover, A. (1995). Children's conceptions of sociomoral affect: Happy victimizers, mixed emotions, and other expectancies. In M. Killen & D. Hart (Eds.), *Morality in Everyday Life* (pp. 87–128). Cambridge: Cambridge University Press.

Bar-Tal, D., Raviv, A. & Leiser, T. (1980). The development of altruistic behavior: Empirical evidence. *Developmental Psychology*, 16, 516–24.

Boer, F. & Dunn, J. (1990). *Children's Sibling Relationships: Developmental and Clinical Issues.* Hillsdale, NJ: Lawrence Erlbaum Associates.

Bretherton, I., Fritz, J., Zahn-Waxler, C. & Ridgeway, D. (1986). Learning to talk about emotions: A functionalist perspective. *Child Development*, 57, 529–48.

Coie, J.D. & Dodge, K.A. (1998). Aggression and antisocial behavior. In W. Damon (Ed.), *Handbook of Child Psychology*, (Vol. 3, pp. 779–862). New York: John Wiley & Sons.

Crick, N.R. (1995). Relational aggression. The role of intent attributions, feelings of distress, and provocation type. *Development and Psychopathology*, 7, 313–22.

Crick, N.R., Casas, J.F. & Mosher, M. (1997). Relational and overt aggression in preschool. *Developmental Psychology*, 33, 570–88.

Crick, N.R. & Dodge, K.A. (1994). A review and reformulation of social information processing mechanisms in children's social adjustment. *Psychological Bulletin*, 115, 74–101.

Crick, N.R. & Grotpeter, J.K. (1995). Relational aggression, gender, and social psychological adjustment. *Child Development*, 66, 710–22.

Cummings, E.M. & Davies, P. (1994). *Children and Marital Conflict: The Impact of Family Dispute and Resolution.* New York: Guilford.

Dodge, K. (1986). A social information processing model of social competence in children. In M. Perlmutter (Ed.), *Minnesota Symposium on Child Psychology*, Vol. 18. Hillsdale, NJ: Lawrence Erlbaum Associates.

Dunn, J., Brown, J.R. & Maguire, M. (1995a). The development of children's moral sensibility: Individual differences and emotion understanding. *Developmental Psychology*, 31, 649–59.

Dunn, J., Creps, C. & Brown, J. (1996). Children's family relationships between two and five: Developmental changes and individual differences. *Social Development*, 5, 230–50.

Dunn, J. & Herrera, C. (1997). Conflict resolution with friends, siblings, and mothers: A developmental perspective. *Aggressive Behavior*, 23, 343–57.

Dunn, J., Slomkowski, C., Donelan, N. & Herrera, C. (1995b). Conflict, understanding, and relationships: Developments and differences in the preschool years. Special Issue: Conflict resolution in early social development. *Early Education and Development*, 6, 303–16.

Eisenberg, N. (1986). *Altruistic Emotion, Cognition and Behaviour.* Hillsdale, NJ: Lawrence Erlbaum Associates.

Eisenberg, N. & Fabes, R. (1998). Prosocial development. In W. Damon (Ed.), *Handbook of Child Psychology*, (Vol. 3, pp. 701–78). New York: John Wiley & Sons.

Eisenberg, N., Fabes, R., Nyman, M., Bernzweig, J. & Pinuelas, A. (1994). The relations of emotionality and regulation to children's anger-related reactions. *Child Development*, 65, 109–28.

Fabes, R. & Eisenberg, N. (1996). *An examination of age and sex differences in prosocial behaviour and empathy.* Unpublished data, Arizona State University.

Farrington, D.P. (1995). The development of offending and antisocial behavior from childhood: Key findings from the Cambridge study in delinquent development. *Journal of Child Psychology and Psychiatry*, 36, 1–36.

Gilligan, C. & Wiggins, G. (1987). The origins of morality in early childhood relationships. In J. Kagan & S. Lamb (Eds.), *The Emergence of Morality in Young Children* (pp. 277–305). Chicago: University of Chicago Press.

Goodenough, F.L. (1931). *Anger in Young Children.* Minneapolis: University of Minnesota Press.

Grych, J.H. & Fincham, F.F. (1990). Marital conflict and children's adjustment: A cognitive contextual framework. *Psychological Bulletin*, 108, 267–90.

Hay, D.F. (1979). Cooperative interactions and sharing between very young children and their parents. *Developmental Psychology, 15*, 647–53.

Hay, D.F. (1994). Prosocial development. *Journal of Child Psychology and Psychiatry, 35*, 29–71.

Hay, D.F., Nash, A. & Pedersen, J. (1983). Interactions between 6-month-olds. *Child Development, 54*, 557–62.

Herrera, C. & Dunn, J. (1997). Early experiences with family conflict: Implications for arguments with a close friend. *Developmental Psychology, 33*, 869–81.

Hoffman, M.L. (1991). Towards an integration of Kohlberg's and Hoffman's moral development theories. *Human Development, 34*, 105–10.

Hume, D. (1751/1966). *An Enquiry Concerning the Principles of Morals*. La Salle, IL: Open Court.

Kochanska, G. (1991). Socialization and temperament in the development of guilt and conscience. *Child Development, 62*, 1379–92.

Krebs, D.L. & Van Hesteren, F. (1994). The development of altruism: Toward an integrative model. *Developmental Review, 14*, 103–58.

Lahey, B. & Loeber, R. (1994). Framework for a developmental model of oppositional defiant disorder and conduct disorder. In D. Routh (Ed.), *Disruptive Behavior Disorders in Childhood*. New York: Plenum Press.

Loeber, R., Lahey, B. & Thomas, C. (1991). Diagnostic conundrum of oppositional defiant disorder and conduct disorder. *Journal of Abnormal Psychology, 100*, 379–90.

Maccoby, E.E. (1986). Social groupings in childhood: Their relationship to prosocial and antisocial behaviour in boys and girls. In D. Olweus, J. Block & M. Radke-Yarrow (Eds.), *The Development of Antisocial and Prosocial Behaviour* (pp. 263–84). New York: Academic Press.

Mischel, W. (1974). Processes in delay of gratification. In L. Berkowitz (Ed.), *Advances in Experimental Social Psychology*, Vol. 7. New York: Academic Press.

Patterson, G.R. (1981). *Coercive Family Process*. Eugene, OR: Castalia Press.

Ross, H.S. & Conant, C.L. (1992). The social structure of early conflict. Interaction, relationships, and alliances. In C.U. Shantz & W.W. Hartup (Eds.), *Conflict in Child and Adolescent Development* (pp. 153–85). Cambridge: Cambridge University Press.

Shantz, C.U. & Hartup, W.W. (1992). *Conflict in Child and Adolescent Development*. Cambridge: Cambridge University Press.

Slomkowski, C.L. & Dunn, J. (1992). Arguments and relationships within the family: Differences in young children's disputes with mother and sibling. *Developmental Psychology, 28*, 919–24.

Smith, A. (1759/1956). *The Theory of Moral Sentiments*. Oxford: Clarendon Press.

Spitz, R.A. (1957). *No and Yes: On the Genesis of Human Communication*. New York: International Universities Press.

Tesla, C. & Dunn, J. (1992). Getting along or getting your own way: The development of young children's use of argument in conflicts with mother and sibling. *Social Development, 1*, 107–21.

Tomada, G. & Schneider, B.H. (1997). Relational aggression, gender, and peer acceptance: Invariance across culture, stability over time, and concordance among informants. *Developmental Psychology, 33*, 601–9.

Turiel, E. (1998). The development of morality. In W. Damon (Ed.), *Handbook of Child Psychology*, (Vol. 3, pp. 863–932). New York: John Wiley & Sons.

Whiting, B.B. & Edwards, C.P. (1973). A cross-cultural analysis of sex differences in the behaviour of children aged 3 through 11. *Journal of Social Psychology*, *91*, 171–88.

4

Neural mechanisms underlying aggressive behaviour

Joe Herbert and Manuela Martinez

Introduction

Inappropriate aggression and violence is a pervasive feature of contemporary society. In humans, it affects all ages; violent behaviour in children (e.g. conduct disorder) is relatively common. Understanding, prevention and treatment of these conditions is frequently incomplete and unsatisfactory. At a research level, there is often little integration between sociological, psychological and neurobiological approaches, even though the three address the same topic. An additional problem with aggression is that it is a compendium of different behaviours.

The great advances in our knowledge of brain function have helped our understanding of the neural mechanisms underlying behaviour. This chapter focuses on what we know of these as they apply to aggression. It draws evidence both from studies on experimental animals, and investigations of normal humans or those with a variety of illnesses. Experimental and clinical studies give very different information, but must be integrated if rational therapy for unwanted or excessive aggression is to be developed.

First, we define aggression and its relation to other social behaviours. Next, we discuss the structure of the brain as it relates to aggression, with particular emphasis on the limbic system. This anatomical view of the brain is complemented by its neurochemical architecture, and we discuss this in relation to aggressive behaviour. We draw our evidence both from experimental studies, which give information about the role of different neural systems, but often under the constraints of laboratory conditions, and from clinical studies that allow direct observation of aggression on humans, but often lack the precise neurobiological information available from animals. The wide variety of methods and approaches used both in animals and humans is nowhere more evident than on studies on aggression. This increases the difficulties of integrating results across disciplines.

Aggression: its relation to other behaviours

Behaviour is complex, and is initiated by complex sets of stimuli and circumstances. Different categories of behaviour may occur during comparatively short spans of time. All this has led to experimental efforts to simplify behaviour. Thus, sexual behaviour is commonly studied by providing circumstances in which it, rather than – say – eating, occurs at high intensity. Furthermore, the essential stimuli that elicit such behaviour can be reduced to the minimum; for example, by the pairing of a potent male with a sexually receptive female in an otherwise empty cage. Parallel studies have been made on other categories of behaviour; eating can be studied by placing food-deprived animals in cages containing either food, or the means (e.g. an operant response) of obtaining food. The rationale for this approach is that such behaviours have definable characteristics, and equally distinct biological or motivational boundaries. Manipulations of the brain can be made to see what effect this has on these distinct behaviours, with the reasonable assumption this will yield information relevant to the neural mechanisms responsible for the behaviour.

The problem with similar approaches to aggression is that some of these assumptions do not apply to this behaviour. Aggression, unlike some other behaviours, has no biological function or purpose in isolation (Attili & Hinde, 1986). Aggressive interactions occur mostly as part of some other pattern of behaviour; for example, as a strategy to achieve sexual goals, or access to preferred foods, or – more generally – as part of the process whereby individuals define their position in the social groups to which they belong, and hence ensure access to restricted resources without the need for constant conflict; a form of social control. So, the attempts to elicit 'aggression' under experimental conditions must be viewed in this light; the underlying reasons why animals fight may be related to different motivational systems, depending on the circumstances under which this occurs. This will be reflected in the neural mechanisms brought into play; different mechanisms may underlie aggressive behaviour when the circumstances and contexts of the aggression change. We have to make a careful distinction between neural mechanisms that underlie the display of aggression (that is, as an identifiable motor pattern) and those that influence whether or not it will be used as a strategy (offence), or determine how one animal responds to aggression from another (defence).

The classification of aggression continues to be unsatisfactory, partly for these reasons. It has been defined as a behaviour characterized by the intent to inflict noxious stimulation on another individual, but this underestimates its subtlety and omits some important features. It is well-known that aggression is not a unitary concept. Several classifications of aggression have been proposed, some elaborate, others more simple. On the basis of functional criteria, aggression has been classified as (a) competition for resources and (b) defence (Archer, 1988). Within this classification different subtypes can be differentiated depending on the stimuli that elicit them and the pattern of behaviour displayed (Brain, 1981; Moyer, 1968). Distinctions have been made between the different types of aggression, largely on the basis of context or stimuli eliciting this behaviour: (a) intermale (or interfemale) (territorial, social conflict etc), (b) maternal, (c) self-defence and (d) infanticide. Predation (interspecific aggression), sometimes included in discussions of aggressive behaviour, more properly belongs to a different category of behaviour (feeding). This chapter is limited to intraspecific aggression (i.e. that occurs between members of the same species), and this has been divided more simply into 'offence' and 'defence' on the basis of the structure of the behaviour (Adams, 1979; Blanchard & Blanchard, 1988). Human physical aggression has also been separated into 'emotional' or 'reactive' (angry outbursts in response to provocation, or aggression carried out with the main intention to harm someone) and 'instrumental' or 'proactive' (goal-oriented, aggression carried out with some other objective that is more important than their victim's injury) (Berkowitz, 1993). In general, both the form of the aggressive act and the context in which it occurs has to be taken into account if a coherent relation to brain function is to be made. Finally, aggression varies over time and place in the real world; this means that there is a constant process of social adaptation to aggression or its consequences – animals and people learn whether or not aggression pays off, and the contexts in which to use it or how best to respond to it. These processes also involve neural mechanisms that lie at the heart of understanding why some individuals use aggression either effectively or inappropriately. It is clear that adequate and theoretically satisfying definitions of aggression are still lacking; the reasons for this are the multiple roles of aggression and a parallel plethora of causative factors (see above). Furthermore, there is often little communication between those studying aggression experimentally, and those concerned with this behaviour in social or clinical contexts in humans.

Most species, including human beings, live in social groups whose structure affects access by individuals to items in short supply (e.g. food, mates, shelter). Direct aggressive confrontation may be used to determine which individual has priority, but it is more usual that animals come to know, through a process of social learning, who is likely to win such an encounter. This determines their strategy, and also gives the group its dominance structure. Animals (or people) low in the hierarchy may not challenge those higher in the scale, presumably because of the perceived cost in terms of potential injury. This mechanism of social control, based on previous aggressive interactions, functions to reduce aggression; but it does have potent effects on individuals. If it is to be effective, social control by hierarchy requires extremely sophisticated neural processing; indeed, there are those who claim that the primary function of the primate brain is to facilitate social interaction (see Herbert, 1987). To understand the role of the brain in aggression requires consideration not only of the means whereby aggression is expressed, but also how individuals respond to aggressive actions by others, and regulate aggression in accordance with social needs.

An important aspect is that physical aggression is displayed mainly by males both in human and other species. This is responsible for the fact that most research both in experimental and clinical studies has been conducted in males. However, it is not true to say that females lack aggressive behaviour. For example, maternal aggression (that is, defence of the young) is commonplace, and, in humans, verbal aggression is part of the behaviour of both sexes.

The brain and aggression

It is axiomatic that the brain plays a central role in aggression, both by recognizing aggression-provoking stimuli, and formulating aggressive responses. Neurons consist of three major elements: dendrites, that collect input information; axons that transmit integrated information using electrical conduction, and synapses that release chemical signals as the result of this action potential. Neurons themselves are gathered together into recognizable structures ('nuclei') and it has long been known that these have functional significance. Nuclei project to other nuclei, and a collection of interconnected regions of the brain forms a neural 'system'.

Thus we can look at the brain as a neuroanatomical structure in which different parts play different roles in aggression. However, we can also look at the brain as formed by neurochemical systems, some of which are more involved in aggression than others. Clinical approaches reflect this: attempts to treat abnormal aggression by localized lesions (e.g. of the amygdala) reflect the first view; the development of drugs that act on aggression relate to the second. Our objective is to draw a picture in which the neuroanatomy and neurochemistry of the brain will be specifically related to the different aspects of aggression.

Although we are not specifically concerned here with the development of the brain, it is important to note that the clues to later aggression may lie in the brain's developmental history. Whether or not there are genetic predisposi-

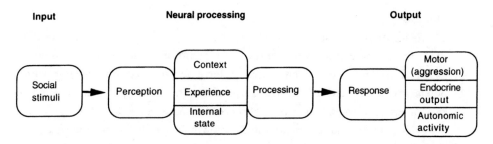

Fig. 4.1. Flow chart showing the process by which social stimuli give rise to aggressive responses. There are three major components: the complex formed by social stimuli (from con-specifics); the reception and processing of this information by the brain, and the formulation of the aggressive response (also by the brain). Each component has several subcomponents, as shown, which together make up the processing step.

tions for aggression, these will be modfied by experience or the environment – particularly during early life. The integrated results of these formative influen- ces have their counterpart in changes in the structure or neurochemical architecture of the brain, whether or not this is apparent at present. One objective of research is to identify critical genetic and environmental factors that influence aggressive behaviour, and to understand more about the way they alter the brain function in relation to this behaviour.

Neuroanatomical basis of aggressive behaviour

The brain is the organ where behaviour – including aggression – is produced. Although the brain works as a whole, it is constructed so that different parts are involved in specific tasks. For aggression, this implies that different parts of the brain are involved from sensory reception of the aggression-provoking stimu- lus to the appropriate (or inappropriate) motor display. Neural mechanisms are required to recognize in others social stimuli that elicit aggression, or aggres- sive acts on their part; to determine the context in which these occur, to formulate the motor, endocrine and autonomic responses that characterize the typical aggressive act and to learn from the results of the aggressive encounters (see Fig. 4.1). Intraspecific aggressive responses depend upon the reception and processing of complex social stimuli. These stimuli are carried by the visual, auditory, tactile and olfactory sensory systems. Thus, it should be noted that it is unwise to draw too precise a boundary round a neural system involved in aggression; clearly, many parts of the brain contribute to this complex behav- iour. In all these processes past experiences, state of the individual and the social context influence the way the individual perceives the stimuli and responds to them.

Methods

There are many methods for studying the brain, and most have been used in the study of aggression. A few of the more common techniques are as follows. Classical studies in experimental animals have been carried out by using lesions or electrical stimulation as the main methods of altering the functioning of specific areas of the brain and to observe the changes produced in aggressive behaviour. In humans, similar information has mainly been obtained from clinical cases in which lesions in specific brain areas (e.g. damage) or electrical stimulation (e.g. epilepsy) are related to changes in aggressive behaviour. A refinement of these techniques involves chemical activation of the brain either generally (i.e. using systemic drugs altering neurochemical systems) or locally (i.e. using injection of neuroactive substances into specific areas of the brain).

More recently, new techniques have allowed us to study the role of specific areas of the brain without the need to alter them. In animals, mapping the brain activity related to aggressive behaviour is possible by the use of the immediate-early gene (IEG) technique (Kollack-Walker & Newman, 1995; Martinez et al., 1998). This technique is based on the fact that the activation of neurons results in the rapid expression of a number of genes, such as c-fos, that act as transcriptional (DNA) regulators. Whilst the identity of the downstream genes are, in most cases, still obscure, this technique can be used to show which brain areas are active during aggression. For other genes with known functions, such as peptides, the product of the gene (either the mRNA or the protein) can be identified by immunohistochemical processes and quantified by image analysis. In humans, brain-imaging techniques allow us to get information about both the structure and the functioning of specific areas of the brain in people with disorders in aggressive behaviour. The main techniques that give information about the structure are computerized tomography (CT) and magnetic resonance imaging (MRI), while those informing on function are positron emission tomography (PET) and regional cerebral blood flow (RCBF).

The modular limbic system and aggression

If we are to map neural systems onto specific patterns of behaviour – like aggression – then we must discuss how we classify neural systems. The limbic system (see Fig. 4.2) has been particularly associated with aggressive behaviour. This system, like many others (e.g. the motor system), is recognized as being composed of anatomically discrete structures, such as the amygdala, hypothalamus, septum, ventral striatum, hippocampus, orbital frontal and cingulate cortex and certain parts of the brain stem (Nieuwenhuys, 1996). This definition relies on two anatomical features; the structures in question can be delineated

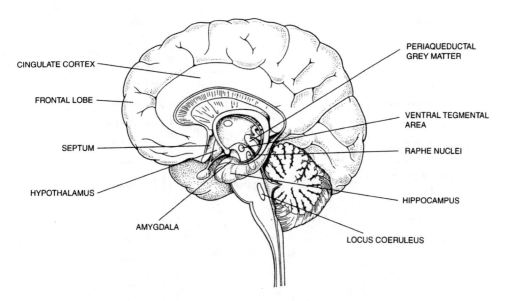

Fig. 4.2. The limbic system in the human brain. The regions referred to in the text are indicated.

from other, nearby ones (e.g. the amygdala can be separated from the striatum); and there are particularly profuse neural connections between components of the system in question. For example, it is well-known that the amygdala has strong projections to the hypothalamus, many of them routed via the septum. The essential corollary is that there is a function, or set of functions, that can be ascribed to a system. In the case of the motor system, this is the generation and control of movement. For the limbic system, there is considerable controversy, but the function we will assume is that this system is concerned with organizing appropriate responses to defined biological needs (e.g. food, water, reproduction, self-defence), a process that includes both homeostasis and adaptation. Aggression, by its nature and function, is an important part of this process. If this is so, then our task will be to try to map the different components of aggression onto the various structures of the limbic system and also to see whether other systems may contribute to this behaviour. We need, therefore, to try to define the special role of the limbic system in aggression, recognizing that this system operates in concert with all the other parts of the brain and that the limbic system has functions other than the regulation of aggression.

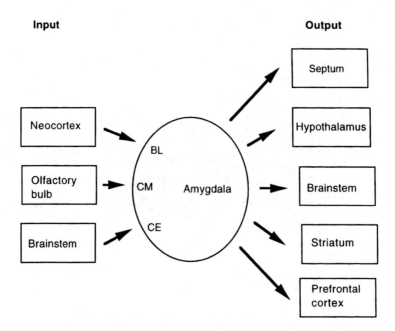

Fig. 4.3. Information flow through the amygdala. Major sources of input are shown on the left; these terminate in regions of the amygdala (BL: basolateral; CM: cortico-medial; CE: central nuclei). Outputs are shown on the right. The functions of these areas in the context of aggressive behaviour are discussed in the text.

The amygdala

Stimuli involved in aggression are analysed by neocortical areas. There must be a pathway that allows this information to gain access to those neural structures that compose aggressive responses. The evidence strongly suggests that the amygdala is an essential component of this pathway. The amygdala receives extensive sensory input from the neocortex (see Fig. 4.3). The cortical association area for visual, auditory, tactile and gustatory information all project to the amygdala through the temporal neocortex. The amygdala also receives direct input from the olfactory bulbs and projections from polysensory convergence areas in frontal and temporal neocortex.

The amygdaloid complex is involved in processes determining the way in which the individual's brain perceives and interprets a given stimulus or situation. Its central function is to associate a sensory stimulus with an emotional response. Thus, the amygdala plays an important role in aggressive behaviour (reviewed by Albert et al., 1993; Blanchard & Blanchard, 1988; Eichelman, 1983; Kling & Brothers, 1992; Miller, 1994; Ursin, 1981; Weiger & Bear, 1988). Damage to the amygdala produces a range of difficulties with the identification of complex natural stimuli, such as losing the capacity to respond to important external cues and it has long been known to induce 'tameness' (that is, loss of an expected aggressive or fearful response to a given situation). Conversely, electrical stimulation of the amygdala can induce aggressive reactions. These are not random, but are mainly directed towards objects that might be expected to elicit them under more normal conditions (e.g. another con-specific – member of the same species – rather than an inanimate object). Similarly, localized seizures in the temporal lobe and sometimes specifically in the amygdala are associated in human beings with aggressive outbursts. These violent episodes occur before as well as during episodes of abnormal electrical activity. Patients with temporal lobe tumours exhibit assaultive rages (see references above).

One conclusion is that the amygdala is part of the system that classifies a set of stimuli on the basis of cortical processing, and passes this emotionally classified information to other parts of the limbic system (e.g. the hypothalamus) that compose the behavioural, endocrine and autonomic responses characteristic of aggression (see Fig. 4.4). However, a large body of experimental work shows that the amygdala is also concerned with the generation of fear, including conditioned fear (that is, learning that previously neutral events may signal aversive events) (Kagan & Schulkin, 1995; Maren & Fanselow, 1996). If an animal loses the capacity to experience fear, then one correlate will be loss of aggression – since many aggressive episodes are born from fear or anticipated fearful events. Similar findings are reported for humans; the amygdala is activated by fearful stimuli in humans (LaBar et al., 1998) and bilateral amygdaloid lesions impair the recognition of fear in others (Adolphs et al., 1995). So whilst there is little doubt that the amygdala is critical for the expression of aggression, its exact role remains enigmatic. However, this has not prevented attempts to control aggression in humans by amygdalectomy (Narabayashi et al., 1963). Furthermore, it is important to remember that the amygdala is also concerned with classifying other categories of response, such as sexual and ingestive behaviours (McGregor & Herbert, 1992) which excludes it being concerned solely with aggression (or fear). Thus, we need to understand how the amygdala provides an essential 'label' on complex social stimuli, how this information is coded, and how it is passed to the executive parts of the limbic system. This includes the septum and the hypothalamus.

The septum
The septum (see Fig. 4.2), the bed nucleus of stria terminalis and the nucleus accumbens have been considered as a 'defence inhibitory system' (reviewed by

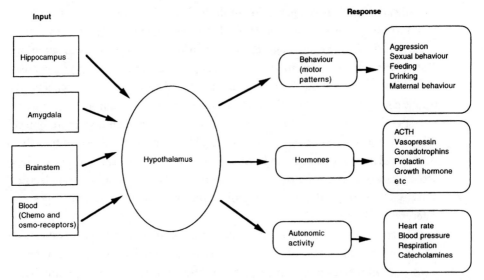

Fig. 4.4. Inputs and outputs of the hypothalamus. The major source of inputs is shown on the left; the three categories of output on the right. Specific patterns of the latter constitute aggressive responses. ACTH: adrenocorticotrophic hormone.

Blanchard & Blanchard, 1988). Damage to these structures produces a transient or longer-lasting 'release' of defensive aggression but also many other behavioural effects such as hyper-reactivity and increased responsiveness to a variety of situations which include alteration in ingestion and sexual behaviour. In humans, stimulation of the septum reduces violent behaviour, and the individual becomes happy and euphoric. On the contrary, tumours in this area are associated with a heightened defensiveness (reviewed by Albert et al., 1993; Ursin, 1981). Altogether, these results indicate that the septum is important in aggression, though its role may not be limited to this behaviour.

The hypothalamus

The hypothalamus is involved in the generation of responses related to the survival of the individual and the species that include motor, endocrine and autonomic reactions (see Fig. 4.4) (Herbert, 1993). It receives internal sensory information directly through chemo- and osmoreceptors, and processed information from the external environment through inputs from the amygdala and other structures. The classical experiments of Bard (1928) showed that section of all brain structures anterior to the hypothalamus resulted in cats showing 'sham rage' with high sympathetic arousal and extreme anger elicited by previously unimportant stimuli. However, when the hypothalamus was also sectioned the animals did not exhibit 'sham rage'.

There is some evidence that different nuclei of the hypothalamus may be concerned with separate forms of aggression such as offence and defence (as well as predation) (reviewed by Blanchard & Blanchard, 1988; Kruk, 1991; Ursin, 1981). Lesions or stimulation in several areas of the hypothalamus have altered aggressive interactions and it is difficult to ascribe specific functions to individual hypothalamic nuclei. For example, Hess (1954) showed that stimulating the lateral hypothalamus in cats caused aggressive behaviour. This stimulation also led to either predatory attack in the presence of a prey or an offence attack when a conspecific male was present. Lesions in the medial hypothalamus (ventromedial nucleus) induced both defence and offence, and resulted in animals that were highly reactive to aggression-provoking stimuli. Defensive aggression seems to be also represented in the anterior hypothalamus, as stimulation of this area resulted in this behaviour only in cornered rats. The preoptic area is also involved with the initiation, modulation, integration and organization of defensive aggression. However, it should be noted that these areas are also implicated in other behaviours. For example, the preoptic area has well-established roles in sexual and maternal behaviour in experimental animals, and the ventromedial hypothalamus is known to be concerned with feeding. Bearing in mind the relation between aggression and other categories of adaptive behaviour, it is clear that there is still uncertainty about the exact role of the hypothalamus in aggression, and whether this can be truly separated from its other adaptive and homeostatic functions.

There are well-documented cases describing humans with tumours in the medial or anterior hypothalamus who became highly aggressive (reviewed by Albert et al., 1993; Eichelman, 1983; van de Poll & van Goozen, 1992). They respond with aggression to stimuli they would have previously considered only annoying (reactive aggression). Damage to the anterior part of the hypothalamus also leads to a dramatic change of character and very aggressive and irritable episodes. 'Sedative' surgical interventions, involving lesions of the posterior hypothalamus have been used in the surgical treatment of aggressive patients. They were said to show remarkable success in patients with intractable violent behaviour (Sano et al., 1970). So it seems that the experimental and clinical evidence are in reasonable agreement about the fundamental role of the hypothalamus in aggressive behaviour.

The midbrain

The hypothalamus controls aggressive display in part through its projections to the brainstem. For example, if the connection between the hypothalamus and the midbrain is interrupted, the stimulation of the hypothalamus does not induce aggression (Ellison & Flynn, 1968). The periaqueductal grey matter (PAG) is a crucial structure for the motor pattern of defensive aggression, although is not involved in offence (see Fig. 4.2). Lesions in this structure in rats attenuate or even abolish defence reactions, whether they be provoked either by a natural threat or by electrical stimulation of the hypothalamus. On the contrary, a lesion in the medial hypothalamus does not in any way prevent such a reaction being triggered by stimulation of the PAG (Mos et al., 1983). This indicates the direction of the neural pathways connecting the two structures. Stimulation of the PAG can elicit highly characteristic defence reactions (including attack or flight) (Bandler et al., 1991). However, it should be noted that the PAG has been implicated in other behavioural functions in addition to aggression or fearful responses (Nieuwenhuys, 1996).

The ventral tegmental area (VTA) is involved in the motor patterns of offence (see Fig. 4.2). Experimental lesions here reduced offence but did not alter defence (or predation) (Adams, 1986). This finding suggests that offence has a discrete substrate in the midbrain and that this is different from that of the defence system. However, it is important to note that VTA lesions interfere with many other behaviours, particularly those that require an active reponse, so it is unlikely that the VTA is specifically concerned with aggression. The VTA is also a major source of forebrain dopaminergic neurons, and the role of the monoamines in aggression is discussed further below.

The frontal neocortex

We have seen that aggression forms an important part of social regulation and social interaction. Cortical regions are essential for social learning, anticipation of the consequences of behaviour and response selection. However, decortication does not affect the ability to express aggression. Completely decorticated rats retain the vast majority of motor patterns of aggression. The frontal neocortex is intimately connected with both the amygdala and the hypothalamus and is therefore in a position to influence these other brain centres which control aggression. More specifically, the prefrontal cortex has an inhibitory influence on the expression of aggressive behaviour (see Fig. 4.2). The orbitofrontal cortex receives information from both external sensory source and from the lower centres which control aggression, and it projects back onto these lower centres (Fuster, 1989). Therefore, this part of the cortex qualifies anatomically as a potential higher level in the control of aggression and this is supported by both experimental and clinical evidence. Stimulation of the deeper orbital layers of the prefrontal cortex inhibits attacks elicited from the hypothalamus in the rat. As a corollary, bilateral lesions of the orbitofrontal cortex resulted in an enhancement of offensive aggression (de Bruin, 1990; de Bruin et al., 1983). In humans, aggression can occur as a feature of frontal lobe damage (reviewed by Giancola, 1995; Miller, 1994). Humans with lesions in the orbitofrontal cortex reacted with impulsivity, without planning or taking into account the consequences of their behaviour. These patients were irritable and had short tempers, responding to minor provocation. They experienced brief outbursts of anger during which they might take impulsive action and, after committing an aggressive act, they were usually indifferent to the consequences (Luria, 1980). Thus, this region is implicated in the process that decides the time, place and strategy of response appropriate to the anger induced by the environment. Techniques determining the activity of the frontal lobes (e.g. glucose uptake by PET) show this is reduced in the frontal lobes (but also other areas, including the amygdala) of violent murderers (Raine et al., 1994, 1997) Recently, the orbitofrontal cortex and dorsolateral cortex have been suggested to be involved in the expression of different categories of aggressive behaviour in humans (Giancola, 1995). It seems likely that the frontal cortex plays a major part in the social regulation of aggression, and the way that aggressive interactions are used to determine social relationships.

Neurochemical modulation of aggressive behaviour

The brain is a chemical machine, and the recognition that neural systems can be defined by the chemical transmitters they use offers a different perspective from the neuroanatomical one. Neurons release a range of chemicals (neurotransmitters) into synapses; these stimulate or suppress the activity of the next set of neurons in the chain, and so on. The release of transmitters is the result of electrical impulses travelling down axons, and the effect of released transmitters is dependent on their binding to specific receptors on the membranes of the next neuron. An important point is that a given neurotransmitter can have many effects, depending on the nature of the receptor with which it comes into contact. This is particularly relevant to the limbic system, which contains a profusion of such neurochemicals and receptors. We will focus on the major chemical groups implicated in neurotransmission: amino acids, monoamines, peptides and steroid hormones; all have been found to be involved in aggression. Chemical neuroanatomy shows us that chemically identifiable systems are organized in the brain as structures that cut across the conventional, modular (anatomical) definitions – the 'systems' referred to above. If we are to understand how the brain controls aggression, then we have to understand the relation between modular and chemical views of the brain. The vast majority of pharmacological treatments to control pathologically aggressive behaviours in humans are based on drugs that are agonists or antagonists to the receptors of the dopaminergic, noradrenergic, serotonergic, GABAergic and opioidergic systems (Miczek et al., 1994).

We should bear in mind that neurochemicals interact and thus we should not expect one neurochemical system to be solely responsible for aggression. Any alteration in one system can affect other systems. Furthermore, the complexity of aggression (see Fig. 4.1) ensures that there may be many roles for each neurochemical, and each component of aggression may be subjected to multiple neurochemical control. However, most studies are conducted on a selected neurochemical and its effect on aggression without paying attention to the possible changes produced in other neurochemical systems. For example, serotonin interacts with dopamine, noradrenaline, acetylcholine, glutamate and neuropeptides.

Amino acids

Amino acids, such as glutamate and g-amino-butyric acid (GABA), represent the simplest transmitters (see Fig. 4.5). They are used throughout the brain, together with a few other candidates, such as glycine (and possibly others); there is nothing special about their role in the limbic system, so far as we know at present, though they clearly play a significant role here as elsewhere. Their apparent chemical simplicity is complicated by a profusion of receptors and post-receptor cellular events. These enable amino-acid transmitters to act as chemical switches in the neural networks that are characteristic, for example, of the cortex as well as in longer-term changes such as those underlying some forms of learning.

GABA

The GABAergic system has a role in the inhibitory control of aggression. A negative correlation between low levels of GABA in some brain areas (such as striatum, hippocampus and amygdala) and aggressive behaviour has been found in animals. Pharmacological studies confirm this inhibitory role (reviewed by Brain & Haug, 1992; Miczek et al., 1994; Paredes & Agmo, 1992). For example, the intraperitoneal injection of GABA transaminase inhibitors (e.g. valproic acid) reduced aggressive behaviour and this was associated with enhanced GABA concentrations in olfactory bulb, striatum and septum.

In humans, benzodiazepines (such as chlordiazepoxide, which acts principally on GABA receptors) are used in conjunction with antipsychotics to sedate and control disturbed behaviour, but their wider effects on aggressive behaviour are difficult to assess. Early work showed benzodiazepines to be useful in

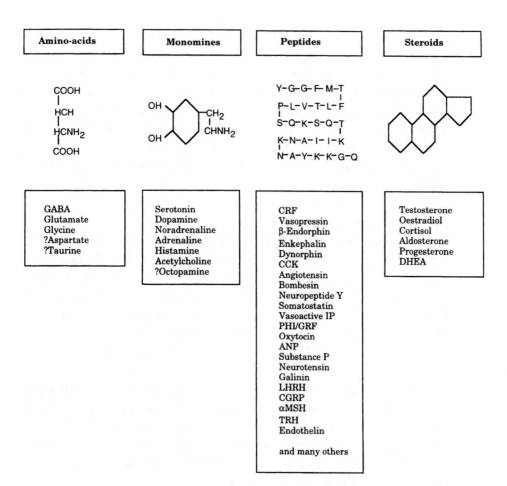

Fig. 4.5. The principal chemical signals in the limbic system. An example of the biochemical structure for each group is shown above (the letters designating the peptide refer to individual amino-acids), and a list of the major components of the groups is given below. GABA: γ-amino-butyric acid; CRF: corticotropin-releasing factor; CCK: cholecystokinin; vasoactive IP: vasoactive intestinal peptide; ANP: atrial natriuretic peptide; LHRH: luteinizing hormone releasing hormone; CGRP: calicotonin-gene related peptide; α-MSH: melanocyte stimulating hormone; TRH: thyrotropin-releasing hormone; DHEA: dehydroepiandrosterone.

controlling aggression but in direct contradiction to this there are reports of rage reactions and a generally increased level of hostility and irritability. Similarly, the biphasic effects of benzodiazepine receptor agonists such as diazepam and chlordiazepoxide have been observed in animals in which aggression is reduced at moderate to high doses, but enhanced at low doses. The pro-aggressive effects of lower doses of benzodiazepines in animals may be of particular relevance to the clinical problems with these substances in the management of aggressive and violent patients. Thus, while these agents rapidly alleviate the feelings of anxiety that often trigger violence, their use in the treatment of aggression has been only moderately successful. These studies emphasize the fact that aggression may be a secondary consequence of primary alterations in other states (in this case, anxiety). Furthermore, there may be differences among compounds; for example, oxazepam has been recommended for use in people with low impulse control (Bond, 1992). There is little information on the use of benzodiazepines in controlling aggression in children.

Monoamines and aggression

The monoamines (e.g. serotonin, noradrenaline and dopamine) represent a family of systems with common features but definable differences. Their comparatively simple chemical nature (see Fig. 4.5) is also counterbalanced by complex arrays of receptors. Whilst they are found throughout the brain, the limbic system has particularly profuse monoaminergic plexuses (see Fig. 4.6). Monoamines have been implicated in a wide variety of functions that range from basic ones (e.g. sleep), as well as more complex attributes such as mood, memory and cognition.

Most current pharmacological evidence linking monoamines with aggression originates from experimental and clinical studies that attempt to specify either a particular neurochemical system in the control of aggression, or a receptor subtype within a given system. Although noradrenaline and dopamine appear to be involved in aggression (Eichelman, 1990), the serotonin (5-HT) system has been thought to play a key role.

Serotonin

Serotonin is broadly distributed throughout the central nervous system (see Fig. 4.6) and is involved in a wide range of psychological functions including sleep, appetite, pain perception, sexual activity, memory and mood control. It has been suggested that it exerts an inhibitory effect over behaviour. One of its characteristic effects seems to be to regulate reactivity to environmental stimuli. If serotonin activity is reduced, there is decreased impulse control and hyper-responsivity to external stimuli. Serotonin has also been involved in a number of mood disorders such as depression and anxiety. Valzelli (1969) reported that reduced turnover in serotonin is typical of spontaneously aggressive rats or rats that had become aggressive after a period of isolation. Furthermore, genetic differences in isolation-induced aggressive behaviour in mice may parallel differences in serotonin synthesis (Valzelli, 1981).

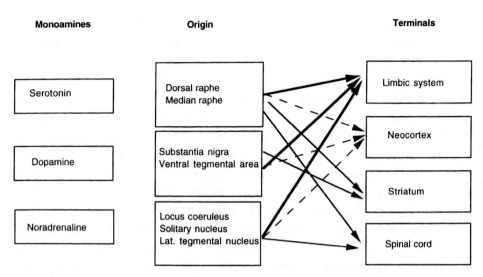

Fig. 4.6. Diagrammatic representation of the origin and distribution of the main monoaminergic systems. The diagram emphasizes their common origin from a few, but distinct, nuclei in the brainstem and widely distributed terminals throughout the cortex, subcortical systems, and spinal cord. All three systems terminate in the limbic system, but the considerable regional differences in the density of innervation by the three categories of fibres in this and other projection areas are not shown, though this is likely to be important in the context of aggression.

In humans, changes in the level and metabolism of serotonin have been correlated with affective behaviour in general and more specifically with aggressive behaviour. Many studies have been carried out to correlate the level of serotonergic functioning with the aggressive behaviour of subjects. Among the measures commonly used as 'markers' (indices) of central 5-HT function are the following: cerebrospinal fluid (CSF) concentrations of 5-hydroxy-indoleacetic acid (5-HIAA; the major metabolite of serotonin); peripheral serotonergic markers such as tritiated imipramine (^{3}H-IMI) binding to platelet membranes (a measure of presynaptic 5-HT functioning); monoamine-oxidase enzyme type B (MAO-B) in platelets, and functional probes with fenfluramine (a drug that releases central serotonin). There is uncertainty about the relevance of peripheral measures (e.g. platelets) to levels of serotonin in the brain. Direct measurement of serotonin levels in the brain and the density of receptors postmortem have also been made. Most recently, individual differences in genes regulating serotonin (e.g. polymorphisms) have been related to emotional traits, or to the prevalence of psychopathology.

Serotonin has become the major focus of biological studies of suicidal behaviour (defined as 'self-aggression') and impulsive aggressive behaviour in humans (reviewed by Coccaro et al., 1992; Mann, 1998). In general, there is a relatively consistent association between serotonin and violent and aggressive acts. Decreased serotonergic function has been found in those individuals with a past history of aggressive acts including violent offences and suicide (reviewed by Asberg, 1994). Specific measures of the risk of impulsive aggression have been correlated with low activity of the central serotonin in individuals with psychiatric and personality disorders as well as in healthy volunteers. An association has been reported between low CSF 5-HIAA concentration and impulsive, destructive behaviours, particularly when aggression and violence are involved (reviewed by Brown & Linnoila, 1990). This has been found in individuals with a past history of suicide attempts; in violent offenders; in subjects suffering from personality disorders characterized by aggressive traits; in alcoholics with aggressive behaviour while sober; in normal adults acting out self-reported hostility; in children with cruelty to animals; in children with disruptive behaviour disorder; in 47XYY syndrome with a history of criminal violence and in parents who had killed or tried to kill a child and then went on to attempt suicide. Furthermore, low binding capacity of imipramine to platelet membranes has been reported in severely aggressive subjects institutionalized since childhood for mental retardation and in suicide attempters in comparison with healthy controls (Marazziti et al., 1993).

It is important to bear in mind that low CSF concentrations of 5-HIAA or a low-activity tryptophan hydroxylase genotype are found in a sizeable proportion of the normal population. There are also polymorphisms in the serotonin transporter and receptors, molecules that determine the efficacy and duration of action of serotonin at the synapse (Collier et al., 1996). It is clearly important to know whether decreased serotonin, however caused, is related to heightened aggression or to problems with impulse control.

Effect of manipulations of the serotonergic system on aggression   The causal relation between serotonin and aggression can only be established from experimental studies in which the effect of the manipulation of the serotonergic system on aggressive behaviour is observed. Studies in animals show that a wide range of aggressive behaviours are sensitive to manipulations of the serotonergic system (reviewed by Bell & Hobson, 1994; Brain & Haug, 1992; Miczek et al., 1994). Depletion of brain serotonin increases aggression. The intracerebroventricular administration of the neurotoxin 5,7-dihydroxytryptamine (5,7-DHT), which causes selective degeneration of the serotonergic terminals, increases offensive, defensive and predatory aggression in rats without change in other social and nonsocial behaviours. A diet without tryptophan or the blockade of the synthesis of serotonin which lower central serotonin increase aggression in rats (Vergnes et al., 1986). Conversely, serotonergic enhancing drugs including the specific serotonin-uptake inhibitors (SSRIs) (such as sertraline, fluvoxamine and fluoxetine) reduce aggression (Olivier et al., 1989; Sanchez & Meier, 1997). In humans, tryptophan depletion in individuals with high trait aggression made them more angry, aggressive, annoyed and hostile whereas this procedure had no effect on individuals with low trait aggression. Thus, in those with pre-existing aggressive traits, acute falls in central serotonin can cause increased subjective and objective aggression (Cleare & Bond, 1995). There are studies suggesting clinical potential for SSRI drugs in the treatment of aggressive behaviour (Castrogiovanni et al., 1992; Cornelius et al., 1990). In children the results are controversial. While, in one study, SSRIs were reported to have little beneficial effect (Constantino et al., 1997), in another fluoxetine (paradoxically) increased aggression in children with obsessive-compulsive disorder (King et al., 1991 but see Coccaro & Kavousi, 1997).

Serotonin receptors and aggression   Subtypes of serotonin receptors may mediate aggressive behaviour differentially. Among those that are more directly involved in aggressive behaviour are the 5-HT$_1$ and 5-HT$_2$ receptors. In general, a class of 5-HT$_1$ agonists, termed 'serenics' (such as eltoprazine [a 5-HT1B receptor agonist], piperazine and fluprazine) have anti-aggressive properties. Studies on rodents have shown that these agonists specifically inhibit offensive aggression without any interference with social functioning, adaptive defensive behaviour or other elements of normal behaviour such as sexual or eating behaviours (reviewed by Miczek et al., 1994; Olivier et al., 1994). The clinician working with aggressive patients needs psychoactive drugs that specifically inhibit destructive behaviour without having other significant behavioural, psychiatric or somatic effects. In this sense, serenics reduce aggressive behaviour without inducing severe adverse effects or diminishing social relationships (reviewed by Ratey & Chandler, 1995). However, the complex relation between fear and aggression has already been noted. Fluprazine and eltoprazine may potentiate fear and anxiety reactions in rodents. Thus, the anti-aggressive effects of serenic substances may be ancillary to an anxiogenic effect; if so, this may limit their clinical usefulness (Miczek et al., 1994).

Studies on rodents suggest that 5-HT$_{1A}$ receptor stimulation results in a decrease in aggressive behaviour (reviewed by Bell & Hobson, 1994). Treatment with agonists of this receptor (such as buspirone, gepirone, ipsapirone, tandospirone and 8-hydroxy-N,N dipropyl-2-aminotetralin (8-OH-DPAT)) reduced offensive aggression without sedative or anxiolytic activity. In humans, buspirone administered to mentally retarded individuals allows maintenance of gains in adaptive functioning while alleviating aggressive tendencies (reviewed by Ratey & Chandler, 1995). Buspirone has also been found to be moderately effective in some aggressive children (Pfeffer et al., 1997). As a corollary, reduced sensitivity of 5-HT_{1A} receptors (determined by the prolactin response to the administration of buspirone) is associated with impulsive aggressive behaviours in personality disorder patients (Coccaro et al., 1990). The 5-HT_{1B} receptor is also involved in aggression (see above). Treatment with the 5-HT_{1B} agonist 1-(3 trifluoromethylphenyl piperazine) reduces offensive aggression (Olivier & Mos, 1992). Mutant mice lacking the 5HT_{1B} receptor attacked another male faster and more intensely than wild-type mice (Ramboz et al., 1996). On the other hand, stimulation of the 5-HT_2 receptor with agonists such as dimethoxy-4-bromo-amphetamine reduces both offensive and defensive aggression (Muehlenkamp et al., 1995).

In the context of animal studies it is important to note that a wide range of behaviours is regulated by changing serotonin, so that it seems as likely that altered aggression is part of this more general effect as that there is a special relation between central serotonin and aggression. In humans, aggression may occur as part of a range of psychiatric disorders, so that alterations in serotonin may be related to the underlying illness, rather than the expression of aggression per se. Nevertheless, if aggression is a prominent part of disinhibited behaviour, then increasing serotonergic activity is a promising and logical therapeutic approach.

Dopamine
Brain dopamine originates largely from two groups of neurons: the substantia nigra, innervating the striatum, and the ventral tegmental area (VTA) innervating the accumbens and the frontal cortex (see Fig. 4.6). The dopaminergic system also plays a role in the genesis of aggressive behaviour. Damage to the VTA reduces aggression, but also many other active behaviours (e.g. sexual behaviour, feeding) (Pucilowski et al., 1980). The striatum is concerned, inter alia, with the expression of motor acts; thus, procedures (such as altering its major dopaminergic input) would be expected to interfere with motor behaviour, such as that necessary for the display of aggressive behaviour.

Studies on rodents suggest that increasing brain dopamine activity creates a state in which animals are more prepared to respond aggressively to stimuli in the environment. Studies with selectively acting D1 and D2 receptor antagonists demonstrate that these substances are potent in suppressing a range of active behaviours that include – but are not specific to – attack and threat (reviewed by Miczek et al., 1994). Thus, in spite of their widespread clinical use in the management of aggressive and violent patients with varying diagnoses, experimental studies have not established a cogent rationale for a specific role of brain dopamine systems and dopamine receptor subtypes in specific types of animal aggression. Although antagonists of receptor D1 decrease aggressive behaviour, the antagonists of receptor D2 are the most frequently used therapeutic agents in the management of violent patients. However, antagonists such as chlorpromazine and haloperidol lack significant behavioural specificity with regard to the decrease in aggressive behaviour. Studies that focus exclusively on aggressive behaviour may fail to take into account the more general behavioural role of dopamine (and other monoamines) on functions such as reward or punishment (Le Moal & Simon, 1992; Ljungberg et al., 1992). On the other hand, experiencing aggression (social defeat) selectively activates the mesolimbic DA system (Tidey & Miczek, 1996).

Noradrenaline

Noradrenaline (like dopamine) is found only in a few neurons. These noradrenergic neurons are located principally in the brainstem, in such nuclei as the solitary nucleus or the locus coeruleus. From these small collections of neurons, noradrenaline-containing fibres spread throughout the brain, though the distribution is not even (some areas receive a richer supply of noradrenaline than others) (Fig. 4.6).

The noradrenergic system also appears to play a role in the genesis of aggressive behaviour. Some studies suggest that abnormalities in noradrenaline function play a role in the vulnerability to aggressive episodes. Hyperactivity of noradrenergic functioning has been found to correlate with aggressive behaviour in human beings. CSF concentrations of the noradrenaline metabolite 3-methoxy-4-hydroxyphenylglycol were positively correlated with a life story of significant aggressive behaviour (Brown et al., 1979). There is increased beta-adrenergic receptor binding in the prefrontal and temporal areas of the cortex in the brains of violent suicide victims compared with accident victims (Mann et al., 1986). Involvement of the noradrenergic system in impulsive aggression is further supported by the finding that noradrenergic receptor blockade is clinically useful in the treatment of aggressive behaviour. Beta-adrenergic blockers such as propranolol and nadolol are effective in reducing aggressive behaviour in chronic psychiatric inpatients, in patients with brain injuries, in adult patients with attention deficit disorder and temper outburst and in organically impaired children (reviewed by Eichelman, 1990; Kavoussi et al., 1997). Clonidine (a presynaptic alpha-2 receptor agonist which decreases overall noradrenergic activity) reduces aggression in children (Kemph et al., 1993). Similarly, antidepressant medications that inhibit noradrenergic uptake or stimulate noradrenergic output increase aggressive behaviours in rodents, and this effect can be blocked by pretreatment with a selective noradrenaline neurotoxin (Cai et al., 1993; Matsumoto et al., 1995).

Peptides

Peptides are altogether more complex chemically, and there are dozens (perhaps hundreds) known to be released in the brain (see Fig. 4.5). Here they act as elsewhere in the body – as complex intercellular signals that allow one cell to influence the activity of others (Herbert, 1993). Peptide-containing neurons are found in all parts of the brain, though the distribution is not even; they are particularly profuse in the limbic system. Peptides are an excellent example of the fact that the neurochemical structure of the limbic system does not correspond to the traditional modular arrangement, suggesting a series of parallel or complementary pathways, each distinguished from the others by its specific content of peptides. In some cases a local group supplies terminals to a wide area (e.g. pro-opiomelanocorticotrophin-expressing neurons: POMC). In others, neurons and terminals are found in several, relatively dispersed areas (e.g. those containing corticotropin-releasing factor: CRF) (Palkovits & Brownstein, 1985). Peptides differ from other neurochemicals (such as the monoamines) in that their behavioural effects can be quite specific; for example, we have seen that altering serotonin can affect many behaviours; but infusions of the peptide angiotensin II induces the very specific behaviour of drinking, which is part of a directed and coordinated response to hypovolaemia (Herbert, 1993). Other peptides invoke other patterns of response; is there a set of peptides specifying aggression?

Peptides, like other neurotransmitters, may have multiple roles in the control of aggression at several levels. These include the neural process (see Fig. 4.1) by which aggression is used as a strategy in the pursuit of defined objectives, such as food, mates etc., or as a means of establishing a social structure (in species that live in groups); or the neural mechanism by which an aggressive strategy is translated into displays of aggressive behaviour and the accompanying autonomic and endocrine activity. The complex behavioural and physiological pattern that forms the response to aggression from others may also involve peptides.

In this chapter, we focus on three peptides that have been particularly associated with aggression. We do not mean to imply that there are not many others; but these are offered as a template for current and future studies in this rapidly developing area. The three are: corticotropin-releasing factor (CRF); vasopressin (AVP) and the opioid peptides.

CRF and aggression

CRF is a 41 amino-acid peptide expressed in neurons and terminals in a number of cell groups in the brainstem associated with autonomic function (such as the parabrachial nucleus, locus coeruleus and dorsal vagal complex) as well as in many areas of the cortex, but particularly in the limbic system (Lewis et al., 1989; Merchenthaler et al., 1982; Sakanaka et al., 1987). There are also high affinity binding sites for CRF scattered throughout those areas containing terminals, though, as for other peptides, there is a limited relation between the relative densities of terminals immunoreactive for CRF and receptors (De Souza 1987; Hauger et al., 1988). CRF seems to have an integrative role in organizing the behavioural, endocrine and autonomic responses to stressful stimuli (such as aggression). Intracerebral infusions of this peptide increased anxiety (fear) in rats. Because the amygdala has been implicated in fear and aggressive behaviour (see above), there is particular interest in the role of CRF in this region. Aggressive and other behavioural responses to another, strange male (a biologically relevant social stressor) were reduced in male rats by intracerebroventricular infusions of CRF but, conversely, these behavioural responses were accentuated when CRF was injected in the amygdala (Elkabir et al., 1990). Thus the role of CRF may depend upon its site of action. CRF under basal conditions has been found to induce a highly localized pattern of *c-fos* expression (Arnold et al., 1992), similar to that observed in rats experiencing acute aggression.

Vasopressin (AVP) and aggression

AVP is widely distributed throughout the central nervous system including hypothalamic and extrahypothalamic nuclei (e.g. bed nucleus of stria terminalis, medial amygdala). Microinjections of AVP into the ventrolateral and anterior hypothalamus and medial amygdala increased offensive aggression in rodents (Ferris & Delville, 1994; Koolhaas et al., 1990). On the contrary, microinjections of AVP V_1-receptor antagonists into the anterior hypothalamus prevented this behaviour (Ferris & Delville, 1994; Ferris & Potegal, 1988; Potegal & Ferris, 1990). However, a negative correlation between AVP in lateral septum and offensive aggression has been found in mice and rats (Compaan et al., 1993; Everts et al., 1997). It should be noted that AVP levels in the septum, medial amygdala and part of the hypothalamus are testosterone-dependent, which may be relevant to the role of testosterone on some forms of aggression (see below) (Delville et al., 1996; Everts et al., 1997; Koolhaas et al., 1991). AVP also potentiated the action of CRF in several contexts, including the expression of aggressive behaviour (Elkabir et al., 1990). Intracerebroventricular infusions of AVP induced *c-fos* immunoreactivity in specific regions of the basal forebrain and brainstem similar (but not identical) to the pattern observed after CRF infusions (Andreae & Herbert, 1993).

Opioids and aggression

The three types of opioids (enkephalin, endorphin and dynorphin) are involved in many neural functions. Their role in aggression, and other aspects of social behaviour, is only just beginning to be studied. Enkephalin-deficient mice showed more offensive aggression and were also more anxious that wild-type controls (Konig et al., 1996). Infusions of enkephalin in the PAG suppressed defensive responses, an effect apparently dependent on changes in the activity of the amygdala (Shaikh et al., 1991). In humans, studies on the role of opioids in aggression are very scanty. Evidence has been obtained in young suicide victims in which an increased number of opiate receptors in the brain have been found (Gross-Isseroff et al., 1990).

Interactions between amines and peptides

Peptides and monoamines interact to regulate behaviour, including aggression. For example, treatment with fluoxetine (a SSRI – see above) prevented the aggression-promoting actions of AVP when microinjected in the hypothalamus (Ferris & Delville, 1996), suggesting a direct interaction between this peptide and the serotonergic system. In humans, a significant positive correlation has been found between CSF levels of AVP and aggression in personality disordered subjects with a history of fighting and assault, in addition to a hyporeactive 5-HT system as assessed by fenfluramine challenge (Coccaro, 1996). Thus, in humans, a hyporeactive 5-HT system may result in enhanced brain levels of AVP and the facilitation of impulsive, aggressive behaviour.

Studies on the role of peptides in aggression are still at an early stage. Peptides other than those discussed here (e.g. oxytocin) have also been implicated in aggressive behaviour (Herbert, 1993). Given the variety of contexts in which this behaviour occurs, this is hardly surprising. We still lack evidence for a precise role for peptides in aggressive behaviour; in particular, whether peptides acting within defined areas of the brain (e.g. the amygdala) may have equally definable roles in the selection, operation or response to aggression. However, there are clear differences between the respective roles of amines, peptides and steroids (see below) in this behaviour (as in others) so that we can expect further clarification within the near future.

Steroids and aggression with special reference to testosterone

Finally, there are chemical signals from outside the brain that act as neural messengers; the most obvious of these are the steroid hormones (Fig. 4.5). The limbic system contains the highest concentrations of steroid receptors (Nieuwenhuys, 1996). The actions of steroids have traditionally been studied experimentally by removing steroids, or administering them. It has become apparent that the age of the animal is a critical factor. In some cases, steroids have been applied locally in the brain, thus combining neuroanatomical and chemical specificity. In humans, most studies (mainly on men) are correlational, though advantage has been taken from studying genetic aberrations or endocrine dysfunction.

Many species have restricted breeding seasons during which sexual behaviour occurs and when levels of gonadal hormones increase. Depending on their social structure, such species may show parallel increases in aggression, prominently between males (Wilson & Boelkins, 1970). In most mammalian species aggression is more common between males than between females. These sex differences have been associated with the organizing and sensitizing effects of androgens during development and their activating effects during puberty and adulthood (Brain, 1981). There are structural changes in the brain in response to exposure to steroids (e.g. testosterone) in early life, though it has proved difficult to relate these to behaviour. These effects are seen in areas of the limbic system where there are androgen receptors, including the anterior hypothalamus, the medial amygdala and the septum, all of them implicated in aggression (Wood & Newman, 1995). In humans, the majority of aggressive, criminal acts are committed by men (they have higher levels of androgens than women). Furthermore, there is a supposition that 'roid rage' (explosive aggressive outbursts) can occur in those who take massive doses of testosterone (Parrott et al., 1994; Yesalis et al., 1993). All this points to testosterone as an aggression-promoting hormone. What is the evidence?

Steroids and aggression during development: organizational effects
The presence of androgens during a critical phase of early life masculinizes and defeminizes the brain. This is thought to be primarily responsible for the organization of particular parts of the brain which renders a male more sensitive to the aggression-inducing action of testosterone in adulthood.

Neonatal administration of androgens to female rats produced an adult in which aggression can be induced after ovariectomy and administration of androgens. Treating female monkeys prenatally with testosterone increased rough-and-tumble play (Goy, 1978). Intrauterine position influences inter-female aggression in mice. Females that develop in utero between two male fetuses are exposed to higher levels of testosterone secreted by male fetuses than females that develop between two females. The former were highly aggressive toward other females but not males in adulthood (Vom Saal, 1983). However, the activational property of testosterone can still be observed in males castrated neonatally when injected with testosterone in adulthood. Thus, prior organization of the neural substrate is not a necessary prerequisite for adult males to exhibit aggression when treated with testosterone, although exposure to testosterone during early life renders a male more sensitive to this action.

The effect of prenatal androgen on aggression in humans has been studied in clinical cases in which the normal levels of androgens are altered by either endocrine disorders (e.g. partial androgen insensibility in genetic males; congenital adrenal hyperplasia in genetic females which involves prenatal androgenization) or by exposure to exogenous hormone manipulations when pregnancy was threatened (e.g. progestagens which have androgenic and estrogenic properties). In general, exposure to androgens prenatally influenced aggressive behaviour during childhood or later life in a manner parallel to that observed in other mammals: an increase in aggression was found in girls exposed prenatally to abnormally high levels of androgens (Berenbaum & Resnick, 1997). However, these observations are complicated by the fact that the girls were not exposed to androgens during adult life (that is, these studies are not strictly comparable to those in animals) so the results are not conclusive (Archer, 1991; Brain, 1994; Meyer-Bahlburg & Ehrhardt, 1982; Rainish & Sanders, 1987). It is important to bear in mind that substances other than hormones may have the capacity to affect the level of prenatal androgens; for example, barbiturates decrease the level of testosterone (Rainish & Sanders, 1982).

Steroids and aggression post-pubertally: activational effects
Aggression increases during puberty in both primate and nonprimate (e.g. rodent) species, particularly in males, and there is a positive correlation between testosterone levels in both blood and CSF in captive monkeys and aggression (Higley et al., 1996). However, treating adult nonhuman primates with testosterone has had variable effects on aggressive interactions (Dixson, 1980). In humans, a number of attempts have been made to relate levels of

testosterone in puberty and adulthood with aggressive behaviour (reviewed by Albert et al., 1993; Archer, 1991, 1994; Brain, 1994). The question is whether individual differences in the level of aggressiveness are related to differences in testosterone levels. In adults, higher testosterone levels have been reported in groups selected for high levels of aggressiveness. For example, salivary testosterone (a measure of 'free' testosterone) correlated positively with violent crimes in male prison inmates (Dabbs et al., 1987). Similar correlates were found in adolescent boys and adult men between testosterone and a variety of aggressive behaviours (Christiansen & Knussmann, 1987; Olweus et al., 1988) though this association has been questioned (Campbell et al., 1997). However, testosterone given to men has not, in all cases, had the expected effects on aggression. For example, supraphysiological doses of testosterone neither increased self-estimated anger or irritability (Bjorkvist et al., 1994), nor anger or hostility (Tricker et al., 1996). However, both testosterone (in boys) and oestrogens (in girls) increased physical aggressivity (as measured by questionnaires) in hypogonadal adolescents (Finkelstein et al., 1997). Men using anabolic steroids scored more highly on an aggressive scale than controls (Yates et al., 1992). Nevertheless, there is general scepticism about a direct relation between testosterone levels and aggression in men (Archer et al., 1998; Hines, 1998).

How can we make sense of these disparate findings? There are two important considerations: the first, that (as pointed out above) testosterone is related to sexual behaviour, which is, in turn, related to intramale aggressivity. So the stimulating effect of testosterone on aggression may only make sense (and be properly studied) in the context of reproductive behaviour and competition. Second, the social structure of primate groups (including humans) is reflected in the pattern of their aggressive interactions. But social status also alters testosterone, so the relation between individual differences in aggressivity and testosterone may be also indirect. A variety of studies, in both human and nonhuman primates, has shown that social 'stress' (that is, demands made by the social or working environment) lowers testosterone and that 'dominant' males have higher levels (Dixson & Herbert, 1977; Kreuz et al., 1972; Rose et al., 1971). A study in adolescent boys showed that those who were rated by their peers as 'tough' and popular 'leaders' had the highest testosterone levels; they were not particularly aggressive. Those who were tough, not leaders, but were aggressive (and unpopular) had lower levels (Schaal et al., 1996). There seems to be a triangular relation between social structure, testosterone and aggression in male primates that needs to be clearly understood if the contribution of testosterone to aggressive behaviour is to be assessed properly. There are also problems about measuring aggression. For example, a distinction must be made between aggressive acts (violence) and aggressive tendencies as revealed by self-report questionnaires.

Lest it should be thought that testosterone is the 'aggressive' steroid, it should be noted that other steroid hormones may play a role in different contexts. For example, lactating rats are highly aggressive to intruding males (rather than females). This aggressive reaction seems to depend upon suckling, and has obvious biological functions (e.g. to protect the young). Testosterone given to lactating females reduces their aggressive reaction to males (see Herbert, 1990). On the other hand, there is some evidence that dehydroepiandrosterone (DHEA; a steroid that is very high in the blood of humans but reduces with age) can reduce aggression in mice (Schlegel et al., 1985). Thus hormones regulate aggression in a context-specific manner; change the context, and the nature of the hormonal control changes as well.

Conclusion

The regulation of aggression is a distributed function of the brain. There are many anatomical areas associated with aggression, though whether there are specific 'aggressive' nuclei remains doubtful. There are also a plethora of neurochemical systems implicated in aggression. The interaction between the types of aggressive behaviour outlined in this chapter goes some way towards explaining the complex and varied expression of this behaviour, and its multiple role in social behaviour. There are many circumstances and contexts in which brain function is altered, and these may have primary or secondary consequences for aggression.

The complexity of aggression – the behaviour pattern, the contexts in which it occurs, and the uses to which it is put – means that there can never be a single, definable neural system underlying this behaviour. Neither can those neural systems implicated in aggression be clearly separated from those more closely associated with other behaviours or other functions. Nevertheless, attempts should continue to define aggression more precisely in terms that allow more exact analysis of its neurobiological basis, since this offers not only greater understanding of the relation between the brain and this crucial category of behaviour, but also direct help to those who try to control unwanted aggression in either animals or humans. The challenge to those studying aggression in children is to identify the interplay between specific genes and critical elements of the social and physical environment that, together, determine long-lasting patterns of aggressive behaviour.

Acknowledgements

The research in our labs is supported by grants from the Wellcome Trust, MRC and BBSRC (JH), by the University of Valencia (MM), a fellowship from the BBV Foundation (MM) and by a joint grant (Acciones Integradas) from the British Council and the Spanish Ministry of Education and Culture (No. 160B). We are grateful to Rachel Chesterton for art work and our many colleagues for their collaboration, and to the editors of this book for many valuable suggestions.

REFERENCES

Adams, D.B. (1979). Brain mechanisms for offense, defense and submission. *Behavioral Brain Science*, 2, 210–41.

Adams, D.B. (1986). Ventromedial tegmental lesions abolish offense without disturbing predation or defense. *Physiology and Behavior*, 38, 165–8.

Adolphs, R., Tranel, D., Damasio, H. & Damasio, A.R. (1995). Fear and the human amygdala. *Journal of Neuroscience*, 15, 5879–91.

Albert, D.J., Walsh, M.L. & Jonik, R.H. (1993). Aggression in humans: What is its biological foundation? *Neuroscience and Biobehavioral Reviews*, 17, 405–25.

Andreae, L.C. & Herbert, J. (1993). Expression of *c-fos* in restricted areas of the basal forebrain and brainstem following single or combined intraventricular infusions of vasopressin and corticotropin-releasing factor. *Neuroscience*, 53, 735–48.

Archer, J. (1988). *Behavioural Biology of Aggression*. Cambridge: Cambridge University Press.

Archer, J. (1991). The influence of testosterone on human aggression. *British Journal of Psychology*, 82, 1–28.

Archer, J. (1994). Testosterone and aggression. *Journal of Offender Rehabilitation*, 21, 3–25.

Archer, J., Birring, S.S. & Wu, F.C.W. (1998) The association between testosterone and aggression among young men: empirical findings and a meta-analysis. *Aggressive Behavior*, 24, 411–20.

Arnold, F.J.L., de Lucas Bueno, M., Shiers, H., et al. (1992). Expression of *c-fos* in regions of the basal limbic forebrain following intra-cerebroventricular corticotropin-releasing factor (CRF) in unstressed or stressed male rats. *Neuroscience*, 51, 377–90.

Asberg, M. (1994). Monoamine neurotransmitters in human aggressiveness and violence: a selective review. *Criminal Behaviour and Mental Health*, 4, 303–27.

Attili, G. & Hinde, R.A. (1986). Categories of aggression and their motivational heterogeneity. *Ethology and Sociobiology*, 7, 17–27.

Bandler, R., Carrive, P. & Zhang, S.P. (1991). Integration of somatic and autonomic reactions within the midbrain periaqueductal grey: viscerotopic, somatotopic and functional organisation. *Progress in Brain Research*, 87, 269–305.

Bard, P. (1928). A diencephalic mechanism for the expression of rage with special reference to the sympathetic nervous system. *American Journal of Physiology, 84*, 490–515.

Bell, R. & Hobson, H. (1994). 5-HT1A receptor influences on rodent social and agonistic behavior: a review and empirical study. *Neuroscience and Biobehavioral Review, 18*, 325–38.

Berenbaum, S.A. & Resnick, S.M. (1997). Early androgen effects on aggression in children and adults with congenital adrenal hyperplasia. *Psychoneuroendocrinology, 22*, 505–15.

Berkowitz, L. (1993). *Aggression. Its Causes, Consequences and Control.* McGraw-Hill, Inc.

Bjorkvist, K., Nygren, T., Bjorklund, A.C. & Bjorkvist, S.E. (1994). Testosterone intake and aggression – real effect or anticipation. *Aggressive Behavior, 20*, 17–26.

Blanchard, D.C. & Blanchard, R.J. (1988). Ethoexperimental approaches to the biology of emotion. *Annual Review of Psychology, 39*, 43–68.

Bond, A.J. (1992). Pharmacological manipulation of aggressiveness and impulsiveness in healthy volunteers. *Progress in Neuro-Psychopharmacology and Biological Psychiatry, 16*, 1–7.

Brain, P.F. (1981). Hormones and aggression in infra-human vertebrates. In P.F. Brain & D. Benton (Eds.), *The Biology of Aggression* (pp. 181–213). The Netherlands: Sythoff and Noordhoof International Publishers.

Brain, P.F. (1994). Hormonal aspects of aggression and violence. In A.J. Reiss, K.A. Miczek & J.A. Roth (Eds.), *Understanding and Preventing Violence*, Vol. 2 (pp. 177–244). Washington DC: National Academic Press.

Brain, P.F. & Haug, M. (1992). Hormonal and neurochemical correlates of various forms of animal 'aggression'. *Psychoneuroendocrinology, 17*, 537–51.

Brown, G.L., Goodwin, F.K. & Ballenger, J.C. (1979). Aggression in humans correlates with cerebrospinal fluid amine metabolites. *Psychiatry Research, 1*, 131–9.

Brown, G.L. & Linnoila, M.I. (1990). CSF serotonin metabolite (5-HIAA) studies in depression, impulsivity and violence. *Journal of Clinical Psychiatry, 51*, 31–41.

Cai, B., Matsumoto, K., Ohta, H. & Watanabe, H. (1993). Biphasic effects of typical antidepressants and Mianserin, an atypical antidepressant, on aggressive behavior in socially isolated mice. *Pharmacology Biochemistry and Behavior, 44*, 519–25.

Campbell, A., Muncer, S. & Odber, J. (1997). Aggression and testosterone: testing a bio-social model. *Aggressive Behavior, 23*, 229–238.

Castrogiovanni, P., Di-Muro, A. & Maremanni, I. (1992). Fluoxetine reduces aggressive behavior in depressive outpatients. *New Trends in Experimental and Clinical Psychiatry, 8*, 57.

Christiansen, K. & Knussmann, R. (1987). Androgen levels and components of aggressive behavior in men. *Hormones and Behavior, 21*, 170–80.

Cleare, A.J. & Bond, A.J. (1995). The effect of tryptophan depletion and enhancement on subjective and behavioural aggression in normal male subjects. *Psychopharmacology, 118*, 72–81.

Coccaro, E.F. (1996). Neurotransmitter correlated of impulsive aggression in humans. In C.F. Ferris & T. Grisso (Eds.), *Understanding Aggressive Behavior in Children*, Vol. 794 (pp. 82–9). New York: New York Academy of Sciences.

Coccaro, E.F., Gabriel. S. & Siever, L.J. (1990). Buspirone challenge: preliminary evidence for a role for central $5\text{-}HT_{1A}$ receptor function in impulsive aggressive behavior in humans. *Psychopharmacology Bulletin, 26*, 393–405.

Coccaro, E.F. & Kavousi, R.J. (1997). Fluoxetine and impulsive aggressive behavior in personality-disordered subjects. *Archives of General Psychiatry, 54*, 1081–8.

Coccaro, E.F., Kavousi, R.J. & Lesser, J.C. (1992). Self- and other-directed human aggression: the role of the central serotonergic system. *International Clinical Psychopharmacology, 16 Suppl. 6*, 70–83.

Collier, D.A., Arranz, M.J., Sham, P. et al. (1996). The serotonin transporter is a potential susceptibility factor of bipolar affective disorder. *NeuroReport, 7*, 1675–9.

Compaan, J.C., Buijs, R.M., Pool, C.W., De Ruiter, A.J.H. & Koolhaas, J.M. (1993). Differential lateral septal vasopressin innervation in aggressive and nonaggressive male mice. *Brain Research Bulletin, 30*, 1–6.

Constantino, J.N., Liberman, M. & Kincald, M. (1997). Effect of serotonin reuptake inhibitors on aggressive behavior in psychiatrically hospitalized adolescents: results of an open trial. *Journal of Child and Adolescent Psychopharmacology, 7*, 31–44.

Cornelius, J.R., Soloff, P.H., Perel, J.M. & Ulrich, R.F. (1990). Fluoxetine trial in borderline personality disorder. *Psychopharmacology Bulletin, 26*, 151–4.

Dabbs, J.M., Frady, R.L., Carr, T.S. & Besch, N.F. (1987). Saliva testsoterone and criminal violence in young adult prison inmates. *Psychosomatic Medicine, 49*, 174–82.

de Bruin, J.P.C. (1990). Orbital prefrontal cortex, dopamine and social-agonistic behavior in male Long Evans rats. *Aggressive Behavior, 16*, 231–48.

de Bruin, J.P.C., van Oyen, H.G.M. & van de Poll, N. (1983). Behavioural changes following lesions of the orbital prefrontal cortex in male rats. *Behavioural Brain Research, 10*, 209–32.

Delville, Y., Mansour, K.M. & Ferris, C.F. (1996). Testosterone facilitates aggression by modulating vasopressin receptors in the hypothalamus. *Physiology and Behavior, 60*, 25–9.

De Souza, E.B. (1987). Corticotropin-releasing factor receptors in the rat central nervous system: characterisation and regional distribution. *Journal of Neuroscience, 7*, 88–100.

Dixson, A.F. (1980). Androgens and aggressive behaviour in primates: a review. *Aggressive Behavior*, 637–47.

Dixson, A.F. & Herbert, J. (1977). Testosterone, aggressive behaviour and dominance rank in captive male talapoin monkeys. *Physiology and Behaviour, 18*, 539–43.

Eichelman, B. (1983). The limbic system and aggression in humans. *Neuroscience and Biobehavioural Reviews, 7*, 391–4.

Eichelman, B.S. (1990). Neurochemical and psychopharmacological aspects of aggressive behavior. *Annual Reviews of Medicine, 41*, 149–58.

Elkabir, D.R., Wyatt, M.E., Vellucci, S.V. & Herbert, J. (1990). The effects of separate or combined infusions of corticotropin-releasing factor and vasopressin either intraventricularly or into the amygdala on aggressive and investigative behaviour in the rat. *Regulatory Peptides, 28*, 199–214.

Ellison, G.D. & Flynn, J.P. (1968). Organized aggressive behavior in cats after surgical isolation of the hypothalamus. *Archives Italiennes de Biologie, 106*, 1–20.

Everts, H.G.J., De Ruiter, A.J.H. & Koolhaas, J.M. (1997). Differential lateral septal vasopressin in wild-type rats: correlation with aggression. *Hormones and Behavior, 31*, 136–44.

Ferris, C.F. & Delville, Y. (1994). Vasopressin and serotonin interactions in the control of agonistic behavior. *Psychoneuroendocrinology, 19*, 593–601.

Ferris, C.F. & Potegal, M. (1988). Vasopressin receptor blockade in the anterior hypothalamus suppresses aggression in hamsters. *Physiology and Behaviour, 44*, 235–9.

Finkelstein, J.W., Susman, E.J., Chinchilli, V.M., et al. (1997). Estrogen or testosterone increases self-reported aggressive behaviors in hypogonadal adolescents. *Journal of Clinical Endocrinology and Metabolism, 82*, 2433–8.

Fuster, J.M. (1989). *The Prefrontal Cortex: Anatomy, Physiology and Neuropsychology of the Frontal Lobe*. New York: Raven.

Giancola, P.R. (1995). Evidence for dorsolateral and orbital prefrontal cortical involvement in the expression of aggressive behavior. *Aggressive Behavior, 21*, 431–50.

Goy, R.W. (1978). Development of play and mounting behavior in female rhesus virilized prenatally with esters of testosterone or dihydrotestosterone. In D.J. Chivers & J. Herbert (Eds.), *Recent Advances in Primatology*, Vol. 1 (pp. 449–62). London: Academic Press.

Gross-Isseroff, R., Dillon, K.A., Israeli, M. & Biegon, A. (1990). Regionally selective increases in mu opioid receptor density in the brains of suicide victims. *Brain Research, 530*, 312–16.

Hauger, R.L., Millan, M.A., Lorang, M., Harwood, J.P. & Aguilera, G. (1988). Corticotropin-releasing factor receptors and pituitary adrenal responses during immobilisation stress. *Endocrinology, 123*, 396–405.

Herbert, J. (1987). Neuroendocrine responses to social stress. *The Neuroendocrinology of Stress. Baillere's Clinical Endocrinology and Metabolism*, Vol. l, No. 2, 467–90.

Herbert, J. (1990). The physiology of aggression. In J. Groebel & R.A. Hinde (Eds.), *Aggression and War* (pp. 58–71). Cambridge: Cambridge University Press.

Herbert, J. (1993). Peptides in the limbic system: chemical codes co-ordinating adaptive responses to behavioural or physiological demand. *Progress in Neurobiology, 41*, 723–91.

Herbert, J. (1996). Sexuality, stress and the chemical architecture of the brain. *Annual Review of Sex Research, 7*, 1–43

Hess, W.R. (1954). *Diencephalon: Autonomic and Extrapyramidal Functions*. New York: Grune and Stratton.

Higley, J.D., Mehlman, P.T., Poland, R.E., et al. (1996). CSF testosterone and 5-HIAA correlate with different types of aggressive behaviors. *Biological Psychiatry, 40*, 1067–82.

Hines, M. (1998). Adult testosterone levels have little or no significance on dominance in men. *Behavioral Brain Sciences, 21*, 377.

Kagan, J. & Schulkin, J. (1995). On the concepts of fear. *Harvard Review of Psychology, 3*, 231–4.

Kavoussi, R., Armstead, P. & Coccaro, E. (1997). The neurobiology of impulsive aggression. *Psychiatric Clinics of North America, 20*, 395–403.

Kemph, J.P., Devane, C.L., Levin, G.M., Jarecke, R. & Miller, R.L. (1993). Treatment of aggressive children with clonidine – results of an open pilot. *Journal of the American Academy of Child and Adolescent Psychiatry, 32*, 577–81.

King, R.A., Riddle, M.A., Chappell, P.B., et al. (1991). Emergence of self-destructive phenomenon in children and adolescents during fluoxetine treatment. *Journal of the American Academy of Child and Adolescent Psychiatry, 30*, 179–86.

Kling, A.S. & Brothers, L.A. (1992). The amygdala and social behavior. In J.P. Aggleton (Ed.), *The Amygdala: Neurobiological Aspects of Emotion, Memory and Mental Dysfunction*, pp. 353–77. New York: Wiley-Liss, Inc.

Kollack-Walker, S. & Newman, S.W. (1995). Mating and agonistic behavior produce different patterns of fos immunolabeling in the male syrian hamster brain. *Neuroscience, 66,* 721–36.

Konig, M., Zimmer, A.M., Steiner, H., et al. (1996). Pain responses, anxiety and aggression in mice deficient in pre-proenkephalin. *Nature, 383,* 535–8.

Koolhaas, J.M., Moor, E., & Hiemstra, Y. (1991). The testosterone-dependent vasopressinergic neurons in the medial amygdala and lateral septum: involvement in social behaviour in male rats. In S. Jard & R. Jamison (Eds.), *Vasopressin* (pp. 213–19). Paris: INSERM/Libbey.

Koolhaas, J.M., van den Brink, T.H.C., Roozendaal, B. & Boorsma, F. (1990). Medial amygdala and aggressive behavior: interaction between testosterone and vasopressin. *Aggressive Behavior, 16,* 223–9.

Kreuz, L.E., Rose, R.M. & Jennings, J.R. (1972). Suppression of plasma testosterone levels and psychological stress. *Archives of General Psychiatry, 26,* 479–83.

Kruk, M.R. (1991). Ethology and pharmacology of hypothalamic aggression in the rat. *Neuroscience and Biobehavioral Reviews, 15,* 527–38.

LaBar, K.S., Gatenby, J.C., Gore, J.C., LeDoux, J.E. & Phelps, E.A. (1998). Human amygdala activation during conditioned fear acquisition and extinction: a mixed-trial MRI study. *Neuron, 20,* 937–45.

Le Moal, M. & Simon, H. (1992). Mesolimbic dopaminergic network: functional and regulatory roles. *Physiological Reviews, 71,* 155–234.

Lewis, D.A., Foote, S.L. & Cha, C.I. (1989). Corticotropin-releasing factor immunoreactivity in monkey neocortex: an immunohistochemical analysis. *Journal of Comparative Neurology, 290,* 599–613.

Ljungberg, T., Apicella, P. & Schultz, W. (1992). Responses of monkey dopamine neurons during learning of behavioral reactions. *Journal of Neurophysiology, 67,* 145–63.

Luria, A.R. (1980). *Higher Cortical Functions in Man.* New York: Basic Books.

Mann, J.J. (1998). The neurobiology of suicide. *Nature Medicine, 4,* 25–30.

Mann, J.J., Standley, M., McBride, P.A. & McEwen, B.S. (1986). Increased serotonin 2 and beta adrenergic receptor binding in frontal cortices of suicide victims. *Archives of General Psychiatry, 43,* 954–9.

Marazziti, D., Rotondo, A., Presta, S., et al. (1993). Role of serotonin in human aggressive behaviour. *Aggressive Behavior, 19,* 347–53.

Maren, S. & Fanselow, M.S. (1996). The amygdala and fear conditioning: has the nut been cracked? *Neuron, 16,* 237–40.

Martinez, M., Phillips, P.J. & Herbert, J. (1998). Adaptation in patterns of c-fos expression in the brain associated with exposure to either single or repeated social stress in male rats. *European Journal of Neuroscience, 10,* 20–33.

Matsumoto, K., Ojima, K. & Watanabe, H. (1995). Noradrenergic denervation attenuates desipramine enhancement of aggressive behavior in isolated mice. *Pharmacology Biochemistry and Behavior, 50,* 481–4.

McGregor, A. & Herbert, J. (1992). Differential effects of excitotoxic basolateral and corticomedial lesions of the amygdala on the behavioural and endocrine responses to either sexual or aggression-promoting stimuli in the male rat. *Brain Research, 574*, 9–20.

Merchenthaler, I., Vigh, S., Petrusz, P. & Schally, A.V. (1982). Immunocytochemical localisation of corticotrophin-releasing factors (CRF) in the rat brain. *American Journal of Anatomy, 165*, 385–96.

Meyer-Bahlburg, H.F.L. & Ehrhardt, A.A. (1982). Prenatal sex hormones and human aggression: a review and new data on progestogen effects. *Aggressive Behavior, 8*, 39–62.

Miczek, K.A. (1991). Tolerance to the analgesic, but not discriminative stimulus of morphine after brief social defeat in rats. *Psychopharmacology, 104*, 181–6.

Miczek, K.A., Weerts, E., Haney, M. & Tidey, J. (1994). Neurobiological mechanisms controlling aggression: preclinical developments for pharmacotherapeutic interventions. *Neuroscience and Biobehavioral Reviews, 18*, 97–110.

Miller, L. (1994). Traumatic brain injury and aggression. *Journal of Offender Rehabilitation, 21*, 91–103.

Mos, J., Lammers, J.H., van der Poel, A.M., et al. (1983). Effects of midbrain central gray lesions on spontaneously and electrically induced aggression in the rat. *Aggressive Behavior, 9*, 133–55.

Moyer, K.E. (1968). Kinds of aggression and their physiological basis. *Communications in Behavioral Biology, 2*, 65–87.

Muehlenkamp, F., Lucion, A. & Vogel, W.H. (1995). Effects of selective serotonergic agonists on aggressive behavior in rats. *Pharmacology Biochemistry and Behavior, 50*, 671–4.

Narabayashi, H., Nagao, T., Saito, Y., Yosluda, M. & Nagahata, M. (1963). Stereotaxic amygdalectomy for behavior disorders. *Archives of Neurology, 9*, 1–16.

Nieuwenhuys, R. (1996). The greater limbic system, the emotional motor system and the brain. *Progress in Brain Research, 107*, 551–80.

Olivier, B. & Mos, J. (1992). Rodent models of aggressive behavior and serotonergic drugs. *Progress in Neuropsychopharmacology and Biological Psychiatry, 16*, 847–70.

Olivier, B., Mos, J. & Raghoebar, P. (1994). Serenics. *Progress in Drug Research, 42*, 167–308.

Olivier, B., Mos, J., van der Heyden, J. & Hartog, J. (1989). Serotonergic modulation of social interactions in isolated male mice. *Psychopharmacology, 97*, 154–6.

Olweus, D., Mattsson, A., Schalling, D. & Low, H. (1988). Circulating testosterone levels and aggression in adolescent males; a causal analysis. *Psychosomatic Medicine, 50*, 261–72.

Palkovits, M. & Brownstein, M.J. (1985). Distribution of neuropeptides in the central nervous system using biochemical micromethods. In A. Bjorklund & T. Hokfelt (Eds.), *Handbook of Chemical Neuroanatomy, 4*, 1–71. Amsterdam: Elsevier.

Paredes, R.G. & Agmo, A. (1992). GABA and behavior: the role of receptor subtypes. *Neuroscience and Biobehavioral Review, 16*, 145–70.

Parrott, A.C., Choi, P.Y.L. & Davies, M. (1994). Anabolic-steroid use by amateur athletes – effects upon psychological mood states. *Journal of Sports Medicine and Physical Fitness, 43*, 292–8.

Pfeffer, C.R., Jiang, H. & Domeshek, L.J. (1997). Buspirine treatment of psychiatrically hospitalized prepubertal children with symptoms of anxiety and moderately severe aggression. *Journal of Child and Adolescent Psychopharmacology, 7*, 145–55.

Potegal, M. & Ferris, C.F. (1990). Intraspecific aggression in male hamsters is inhibited by intrahypothalamic VP-receptor antagonist. *Aggressive Behavior, 15*, 311–20.

Pucilowski, O., Kostowski, W., Bidinski, A. & Hauptmann, M. (1980). Effect of 6-hydroxy-dopamine-induced lesions of A10 dopaminergic neurons on aggressive behaviour in rats. *Pharmacology Biochemistry and Behavior, 16*, 547–51.

Raine, A., Buchsman, M. & LaCasse, L. (1997). Brain abnormalities in murderers indicated by positron emission tomography. *Biological Psychiatry, 42*, 495–508.

Raine, A., Buchsman, M.S., Stanely, G., et al. (1994). Selective reductions in frontal glucose-metabolism in murderers. *Biological Psychiatry, 36*, 365–73.

Rainish, J.M. & Sanders, S.A. (1982). Early barbiturate exposure: the brain, sexuality dimorphic behavior, and learning. *Neuroscience and Biobehavioral Reviews, 6*, 311–19.

Rainish, J.M. & Sanders, S.A. (1987). Behavioral influences of prenatal homones. In C.B. Nemeroff & P.T. Loosen (Eds.), *Handbook of Clinical Psychoneuroendocrinology* (pp. 431–48). New York: Guilford Press.

Ramboz, S., Saudou, F., Amara, D.A., et al. (1996). 5-HT$_{1B}$ receptor knock out-behavioral consequences. *Behavioural Brain Research, 73*, 305–12.

Ratey, J.J. & Chandler, H.K. (1995). Serenics. Therapeutic potential in aggression. *CNS Drugs, 4*, 256–60.

Rose, R.M., Holaday, J.W. & Bernstein, I.S. (1971). Plasma testosterone, dominance rank and aggressive behavior in male rhesus monkeys. *Nature, 231*, 366–8.

Sakanaka, M., Shibasaki, T. & Lederis, K. (1987). Corticotropin releasing factor-like immunoreactivity in the rat brain as revealed by a modified cobalt-glucose oxidase-diaminobenzidine method. *Journal of Comparative Neurology, 260*, 256–98.

Sanchez, C. & Meier, E. (1997). Behavioral profiles of SSRIs in animal models of depression, anxiety and aggression. *Psychopharmacology, 129*, 197–205.

Sano, K., Mayanagi, Y., Sekino, H., Ogashiwa, M. & Ishyima, B. (1970). Results of stimulation and destruction of the posterior hypothalamus in man. *Journal of Neurosurgery, 33*, 689–707.

Schaal, B., Tremblay, R.E., Soussignan, R. & Susman, E.J. (1996). Male testosterone linked to high social dominance but low physical aggression in early adolescence. *Journal of the American Academy of Child and Adolescent Psychiatry, 34*, 1322–30.

Schlegel, M.L., Spetz, J.F., Robel, P. & Haug, M. (1985). Studies on the effects of dehydroepi-androsterone and its metabolites on attack by castrated mice on intruders. *Physiology and Behaviour, 34*, 867–70.

Shaikh, M.B., Lu, C.L. & Siegel, A. (1991). An enkephalinergic mechanism involved in amygdaloid suppression of affective defence behavior elicited from the midbrain periaqueductal grey in the cat. *Brain Research, 559*, 109–17.

Tidey, J.W. & Miczek, K. (1996). Social defeat selectively alters mesocorticolimbic dopamine release: an in vivo microdialysis study. *Brain Research, 721*, 140–9.

Tricker, R., Casaburi, R., Storer, T.W., et al. (1996). The effects of supraphysiological doses of testosterone on angry behavior in healthy eugonadal men – a clinical research-center study. *Journal of Clinical Endocrinology and Metabolism, 81*, 3754–8.

Ursin, H. (1981). Neuroanatomical basis of aggression. In P.F. Brain & D. Benton (Eds.),

Multidisciplinary Approaches to Aggression Research (pp. 269–95). Amsterdam: Elsevier/North-Holland Biomedical Press.

Valzelli, L. (1969). Aggressive behaviour induced by isolation. In S. Garattini & E.B. Sigg (Eds.), *Excerpta Medica* (pp. 70–6). Amsterdam: Elsevier Publishers.

Valzelli, L. (1981). *Psychobiology of Aggression and Violence*. London: Raven Press.

Van de Poll, N.E. & van Goozen, S.H.M. (1992). Hypothalamic involvement in sexuality and hostility: comparative psychological aspects. In D.F. Swaab, M.A. Hofman, M. Mirmiran, R. Ravid & F.W. van Leeuwen (Eds.), *Progress in Brain Research*. Vol. 93 (pp. 343–60). Amsterdam: Elsevier Science Publishers.

Vergnes, M., Depaulis, A. & Boehrer, A. (1986). Parachlorophenylalanine-induced serotonin depletion increases offensive but not defensive aggression in male rats. *Physiology and Behavior, 36*, 653–8.

Vom Saal, F.S. (1983). Models of early hormonal effects on intrasex aggression in mice. In B.B. Svare (Eds.), *Hormones and Aggressive Behavior* (pp. 234–45). New York: Plenum Press.

Weiger, W.A. & Bear, D.M. (1988). An approach to the neurology of aggression. *Journal of Psychiatric Research, 22*, 85–98.

Wilson, A.P. & Boelkins, R.C. (1970). Evidence for seasonal variation in aggressive behaviour by *Macaca mulatta*. *Animal Behaviour, 18*, 719–24.

Wood, R.I. & Newman, S.W. (1995). Androgen and estrogen receptors co-exist within individual neurons in the brain of the Syrian hamster. *Neuroendocrinology, 62*, 487–97.

Yates, W.R., Perry, P. & Murray, S. (1992). Aggression and hostility in anabolic steroid users. *Biological Psychiatry, 31*, 1232–4.

Yesalis, C., Kennedy, N., Kopstein, A. & Bahrke, M. (1993). Anabolic-androgenic steroid use in the United States. *Journal of the American Medical Association, 270*, 1217–21.

5

Biosocial influences on antisocial behaviours in childhood and adolescence

Jonathan Hill

Introduction

It is evident from many chapters in this volume that the origins and mainten-ance of conduct problems in childhood entail transactional processes between the individual and the environment (see also Caspi & Moffitt, 1995). Equally it is clear that many of the children who are at highest risk have problems that appear early and are remarkably predictive of antisocial behaviour in adoles-cence and early adult life, which suggests that stable individual vulnerabilities may be important. These have been characterized in terms of genetic influen-ces (Simonoff, chapter 8, this volume), neuropsychological deficits (Lynam & Henry, chapter 9, this volume) perceptual processes (Pettit et al., chapter 11, this volume) and attachment status (DeKlyen & Speltz, chapter 12, this vol-ume). At this stage we cannot be sure to what extent these accounts reflect different processes that might contribute independently or in combination to risk, or overlapping processes viewed from different standpoints. If they are different, and they do contribute independently, we need models of the way in which this might happen, and one route is via consideration of biosocial and biopsychological processes.

The distinction between the 'bio' and the 'social' is in many respects artificial. There is nothing intrinsically less biological about social interactions than physiological processes (Bolton & Hill, 1996). We will take 'biological' to refer principally to neuroanatomy, neurochemistry and neurophysiology, and 'social' to family, peer and wider social processes. Psychological processes may be seen as mediating between the biological and the social.

The purpose of this chapter is to link some of the perspectives reviewed in other chapters to the development of the brain and influences on it, and then to consider some findings on the psychobiology of conduct problems. Reference will be made to features of neuroanatomy and neurochemistry that are covered in more detail in the preceding chapter (Herbert & Martinez, chapter 4) and illustrated in the figures in that chapter.

The outcomes assessed in the studies to be reviewed have varied

considerably, ranging from scores on behaviour checklists in children to officially recorded crime in young adults. Two key points reviewed extensively by
Angold & Costello (chapter 6, this volume) should be borne in mind. Firstly
different antisocial behaviours seen at different ages may reflect the same
underlying processes, and equally similar behaviours may reflect different
processes. Secondly it is likely that conduct problems, including those that are
currently subsumed within particular diagnostic categories are likely to be
heterogeneous. Age of onset of antisocial behaviours, associated comorbid
conditions and gender are three sources of heterogeneity that have received
considerable attention. It follows that there may be substantial variability in the
extent and nature of biosocial influences on antisocial behaviours in relation to
these factors.

Key issues in the development of the brain

Background

There is growing evidence that events early in development are related to
persistent conduct problems, and that therefore an understanding of factors
that influence early brain development will be important. For instance an
increased risk associated with smoking in pregnancy may result from an effect
of nicotine on brain development (Fergusson et al., 1998; Wakschlag et al.,
1997). The association of the temperamental characteristic 'lack of control' at
age 3 years with the likelihood of violent convictions at age 18, suggests that
early childhood variations in the functioning of the relevant neural systems
may influence vulnerability (Henry et al., 1996).

Identification of early causes and indicators of altered neuronal function that
might contribute to conduct problems requires an understanding of the development of normal structures. It is becoming increasingly clear that the young
brain is a dynamic structure in which there are spurts and plateaux of development which are influenced by a complex interplay of genetic and social
influences. The impact of biological or social risk factors is likely to be affected
by preceding vulnerability, timing and additive or interactional effects of other
risk or protective factors. Some influences on neural systems appear to have
transient effects whilst others are more persistent, some are reversible and
others more permanent.

Brain development

The central nervous system is composed of neurones and glial cells. Neurones
are cells that transmit information along their axons in the form of electrical

impulses. Information is transmitted from one neurone to another at synapses via neurotransmitters. Dendrites are specialized branches of the neurone that receive information from other neurones. Most neurones have around 1000 contacts with other neurones, although the elaborate dendritic network of the cerebellar Purkinje cells receive around 150 000 contacts through their dendrites. Glial cells serve predominantly a physical and nutritional support role, although they also have a role in the re-uptake of neurotransmitters.

Most of the specialized structures of the brain outlined in the previous chapter (Martinez & Herbert, chapter 4) can be identified in the human brain during gestation. The formation of the structures entails division of neuronal precursor cells, followed by migration and the formation of selective connections. Selective connections occur in two ways, through cellular competition and death, and through 'process elimination'. Neuronal competition and death involves immature neurones early in prenatal development (Hamburger & Oppenheim, 1982). Neurites (precursors of axons and dendrites) are sent out to target cells which secrete a trophic substance that promotes neuronal survival. Cells that do not compete successfully for the trophic substance from the target cell either obtain it from another target cell or die. The neurites of successful cells establish synaptic connections with target cells. Process elimination occurs in the late prenatal period and extends into the postnatal period as neurones develop extensive dendrites and axons (Carlson et al., 1988). Dendrites and axons extend towards other target cells apparently guided by a combination of processes intrinsic to the neurone and extrinsic factors. More synapses are formed than survive in the mature brain, and the consolidation or elimination of synapses in development appear to be related to the extent of synaptic activity. It is thought that the selective loss of synapses fine tunes the developing brain structure. In humans this process continues throughout childhood. For instance in the frontal cortex synaptic density peaks in the early postnatal period and then declines up to the age of 16 years (Huttenlocher, 1979).

The interplay between brain development and experience

It seems likely that in some brain structures synaptic formation and loss are uninfluenced by environmental stimuli, and in others these are powerful. The interaction between genetically programmed synaptic developments and environmental experiences provide the basis for plasticity and fine tuning. Clear evidence for an effect of experience on synapse formation and dendritic growth comes from studies of the visual system. In the mature visual cortex there are alternating columns of cells that respond preferentially to one eye or the other. These columns develop through pruning of dendrites which is driven by visual experience. If one eye is blocked the stripes in the column corresponding to the blocked eye become narrower, and those linked to the unblocked eye become wider (Shatz, 1990). This effect is seen only over a certain critical period. If visual input is blocked after that period there is no effect, and if it is unblocked before the critical period there is no effect. It is likely that this is a widespread mechanism whereby 'the normal development of the nervous system unfolds as a series of timed genetic events whose expression depends on properly timed and delivered environmental stimuli' (Ciaranelo et al., 1995).

Such interactions at the cellular level between genetically timed events and experience are mirrored in physiological and behavioural processes. A physiological example is provided by spontaneously hypertensive rats (SHR); strains in which hypertension is passed from one generation to another. If SHR rat pups are raised by normal rat mothers they do not develop hypertension, and if SHR rat mothers rear non-SHR rat pups they do not develop hypertension (Myers et al., 1989). It appears therefore that SHR rat mothers confer a genetic risk to their offspring, which is manifest only when the pup is also exposed to the SHR mother's behaviour. A similar point is made in relation to aggressive behaviours in a series of studies carried out by Cairns and colleagues. Selective breeding produced two lines of mice, one that was highly aggressive and one that had a strong tendency to freeze upon social contact (Gariepy et al., 1988). In the low aggressive line, dopamine concentrations were lower in the caudate nucleus and nucleus accumbens which are associated with emotional responding, motivational states and initiation of action. (See also Herbert & Martinez, chapter 4, this volume.) As we shall see later in this chapter dopaminergic pathways from the ventral tegmental area of the brain stem to the nucleus accumbens have been implicated in models of a 'Behavioural Activation System' (Gray, 1987). However in a series of experiments involving social contact with other mice, many of the low aggressive mice could achieve dominance over the high aggressive mice, and this was accompanied by an increase in dopaminergic activity (Gariepy, 1996). Thus, notwithstanding marked genetic differences accompanied by predictable differences in neurotransmitter levels, there were profound effects of social experience on patterns of behaving. The extent to which such processes occur in humans is not known, however given the prolonged period of fine tuning through synapse elimination in human development, it seems that they may be important.

Sex differences

Sex differences in rates of aggression and disruptive behaviours within the normal range and at the extremes are very striking, and a biosocial model of conduct disorder will have to account for these. Neurobiological differences may have an effect directly by increasing risk, or through a general vulnerability to physical or psychological stressors, or through particular features which add to risk through transactional processes with environmental factors.

Differences between the brains of males and females appear to be governed by the action of circulating sex hormones (androgens and oestrogens) on neurones, and are not primarily the result of genetic differences acting within nerve cells. These hormones affect nerve cell division, migration and survival. Males and females are morphologically indistinguishable until the sixth week of in utero development, when in males the testes start to secrete testosterone. In humans testosterone levels reach peaks at between 3–5 months of gestation and in the first six weeks postnatally, when they are several times higher than in the adult male. As Herbert & Martinez (chapter 4, this volume) point out there are androgen receptors in areas of the limbic system including the anterior hypothalamus, the medial amygdala and the septum, and these structures have been implicated in aggression. If there are links between hormonally mediated sex differences in these structures and aggression, these could operate either through hormonal effects on structure, or hormonal activation of these structures. There is evidence that both mechanisms occur. Specific areas of the mammalian nervous system are thought to be sensitive to gonadal hormones during critical developmental periods before birth and in infancy, resulting in relatively permanent organizational changes in neural structure that are not dependent on hormonal stimulation (Todd et al., 1995). Intriguingly it has been argued that prenatal testosterone may contribute to the increased risk of language delay in boys, either through interfering with neuronal development (Geschwind & Galaburda, 1985), or through reduction of selective neuronal death (Galaburda et al., 1987). Given the links between language delay and conduct problems (Lynam & Henry, chapter 9, this volume), this might provide a mechanism linking effects of testosterone on the developing brain structure to antisocial behaviours in childhood. Other structures, notably female hypothalamic cells are very sensitive to changes in levels of oestrogen.

In spite of the presence of these mechanisms, the evidence for an effect of androgens on aggression is conflicting, and complex. Herbert & Martinez review the recent evidence in chapter 4, this volume. In relation to aggression in adolescence they refer to the work of Tremblay and colleagues showing that at age 13 testosterone levels were associated with social status and not with aggressiveness (Schaal et al., 1996). By age 16 there appeared to be a strong association between aggression and testosterone levels, suggesting that there may be a developmental change in the role of testosterone (Tremblay et al.,

1997). As Herbert & Martinez comment, there appears to be a triangular relationship between social structure, testosterone and aggression in male primates, and this relationship may change over time.

Sex differences in risk may also arise from a more general vulnerability to physical insult or stressor in the immature male central nervous system (Goodman, 1991). For instance as we shall see, the long-term impact of maternal smoking in pregnancy on the risk of later antisocial behaviours appears to be stronger in males than in females (Fergusson et al., 1998).

Whilst the structural differences in the brains of males and females may contribute directly to an increased risk of conduct problems, they may also lead to gender differences in the normal range, which in turn contribute to variations in responses from parents and caretakers, and hence lead to differences in risk through interactional and transactional processes. For instance in monkeys testosterone increases rough and tumble play (Herbert & Martinez, chapter 4, this volume), and such an effect in humans in conjunction with family stress may increase the likelihood of inconsistent or harsh parenting and hence affect the risk of oppositional or aggressive behaviours.

Psychobiological theories of risk

Temperament

With these neurodevelopmental considerations in mind we turn to some specific theories of relevance to the development of antisocial behaviours in childhood. Individual differences in infancy that might contribute to subsequent risk of psychopathology were conceptualized by Thomas and Chess in terms of temperament. Their pioneering work in the New York Longitudinal Study (NYLS) indicated that individual differences were predictive of subsequent adaptation (Thomas et al., 1968). In general cross-sectional studies of parent-reported temperament and parent-reported behavioural problems have found associations (e.g. Barron & Earls, 1984, Prior et al., 1987). However these studies are difficult to interpret for a variety of reasons including the possibility that items referring to behaviour problems and to aspects of temperament are confounded, because they are measured at the same time. A major strength of the New York Longitudinal Study was that it attempted to predict behaviour problems longitudinally. However Cameron (1978) in a reanalysis of the NYLS data found that difficult temperament in the first year predicted only mild behavioural problems subsequently and paradoxically, in boys, scores reflecting less difficult temperament were associated with subsequent more severe problems. Bates et al. (1985) did not find a relationship between home observations of temperament in infancy and mother-reported behaviour problems at age 3, and Amaziadae et al. (1989) found no association between mothers' ratings of infant temperament and behaviour problems at 4 years of age.

One reason that temperament has proved an inconsistent predictor may be that the dimensions of temperament identified by Thomas and Chess included a wide range of qualities with substantial conceptual overlap, many of which are highly correlated (Rothbart et al., 1995). Subsequent studies have identified a smaller group of factors and have attempted to link them to possible underlying neural systems. The aim of this work has been to identify processes that, separately or in combination, are adaptive or maladaptive, and to relate these processes to brain structures and neurochemistry. We will focus on behavioural activation and inhibition, attention and affect regulation.

Approach and inhibition

The successful regulation of approach behaviours to rewarding stimuli and avoidance of harmful stimuli has been central to the evolutionary success of most living organisms (Schneirla 1959). The idea that humans vary in the extent to which approach or avoidance predominate has a long history going back at least to Hippocrates and Galen (Windle, 1995). Recent formulations of an appetitive/approach system that mobilises approach behaviour to stimuli that predict positive events, are known variously as the Behavioural Activation System (Gray, 1987), Behavioural Facilitation System (Depue & Iacono, 1989), the Expectancy Foraging System (Panksepp, 1992) and Novelty Seeking (Cloninger, 1986). Depue & Iacono also have proposed that this system promotes irritative aggression when goals are blocked. The neural system associated with these processes is believed to comprise areas of the basolateral amygdala that respond to reward-related inputs by activating dopaminergic neurones within the brain stem's ventral tegmental area, which in turn projects to the nucleus accumbens where they facilitate approach responses. Relatively stable individual differences in the propensity to approach objects are evident from around 6 months (Rothbart, 1988).

Gray (1987) has proposed that a Behavioural Inhibition System motivates responses to signals that predict punishment or threats, including inhibition of ongoing motor activity, increase of arousal, and direction of attention toward relevant information in the environment. This is very similar to Cloninger's concept of Harm Avoidance (Cloninger, 1986). The neuronal circuitry is thought to involve the hippocampus, and the lateral nucleus of the amygdala, both of which are involved in labelling fearful stimuli (Davis, 1992; LeDoux,

1995, 1996; Herbert & Martinez, chapter 4 and Fig. 4.2, this volume). Further circuits connect eventually to the brain stem to regulate aspects of fearful behaviour including freezing, facial and vocal expression and heart rate changes, and to reticular and cortical circuits to regulate attention. Regulation of the behavioural inhibitory system appears to be both noradrenergic and serotonergic (Rogeness & McLure, 1996). Individual differences in fearful inhibition appear towards the end for the first year, and stability from the second to eighth years of life has been shown (Kagan et al., 1988).

Cloninger (1986) has proposed a third motivational system which he has termed Reward Dependence. This refers to the extent to which the individual is motivated by rewards, including social interactions and approval from others. Cloninger has hypothesized that reward dependence is associated with noradrenergic activity.

Attention

Attentional systems are critical to responses to rewarding or aversive stimuli. Accurate appraisal requires adequate attention and, equally, prolonged attention to a stimulus may lead to an overestimate of its significance or to failure to gather information from other relevant sources. There is evidence that the Posterior Attentional System involving the mid brain superior colliculus, the thalamus and the parietal lobe is responsible for influencing the extent of focus on particular aspects of experiences (Derryberry & Rothbart, 1997). The analogy of the zoom lens of a camera has been used. If attention is limited to a particular location in visual space considerable detail is seen, however this is at the expense of the bigger picture. Disruption to the effective functioning of this system could lead to failure to appraise stimuli in enough detail, or of overemphasis of some stimuli at the expense of others. Either could lead to inaccurate appraisal of potentially rewarding or threatening stimuli (Posner & Raichle, 1994). Whilst the posterior attentional system is thought to operate unconsciously, the Anterior Attentional System, associated with the anterior cingulate cortex (Fig. 4.2, this volume) has been hypothesized to influence conscious 'effortful control' of behaviour. Derryberry and Rothbart used a test of ability to use a rule to inhibit a response as an index of this attentional system in children between the ages of 27 and 36 months. Children who performed well on this task were described by their parents as more skilled at attentional shifting and focusing, less impulsive and less prone to frustration reactions (Gerardi et al., 1996).

Possible links with conduct problems

The role of these motivational and attentional systems in the genesis of conduct problems is inevitably in many respects speculative. However the general principles make links with areas covered in other chapters of the book. Derryberry & Rothbart (1997) have hypothesized that there is an interaction between the neural systems referred to earlier which mainly involve the limbic system and brain stem (their Figures 2 and 3), and cortical structures and the environment. Cortical processes involving perception and cognition provide representations of the physical and social world to the subcortical motivational systems. These representations also refer to the self in relation to others. In turn these representations are influenced by appetitive and defensive needs. In the presence of a supportive environment with clear and consistent reinforcers the quality of the information provided by the cortical structures is likely to improve with age, thus leading to increasingly effective regulation of the motivational systems. For instance a child who has a strong appetitive/ approach system is likely to develop a well socialized outgoing personality provided complementary inhibition in relation to inappropriate approaches has been established. This depends not only on the activation of behavioural systems, but also on the establishment of representational links between punishment and those aspects of the environment for which approach is not appropriate, and these are likely to result from effective learning.

Equally, combinations of threatful or confusing environmental experiences may contribute to inaccurate information processing and to extreme activation or frustration of motivational systems leading to emotional or behavioural disturbances. For instance inconsistent parenting may lead to failure to associate inhibition of reward seeking with objects that do not belong to the child and hence increase the risk of stealing. In turn the relative strengths of the reward seeking and the behavioural inhibition systems might also affect the way the child represents situations, and his/her capacity to anticipate various consequences. 'If a child's representations emphasise rewards at the expense of punishment, it will be easy to anticipate the positive consequences of approach behaviour but more difficult to predict the negative outcomes that might occur' (Derryberry & Rothbart, 1997).

The relationship of motivational systems to aggression is complex because, as Herbert & Martinez (chapter 4, this volume) outline, 'aggression, unlike some other behaviours, has no biological functional purpose in isolation'. Gray (1987) has argued that predatory or instrumental aggression is a function of the appetitive system. Clearly the question arises as to why emotions such as anger should be associated with a motivational system that is oriented towards stimuli that predict positive events. One possibility is that where there is a strong approach motivation that is frustrated this leads to distress involving frustration and anger. This is supported by the findings that aggression in 6–7-year-olds is related both to activity and smiling and to anger/frustration in infancy (Rothbart et al., 1994). Alternatively aggressive behaviours may result from a failure of the inhibitory system to control aggression (Quay, 1993), and support for this comes from studies reviewed later in the chapter.

Consideration of the role of attentional systems leads to further predictions regarding the representation of the external world and motivational systems. The response to high and persistent levels of threat may be important to the origins of conduct problems for some children. Pettit et al. (chapter 11, this volume) have reviewed the evidence that children who have been physically abused are more likely to perceive threats in everyday experiences than those who have not. This suggests that the child will give high salience to threatening aspects of the environment and hence will have difficulty shifting attention either through the posterior or the anterior attentional systems to other aspects of the environment. The child may then be unable to assess situational sources of relief and safety, and self-concepts relating to success and efficacy, with the result that the behavioural inhibition system may be overwhelmingly activated leading to withdrawn or anxious behaviour. Alternatively the child may use an avoidant strategy, disengaging attention from the threatening situation without attending to sources of relief and coping options. This may reduce fear leaving the appetitive/aggressive system uninhibited, thus leading to an aggressive response to actual or perceived threats.

Frontal cortex

Herbert & Martinez (chapter 4, this volume) have referred to the intimate connection between the frontal lobe and the amygdala and the hypothalamus, and its role in the control of aggression. More generally a range of functions including sustaining attention, goal formation, anticipation and planning, self-monitoring and self-awareness, often referred to under the heading 'executive functions' are subserved by the frontal lobe and its connections to the limbic structures (Stuss & Benson, 1986). Lynam & Henry (chapter 9, this volume) have reviewed the evidence for specific deficits in frontal lobe functioning in relation to conduct problems. Here we refer briefly to the role of frontal activity in relation to the regulation of emotions and temperamental characteristics. Fox and colleagues (Fox et al., 1996) have proposed that the combination of reactivity to novelty and the expression of negative affect puts infants at risk for subsequent externalizing problems. They argue that areas in the right frontal lobe are involved in the expression of negative affect and in the left frontal lobe with positive affect. This is based on evidence from studies of localized brain lesions, affective reactions of patients undergoing sodium amytal examination, and electrical activity patterns in clinical populations. In support of this hypothesis Fox et al. (1995) found that 4-year-old children with resting right frontal asymmetry on EEG were more likely to exhibit reticent and anxious behaviour during a peer play session compared with children exhibiting greater left frontal asymmetry. Links with serious conduct problems remain to be established, however in a low risk sample Fox et al. (1996) found that externalizing problems were predicted by the combination of high sociability and greater right frontal lobe activation on EEG, whilst there were no elevations of scores for externalizing behaviours in groups that had right activation and were not highly sociable, nor those who were sociable and had left activation.

Neurotransmitters

Background

Considerable attention has been paid to the possibility that alterations in neurotransmitter levels underpin psychiatric conditions such as depression and attention deficit hyperactivity disorder (ADHD). As Herbert & Martinez (chapter 4, this volume) make clear neurotransmitters in the brain serve many contrasting and interacting functions, and frequently measures of their levels are crude indicators of activity. The interdependence of neurotransmitter systems suggests that the balance among them, as much as the absolute levels of transmitters, may be important to the regulation and expression of behaviour. Nevertheless the investigation of neurotransmitter function is of relevance to an understanding of neural systems, and the interplay between the developing child and the environment. In this chapter we focus on the biogenic amines, dopamine, noradrenaline and serotonin (5HT). As we saw earlier Gray has postulated that the behavioural activation system is associated with dopamine and the behavioural inhibition system with noradrenalin and serotonin activity. Cloninger in outlining a parallel model proposed that novelty seeking is associated with dopamine activity, reward dependence with noradrenalin, and harm avoidance with serotonin. Significant genetic influences on levels of all three monoamines have been demonstrated in studies of monkeys and humans (Clarke et al., 1995; Higley et al., 1993; Oxenstierna et al., 1986). Equally there is substantial evidence that there are neurotransmitter–environment interactions.

Monamines, development and experience

The developmental patterns of activity of noradrenalin (NA), dopamine (DA) and serotonin (5HT) are different. Levels of metabolites of dopamine decrease with age, and the density of dopamine receptors (D1 and D2) rises from birth to 2 years, and then declines through childhood (Rogeness & McClure, 1996; Seeman et al., 1987). By contrast levels of the enzyme dopamine-β-hydroxylase which is involved in the conversion of dopamine to noradrenalin increases in activity from birth to around 7 years of life, when it reaches adult levels (Weinshilboum, 1983). It is tempting to conclude that this increase in noradrenalin activity relative to dopamine activity may be associated with an increased role for behavioural inhibition in relation to behavioural activation, and hence increased behavioural control, as development proceeds.

Clear effects of early social and maternal deprivation on the development of the brain biogenic amine system in rats and monkeys have been demonstrated (Kraemer et al., 1991). Studies in rats have demonstrated that stress in pregnancy has persistent behavioural effects in the offspring, and these are associated with altered dopamine levels (Fride & Weinstock, 1988). Schneider et al. (1998) compared the behavioural responses and CSF concentrations of biogenic amines following social isolation at age 8 months, of monkeys derived from either stressed or undisturbed pregnancies. Those who had experienced stressed pregnancies showed behavioural differences when reunited with their peers, and had altered levels of CSF metabolites of brain monoamines. As we saw earlier genetically determined dopamine levels associated with low aggression in mice are altered following social experience. In monkeys maternal deprivation appears to be associated specifically with altered noradrenaline activity and with altered patterns of correlation among neurotransmitter levels. Studies by Kraemer and colleagues have indicated that the effects may be persistent and stress related. They compared monkeys who were mother deprived during infancy with monkeys who were socially reared. By 36 months there were no behavioural differences and the measures of CSF neurotransmitter metabolites did not differ. However, after administration of d-amphetamine, deprived monkeys showed more clinging, submission and aggression, and higher levels of CSF noradrenalin (Kraemer et al., 1984). Kraemer et al. conclude that following deprivation the noradrenalin system apparently matures but remains vulnerable to stressors.

Possible associations with conduct problems

Rogeness and colleagues (Rogeness & McClure, 1996) have provided some evidence that in children referred for psychiatric treatment, levels of dopamine-β-hydroxalase (an index of noradrenalin synthesis) were lower in those who had been neglected. Low dopamine-β-hydroxalase levels were also associated with conduct disorder. The findings are consistent with other reports of associations between conduct disorder and low dopamine-β-hydroxalase (Bowden et al., 1988) and could be seen as support for the role of an ineffective behavioural inhibition system mediated by an effect of neglect on the noradrenalin system. While such a possibility is intriguing it also runs counter to much of the evidence reviewed by Herbert & Martinez (chapter 4, this volume) that aggression is associated with increased noradrenergic activity. There are at least two key differences between these conflicting groups of findings. Studies documenting links between increased levels of noradrenalin and aggression have generally been carried out with adults and have involved measurement of central nervous system noradrenalin metabolites or the use of drugs that affect noradrenalin action. By contrast studies that have found an association between reduced noradrenalin and aggression have generally been carried out with children and have assessed noradrenalin metabolites in the blood. Furthermore, a substantial number of studies of adults and children have failed to find these associations (Berman et al., 1997).

Similar considerations apply to the relationship of serotonin to the development of conduct problems. Herbert & Martinez (chapter 4, this volume) have summarized the evidence that serotonin depletion is associated with increased impulsiveness and aggression. Some of the limited evidence on children supports this view. Kruesi et al. (1990) found that in children with disruptive behaviours concentrations of a CSF serotonin metabolite (5HIAA) were inversely correlated with ratings of aggressive behaviour, and at two years follow-up lower 5HIAA levels were predictive of aggressive behaviour (Kruesi et al., 1992).

By contrast in a study of the younger brothers of delinquents, Pine et al. (1997) found associations between aggressive and oppositional behaviours and increased serotonin levels. Serotonin levels were assessed by measuring the prolactin response to fenfluramine hydrochloride. Fenfluramine increases synaptic serotonin release and decreases re-uptake, and the resulting increase in synaptic serotonin stimulates a rise in circulating prolactin. There was some variability in the results, depending on which index of prolactin response to fenfluramine was used, however there was consistent evidence that aggression was associated with increased serotonin levels as reflected in the prolactin response. Increased prolactin response was related to DSM Oppositional Defiant Disorder or Conduct Disorder but not ADHD, although small numbers precluded any firm conclusions. Increased serotonin activity was also independently associated with lack of maternal support. Halperin et al. (1994) also found a higher average prolactin response in 10 aggressive boys with ADHD compared to 14 boys with ADHD who were not aggressive. Castellanos et al. (1994) found that CSF 5HIAA was positively correlated with aggression in 29 boys with ADHD.

In their general population longitudinal study Moffitt et al. (1997) demonstrated that violence in 21-year-old males was independently associated with higher levels of whole blood serotonin. Whole blood serotonin is an indirect index of central nervous system serotonergic activity in the brain, and there is moderately consistent evidence that high blood levels are associated with low levels of serotonin release in the brain. In this study violence was also associated with family conflict but serotonin levels did not mediate this association. However there was an interaction whereby higher serotonin (taken to reflect low CNS serotonin activity) and family conflict were together associated with a greatly increased likelihood of violence. In turn violence at age 18 had been predicted from measures of the temperamental characteristic 'lack of control' at age 3 (Henry et al., 1996, and see later in this chapter).

Thus the findings from within childhood are contradictory, and those that have identified increased serotonin activity in childhood are in contrast to those from adult life that indicate more consistently that aggression is associated with low serotonin activity. This may result from developmental changes, or may reflect the different ways in which serotonin activity is assessed. Equally it is important to recall that as Martinez & Herbert outline (chapter 4, this volume) there are at least a dozen receptors for serotonin and these may mediate aggressive behaviours differentially. Variations in relation to comorbid conditions such as ADHD and depression, developmental differences, and unmeasured aspects of environmental stressors may also be relevant, and await investigation.

The prediction of antisocial behaviours from hypothesized biosocial systems

Heart rate

A low resting pulse rate has been found consistently to be associated with antisocial behaviour (Raine, 1993). Farrington (1997) assessed heart rate at age 18 in the Cambridge Study in Delinquent Development, a prospective longitudinal survey of the development of antisocial behaviour which has followed 411 London (UK) males from the age of 8. He found that it was associated with prior and subsequent convictions for violence after controlling for other variables. Raine has reported that the association is stronger among boys who do not come from backgrounds with adverse social circumstances (Raine et al., 1997). He argues that this means there is a greater biological contribution to risk of antisocial behaviour where psychosocial stressors are less likely also to contribute to the risk. However Farrington found interactions in the opposite direction. That is to say that the combination of low heart rate and psychosocial risk factors, particularly large family size and poor relationship with a parent, disproportionately increased the risk of violence. The nature of the link between low heart rate and antisocial behaviour remains unclear. It may be that low heart rate is a reflection of low autonomic activity resulting in less effective inhibition of aggression or antisocial behaviour. Equally it could reflect habituation to social controls and punishments consequent upon repeated antisocial behaviour from an early age. 'The challenge to future researchers to measure heart rate and violence more frequently, to specify changes and to developmental sequences in both, and to explain precisely why heart rate and violence are associated.' (Farrington, 1997).

Temperament

As we saw earlier the evidence regarding the link between temperament as defined by Thomas and Chess and the development of behaviour problems has been inconsistent. Research based on temperament has attempted to define the dimensions more precisely and relate them to biological systems. We do not yet know whether assessments in infancy based on these more defined hypothesized neural mechanisms will predict subsequent significant conduct problems. However longitudinal studies based on broader assessments of young children are promising.

Henry et al. (1996) have demonstrated substantial persistence of early appearing conduct problems into early adult life based on the Dunedin Multidisciplinary Health and Development Study of consecutive births between 1 April 1972 and 31 March 1973. Repeated assessments with a battery of psychological, medical and sociological measures have enabled predictions from a range of risk factors, after controlling for other relevant factors, to be examined. Measures of a number of aspects of temperament were obtained at ages 3 and 5 and yielded an index of 'lack of control', which reflected an inability to modulate impulse expression, impersistence in problem solving, and reactivity to stress and challenge expressed in affectively charged negative reactions (Henry et al., 1996). Whilst this definition is not as narrow as those we reviewed earlier, it includes difficulty in inhibiting inappropriate responses and negative affect. In males the likelihood of conviction for a violent offence by age 18 compared to that of no offence was predicted by lack of control and by number of changes of parental figures experienced up to the age of 13. There was a statistical interaction between these two factors, meaning that the combination added to the risk above that expected from the sum of the separate risks. However among the convicted groups violence at age 18 was predicted only by lack of control. Raine et al. (1998) have reported an association between fearlessness and stimulation seeking at age 3 years and aggression at age 11 years. Their sample was comprised of all children born in 1969 in two towns in Mauritius. Laboratory based assessments of stimulation seeking and fearfulness were made at age 3, and modified scales of aggression and nonaggressive antisocial behaviours from the Child Behaviour Checklist were used at age 11. In a comparison of children scoring one standard deviation above and below the mean at age 11 on each of the scales, the aggressive group of children had shown significantly higher levels of fearlessness and stimulation seeking at age 3. Apart from socioeconomic status the study did not control for environmental psychosocial factors that might either be associated with fearlessness and stimulation seeking, or that are likely to be associated with aggression at age 11.

Kerr et al. (1997) examined the role of behavioural inhibition, referring to signs of anxiety in the children, contrasted with non-anxious social withdrawal or avoidance. Subjects came from the Montreal Longitudinal Experimental Study which followed boys of low socioeconomic status from kindergarten. Peer nomination techniques were used at ages 10–12 to assess disruptiveness, inhibition and withdrawal. Four groups of disruptive children were created according to whether they had both inhibition and avoidance, one of those characteristics, or neither. The two disruptive groups that were not also inhibited, one of which was also withdrawn, had increased rates of delinquency at ages 13–15, whilst the two inhibited groups were not at increased risk. This provided some support for Cloninger's distinction between harm avoidance (anxious inhibition) and reward dependence (responsiveness to social rewards).

The antenatal and perinatal periods

The extent of environmental influences on brain development that we reviewed earlier suggests potential both for vulnerability and plasticity. We consider in this section the impact of obstetric complications and smoking in pregnancy. Moffitt (1993) proposed that birth complications might be a contributory factor to neuropsychological deficits associated with conduct problems. Recent reports from two large scale general population studies support this proposal. Allen et al. (1998) assessed a representative sample of 579 adolescents in Oregon, USA for current psychiatric disorders, including disruptive behaviour disorders, and obtained retrospective information on the pregnancy and birth from their mothers. After controlling for current family relationships and for other prenatal and perinatal events such as maternal smoking and prematurity, obstetric complications were associated with risk of disruptive behaviours. Raine et al. (1997) have reported findings from a study of 4269 males, consecutive births in Copenhagen, Denmark, between September 1959 and December 1961, and their histories of recorded crime up to the age of 34. Standardized assessments of complications were made at the time of delivery and measures of maternal rejection, maternal psychiatric illness and socioeconomic status were obtained at age 1 year. Convictions for violent offences were predicted by a combination of birth complications and maternal rejection but not by either of these separately. Poor social circumstances predicted independently and did not interact with either birth complications or maternal rejection. The combination of birth complications and maternal rejection also distinguished between violent and nonviolent offenders. Furthermore this combination also predicted the most serious form of violent crimes, robbery, rape or murder in comparison with all other subjects, and was associated with violent offending that started before the age of 18.

These findings may support a biosocial model of vulnerability arising in part from perinatal complications. Equally it may be that birth complications are correlates of other possible causal factors that have not been assessed. This is particularly important in relation to antenatal and perinatal factors where several risks are highly associated. Obstetric complications are known to be associated with young maternal age, poor antenatal care, poor socioeconomic conditions, alcohol and drug use in pregnancy and maternal smoking (Fraser et al., 1995; Seamark & Gray, 1998), which may carry the risk for subsequent antisocial behaviours. These risks may also be associated with subsequent risks, such as hostile or inconsistent parenting, that in turn increase the likelihood of disruptive behaviours.

Findings from the Christchurch Health and Development Study indicate that smoking in pregnancy adds to the risk of conduct problems in adolescence (Fergusson et al., 1998). Subjects were born during mid-1977 in Christchurch, New Zealand, and were assessed at birth, at age 4 months and at annual intervals up to age 16, and again at age 18. The prediction to DSM–IV symptoms at age 18 was examined after controlling for mother's education and age, whether the pregnancy was planned, alcohol and drug use during pregnancy, child rearing practices, and child sexual abuse recalled at age 18. Smoking in pregnancy was an independent predictor of conduct problems in boys together with parental criminal behaviour, the use of physical punishment and a history of child sexual abuse. Smoking did not predict depression or anxiety, and there was an interaction with gender indicating that effect was substantially stronger for males than females. However the prediction held for mean number of DSM symptoms of conduct problems and not for DSM diagnosis of conduct disorder. Wakschlag et al. (1997) also found evidence for risk associated with smoking in pregnancy within a clinical population of boys. They compared children referred to a mental health service who were assessed over a 6-year period as having conduct disorder, and those who were not conduct disordered. Maternal smoking and other pregnancy factors were assessed in interview at the time of referral when their children were between 7–12 years of age. After controlling for socioeconomic status, pregnancy and perinatal variables, parental psychopathology, and family and parenting risk factors, smoking more than one half packet of cigarettes daily during pregnancy was an independent predictor of conduct disorder. Maternal age, low parental supervision and harsh discipline were also independently associated with conduct disorder.

Perinatal complications and smoking in pregnancy may share common effects on the baby for instance through reduced oxygen to the brain. Animal experiments on smoking have also shown that there are effects on peripheral and central noradrenergic activity, on uptake of serotonin and on dopaminergic systems, probably due to effects of nicotine. In other words all of the mono-amine neurotransmitter systems known to be implicated in the regulation of activity and affect are vulnerable to the effects of smoking in pregnancy. Although interaction effects were not evident in these studies, additive effects of biological and psychosocial influences were clear.

Conclusion

In concluding it is important to reiterate the need for caution. Neuronal structures and neurotransmitters serve many interlocking and contrasting functions, which probably reflect genetic and environmental influences that change with development. Even where associations appear to be consistent, unravelling the causal story is frequently demanding (see Lynam & Henry, chapter 9, this volume). For instance if it were possible to show consistent associations between serotonin and aggression, evidence for a causal role would require that serotonin differences could be shown to precede the onset of aggression, and that this link had specificity. Then it would be important to establish mechanisms. These might include a direct effect of the neurotransmit-ter (a) on aggression, (b) on other relevant affective or behavioural systems, (c) on an aspect of behaviour that in turn increased the likelihood of adverse responses in the environment, or (d) in increasing vulnerability to particular experiences. Possible 'third variable' explanations would need to be explored. For instance studies of nonhuman primates have shown that disruption of the parent–child relationship may produce behavioural changes in the offspring and alteration in central serotonin activity. Whilst the mediating role for serotonergic systems is a possibility, so also is a mechanism mediated via learning processes that does not involve serotonin. Correlations between aspects of parenting and serotonin activity do not demonstrate causal links. In animal experiments a congenital monoamine oxidase deficiency has been shown to produce familial serotonin abnormalities and impulsive aggression (Brunner et al., 1993), which might be reflected in poor parenting and aggressiveness in children.

Nevertheless the study of the biological bases of aggressive and disruptive behaviours promises to be fruitful, and may serve rather contrasting functions. On the one hand it could offer the possibility of a simple reductionist explanation of disorder. On the other hand, by highlighting the complexity of the interplay between the biological and the social it creates the possibility of a genuine integration of an understanding of such factors within a developmental framework. At this stage the enterprise resembles that of an early cartography, in which particular features of the landscape have been added to the map and in turn perusal of the map will lead to the search for further details of the landscape.

REFERENCES

Allen, N.B., Lewinsohn, P.M. & Seeley, J.R. (1998). Prenatal and perinatal influences on risk for psychopathology in childhood and adolescence. *Development and Psychopathology*, 10, 513–29.

Amaziadae, M., Cote, R., Bernier, H., Bout, I.N.P. & Thiverge, J. (1989). Significance of extreme temperament in infancy for clinical status in preschool years. 1: Value of extreme temperament at 4–8 months for predicting diagnosis at 4.7 years. *British Journal of Psychiatry*, 154, 535–43.

Barron, A.P. & Earls, F. (1984). The relation of temperament and social factors to behaviour problems in three year-old children. *Journal of Child Psychology and Psychiatry*, 25, 23–33.

Bates, J.E., Maslin, C.A. & Franke, K.A. (1985). Attachment security, mother-child interaction, and temperament as predictors of behaviour problem ratings at age 3 years. In I. Bretherton and E. Waters (Eds.), *Growing Points in Attachment Theory and Research* (pp. 167–93). Society for Research in Child Development Monographs, Serial number 209.

Berman, M.E., Karoussi, R.J. & Coccaro, E.F. (1997). Neurotransmitter correlates of human aggression. In D.M. Stoff, J. Breiling & J.D. Maser (Eds.), *Handbook of Antisocial Behaviour* (pp. 305–13). New York: John Wiley & Sons.

Bolton, D. & Hill, J. (1996). *Mind, Meaning and Mental Disorder: The Nature of Causal Explanation in Psychology and Psychiatry.* Oxford: Oxford University Press.

Bowden, C.L., Deutsch, C.K. & Swanson, J.M. (1988). Plasma dopamine-β-hydroxylase and platelet monoamine oxidase in attention deficit disorder and conduct disorder. *Journal of the American Academy of Child and Adolescent Psychiatry, 27,* 171–4.

Brunner, H.G., Nelen, M., Breakefield, X.O., Ropers, H.H. & van Oost, B.A. (1993). Abnormal behaviour associated with a point mutation in the structural gene for monoamine A. *Science, 262,* 578–80.

Cameron, J.R. (1978). Parental treatment, children's treatment and the risk of childhood behavioural problems: 2. Initial temperament, parental attitudes, and the incidence and form of behavioural problems. *American Journal of Orthopsychiatry, 48,* 140–7.

Carlson, M., Earls, F. & Todd, R.D. (1988). The importance of regressive changes in the development of the nervous system: towards a neurobiological theory of child development. *Psychiatric Developments 1,* 1–22.

Caspi, A. and Moffitt, T.E. (1995). The continuity of maladaptive behaviour: from description to understanding in the study of antisocial behaviour. In D. Cicchetti & D.J. Cohen (Eds.), *Developmental Psychopathology,* Vol. 2. New York: John Wiley & Sons.

Castellanos, J., Elia, J., Kruesi, M.I. et al. (1994). Cerebrospinal fluid monoamine metabolites in boys with Attention Deficit Hyperactivity Disorder. *Psychiatry Research, 52,* 305–16.

Ciaranello, R.D., Aimi, J., Dean, R.R., et al. (1995). Fundamentals of molecular neurobiology. In D. Cicchetti & D.J. Cohen (Eds.), *Developmental Psychopathology,* Vol. 1 (pp. 109–60). New York: John Wiley & Sons.

Clarke, A.S., Kammerer, C., George, K. et al. (1995). Evidence of heritability of norepinephrine, HVA, and 5HIAA values in cerebrospinal fluid of rhesus monkeys. *Biological Psychiatry, 38,* 572–7.

Cloninger, C.R. (1986). A unified biosocial theory of personality and its role in the development of anxiety states. *Psychiatric Developments, 3,* 167–226.

Davis, M. (1992). The role of the amygdala in fear and anxiety. *Annual Review of Neuroscience, 15,* 353–75.

Depue, R.A. & Iacono, W.G. (1989). Neurobehavioural aspects of affective disorders. *Annual Review of Psychology, 40,* 457–92.

Derryberry, D. & Rothbart, M.K. (1997). Reactive and effortful processes in the organisation of temperament. *Development and Psychopathology, 9,* 633–52.

Farrington, D.P. (1997). The relationship between low resting heart rate and violence. In A. Raine, P.A. Brennan, D.P. Farrington & S.A. Mednick (Eds.), *Biosocial Bases of Violence* (pp. 89–105). New York: Plenum Press.

Fergusson, D.M., Woodward, L.J. & Horwood, L.J. (1998). Maternal smoking during pregnancy and psychiatric adjustment in late adolescence. *Archives of General Psychiatry, 55,* 721–7.

Fox, N.A., Rubin, K.H., Calkins, S.D., et al. (1995). Frontal activation asymmetry and social competence at four years of age. *Child Development, 66,* 1770–84.

Fox, N.A., Schmidt, L.A., Calkins, S.D., Rubin, K.H. & Coplan, R.J. (1996). The role of frontal activation in the regulation and dysregulation of social behaviour during the preschool years.

Development and psychopathology, 8, 89–102.

Fraser, A.M., Brockert, J.E. & Ward, R.H. (1995). Association of young maternal age with adverse reproductive outcomes. *New England Journal of Medicine, 332,* 1113–17.

Fride, E. & Weinstock, M. (1988). Prenatal stress increases anxiety related behaviour and alters cerebral lateralisation of dopamine activity. *Life Sciences, 42,* 1059–65.

Galaburda, A.M., Corsiglia, J., Rosen, G.D. & Sherman, G.F. (1987). Planum temporale asymmetry, reappraisal since Geschwind and Levitsky. *Neuropsychologia, 25,* 853–68.

Gariepy, J.-L. (1996). The question of continuity and change in development. In R.B. Cairns, G.H. Elder & E.J. Costello (Eds.), *Developmental Science* (pp. 78–96). Cambridge: Cambridge University Press.

Gariepy, J.-L., Hood, K.E. & Cairns, R.B. (1988). A developmental–genetic analysis of aggressive behaviour in mice: 3. Behavioural mediation by heightened reactivity or increased immobility? *Journal of Comparative Psychology, 102,* 392–9.

Gerardi, G., Rothbart, M.K., Posner, M.I. & Kepler, S. (1996). *The development of attentional control: performance on a spatial Stroop-like task at 24, 30 and 36–38 months of age.* Poster session presented at the Annual Meeting at the International Society for Infant Studies. Providence RI.

Geschwind, N. & Galaburda, A.M. (1985). Cerebral lateralisation: biological mechanisms, associations and pathology: I. A hypothesis and a program for research. *Archives of Neurology, 42,* 428–59.

Goodman, R. (1991). Developmental disorders and structural brain development. In M. Rutter & P. Caesar (Eds.), *Biological Risk Factors for Psychosocial Disorders* (pp. 20–39). Cambridge: Cambridge University Press.

Gray, J.A. (1987). *The Psychology of Fear and Stress* (2nd Edn). New York: McGraw-Hill.

Halperin, J.M., Sharma, V., Siever, L.J., et al. (1994). Serotonergic function in aggressive and nonaggressive boys with attention deficit hyperactivity disorder. *American Journal of Psychiatry, 151,* 243–8.

Hamburger, V. & Oppenheim, R.W. (1982). Naturally occurring neuronal death in vertebrates. *Neuroscience Commentary, 1,* 35–55.

Henry, B., Caspi, A., Moffitt, T.E. & Silva, P.A. (1996). Temperamental and familial predictors of violent and non-violent criminal convictions: age 3 to age 18. *Developmental Psychology, 32,* 614–23.

Higley, J.D., Thompson, W.W., Champoux, M. et al. (1993). Paternal and maternal genetic and environmental contributions to cerebrospinal fluid monoamine metabolites in rhesus monkeys (*Macaca mulatta*). *Archives of General Psychiatry, 50,* 615–23.

Huttenlocher, P.R. (1979). Synaptic density in human frontal cortex: developmental changes and effects of ageing. *Brain Research, 163,* 195–205.

Kagan, J., Reznick, J.S. & Snidman, N. (1988). Biological bases of childhood shyness. *Science, 240,* 167–73.

Kerr, M., Tremblay, R.E., Pagini, L. & Vitaro, F. (1997). Boys' behavioural inhibition and the risk of later delinquency. *Archives of General Psychiatry, 54,* 809–16.

Kraemer, G.W., Ebert, M.H., Lake, C.R. & McKinney, W.T. (1984). Hypersensitivity to d-amphetamine several years after early social deprivation in rhesus monkeys. *Psychopharmacology, 82,* 266–71.

Kraemer, G.W., Ebert, M.H., Schmidt, D.E. & McKinney, W.T. (1991). Strangers in a strange land: a psychobiological study of mother–infant separation in rhesus monkeys. *Child Development, 62,* 548–66.

Kruesi, M.J.P., Hibbs, E.D., Zahn, T.P., et al. (1992). A 2-year prospective follow up study of children and adolescents with disruptive behaviour disorders. *Archives of General Psychiatry, 49,* 429–35.

Kruesi, M.J.P., Rapoport, J.L., Hamburger, S., et al. (1990). Cerebrospinal fluid monamine metabolites, aggression, and impulsivity in disruptive behaviour disorders of children and adolescence. *Archives of General Psychiatry, 47,* 419–26.

LeDoux, J.E. (1995). In search of an emotional system in the brain: leaping from fear to emotion and consciousness. In M.S. Gazzaniga (Ed.), *The Cognitive Neurosciences* (pp. 1049–62). Cambridge, MA: MIT Press.

LeDoux, J.E. (1996). *The Emotional Brain.* New York: Simon and Schuster.

Moffitt, T.E. (1993). The neuropsychology of conduct disorder. *Development and Psychopathology, 5,* 135–51.

Moffitt, T.E., Caspi, A., Fawcett, P. et al. (1997). Whole blood serotonin and family background relate to male violence. In A. Raine, P.A. Brennan, D.P. Farrington & S.A. Mednick (Eds.), *Biosocial Bases of Violence* (pp. 321–40). New York: Plenum Press.

Myers, M.M., Brunelli, S.A., Shair, H.M., Squire, J.M. & Hofer, M.A. (1989). Relationships between maternal behaviour of SHR and WKY dams and adult blood pressures of cross-fostered F1 pups. *Developmental Psychobiology, 22,* 55–67.

Oxenstierna, G., Edman, G., Iselius, L., et al. (1986). Concentrations of monoamine metabolites in the cerebrospinal fluid of twins and unrelated individuals – a genetic study. *Journal of Psychiatric Research, 28,* 19–29.

Panksepp, J. (1992). A critical role for 'affective neuroscience' in resolving what is basic about basic emotions. *Psychological Review, 99,* 554–60.

Pine, D.S., Caplan, J.D., Wasserman, G.A., et al. (1997). Neuroendocrine response to fenfluramine challenge in boys. *Archives of General Psychiatry, 54,* 839–46.

Posner, M.I. & Raichle, M.E. (1994). *Images of Mind.* New York: Scientific American.

Prior, M.R., Sanson, A., Oberklaid, F. & Northam, E. (1987). Measurement of temperament in 1–3 year old children. *International Journal of Behavioural Development, 10,* 131–2.

Quay, H.C. (1993). The psychobiology of under-socialised aggressive conduct disorder: a theoretical perspective. *Development and Psychopathology, 5,* 165–80.

Raine, A. (1993). *The Psychopathology of Crime: Criminal Behaviour as a Clinical Disorder.* San Diego: Academic Press.

Raine, A., Brennan, P. & Mednick, S.A. (1997). Interaction between birth complications and early maternal rejection in predisposing individuals to adult violence: specificity to a serious, early-onset violence. *American Journal of Psychiatry, 154,* 1265–71.

Raine, A., Reynolds, C., Venables, P.H., Mednick, S.A. & Farrington, D.P. (1998). Fearlessness, stimulation-seeking, and large body size at age 3 years as early predispositions to childhood aggression at age 11 years. *Archives of General Psychiatry, 55,* 745–51.

Rogeness, G.A. & McClure, E.B. (1996). Development and neurotransmitter–environmental interactions. *Development and Psychopathology, 8,* 183–99.

Rothbart, M.K. (1988). Temperament and the development of inhibited approach. *Child Development, 59*, 1241–50.

Rothbart, M.K., Derryberry, D. & Posner, M.I. (1994). A psychobiological approach to the development of temperament. In J.E. Bates & T.D. Wachs (Eds.), *Temperament: Individual Differences at the Interface of Biology and Behaviour* (pp. 83–116). Washington DC: American Psychological Association.

Rothbart, M.K., Posner, M.I. & Hershey, K.L. (1995). Temperament, attention, and developmental psychopathology. In D. Cicchetti & D.J. Cohen (Eds.), *Developmental Psychopathology* (pp. 315–40). New York: John Wiley & Sons.

Schaal, B., Tremblay, R.E., Soussignan, R. & Susman, E.J. (1996). Male testosterone links to high social dominance but low physical aggression in early adolescence. *Journal of the American Academy of Child and Adolescent Psychiatry, 35*, 1322–30.

Schneider, M.L., Clarke, A.S., Kraemer, G.W., et al. (1998). Prenatal stress alters brain biogenic amine levels in primates. *Development and Psychopathology, 10*, 427–40.

Schneirla, T.C. (1959). An evolutionary and developmental theory of biphasic process underlying approach and withdrawal. In M.R. Jones (Ed.), *Nebraska Symposium on Motivation* (pp. 297–339). Lincoln, NE: University of Nebraska Press.

Seamark, C.J. & Gray, D.J.T. (1998). Teenagers and risk-taking: pregnancy and smoking. *British Journal of General Practice, 48*, 985–6.

Seeman, P., Bzowej, M.H., Guan, H.C., et al. (1987). Human brain dopamine receptors in children and ageing adults. *Synapse, 1*, 399–404.

Shatz, C.J. (1990). Impulse activity and the patterning of connections during CNS development. *Neuron, 5*, 745–56.

Stuss, D.T. & Benson, D.F. (1986). *The Frontal Lobes.* New York: Raven Press.

Thomas, A., Chess, S. & Birch, H.G. (1968). *Temperament and Behaviour Disorders in Children.* New York: New York University Press.

Thomas, A., Chess, S., Birch, H.G., Hertzig, M.E. & Korn, S. (1963). *Behavioural Individuality in Early Childhood.* New York: New York University Press.

Todd, R.D., Swarzenski, B., Crossi, P.G. & Visconti, P. (1995). Structural and functional development of the human brain. In D. Cicchetti & D.J. Cohen (Eds.), *Developmental Psychopathology*, Vol. 1 (pp. 161–94). New York: John Wiley & Sons.

Tremblay, R.E., Schaal, B., Boulerice, B., et al. (1997). Male physical aggression, social dominance and testosterone levels at puberty: a developmental perspective. In A. Raine, P.A. Brennan, D.P. Farrington & S.A. Mednick (Eds.), *Biosocial Bases of Violence* (pp. 271–91). New York: Plenum Press.

Wakschlag, L.S., Lahey, B.B., Loeber, R.L., et al. (1997). Maternal smoking during pregnancy and the risk of conduct disorder in boys. *Archives of General Psychiatry, 54*, 670–6.

Weinshilboum, R.M. (1983). Biochemical genetics of catecholamines in man. *Mayo Clinic Proceedings, 58*, 319–30.

Windle, M. (1995). The approach/withdrawal concept: associations with salient constructs in contemporary theories of temperament and personality development. In K.E. Hood, G. Greenberg, E. Tobach (Eds.), *Behavioural Development: Concepts of Approach/Withdrawal and Integrative Levels* (pp. 329–70). New York: Garland.

6

The epidemiology of disorders of conduct: nosological issues and comorbidity

Adrian Angold and E. Jane Costello

Is conduct disorder a disorder?

Epidemiology is the study of the distribution of diseases and their causes and correlates in defined populations in time and space. It might be better to say that we study the distribution of 'putative' diseases (hereinafter referred to as 'disorders'), because it often happens that what has been thought of as a single disease at one point in time is later recognized as a group of diseases with certain common clinical characteristics. On the other hand, some originally separate diseases come to be seen as being manifestations of a unitary underlying disease process. By a 'disorder' we mean a grouping of symptoms, signs and pathological findings (a 'syndrome') that is deviant from some standard of 'normality'. Disease status depends on the disorder being shown to have a distinctive genetic basis, etiology, physical pathology, particular prognosis or specific treatment response (Angold, 1988).

Many psychiatric disorders can be characterized as having a core group of key features around which other symptoms and impairments cluster. For instance, depressed mood is a key feature of depressive disorders. It may turn out that there are some individuals who 'have' a disorder but lack its key features, but such cases are anomalous. Conduct disorder (CD) is rather different, because it consists of a group of behaviours, none of which is conceptually central to our understanding of the disorder. The only requirement is that individuals should manifest a lot of these behaviours if they are to be given the diagnosis. Even at the level of conceptual grouping, the items constituting conduct disorder are not immediately and self-evidently coherent. Thus DSM–IV groups the items for Conduct Disorders into four categories: (1) aggressive conduct that causes or threatens physical harm to people or animals, (2) nonaggressive conduct that causes property loss or damage, (3) deceitfulness or theft, and (4) serious violation of rules. To this we must add the four underlying constructs for DSM–IV Oppositional Defiant Disorder (ODD): (5)

negativism, (6) defiance, (7) disobedience and (8) hostility. At best, we might say that conduct disorder consists of a group of behaviours that adults in legally constituted administrative authority do not like children to do. However, as we shall see, these different sorts of behaviour do tend to occur together in the same children, and there is evidence that such problems are associated with at least somewhat distinctive correlates and outcomes. Thus conduct disorder merits treatment as a disorder. The purpose of this chapter is to review the epidemiological evidence for its status as a disease (or group of diseases) and to identify problems that call for further research.

We identify four broad classes of research in the area: (1) early studies of individual behaviours, (2) factor analytic studies of problem behaviour, (3) studies of the diagnosis of conduct disorder or oppositional defiant disorder and (4) developmental studies of behavioural disturbance.

Studies of individual symptoms of behavioural disturbance

The earliest epidemiological studies of behavioural disturbance were simply surveys of the prevalence of individual types of disturbed behaviour. For instance, McFie (1934) questioned teachers about a range of problems in their 12–14-year-old pupils. She was surprised to find that 46.2% of children had at least one problem. The commonest 'behaviour disorders' were 'lying, stealing, begging' (3.4%), 'bullying, quarrelling' (2.4%), 'shifty, unstable' (2.4%), 'restless, fidgety' (2.1%), and 'clowning, in limelight' (2.0%). Cummings (1944) also used teachers as informants about 2–7-year-olds. Besides very high rates of symptoms of what we would now call attention deficit hyperactivity disorder (ADHD) symptoms, she found 'aggressiveness' in 10.9%, 'lying' in 8.4% and cruelty in '7.1%' of these 2–7-year-olds. She also found that cruelty was more common in boys, and that the children of 'parents constantly absent or neglectful' were more likely to display antisocial symptoms. Thus, early on, it was established that individual 'conduct problems' were very common, that aggression was more common in boys than girls (see also Cullen & Boundy, 1966; Griffiths, 1952; Haggerty, 1925; Long, 1941; Olson, 1930; Young-Masten, 1938) and that these symptoms were associated with lax parenting. These two studies also illustrate a point that has perhaps been rather forgotten – that some conduct problems now associated with DSM–IV Conduct Disorder, like lying and some forms of aggression, actually have their peak prevalences by age 5 (not in adolescence), as shown in the California Guidance Study (Macfarlane et al., 1954) and by Griffiths (1952) (see Loeber & Stouthamer-Loeber, 1997 for a summary of more recent work on aggression in this regard). Even earlier work

(Wickman, 1928; Yourman, 1932) had indicated that teachers regarded overt behaviour disturbances as being more serious than withdrawn behaviour, and that such behaviour was associated with poor school performance (Haggerty, 1925; Yourman, 1932).

In the absence of clearly defined diagnostic categories, the authors of the studies considered above sometimes grouped symptoms on an *ad hoc* basis. In general, the presence of any one of a group resulted in the individual being classified as a member of that group. In effect a crude diagnosis was made on the basis of the presence of any one symptom. This was unsatisfactory, because it resulted in children who were obviously not really disturbed getting lumped in with children who gave their teachers, parents and themselves cause for considerable concern. In other words, this system failed to distinguish between naughty normal children and those with serious problems. One obvious solution to this problem was to count as 'disturbed' only those children who had a lot of problems (Haggerty, 1925; Olson, 1930). That required the use of some arbitrary cutpoints in the determination of how many children had conduct problems, but then so does any medical diagnostic system. However, it was also clear that different children had different kinds of problems, so just counting up the total number of symptoms of all types was also unsatisfactory. But how to decide which symptoms to combine together for each 'kind of problem' scale (Olson, 1930)? The next section deals with factor analytic attempts to solve these problems of differentiating normal from abnormal and grouping symptoms for 'diagnostic' purposes.

Factor analytic studies of child behaviour problems

The factor analytic studies of clinical samples beginning in the 1940s (see Achenbach & Edelbrock, 1978 for a scholarly summary of the earlier work) started by focusing on adult (parent, teacher, case worker) reports of child problems, and were constrained by the requirements of the factor analytic methods usually employed – principal components or principal factor analysis with varimax rotation. Items were excluded from scales when they occurred rarely in the sample (in fewer than 5% of individuals for the Child Behavior Checklist (CBCL) for instance; Achenbach & Edelbrock, 1981), so instances of relatively uncommon, but highly problematic, behaviours (such as forced sex) were usually never asked about. We must also suppose that parents, teachers and case workers often did not know about their children's covert antisocial activities, and so will have under-reported these aspects of behaviour.

The first notable finding is that there was a good deal of consistency in findings across informants, measures and samples. The broad distinction between 'overcontrolled', 'internalizing' or emotional disorders, and 'undercontrolled', 'externalizing' or behavioural problems was identified everywhere, though other 'broad band' syndromes were also sometimes identified (Achenbach & Edelbrock, 1978; Achenbach et al., 1989; Crijnen et al., 1997; Verhulst, 1995; Verhulst & Achenbach, 1995). It was also clear that even though subscales were constructed so as to be statistically orthogonal (i.e. uncorrelated) as far as their item content was concerned, the dimensions represented by the factors are positively associated with one another in both clinically referred and nonreferred children (Garnefski & Diekstra, 1997; McConaughy & Achenbach, 1994; Verhulst & van der Ende, 1993).

Among the 'narrow' band factors that underlay the 'broad band' externalizing factor two key syndromes often emerged, which we may call 'aggressive conduct problems' and 'nonaggressive conduct problems', although they have gone by many different names from study to study (Achenbach et al., 1989; DeGroot et al., 1994). The important point is that there has long been evidence that physical aggression involves separate developmental pathways from those relating to nonaggressive behaviour problems, although these pathways are also clearly correlated. This literature, and extensions of it are also responsible for conduct disorder subtyping schemes that rely on patterns of peer relationships and social behaviour (Quay, 1986), such as the ICD–10 distinction between 'unsocialized' and 'socialized' conduct disorder. The former describes children with poor peer and adult relationships, who are also likely to be aggressive, while the latter included children who have good peer relationships and tend to engage in group oriented antisocial activities.

It is also important to note that the behaviour problem scales derived from this factor analytic work were all based on clinical or disturbed samples, rather than general population samples, so we can also expect them to have been biased by the nature of individuals referred to clinical services. For instance the scales of the CBCL were developed through factor analyses in clinical samples, and then nonclinical samples were used only to establish normalized distributions of T scores for each scale (Achenbach, 1978; Achenbach & Edelbrock, 1979). It must also be remembered that the factors extracted depend on the items entered into the factor analysis, and that though different questionnaires often produce similar factors, there are also often notable differences. Consider for example Achenbach and colleagues' conclusion that the CBCL did not produce a factor similar to the DSM category of Oppositional Defiant Disorder (Achenbach, 1980) in three large clinical samples from the USA and Holland. In contrast, the recent revisions of the Conners' rating scale (CRS) found a factor that very closely resembles operational defiant disorder (Conners, 1997), based on factors derived from relatively large nonclinical populations. Inspection of the two questionnaires reveals that the CBCL does not include many items relevant to the DSM construct of Operational Defiant Disorder, but that the CRS includes all the relevant items. On the other hand, the familiar 'aggressive' and 'delinquent' factors from the CBCL do not appear in the factor solutions from the CRS, but this is not surprising because a number of the relevant items are absent from the latter. The point here is that, just as whether a child receives an ICD–10 or DSM–IV diagnosis of Conduct Disorder is dependent on the definitions of Conduct Disorder given in the manuals of those nosologies, so the patterns of disturbance that emerge from factor analytic studies depend on the items included and the populations on which the subscales were developed. Neither method is purely 'empirical' since both depend on a priori conceptualizations of the phenomena that should be included in the original item pool from which either the questionnaire or the diagnostic category are eventually derived.

If the narrow band syndromes are correlated with one another, it is possible that the supposed underlying processes they represent are really just subsets of items that should properly be interpreted as being part of a single overarching process. It must be remembered that there is no unique best solution for a factor analysis – in fact such a solution is not even a theoretical possibility. Rather each factor analyst presents what appears to him or her to be the best solution. Given that factor analytic attempts to parse psychopathology have been directed towards identifying coherent subsets of symptoms, they have emphasized descriptions of narrow band factors, rather than the associations among those factors.

As an example of what we mean here, consider the 48 items from the CBCL that we used as a screening tool in the Great Smoky Mountains Study (GSMS). It was administered to a random sample of 3909 parents of 9-, 11- or 13-year-olds. Inspection of the item frequency tables indicated that 10 items occurred in fewer than 5% of the reports. These were Cruel to animals, Physically attacks people, Prefers older children, Runs away from home, Sets fires, Steals at home, Steals outside home, Truancy, Uses alcohol/drugs and Vandalism. If one adopts the usual factor analytic approach of excluding such relatively 'rare' items, it will not be surprising if a 'conduct disorder' factor fails to emerge – the key items that are involved in the construct will not have been included in the analysis! However, the statistical problem here is not determined by any particular percentage cutoff, but by having enough subjects with positive ratings to generate a reasonable estimate of the factor loadings of the items in

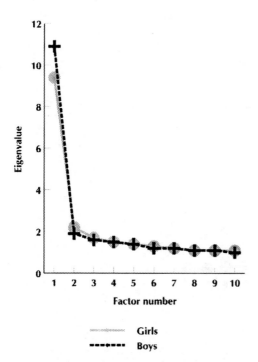

Fig. 6.1. Scree plot from PCA of GSMS screen.

question. We decided that we would only include items that were positively endorsed by at least 30 parents. This meant that four items were excluded: Runs away from home, Uses alcohol or drugs, Vandalism and Truancy. Even so this means that we are still missing three important DSM–IV Conduct Disorder items. Be that as it may, we ran a principal components analysis (PCA), which resulted in the scree plot shown in Fig. 6.1 for the first ten factors for boys and girls separately. The scree plots suggest that a single factor solution may be the solution of choice, since the first factor has a much higher eigenvalue than any of the others and the others are all rather close together. For neither boys nor girls did any factors other than the first explain more than 5% of the common variance. Examination of the factor loadings on this first unrotated factor showed that all but six of the items had loadings of at least 0.3, but each of these loaded positively on the first factor (the lowest loading was 0.17). One could well argue at this point that we are dealing with a unidimensional underlying problem scale involving all the items. However, the intention of previous factor analytic studies has been to identify separate dimensions underlying overall scores, so factor analysts have always gone on to rotate their solutions to produce multiple orthogonal factors. For illustrative purposes,

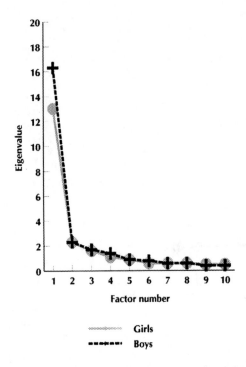

Fig. 6.2. Scree plot from ML FA of GSMS screen.

consider a three factor solution using varimax rotation. Our expectation from the clinical sample analyses from which the 'official' factor structure of the CBCL has been derived is that we should see clear 'ADHD', 'aggressive' and 'delinquent' factors. Items with factor loadings greater than 0.4 in boys are marked with an asterisk on the left hand side of Table 6.1. Factor 3 appears to be a clear 'delinquency' factor, but neither factor 1 nor factor 2 entirely fit the familiar clinical pattern. Factor 2 comes closest to unsocialized aggression, but includes several oppositional defiant disorder behaviours. Factor 1 represents a mixture of oppositional defiant disorder and ADHD behaviours.

Now compare these results with those from a maximal likelihood factor analysis (MLFA – a method that is statistically preferable with a large data set). We note that in males the first unrotated factor accounts for 73% of the common variance (see Fig. 6.2), while in females it accounts for 76% of the common variance. The results of the three factor solutions for boys are given on the right hand side of Table 6.1. Factor 3 certainly appears to be an 'ADHD' factor. Factor 1 appears as an amalgam of 'irritating and irritable behaviours' that is reminiscent of some aspects of DSM–IV Oppositional Defiant Disorder.

Factor 2, however, is a clear mixture of both aggressive and delinquent behaviours, which is very reminiscent of DSM–IV Conduct Disorder.

However, in neither the PCA nor the MLFA do we see clear 'hyperactivity', 'aggression' and 'delinquency' factors. Note also that of the 64 component loadings greater than 0.4 only a minority are common to both three factor solutions, even when the factors most similar to each other are compared (rather than making comparisons between the pairs of first, second and third factors). For instance, the third factor emerges as a 'pure' ADHD dimension in the MLFA, while ADHD symptoms remain mixed in with a rag bag of other items in factor 1 in the PCA. On the other hand, the third component in the PCA is a relatively 'pure' 'delinquency' component, but no such component emerges in the MLFA.

So which is the 'correct' solution? The answer is that none is necessarily more correct than any other. Both one factor solutions are very similar, and we lean towards the MLFA analysis as far as the three factor solutions are concerned because it has some statistical advantages in large samples. However, each analysis provides a particular view of the data. The single factor solutions remind us that all the items are correlated with one another. That we can extract what may be meaningful statistically orthogonal dimensions, which sometimes separate various components of ADHD, aggression and delinquency means that we should take seriously the possibility that these may not be unitary components. But we should also recognize that the phenomena in the real world are not orthogonal. What the diagnostic literature calls comorbidity is equally a phenomenon in the world of questionnaires. We need to realize that PCA and factor analysis are blunt tools for the development of a nosology. They can be very informative in the early stages of exploring the nature of psychopathological phenomena, and for the development of scales, but they will never lead to the identification of indisputable phenomenological dimensions. Much has been made of the advantages of 'empirical' classification based on PCA, but each of the solutions presented above could serve as the basis for such a classification, and in the end, the key factors in what that classification would look like would be (1) the initial choice of items to include in the analysis, (2) the choice of sample upon which to base the analysis, (3) subjective decisions as to which type of analysis produced the best results, and (4) subjective decisions as to what level of factor loading to use as a cutoff in deciding which items to include in each factor-based scale. There is nothing inherently more 'empirical' in this approach than in having a committee of experienced clinicians and researchers meet to decide on the content of the next DSM.

Table 6.1. Three factor principal components analysis and maximum likelihood factor analysis of the GSMS screen

	Principal Components Analysis				Maximum Likelihood Factor Analysis		
	Factor 1	Factor 2	Factor 3		Factor 1	Factor 2	Factor 3
Acts too young	52 *	10	16		28	13	40 *
Argues a lot	48 *	39	−1		55 *	13	22
Bragging, boasting	31	29	11		33	21	14
Can't concentrate	69 *	0	23		17	12	77 *
Can't sit still	67 *	9	16		30	11	60 *
Cruel to animals	0	31	29		12	34	5
Cruelty, bullying, meanness	12	61 *	28		37	52 *	5
Demands attention	52 *	34	4		48 *	17	31
Destroys own things	31	28	37		23	38	28
Destroys others' things	16	40 *	45 *		21	52 *	19
Disobedient at home	42 *	45 *	16		53 *	29	20
Disobedient at school	47 *	28	30		37	32	34
Doesn't get along well with others	26	42 *	25		24	41 *	26
Doesn't feel guilty	26	22	23		24	23	18
Easily jealous	37	43 *	−4		45 *	18	19
Feels unloved	33	50 *	4		42 *	27	22
Others out to get him/her	27	53 *	14		34	40	23
Many fights	15	46 *	23		24	41 *	16
Hangs out with those who get in trouble	33	17	31		22	27	25
Impulsive	64 *	21	21		42 *	20	47 *
Lying or cheating	40 *	30	45 *		34	41 *	30

21	8	2	Bites fingernails	13	6	13
45 *	31	5	Nervous, highly strung, tense	36	19	31
19	38	28	Not liked by other children	14	43 *	25
−4	52 *	34	Physically attacks people	14	53 *	6
53 *	6	34	Poor school work	17	23	53 *
35	16	9	Poorly coordinated, clumsy	20	15	27
19	22	3	Prefers older children	21	12	10
23	56 *	−3	Screams a lot	46 *	25	7
25	31	13	Secretive	33	20	12
2	15	39	Sets fires	8	28	4
49 *	18	6	Showing off, clowning	42 *	10	22
15	13	62 *	Steals at home	10	44 *	18
6	4	67 *	Steals outside home	2	40	12
45 *	44 *	1	Stubborn, sullen, irritable	59 *	16	18
41 *	48 *	6	Sudden mood changes	53 *	24	20
34	51 *	10	Sulks	51 *	28	16
17	47 *	13	Suspicious	29	34	12
18	34	17	Swearing	32	25	7
50 *	12	−2	Talks too much	34	4	26
35	22	0	Teases	34	10	11
37	59 *	0	Temper tantrums	62 *	25	13
4	63 *	32	Threatens people	32	57 *	2
5	−2	42 *	Truancy	6	19	2
47 *	28	3	Unusually loud	42 *	15	24

Rates of conduct disorder using the ICD or DSM diagnostic systems

An alternative to factor analytic approaches to the diagnosis of conduct disorder/oppositional defiant disorder is to predefine the disorder on the basis of current knowledge about the relationships among symptoms, and then to determine the prevalence of this 'clinical syndrome' in the general population. The two principal diagnostic systems in use for the last 20 years have taken substantially different approaches to the diagnosis of disorders of conduct. In 1980 the *Diagnostic and Statistical Manual of Mental Disorders, Third Edition* (DSM–III) (American Psychiatric Association, 1980) introduced the diagnosis of oppositional disorder, requiring that two of five behaviours (violations of minor rules, temper tantrums, argumentativeness, provocative behaviour and stubbornness) be present for the diagnosis to be met (American Psychiatric Association, 1980, p. 35). The DSM–III criterion set included no indication of how often each of its constituent behaviours had to occur. The DSM–III–R (American Psychiatric Association, 1987) introduced such an indication by including the word 'often' in the specification of each criterion in an expanded group of nine criteria (of which five had to be present), and an important clarification in the statement 'Consider a criterion met only if the behavior is considerably more frequent than that of most people of the same mental age'. However, we know of only one study that has reported how often the individual criterion symptoms for oppositional defiant disorder occur in the general population (Angold & Costello, 1996). That study indicated that if 'often' was defined as being above the 90th general population percentile for the frequency of that behaviour, quite different frequency cutoffs were required for different oppositional defiant disorder symptoms. DSM–IV (American Psychiatric Association, 1994) continued to demand that the behaviours 'often' be present, but reduced the number of symptom criteria to eight (of which four must be present). The other criteria remain essentially unchanged except for minor differences in wording, as does the name oppositional defiant disorder introduced in the DSM–III–R. DSM–IV further states that the diagnosis only applies if 'The disturbance in behavior causes clinically significant impairment in social, academic, or occupational functioning'.

ICD–9 diagnoses (Rutter et al., 1979) were vaguely specified, but behaviours that constituted DSM Oppositional Defiant Disorder were included in the diagnosis of conduct disorder. This practice has continued in ICD–10, which, however, specified the diagnostic rules more precisely, so that ICD–10 Conduct Disorder is very similar to what would result from combining DSM–IV CD and ODD symptoms into a single criterion set. However, there is an important difference hiding here. According to the ICD–10 scheme, the presence of any four (of 23) symptoms is sufficient for the diagnosis of the ICD–10 ODD subtype. Three more severe symptoms are required for the ICD–10 CD subtypes. Many ODD behaviours become less common between childhood and adolescence (Campbell, 1990; Loeber et al., 1991), while many CD behaviours (especially covert behaviours) become more common (Farrington, 1986; Farrington et al., 1990; Le Blanc & Fréchette, 1989; Loeber, 1988). Given that the DSM–IV criteria for ODD and CD do not overlap in content, this means that it is possible for an individual who has previously met criteria for DSM–IV ODD, and who will later meet criteria for DSM–IV CD, to meet criteria for neither at an intermediate stage, despite having, say, three ODD symptoms and two CD symptoms at that point – a total of five relevant symptoms when ODD requires only four symptoms and CD only three. ICD–10 would allocate a diagnosis of the ODD subtype in such a case. To examine the effects of these classification rules, we categorized children in the Great Smoky Mountains Study into one of four exclusive categories – (1) those who met full DSM–IV for CD, (2) those who met full DSM–IV criteria for ODD, (3) those who met DSM–IV criteria for neither CD nor ODD, but met ICD–10 criteria for CD–ODD subtype and (4) those who met none of these criteria. Across three waves of data covering ages 10–16 the rates of each of the CD groups was: DSM–IV CD – 2.2%, DSM–IV ODD – 1.6%, and ICD–10 only CD–ODD subtype – 2.8%. Note that all of the individuals in the DSM–III–R CD and ODD groups would also have met criteria for ICD–10 CD. We may, therefore, suppose that other studies that have used the DSM–III, DSM–III–R or DSM–IV rules for diagnosing disorders of conduct will have substantially underestimated (by around 40%) the numbers of individuals who have significant conduct problems according to the ICD–10 rules.

As if this were not sufficiently troublesome, the ICD-based studies also split disorders of conduct into pure conduct disorder and mixed disorders of conduct and emotions. The latter category roughly corresponds to DSM ODD or CD plus an emotional disorder diagnosis. So to arrive at an ICD-based estimate of CD we need to add the rates for pure CD and mixed disorders of conduct and emotions together. The rates for this combination were 3.4 in the Isle of Wight 10–11-year-olds (Rutter & Graham, 1966), and 4% in the Isle of Wight follow-up at ages 14–15. In these studies it was also found that the pure conduct disorders at age 10–11 were more likely to persist into adolescence than mixed disorders or pure emotional disorders (Graham & Rutter, 1973). A study from Mannheim found that 1.8% of 8-year-olds had a conduct disorder, compared with 8.4% at age 13 (Esser et al., 1990). Fombonne's (1994) study in Chartres

Table 6.2. Rate of diagnosis and comorbidity in general population studies

Study (DSM)	N	Age	Time frame	Pop. rate of a (%)	Pop. rate of b (%)	Rate of a in b (%)	Rate of a not in b (%)	Rate of b in a (%)	Rate of b not in a (%)	OR	CI	P
a = CD/ODD	b = ADHD											
1 (III)	792	11	1 yr	9.1	6.7	47.2	7.1	34.7	4.4	11.6	6.3–21.5	***
2 (II)	943	15	1 yr	9.0	2.1	20.0	8.8	4.7	1.9	2.6	0.85–8.0	***
5 (III)	278	7–11	6 mo	9.8	2.3	54.6	8.7	13.0	1.2	12.6	3.6–44.1	***
6 (III)	278	12–18	6 mo	13.9	12.2	46.9	9.4	41.0	7.5	8.6	3.8–48.7	***
10 (III)	222	9–16	6 mo	10.5	10	93.0	—	35.7	—	phi = 0.47	—	***
11 (III-R)	1015	9–13	3 mo	5.2	1.9	33.3	4.7	11.8	1.3	10.2	4.5–22.3	***
12 (IV)	970	10–14	3 mo	4.8	1.0	35.5	4.5	7.5	0.69	11.7	4.9–28.2	***
13 (IV)	928	11–15	3 mo	3.3	0.9	22.1	3.1	5.8	0.7	8.7	2.0–37.9	**
14 (IV)	820	12–16	3 mo	2.9	0.6	13.9	3.6	3.1	0.6	5.6	0.7–44.6	ns
15 (III-R)	323	9–13	3 mo	6.6	1.3	25	6.3	4.8	1.0	4.9	0.49–49.6	ns
16 (IV)	317	10–14	3 mo	8.3	1.3	50.0	7.7	7.7	0.7	11.9	1.6–88.4	*
17 (IV)	304	11–15	3 mo	5.0	1.0	67	4.4	13.3	0.35	43.7	3.7–513	**
18 (IV)	289	12–16	3 mo	4.2	0.4	100	3.9	8.3	0	—	—	—
19 (III-R)	986	15	6 mo	10.8	4.8	—	—	—	—	26.8	13.7–52.4	*
20 (III-R)	2762	8–16	3 mo	4.3	1.4	—	—	—	—	3.2	0.9–8.7	ns

a = CD/ODD		b = Depression										
1 (III)	792	11	1 yr	9.1	1.8	78.6	8.7	15.3	0.47	38.3	10.4–141	***
2 (III)	943	15	1 yr	9.0	4.2	32.5	8.0	15.3	3.15	5.6	2.7–11.2	***
3 (III-R)	930	18	1 yr	5.5	18.0	7.2	5.1	23.5	17.6	1.4	0.74–2.8	ns
4 (III)	150	14–16	1 yr	14.7	8.0	83.3	8.7	45.9	1.6	52.5	10.3–268	***
5 (III)	278	7–11	1 yr	9.8	1.6	13.5	9.7	2.2	1.5	1.5	0.15–14.3	ns
6 (III-R)	278	12–18	6 mo	13.9	4.2	67.7	11.6	20.4	1.6	15.9	4.4–58.0	***
7 (III-R)	776	9–18	1 yr	7.1	3.4	23.7	6.6	10.9	2.8	4.3	1.6–11.5	*
8 (III-R)	776	11–20	1 yr	5.8	2.8	22.7	5.3	11.1	2.3	5.2	1.9–13.9	—
9 (III-R)	1710	14–18	curr	1.8	2.9	8.0	1.6	12.9	2.7	5.3	1.8–15.7	**
10 (III)	222	9–16	6 mo	10.5	8.0	55.8	—	45.4	—	18.4	6.1–55.3	***
11 (III-R)	1015	9–13	3 mo	5.2	1.5	28.9	4.8	8.4	1.1	8.01	2.8–22.6	***
12 (IV)	970	10–14	3 mo	4.9	3.1	25.7	4.3	16.0	2.4	7.8	2.6–23.1	***
13 (IV)	928	11–15	3 mo	3.4	3.2	42.9	2.0	41.4	1.9	36.2	11.1–118	***
14 (IV)	820	12–16	3 mo	2.9	2.7	4.4	2.9	4.0	2.6	1.6	0.38–6.5	ns
15 (III-R)	323	9–13	3 mo	6.5	0.31	0	6.5	0	0.33	—	—	—
16 (IV)	317	10–14	3 mo	8.2	1.6	60.0	7.4	11.5	0.7	18.8	3.0–118	**
17 (IV)	304	11–15	3 mo	5.3	4.3	38.5	3.8	31.3	2.8	15.9	4.5–56.6	***
18 (IV)	289	12–16	3 mo	4.2	1.7	0	4.2	0	1.8	—	—	—
19 (II-R)	986	15	6 mo	10.8	6.6	—	—	—	—	3.4	1.9–6.3	*
20 (II-R)	2762	8–16	3 mo	4.3	1.2	—	—	—	—	11.2	4.6–25.6	*

Table 6.2. (cont.)

Study (DSM)	N	Age	Time Frame	Pop. rate of a (%)	Pop. rate of b (%)	Rate of a in b (%)	Rate of a not in b (%)	Rate of b in a (%)	Rate of b not in a (%)	OR	CI	P
a = CD/ODD		b = Anxiety										
1 (III)	792	11	1 yr	9.1	7.4	32.2	8.1	26.4	6.3	5.4	2.9–9.9	***
2 (III)	943	15	1 yr	9.0	10.7	5.9	9.4	7.1	11.1	0.61	0.26–1.4	ns
3 (III-R)	930	18	1 yr	5.5	19.7	7.1	5.1	25.5	19.3	1.4	0.74–2.7	ns
4 (III)	150	14–16	1 yr	14.7	8.7	69.2	9.5	40.9	3.1	21.5	5.8–79.5	***
5 (III)	278	7–11	1 yr	9.8	15.4	19.4	8.0	30.7	13.8	2.8	1.3–6.12	**
6 (III-R)	278	12–18	6 mo	13.9	14.4	20.8	12.8	21.6	13.3	1.8	0.8–3.9	ns
10 (III)	222	9–16	1 yr	—	—	62.4	—	55.3	—	phi = 1.4	—	*
11 (III-R)	1015	9–13	3 mo	5.2	5.5	18.3	4.4	19.2	4.7	4.81	2.13–10.9	***
12 (IV)	970	10–14	3 mo	4.9	3.8	13.0	4.6	9.9	3.4	3.1	1.4–6.9	**
13 (IV)	928	11–15	3 mo	3.4	2.8	7.9	3.2	6.6	2.7	2.6	0.85–7.7	ns
14 (IV)	820	12–16	3 mo	2.9	0.98	16.2	2.8	5.5	0.9	6.8	1.6–29.6	**
15 (III-R)	323	9–13	3 mo	6.5	5.3	5.9	6.5	4.8	5.3	0.89	0.11–7.1	ns
16 (IV)	317	10–14	3 mo	8.2	3.8	33.3	7.2	15.4	2.8	6.4	1.8–23.0	**
17 (IV)	304	11–15	3 mo	5.3	2.0	33.3	4.7	12.5	1.4	10.1	1.7–60.2	*
18 (IV)	289	12–16	3 mo	4.2	3.8	27.3	3.2	25.0	2.9	11.2	2.5–49.4	**
19 (III-R)	986	15	6 mo	10.8	12.8	—	—	—	—	3.2	1.8–5.5	*
20 (III-R)	2762	8–16	3 mo	4.3	4.4	—	—	—	—	3.7	1.9–6.8	*

Study 1. (Anderson et al., 1987).
Study 2. (McGee et al., 1990) A follow-up of study 1.
Study 3. (Feehan et al., 1994) A follow-up of studies 1 and 2.
Study 4. (Kashani et al., 1987).
Study 5. (Costello et al., 1988).
Study 6. Costello, unpublished DISC DSM–III–R diagnoses from a five-year follow-up of study 5.

Study 7. (Velez et al., 1989).
Study 8. (Velez et al., 1989) A follow-up of study 7.
Study 9. (Rhode et al., 1991).
Study 10. (Lewinsohn et al., 1993).
Study 11. (Bird et al., 1993).
Study 12–15. (Angold et al., 1998) Four annual waves of data collection.

Study 16–19. (Costello et al., 1997) Four annual waves of data collection.
Study 20. (Fergusson et al., 1993a). P values reported only as > or < 0.05.
Study 21. (Simonoff et al., 1997). P values reported only as > or < 0.05.

found that the rate of 'conduct disorders' was 9.3% in boys and 3.2% in girls, but included 'hyperkinetic disorders' in this classification, so we cannot tell how many met criteria for conduct disorder as we usually mean it today.

A number of studies from the mainland USA, Puerto Rico, Holland and New Zealand have reported rates of ODD and CD using one of the DSM nosologies, and Table 6.2 shows these rates for the combined category of ODD or CD, to provide a rough parallel with the ICD studies, from studies that reported rates of association among diagnoses. We should note, in addition, that Verhulst and colleagues (Verhulst et al., 1997) reported that DSM–III–R ODD was present in 1.2% of Dutch 13- to 18-year-olds, while the rate of CD was 2.0%. Across the age range from 8–16 rates vary from 1.8% to 14.7% (so the ICD estimates all fall within this range as well). However, half of the estimates fall between 5.9% and 9.1%, with a median of 5.8%. It seems reasonable to conclude, therefore, that the average rate of the combined category of CD or ODD is between 5% and 10% of the general population aged between 8 and 16 years. It is possible that overall rates will appear to be lower in the future with the adoption of the DSM–IV criteria. On the other hand, we have already seen that adopting ICD–10 type rules for defining CD led to a substantial increase in its apparent prevalence in the Great Smoky Mountains Study. So what is the 'true' prevalence of CD? The answer is that this is a meaningless question at this point, because we have no agreement on what constitutes a 'true' case of CD. We can say, however, that, in general, across the industrialized Western world at any one time, probably between 5% and 10% of 8–16-year-olds have notable behavioural problems of the type commonly considered part of the spectrum of CD/ODD. In other words, CD/ODD represents a gigantic public health problem.

Age and gender effects on conduct disorder

As we have already noted, CD/ODD behaviours have usually been found to be more common in boys than girls for the last 70 years. However, less attention has been paid to the fact that there is probably wide variation in the gender-specific rates of CD/ODD individual symptoms. For instance, very few girls force boys to have sex with them, but we do not expect to see such an extreme gender differentiation in lying! It is also likely that the sex ratio is less for DSM ODD than it is for DSM CD. For instance, in the GSMS, the sex OR for DSM–IV ODD was 1.2, while that for DSM–IV CD was 2.9. It also seems likely that much of the gender difference lies in aggression rather than CD as a whole. There is evidence that differences in rates of nonaggressive CD between males

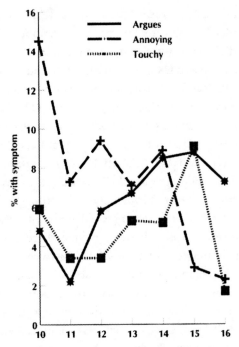

Fig. 6.3. ODD symptom rates by age in the GSMS.

and females are small or even nonexistent (Lahey et al., in press; Zoccolillo, 1993). Adolescent-onset CD (which tends to involve less in the way of aggression) may also be fairly evenly divided in its membership between boys and girls (McGee et al., 1992). We also need to bear in mind that the definition of DSM CD focuses on things that boys do, and we may simply not be measuring important aspects of antisocial behaviour in girls (Zoccolillo, 1993). Zoccolillo et al. (1996) found that the DSM–III–R criteria for CD failed to identify a group of girls with early onset pervasively antisocial behaviour, but that lowering the criteria for diagnosis to two symptoms, and adding violation of rules to the criterion symptoms for CD increased the rate of diagnosis to 35% in the pervasively antisocial girls, but only 1% in girls who did not have persistently antisocial behaviour. Of course, having different criteria for the same disorder in the two sexes raises questions about whether the same disorder is being identified in boys and girls, but perhaps that is better than failing to identify antisocial behaviour in many girls at all.

The issue of age effects on CD/ODD as a diagnosis is a red herring in principle. One can be sure that DSM–IV CD is more common in 15-year-olds than 6-year-olds, but that is because DSM took the path of separating the antisocial acts committed by older children out into DSM CD, while antisocial acts characteristic of younger children were placed in DSM ODD (Campbell, 1990; Farrington, 1986; Farrington et al., 1990; Hinshaw et al., 1993; Le Blanc & Fréchette, 1989; Loeber, 1988; Loeber et al., 1991). No such separation was made in ICD–10, so we would expect to see quite different age distributions depending upon which diagnostic criteria we used. However, the situation is, in reality, even more complicated. Consider, for instance the DSM–IV ODD symptoms 'argues with adults', 'annoying behaviour', and 'touchy easily annoyed'. Figure 6.3 shows the rates of these symptoms by age in the GSMS. Arguing becomes more common with increasing age; there is no significant age effect on touchy or easily annoyed; annoying behaviour becomes significantly less common with age. It should come as no surprise that there is no significant effect of age on the diagnosis of DSM–IV ODD between ages 10 and 16 (the overall odds ratio for age was 0.996). Similar effects occur with the symptoms of DSM CD. The point is that we know that children with conduct problems manifest different symptoms at different ages, so the nature of age effects on fixed sets of symptoms will depend entirely upon which symptoms we decide to include in the diagnosis, regardless of the real effects of age on the underlying processes generating those symptoms. If the diagnosis is meant to reflect the presence of the psychopathological processes underlying the manifest symptomatology, then simply counting symptoms cross-sectionally in the same way at all ages is sure to be a poor way of detecting the 'true' diagnosis, whether one uses questionnaire-based 'empirically-derived' syndromes or DSM or ICD diagnoses.

It will be apparent from Table 6.2 that children under 7 are not represented in the rates of CD/ODD. The reason for this is that both the DSM and ICD systems for diagnosing CD/ODD and distinguishing CD/ODD from other disorders are based upon studies of, and clinical experience with, older children. We simply do not know what the proper criteria for CD/ODD should be in preschoolers, or even whether we can really distinguish ODD from ADHD at this age. Factor analytic studies indicate that the broad distinction between disruptive and emotional (externalizing and internalizing) syndromes holds up in younger children, but there is not much agreement on classification beyond that (see Campbell, 1995 for a helpful review). It has been suggested that the male predominance in disruptive behaviour is low in the preschool years, but as we have already seen, the size of the sex ratio appears to depend on the extent to which disruptive disorders are defined by physical aggression, and that the sex ratio in ODD is not far from unity in later childhood and adolescence. We remain unconvinced that the sex ratios for disruptive behaviours change substantially with age. What we do know is that there is substantial continuity from early temperamental difficulties, through ADHD and oppositionality to conduct problems in later childhood and into adolescence (Campbell, 1995), and that behaviour problems are as common, or perhaps even more common in preschoolers than at later ages (Lavigne et al., 1996).

At the adult end of the age spectrum we again run into definitional problems that complicate the analysis of continuity and discontinuity in antisocial behaviour. The diagnostic criteria for antisocial personality disorder require that conduct problems should have been present in adolescence, and the DSM–IV diagnosis of CD precludes that of ODD, while in ICD–10 the two diagnoses are treated as a single category. All of these diagnostic rules recognize the well-established fact that there is a developmental pathway from oppositional problems in childhood through adolescent conduct disorder to antisocial personality disorder (Farrington, 1995; Fergusson et al., 1996a; Loeber et al., 1991, 1992, 1995; Robins, 1974, 1978). It is also well-established that this pathway grows narrower with time – there are more oppositional children than there are CD adolescents than there are adults with antisocial personality disorder. If we confine ourselves to childhood and adolescence, and thereby to the relationship between ODD and CD, we find that the small literature comparing the correlates of these two disorders finds them to be similar in terms of SES, family history and impairment, but that the relationships of these factors with CD are stronger (Faraone et al., 1997; Frick et al., 1992; Loeber et al., 1991; Rey et al., 1988). There is undeniable evidence that ODD is often a developmental precursor of CD, which has often been regarded as being a later and more severe manifestation of a process that earlier appeared as oppositionality. Methods usually associated with the questionnaire approach to psychopathology, like factor analysis of individual items, have sometimes been applied to the distinction between ODD and CD, with interesting results. For instance, Frick et al. (1991) found that bullying (a symptom of CD) consistently loaded on an ODD factor, while fighting and lying (again both CD symptoms) loaded equally on both the ODD and CD factors. Another report from the same study (Loeber et al., 1995) found that physical fighting was the single symptom of all the symptoms of CD that best predicted the onset of full CD. This suggests that bullying may be misplaced in the diagnostic criteria, while fighting and lying may belong in both sets of criteria, if they are to be kept separate.

Considerations of this sort, and a willingness to consider symptoms that are not included in the DSM definitions of ODD and CD, led Loeber and his colleagues (Loeber et al., 1993; Russo et al., 1994) to suggest that these diagnoses be replaced by three categories ordered both in time and severity, which they called 'modified oppositional disorder', 'intermediate CD' and 'advanced CD'. On the other hand, some (Achenbach & McConaughy, 1993; Quay, 1986, 1993) have argued (with good reason) that both DSM ODD and DSM CD are flawed because both contain mixtures of items from what should be regarded as separate dimensions of 'aggression' and 'delinquency'.

However, we have to remember that a number of individuals begin to manifest notable CD behaviours in adolescence (or even adulthood), without a previous history of antisocial behaviour (Loeber, 1988; Moffitt, 1990; Moffitt et al., 1996), and that this group may well have better adult outcomes than the early onset group. Here age of onset becomes relevant because it is overtly included in the diagnostic criteria, rather than just having a covert effect as a result of the selection of criterial items with particular age distributions.

So much for the distinction between DSM–IV ODD and DSM–IV CD. We now turn our attention to the distinction between oppositional defiant disorder/conduct disorder and other psychiatric disorders and the problems raised by the ubiquity of diagnostic comorbidity.

The problem of comorbidity

We have already seen that the questionnaire-based internalizing and externalizing syndromes are correlated with one another (Garnefski & Diekstra, 1997; McConaughy & Achenbach, 1994; Verhulst & van der Ende, 1993). In other words, there is unassailable evidence of 'comorbidity' between statistically derived syndromes. ICD-based studies also attest to the frequent occurrence of diagnostic comorbidity.

Mixed disorder of conduct and emotions was the third most common diagnosis in the Isle of Wight and its associated studies when the children were first interviewed at age 10–11 (Rutter & Graham, 1966) and also when the children were re-interviewed at age 14–15 (Graham & Rutter, 1973; Rutter et al., 1970). Mixed disorder was diagnosed 14 times more often than would be expected from the prevalence of the separate disorders at age 10–11, and eight times more often at age 14–15. In a similar study carried out in an inner London borough, all disorders were diagnosed more frequently than on the Isle of Wight, while mixed disorders were three times more common than expected by chance. A study from Mannheim found that 1.8% of 8-year-olds had a conduct disorder, compared with 8.4% at age 13 (Esser et al., 1990). Mixed disorders in children from Mannheim were nine times more common than expected by chance at age 8, and four times more common at age 13, when they were the third most common diagnosis (Esser et al., 1990; Laucht &

Schmidt, 1987). Vikan (1985) also reported from Norway that mixed disorders were the third most prevalent diagnosis; more frequent than the prevalence of either conduct or neurotic disorders alone would predict. Fombonne's French study (1994) gives numbers of children with mixed disorders of conduct and emotions which suggest that comorbidity occurred much more frequently than chance would predict.

Rates of diagnostic comorbidity from general population surveys using the DSM

In this section we review the literature on comorbidity with CD/ODD generated by the use of the DSM, in its three most recent editions. Table 6.2 lists recent community studies that have used standardized psychiatric interviews with parents and children to generate diagnoses according to DSM–III, DSM–III–R, or DSM–IV and have reported rates of comorbidity between disorders in such a way as to permit us to determine the joint odds ratios (OR) for the pairs of disorders or types of disorder. Note that the joint odds ratio has the useful property of being invariant to the 'direction' of the comorbidity question – it has the same value whether one adds the question 'what are the relative odds of having A given B or not B' or the question 'what are the relative odds of having B given A or not A'. Thus single values summarizing comorbidity were: 10.7 (95% CI = 7.7–14.8) with ADHD, 6.6 (95% CI = 4.4–11.0) with depression and 3.1 (95% CI = 2.2–4.6) with anxiety. Examination of the 95% confidence intervals around these estimates indicated that the OR for comorbidity with anxiety was significantly lower than that for comorbidity with either depression or ADHD. While it is now clear that comorbidity is not just a result of referral biases, rater halo effects, the use of multiple informants, the presence of nonspecific symptoms in the criterion sets for multiple diagnoses (Angold et al., in press), or individual symptoms giving rise to codings of multiple symptoms from multiple informants, recent evidence suggests that comorbidity between CD/ODD and anxiety disorders may be an epiphenomenon of the relationships between anxiety and depression and anxiety and ADHD, when both of these conditions are also associated with CD/ODD (Angold et al., 1999). In other words, there may be no independent relationship between CD/ODD and anxiety in the absence of comorbid depression or ADHD.

The meaning of comorbidity

Given that high rates of comorbidity represent real associations among symptoms of supposedly different disorders, we have to ask what these associations might mean. One possibility is that apparent comorbidity results from the current diagnostic rules generating spurious multiple diagnoses in highly symptomatic individuals. The idea here is that both the ICD and the DSM diagnostic rules arbitrarily split up symptoms of a generic 'antisocial problem dimension', so that those with many symptoms (i.e. more severe problems) meet criteria for multiple diagnoses.

Comorbidity as a marker of severity

Individuals with both ADHD and ODD or CD have higher levels of CD/ODD symptoms than children with 'pure' CD (Hinshaw et al., 1993; Kuhne et al., 1997; Offord et al., 1979; Walker et al., 1987), greater levels of parental psychopathology, conflictual interactions with parents, peer rejection, school problems and psychosocial adversity (Abikoff & Klein, 1992; Carlson et al., 1997; Fletcher et al., 1996; Johnston & Pelham, 1986; Kuhne et al., 1997; Lahey et al., 1988; Milich & Dodge, 1984; Reeves et al., 1987; Schachar & Wachsmuth, 1990), and worse outcomes than those with either ADHD or conduct problems alone (Barkley, 1990; Lyons et al., 1988; Satterfield & Schell, 1997; see Taylor et al., 1996 for a review).

The indications are that depression has little effect on the course of conduct disorder (Capaldi, 1992; Zoccolillo, 1992), though there are suggestions that conduct disorder may be associated with more severe concurrent depressions (Marriage et al., 1986; Noam et al., 1994; Rudolph et al., 1994), but perhaps with less risk that depression will continue into adulthood (Harrington et al., 1991). On the other hand, the combination of conduct disorder and depression is strongly associated with suicide, especially when combined with alcohol use (Andrews & Lewinsohn, 1992; Brent et al., 1988, 1990, 1993a, 1993b; Lewinsohn et al., 1994; Martunnen et al., 1991; Rhode et al., 1991; Shaffer, 1993; Shaffer & Fisher, 1981).

Conduct disorder with an anxiety disorder has been associated with less impairment (Walker et al., 1991), and perhaps lower rates of aggression and violent crime (Hinshaw et al., 1993), at least in younger children, and with higher levels of evening salivary cortisol than those found in either conduct disorder or anxiety alone (McBurnett et al., 1991). On the other hand, several studies of shyness and social withdrawal indicate that these features have negative implications for children with conduct problems (see Loeber & Keenan, 1994 for a review).

The clearest indication, then, is that the combination of conduct disorder/oppositional defiant disorder with ADHD is a notably malignant combination, but it would be wrong to conclude that comorbidity is nothing more than a marker for the overall severity of antisocial problems.

Comorbidity between conduct disorders and emotional disorders – are the latter simply part of the former, does conduct disorder cause depression, or do conduct disorder and depression have common or correlated causes?

A second group of explanations for comorbidity are based on possible developmental associations among comorbid diagnoses. Zoccolillo's (1992) thoughtful review of the relationships between conduct disorder and depressive and emotional disorders across the life span concluded that in our present state of knowledge separate disorders should be diagnosed when conditions comorbid with conduct disorder are observed, and firmly rejected the ICD–10 category of Depressive Conduct Disorder. In considering the very limited evidence on a variety of explanations for conduct disorder comorbidity he concluded that the best solution might be to regard conduct disorder as a 'disorder of multiple dysfunction', with depression or anxiety representing dysfunctions in affect regulation and conduct disorder presumably being a form of social dysregulation. Given the evidence cited, it seems that this conclusion is only meant to apply to life-course persistent conduct problems. His key lines of evidence were: (1) the more severe the antisocial behaviour, the greater the likelihood of comorbidity with non-antisocial disorders, (2) conduct disorder only predicts adult affective disturbance in individuals who have persistent antisocial behavior in adulthood and (3) conduct disorder is associated with earlier onset of affective disturbances, at around the same time as the first conduct disorder symptoms appear. A good deal of additional work is needed to provide convincing evidence on each of these topics, but they also admit of an alternative explanation – that conduct disorder causes affective disorders. Aggressive and conduct disorder children often interpret the social actions of others as being hostile (Quiggle et al., 1992), have problems in all sorts of social relationships, do poorly at school, get into serious trouble with the authorities and are often told that they are bad. The literatures on life events, chronic difficulties and hassles, and cognitive styles in depression suggest that these correlates of conduct disorder could cause depression (see Capaldi, 1992 for a version of this model). Fergusson and his colleagues (1996b) present a test of this hypothesis. They fit structural equation models to their general population data to test the contrasting hypotheses that the relationship between conduct disorder and depression was the result of correlations among the risk factors for the two disorders or the result of reciprocal causation. They found no support for the idea that either disorder caused the other, but noted that a substantial amount of the covariation between them could be explained by their having common or correlated risk factors. This elegant study underscores the usefulness of having measures of comorbidity on individuals at more than one point in time, and suggests an analytic approach that could be replicated with data from several of the general population studies listed in Table 6.2.

An alternative approach involving direct statistical comparisons among the relationships of risk factors measured in childhood with internalizing, externalizing and substance abuse problems measured eight years later is illustrated by the work of Cohen et al. (1990). This study found that certain risk factors were 'common' to more than one problem outcome. For instance, parental mental illness and remarriage were associated with both internalizing and externalizing problems. Other factors appeared to be relatively 'specific' to only one sort of problem. For instance, residential instability was protective against substance abuse, but had no significant effect on either internalizing or externalizing problems. Family social isolation was related only to internalizing problems. The key strengths of this study are that it involves simultaneous examination of the effects of multiple risk factors on multiple outcomes measured at multiple points in time. Many statistical approaches to complex longitudinal data are now available, and, though it is often difficult to decide exactly how to implement the effects of comorbidity in such models, this general approach is one that deserves to be much more widely implemented.

Subtypes and disorders defined by comorbidity

The two 'combined' conditions for which there is most research support in child and adolescent psychiatry are hyperkinetic conduct disorder, and depressive conduct disorder. However, it is interesting to note that the data typically adduced in favour of these two categories differ. Depressive conduct disorder is supported by arguments that the psychosocial and genetic correlates and outcomes of the combined category are more like those of conduct disorder than they are like those of depression – hence depressive conduct disorder is basically a form of conduct disorder. In essence, the combined form is not distinct from conduct disorder (Esser et al., 1990; Harrington et al., 1991; Renouf et al., 1997; Steinhausen & Reitzle, 1996). Coupled with this is evidence that the depressions in depressive conduct disorder are distinct from other depressions (though there is also evidence that they may not be so distinct as all that; Fleming et al., 1993; Kovacs et al., 1988).

On the other hand the evidence in favour of considering a separate subtype of hyperkinetic conduct disorder (or perhaps it would be better called conduct disordered ADHD; Jensen et al., 1997) is that this condition is distinct both from other forms of ADHD and from other forms of CD. The process began with clinical studies documenting high rates of comorbidity in clinical populations of children with ADHD, which led investigators to suggest that there might be meaningful differences in the nature of comorbid and non-comorbid disorders (Biederman et al., 1991; Jensen et al., 1997; Munir et al., 1987; Schachar & Logan, 1990). The evidence discussed above, that ADHD comorbid with conduct problems had particularly malignant outcomes, strengthened the case (Taylor, 1994). More recently, family studies have lent further weight to the argument. These provide strong evidence that antisocial, substance abuse, and depressive disorders are more common in the parents of children with combined ADHD and conduct disorder/oppositional defiant disorder than in parents of children with 'pure' ADHD, but not unassailable evidence that hyperkinetic conduct disorder is a familially distinct subtype (see Faraone et al., 1997). Results from the Virginia Twin Study of Adolescent Behavioral Development also suggest a common genetic component underlying hyperkinetic disorder and conduct disorder in younger boys (Silberg et al., 1996a, 1996b), but weaker genetic liability for noncomorbid antisocial behaviour. On the other hand, some longitudinal data have not supported the subtype hypothesis (e.g. Taylor et al., 1996), and the presence of conduct problems has little effect on the response of ADHD symptoms to medications or on neuropsychological performance (Abikoff & Klein, 1992; Schachar & Rannock, 1995; Seidman et al., 1995). At least some of the data can also be seen to support the idea that ADHD and antisocial behaviour reflect 'different phases of the manifestation of the same underlying liability' (Rutter, 1997), in other words, heterotypic continuity in a unitary underlying disease.

As a field, we have a fairly noncontroversial approach to deciding whether conditions are separate. It relies on demonstrating differences between putative disorders at multiple levels (Cantwell, 1995; Robins & Guze, 1970; Rutter, 1978). According to this approach, lack of differentiation between pure conduct disorder and depressive conduct disorder is evidence that depressive conduct disorder is not a separate condition from conduct disorder, as Steinhausen & Reitzle (1996) have pointed out. But in the case of hyperkinetic conduct disorder, the argument is that both the ADHD and the conduct disorder components are different in the combined disorder. By the logic that allows a new subcategory to be created when only one of the components is different in the combined form compared with the pure form, a disorder where both components are different should surely be regarded as being a separate disorder. By this rule, the data on comorbid ADHD and conduct disorder is evidence for establishing a separate diagnosis based on comorbidity. This working hypothesis would be consistent with Zoccolillo's 'disorder of multiple dysfunction' (Zoccolillo, 1992).

Comorbidity with substance abuse – timing of onset or comorbidity as predictors of adult outcomes?

Another area where a key issue in the relationship between disorders turns on developmental timing concerns the relationships between substance abuse and other psychiatric disorders. Many retrospective studies have noted the link between reported early onset of drug use and later persistence or problem use (Andreasson et al., 1992; Fleming et al., 1982; Kandel et al., 1986; Kaplan et al., 1986; Mills & Noyes, 1984; Robins & Murphy, 1967; Robins & Przybeck, 1985; Robins & Ratcliff, 1980; Tubman et al., 1990; Welte & Barnes, 1985; Yamaguchi & Kandel, 1984). Anthony & Petronis (1995), for example, made elegant use of the ECA data to show that risk of adult drug problems was linearly related to age at onset, being twice as high in adults reporting first use before age 13 than in those with first use after age 17. The time from first use to problem use was around four years irrespective of age at first use. Remarkably, we could find no prospective study testing Anthony & Petronis's retrospective finding of a linear relationship between age at onset and probability of adult problem drug use. Most of the prospective studies simply compare late drug use of early users with early nonusers, but still point to the negative impact of early use for later problem use (Anderson et al., 1989; Boyle et al., 1992; Stein et al., 1987; Van Kammen et al., 1991; Windle, 1990; Zucker & Gomberg, 1986).

Numerous questionnaire and diagnostic studies have demonstrated associations between adolescent drug and alcohol use and various forms of psychopathology, including low self-esteem, depression scale scores, antisocial behaviour, rebelliousness, aggressiveness, crime, delinquency, truancy and poor school performance, conduct disorder, anxiety disorders, depressive disorders, suicide and ADHD (see Angold et al., 1999). In fact, many studies of antisocial behaviour still include early drug use as one among a range of possible symptoms (Elliott et al., 1984; Farrell & Taylor, 1994; Farrington, 1983; Hammersley et al., 1990; Moffitt, 1993), although it is treated in DSM–IV as an associated symptom. Children who later become problem drinkers or drug users have been found to have high rates of school dropout and poor achievement, rebelliousness, antisocial behaviour, aggressive behaviour, delinquency and family problems (Angold et al., 1999).

Studies of temporal ordering have generally found that onset of other psychiatric disorders precedes that of problem alcohol and drug use (Boyle et al., 1992; Ellickson & Hays, 1991; Elliott et al., 1988; Gittelman et al., 1985; Rohde et al., 1996; Van Kammen & Loeber, 1994), but this may be because it takes longer to reach DSM-level drug abuse or dependence than to manifest other disorders. Loeber (1988, pp. 94–5) summarizes the evidence in relation to delinquency thus: 'Across different delinquent types of offenders, about twice as many initiate drug use after their delinquent involvement compared with initiating delinquency after drug use'. However, one would expect that the trajectory of deviant behaviour would be interwoven with the trajectory of drug involvement (Friedman et al., 1987). Brook et al's (1998) work provides a nice example here. Across the period from middle adolescence to early adulthood, they found no evidence that depressive disorders, anxiety disorders or conduct disorders had any influence on later drug use once adolescents had started to use drugs. On the other hand, drug use was related to the development of later depressive disorders. As the authors of this study pointed out, their findings do not contradict the idea that earlier psychiatric problems (such as conduct disorder in late childhood or early adolescence) are associated with later substance abuse. Indeed, their own earlier work showed pathways from various childhood personality characteristics and aggression to later substance use, mediated by depressive symptoms and unconventionality (Brook et al., 1995a, b, 1996, 1997). General developmental principles (Costello & Angold, 1996) teach us that relationships among disorders may change over time as patterns of reciprocal influence between the causes and effects of different forms of psychopathology become established.

Almost all this research has been on boys only, and we need more work on girls, especially since what has been done suggests that drug use may follow depression or anxiety in girls, but that this order is reversed in boys (Rohde et al., 1996). In passing, we should also note that studies showing that ADHD is probably associated with an increased risk of substance abuse have also found this association to be mediated through the high rates of conduct disorder that occur in ADHD, rather than being a direct effect of ADHD itself (Fergusson et al., 1993b; Gittelman et al., 1985; Loney, 1988) – once again, shades of undersocialized, aggressive conduct disorder.

Robins, using data from two follow-up studies and from the ECA, states

Abuse is extremely rare for those free of (early) conduct problems, no matter how early substance use began. At every other level of conduct problems, however, the earlier that use begins, the greater is the likelihood of substance abuse . . . For those first using substances before age 20, the number of conduct problems was an even better predictor of substance abuse than was age of onset (before or after age 15). Among those beginning substance use before age 15 with seven or more conduct problems, more than half developed substance abuse; with only one conduct problem, only 5% did so. When first use occurred between ages 15 and 19, there is still a large effect from number of conduct problems, but the control for age of first use somewhat reduced their impact. (Robins & McEvoy, 1990, p. 196)

Despite the mass of literature reviewed above, we can find no direct, prospective test of this important conclusion. The data we have presented could also be seen as indicating that it is conduct problem comorbidity that predicts later drug abuse, not age of initiation of use itself, and that the apparent effect of age at initiation results from earlier initiation of substance use by individuals with conduct problems (and perhaps other psychiatric disorders). These contrasting hypotheses are directly testable, though we are aware of no prospective study that has tested them.

Developmental approaches to conduct disorders

The other important advance that is ongoing at the moment is in some ways a return to the focus on individual symptoms that characterized some of the earliest surveys of child behaviour problems. There is a key difference in this modern work in that it focuses upon developmental progressions from one type of antisocial behaviour to others. The focus is now on characteristic antisocial trajectories. Returning to the subject of age effects on conduct disorder/oppositional defiant disorder, we find that there is growing evidence that age of onset of antisocial behaviour is an important factor in differentiating subtypes of conduct disorder/oppositional defiant disorder. Childhood onset antisocial behaviour begins in early childhood with oppositionality, progresses towards early symptoms of conduct disorder, like lying and stealing, and involves a substantial aggressive component (Hinshaw et al., 1993; Lahey et al., 1998; McGee et al., 1992; Moffitt et al., 1996). It is more common in males than females. In many ways this group corresponds to the earlier formulation of 'undersocialized aggressive conduct disorder' (Hewitt & Jenkins, 1946; Quay, 1993), but that formulation has an additional focus on aggression and disturbances of interpersonal relationships. Both approaches also place reliance on evidence that early onset conduct disorder is associated with high rates of neuropsychological disturbances, such as ADHD, lower IQ, and other cognitive deficits (Moffitt, 1993; Moffitt & Lynam, 1992; Quay, 1993). Contrasted with this early onset group is adolescent onset antisocial behaviour, which is characterized by a better prognosis, better social relationships, lower rates of overt aggression, a more even sex ratio, and relative lack of neurocognitive deficits (Hinshaw et al., 1993; Lahey et al., 1998; McGee et al., 1992; Moffitt, 1993; Quay, 1993). This group corresponds in many ways with the idea of 'socialized delinquency' (Hewitt & Jenkins, 1946). However, we must remember that there is good evidence that a minority of violent individuals do not have early histories of aggression (Loeber & Stouthamer-Loeber, 1997), and a simple partition into 'early' and 'late' onset conduct disorder is almost certainly an oversimplification of a complex subtyping problem.

A different developmental pathway distinction that has gained empirical support is that between the development of 'overt' antisocial acts (typically involving direct confrontation or the threat of physical harm) and 'covert' antisocial acts (such as stealing or lying) (Loeber & Hay, 1994; Loeber & Stouthamer-Loeber, 1997). The Pittsburgh Youth Study has provided some very provocative findings in this area. In their latest formulations, Loeber & Stouthamer-Loeber (1997) suggest that there are three basic pathways to be considered for boys; '(a) an overt pathway, starting with minor aggression, followed by physical fighting, and followed in turn by violence; (b) a covert pathway, consisting of a sequence of minor covert behaviors, followed by property damage (firesetting or vandalism), and moderate to serious forms of delinquency; and (c) an authority conflict pathway prior to age 12, consisting of a sequence of stubborn behavior, defiance, and authority avoidance (truancy, running away, staying out late at night)'. More advanced levels in the pathway are reached by progressively smaller numbers of individuals, and the most disturbed show antisocial behaviours characteristic of multiple pathways (shades of undersocialized aggressive conduct disorders). The other important characteristic of these pathways is that, as individuals progress along them, they tend to retain earlier antisocial behaviours, so that there are progressive increases not only in the 'severity' of the behaviours manifested, but also in their diversity within individuals. Loeber's overall tripartite model has recently received quite substantial support from analyses conducted in two other large longitudinal datasets (Tolan & Gorman-Smith, 1997).

There now seems to be little doubt that there is a range of different developmental pathways or 'subtypes' within oppositional defiant disorder/ conduct disorder behaviours and that they are characterized both by differences in patterns of onset, phenomenology and change in conduct disorder/ oppositional defiant disorder symptoms, as well as patterns of diagnostic comorbidity.

Is conduct disorder becoming more common?

There is no doubt that convictions for serious and violent crimes among juveniles are substantially higher now in the USA than they were in the 1950s, and that reports of victimization are also higher (Farrington & Loeber, 1998; Loeber, 1990). It is, therefore, not unreasonable to suppose that more crimes of this sort are being committed by American juveniles. The same holds for other western European countries with adequate statistics. While it is possible to argue that increases in rates of detection, arrest and prosecution of juvenile criminals may be partly responsible for this increase (Loeber et al., 1998), it seems unlikely that this is the whole story. If there is an increase in the numbers of individuals reaching the 'end point' of certain antisocial developmental pathways, then it is reasonable to suppose that there might be more individuals in earlier stages of those pathways; in other words, that increases in juvenile crime reflect increases in juvenile conduct disorder/oppositional defiant disorder. But can the latter contention be supported? Not directly. There are no comparable studies of rates of conduct disorder/oppositional defiant disorder, as a diagnosis, or even clearly comparable sets of symptoms from the 1950s, '60s and '70s to allow us to make direct comparisons. The best approximation to such a comparison is provided by the renorming of the Child Behavior Checklist. Here it was found that American children in 1989 were rated as showing higher externalizing scores by their parents than were children in 1976 (Achenbach & Howell, 1993). Teacher reports between 1981/1982 and 1989 also showed increases in problem behaviours. However, these changes were part of a general pattern of increases in psychopathology of all types, rather than being limited to antisocial behaviour. It is also worth noting that these temporal changes were of a size similar to those observed between nationalities (Achenbach et al., 1990; Crijnen et al., 1997), but these national differences in CBCL scores do not show any obvious correlation with national differences in the rates of juvenile crime.

A third line of evidence derives from general population retrospective recall studies of adults from the USA and Australia. Although these studies are fraught with the potential for recall problems, they also indicate that rates of juvenile conduct problems have been increasing over the last 70 years (see Robins, in press, for a helpful summary).

All the available evidence, therefore, indicates that antisocial behaviour has been increasing over this century in the western world. We know of no evidence to the contrary. Admittedly, none of these three lines of evidence is very strong in itself, and all are vulnerable to serious methodological criticisms. However, the problems are different in the three cases, and it must be admitted that it is striking that there should be such uniformity of conclusions from such very different sorts of study.

Conclusions

Several key points emerge from this epidemiological literature. First, there is almost certainly a set of underlying developmental behavioural dimensions underlying conduct disorder/oppositional defiant disorder. Key factors that have appeared over and over again for years include (1) the distinction between overt (aggressive and violent) and covert behaviours; (2) the distinction between early onset and later onset antisocial behaviour; (3) subgroup differences in relationships with adults and peers; (4) subgroup differences in comorbidity (particularly with ADHD, depression and substance abuse); (5) the need to regard antisocial behaviour as an intrinsically developmental problem; (6) the relative neglect of girls in research on antisocial behaviour.

In boys at least, we also note that all the distinctions labelled (1)–(5) above are linked together. There appears to be a subgroup of antisocial children who begin to have problems early in life, who have attentional and hyperkinetic disorders and neurocognitive deficits, are aggressive, and have poor peer relationships characterized by hostility and suspicion. These children have poor outcomes in adolescence and adulthood since as they age they show diversification of problem behaviours.

DSM–IV states that

the essential feature of a Personality Disorder is an enduring pattern of inner experience and behavior that deviates markedly from the expectations of the individual's culture and is manifested in at least two of the following areas: cognition, affectivity, interpersonal functioning, or impulse control (Criterion A). This enduring pattern is inflexible and pervasive across a broad range of personal and social situations (Criterion B) and leads to clinically significant distress or impairment in social, occupational or other important areas of functioning (Criterion C). The pattern is stable and of long duration, and its onset can be traced back at least to adolescence or early adulthood (Criterion D).

It is our contention that there is overwhelming evidence for the existence of a class of children who have a disorder that meets all of these criteria, including having disturbances in all four areas related to Criterion A. In other words that such children have a disruptive personality disorder. The adult form of this disorder is well known to be antisocial personality disorder – an Axis 2 disorder. One advantage of this interpretation is that it removes the strange discontinuity implied by having a developmentally continuous psychopathological process classified as Axis 1 disorders in childhood and adolescence and as an Axis 2 disorder in adulthood. Separating this diagnostically distinct group out from other forms of antisocial behaviour would also help with the classification of those other forms of behaviour.

It is not yet clear exactly what are the right ways to parse these other possible subtypes or disorders, but we know enough to be sure that lumping them all together and simply counting them up without regard to age (as in ICD–10) hardly does justice to the problem. On the other hand splitting the 'symptoms' into two groups (one for 'mild' symptoms that are seen more often in younger children, and one for 'more severe' symptoms that are seen in older children and adolescents) in the form of DSM–IV Oppositional Defiant Disorder and DSM–IV Conduct Disorder results in symptomatic individuals with mixtures of symptoms not being diagnosed at all and splits some aggressive components of antisocial behaviour between the two. Thus neither current official solution provides us with a very powerful tool for describing the distributions of antisocial behaviour in time and space (the purpose of epidemiology). However, longitudinal epidemiological studies are revealing the ways in which antisocial behaviours emerge over time, and seem to be getting close to the point where it will be possible to produce diagnostic conventions that take into account the developmental dimension so lacking at present.

That said, we may return to the question we opened with – whether conduct disorder/oppositional defiant disorder constitutes a disease or group of diseases. It seems clear that it is not a unitary phenomenon, so it is unlikely that it constitutes a simple disease. On the other hand there is ample evidence supporting conduct disorder/oppositional defiant disorder as a group of syndromes with characteristic patterns of development, comorbidity and outcomes over time. Some or all of these syndromes have a genetic basis and are sources of substantial morbidity and mortality. We have also seen evidence for some specificity in their etiology. Conduct disorder/oppositional defiant disorder can, therefore, be regarded as being a group of diseases that constitute one of the greatest of all public health challenges for the twenty-first century.

REFERENCES

Abikoff, H. & Klein, R.G. (1992). Attention-deficit hyperactivity and conduct disorder: Co-morbidity and implications for treatment. *Journal of Consulting and Clinical Psychology*, 60, 881–92.

Achenbach, T.M. (1978). The Child Behavior Profile: I. Boys aged 6–11. *Journal of Consulting and Clinical Psychology*, 46, 478–88.

Achenbach, T.M. (1980). DSM–III in light of empirical research on the classification of child psychopathology. *Journal of the American Academy of Child and Adolescent Psychiatry*, 19, 395–412.

Achenbach, T.M., Conners, C.K., Quay, H.C., Verhulst, F.C. & Howell, C.T. (1989). Replication of empirically derived syndromes as a basis for taxonomy of child/adolescent psychopathology. *Journal of Abnormal Child Psychology*, 17, 299–323.

Achenbach, T.M., Edelbrock, C.S. (1978). The classification of child psychopathology: A review and analysis of empirical efforts. *Psychological Review*, 85, 1275–1301.

Achenbach, T.M. & Edelbrock, C.S. (1979). The Child Behavior Profile: II. Boys aged 12–16 and girls aged 6–11 and 12–16. *Journal of Consulting and Clinical Psychology*, 47, 223–33.

Achenbach, T.M. & Edelbrock, C.S. (1981). Behavorial problems and competencies reported by parents of normal and disturbed children aged four through sixteen. *Monographs of the Society for Research in Child Development*, 46, 1–82.

Achenbach, T.M., Hensley, V.R., Phares, V. & Grayson, D. (1990). Problems and competencies reported by parents of Australian and American Children. *Journal of Child Psychology and Psychiatry*, 31, 265–86.

Achenbach, T.M. & Howell, C.T. (1993). Are American children's problems getting worse? A 13-year comparison. *Journal of the American Academy of Child and Adolescent Psychiatry*, 32, 1145–54.

Achenbach, T.M. & McConaughy, S.H. (1993). Taxonomy of internalizing disorders of childhood and adolescence. In W.M. Reynolds (Ed.), *Internalizing Disorders in Children and Adolescents* (pp. 19–60). New York: John Wiley & Sons.

American Psychiatric Association (1980). *Diagnostic and Statistical Manual of Mental Disorders* (3rd edn) (DSM–III). Washington, DC: APA.

American Psychiatric Association (1987). *Diagnostic and Statistical Manual of Mental Disorders* (3rd edn, revised) (DSM–III–R). Washington, DC: APA.

American Psychiatric Association (1994). *Diagnostic and Statistical Manual of Mental Disorders* (4th edn) (DSM–IV). Washington, DC: APA.

Anderson, J.C., Williams, S., McGee, R. & Silva, P.A. (1987). DSM–III disorders in preadolescent children: Prevalence in a large sample from the general population. *Archives of General Psychiatry*, 44, 69–77.

Anderson, T., Bergman, L.R. & Magnusson, D. (1989). Patterns of adjustment problems and alcohol abuse in early adulthood: A prospective longitudinal study. *Development and Psychopathology*, 1, 119–31.

Andreasson, S., Allebeck, P., Brandt, L. & Romelsjo, A. (1992). Antecedents and covariates of high alcohol consumption in young men. *Alcoholism, Clinical and Experimental Research*, 16, 708–13.

Andrews, J.A. & Lewinsohn, P.M. (1992). Suicidal attempts among older adolescents: Prevalence and co-occurrence with psychiatric disorders. *Journal of the American Academy of Child and Adolescent Psychiatry*, 31, 655–62.

Angold, A. (1988). Childhood and adolescent depression. I: Epidemiological and aetiological aspects. *British Journal of Psychiatry*, 152, 601–17.

Angold, A. & Costello, E.J. (1996). Toward establishing an empirical basis for the diagnosis of Oppositional Defiant Disorder. *Journal of the American Academy of Child and Adolescent Psychiatry*, 35, 1205–12.

Angold, A., Costello, E.J. & Erkanli, A. (1999). Comorbidity. *Journal of Child Psychology and Psychiatry*, 40, 57–87.

Angold, A., Erkanli, A., Egger, H.M. & Costello, E.J. (submitted), Comorbidity real and 'epiphenomenal' in the Great Smoky Mountains Study. *American Journal of Psychiatry*.

Anthony, J.C. & Petronis, K.R. (1995). Early-onset drug use and risk of later drug problems. *Drug and Alcohol Dependence*, 40, 9–15.

Barkley, R.A. (1990). The adolescent outcome of hyperactive children diagnosed by research criteria: I. An 8-year prospective follow-up study. *Journal of the American Academy of Child and Adolescent Psychiatry, 29*, 546–57.

Biederman, J., Newcorn, J. & Sprich, S. (1991). Comorbidity of attention deficit hyperactivity disorder with conduct, depressive, anxiety, and other disorders. *American Journal of Psychiatry, 148*, 564–77.

Bird, H.R., Gould, M.S. & Staghezza, B.M. (1993). Patterns of diagnostic comorbidity in a community sample of children aged 9 through 16 years. *Journal of the American Academy of Child and Adolescent Psychiatry, 32*, 361–8.

Boyle, M.H., Offord, D.R., Racine, Y.A., et al. (1992). Predicting substance use in late adolescence: Results from the Ontario Child Health Study Follow-up. *American Journal of Psychiatry, 149*, 761–7.

Brent, D.A., Kolko, D.J., Allan, M.J. & Brown, R.V. (1990). Suicidality in affectively disordered adolescent inpatients. *Journal of the American Academy of Child and Adolescent Psychiatry, 29*, 586–93.

Brent D.A., Kolko, D.J., Wartella, M.E., et al. (1993a). Adolescent psychiatric inpatients' risk of suicide attempt at 6-month follow-up. *Journal of the American Academy of Child and Adolescent Psychiatry, 32*, 95–105.

Brent, D.A., Perper, J.A., Goldstein, C.E., et al. (1988). Risk factors for adolescent suicide: A comparison of adolescent suicide victims with suicidal inpatients. *Archives of General Psychiatry, 45*, 581–8.

Brent, D.A., Perper, J.A., Moritz, G., et al. (1993b). Psychiatric risk factors for adolescent suicide: a case-control study. *Journal of the American Academy of Child and Adolescent Psychiatry, 32*, 521–9.

Brook, J.S., Cohen, P. & Brook, D.W. (1998). Longitudinal study of co-occurring psychiatric disorders and substance use. *Journal of the American Academy of Child and Adolescent Psychiatry, 37*, 322–30.

Brook, J.S., Whiteman, M., Balka, E.B. & Cohen, P. (1997). Drug use and delinquency: shared and unshared risk factors in African American and Puerto Rican adolescents. *Journal of Genetic Psychology, 158*, 25–39.

Brook, J.S., Whiteman, M., Cohen, P., Shapiro, J. & Balka, E. (1995a). Longitudinally predicting late adolescent and young adult drug use: childhood and adolescent precursors. *Journal of the American Academy of Child and Adolescent Psychiatry, 34*, 1230–8.

Brook, J.S., Whiteman, M., Finch, S. & Cohen, P. (1995b). Aggression, intrapsychic distress, and drug use: antecedent and intervening processes. *Journal of the American Academy of Child and Adolescent Psychiatry, 34*, 1076–84.

Brook, J.S., Whiteman, M., Finch, S.J. & Cohen, P. (1996). Young adult drug use and delinquency: Childhood antecedents and adolescent mediators. *Journal of the American Academy of Child and Adolescent Psychiatry, 35*, 1584–92.

Campbell, S.B. (1990). *Behavior Problems in Preschool Children: Developmental and Clinical Issues.* New York: Guilford Press.

Campbell, S.B. (1995). Behavior problems in preschool children: A review of recent research. *Journal of Child Psychology and Psychiatry, 36*, 113–49.

Cantwell, D.P.C. (1995). Child psychiatry, introduction and overview. In H.I. Kaplan & B.J. Sadock (Eds.), *Comprehensive Textbook of Psychiatry* (pp. 2151–4). Baltimore: Williams & Wilkins.

Capaldi, D.M. (1992). Co-occurrence of conduct problems and depressive symptoms in early adolescent boys, II. A 2-year follow-up at grade 8. *Development and Psychopathology, 4,* 125–44.

Carlson, C.L., Tamm, L. & Gaub, M. (1997). Gender differences in children with ADHD, ODD, and co-occurring ADHD/ODD identified in a school population. *Journal of the American Academy of Child and Adolescent Psychiatry, 36,* 1706–14.

Cohen, P., Brook, J.S., Cohen, J., Velez, N. & Garcia, M. (1990). Common and uncommon pathways to adolescent psychopathology and problem behavior. In L.N. Robins (Ed.), *Straight and Devious Pathways from Childhood to Adulthood* (pp. 242–58). New York: Cambridge University Press.

Conners, C.K. (1997). *Conners' Rating Scales Revised: Instruments For Use With Children and Adolescents.* North Tonawanda, NY: Multi-Health Systems, Inc.

Costello, E.J. & Angold, A. (1996). Developmental psychopathology. In R.B. Cairns, G.H. Elder & E.J. Costello (Eds.), *Development Science* (pp. 23–56). New York: Cambridge University Press.

Costello, E.J., Costello, A.J., Edelbrock, C. et al. (1988). Psychiatric disorders in pediatric primary care, Prevalence and risk factors. *Archives of General Psychiatry, 45,* 1107–16.

Costello, E., Farmer, E., Angold, A., Burns, B. & Erkanli, A. (1997). Psychiatric disorders among American Indian and white youth in Appalachia: the Great Smoky Mountains study. *American Journal of Public Health, 87,* 827–32.

Crijnen, A.A.M., Achenbach, T.M. & Verhust, F.C. (1997). Comparisons of problems reported by parents of children in 12 cultures: Total problems, externalizing, and internalizing. *Journal of the American Academy of Child and Adolescent Psychiatry, 36,* 1269–77.

Cullen, K.J. & Boundy, C.A.P. (1966). The prevalence of behavior disorders in the children of 1000 Western Australian families. *Medical Journal of Australia, 2,* 805–8.

Cummings, J.D. (1944). The incidence of emotional symptoms in school children. *British Journal of Educational Psychology, 14,* 151–61.

De Groot A., Koot, H.M. & Verhulst, F.C. (1994). Cross-cultural generalizability of the Child Behavior Checklist Cross-Informant Syndromes. *Psychological Assessment, 6,* 225–30.

Ellickson, P.L. & Hays, R.D. (1991). Antecedents of drinking among young adolescents with different alcohol use histories. *Journal of Studies on Alcohol, 52,* 398–408.

Elliott D.S., Huizinga, D. & Ageton, S.S. (1984). *Explaining Delinquency and Drug Use.* Beverly Hills, CA: Sage Publications.

Elliott D.S., Huizinga, D. & Menard, S. (1988). *Multiple Problem Youth: Delinquency, Substance Use and Mental Health Problems.* New York: Springer-Verlag Publishing.

Esser, G., Schmidt, M.H. & Woerner W. (1990). Epidemiology and course of psychiatric disorders in school-age children – results of a longitudinal study. *Journal of Child Psychology and Psychiatry, 31,* 243–63.

Faraone, S.V., Biederman, J., Jetton, J.G. & Tsuang, M.T. (1997). Attention deficit disorder and conduct disorder, Longitudinal evidence for a familial subtype. *Psychological Medicine, 27,* 291–300.

Farrell, M. & Taylor, E. (1994). Drug and alcohol use and misuse. In M. Rutter, E. Taylor & L. Hersov (Eds.), *Child and Adolescent Psychiatry: Modern Approaches*, pp. 529–45. Oxford: Blackwell Scientific Publications.

Farrington, D. (1986). Age and crime. *Crime and Justice: An Annual Review of Research, 7*, 29–90.

Farrington, D.P. (1983). Offending from 10 to 25 years of age. In K.T. VanDusen & S.A. Mednick (Eds.), *Prospective Studies of Crime and Delinquency* (pp. 17–37). Boston, MA: Kluwer-Nijhoff.

Farrington, D.P. (1995). The twelfth Jack Tizard memorial lecture: The development of offending and antisocial behaviour from childhood: key findings from the Cambridge study in delinquent development. *Journal of Child Psychology and Psychiatry, 36*, 929–64.

Farrington, D. & Loeber, R. (1998). Major aims of this book. In R. Loeber & D.P. Farrington (Eds.), *Serious & Violent Juvenile Offenders: Risk Factors and Successful Interventions* (pp. 1–10). Thousand Oaks: Sage Publications.

Farrington, D.P., Loeber, R. & Elliott, D.S. (1990). Advancing knowledge about the onset of delinquency and crime. In B.B. Lahey & A.E. Kazdin (Eds.), *Advances in Clinical Child Psychology* (pp. 283–342). New York: Plenum Press.

Feehan, M., McGee, R., Raja, S.N. & Williams, S.M. (1994). DSM–III–R disorders in New Zealand 18-year-olds. *Australian and New Zealand Journal of Psychiatry, 28*, 87–99.

Fergusson, D.M., Horwood, L.J. & Lynskey, M.T. (1993a). Prevalence and comorbidity of DSM–III–R diagnoses in a birth cohort of 15 year olds. *Journal of the American Academy of Child and Adolescent Psychiatry, 32*, 1127–34.

Fergusson, D.M., Lynskey, M.T. & Horwood, L.J. (1993b). Conduct problems and attention deficit behaviour in middle childhood and cannabis use by age 15. *Australian and New Zealand Journal of Psychiatry, 27*, 673–82.

Fergusson, D.M., Lynskey, M.T. & Horwood, L.J. (1996a). Factors associated with continuity and change in disruptive behavior patterns between childhood and adolescence. *Journal of Abnormal Child Psychology, 24*, 533–53.

Fergusson, D.M., Lynskey, M.T. & Horwood, L.J. (1996b). Origins of comorbidity between conduct and affective disorders. *Journal of the American Academy of Child and Adolescent Psychiatry, 35*, 451–60.

Fleming, J.E., Boyle, M.H. & Offord, D.R. (1993). The outcome of adolescent depression in the Ontario child health study follow-up. *Journal of the American Academy of Child and Adolescent Psychiatry, 32*, 28–33.

Fleming, J.P., Kellam, S.G. & Brown, C.H. (1982). Early predictors of age at first use of alcohol, marijuana, and cigarettes. *Drug and Alcohol Dependence, 9*, 285–303.

Fletcher, K.E., Fisher, M., Barkley, R.A. & Smallish, L. (1996). A sequential analysis of the mother–adolescent interactions of ADHD, ADHD/ODD, and normal teenagers during neutral and conflict discussions. *Journal of Abnormal Child Psychology, 24*, 271–97.

Fombonne, E. (1994). The Chartres Study: I. Prevalence of psychiatric disorders among French school-aged children. *British Journal of Psychiatry, 164*, 69–79.

Frick, P.J., Lahey, B.B., Loeber, R., et al. (1992). Familial risk factors to oppositional defiant disorder and conduct disorder: parental psychopathology and maternal parenting. *Journal of Consulting and Clinical Psychology, 60*, 49–55.

Frick, P.J., Lahey, B.B., Loeber, R., et al. (1991). Oppositional defiant disorder and conduct disorder in boys: patterns of behavioral covariation. *Journal of Clinical Child Psychology, 20,* 202–8.

Friedman, A.S., Utada, A.T., Glickman, N.W. & Morrissey, M.R. (1987). Psychopathology as an antecedent to, and as a 'consequence of', substance use in adolescence. *Drug Education, 17,* 233–44.

Garnefski, N. & Diekstra, R.F.W. (1997). 'Comorbidity' of behavioral, emotional, and cognitive problems in adolescence. *Journal of Youth and Adolescence, 26,* 321–38.

Gittelman, R., Mannuzza, S., Shenker, R. & Bonagura, N. (1985). Hyperactive boys almost grown up: I. Psychiatric status. *Archives of General Psychiatry, 42,* 937–47.

Graham, P. & Rutter, M. (1973). Psychiatric disorders in the young adolescent: a follow-up study. *Proceedings of the Royal Society of Medicine, 6,* 1226–9.

Griffiths, W. (1952). *Behavior Difficulties of Children as Perceived and Judged by Parents, Teachers, and Children Themselves.* Minneapolis: The University of Minnesota Press.

Haggerty, M.E. (1925). The incidence of undesirable behavior in public school children. *Journal of Educational Research, 12,* 102–22.

Hammersley, R., Forsyth, A. & Lavelle, T. (1990). The criminality of new drug users in Glasgow. *British Journal of Addictions, 85,* 1583–94.

Harrington, R., Fudge, H., Rutter, M., Pickles, A. & Hill, J. (1991). Adult outcomes of childhood and adolescent depression: II. Links with antisocial disorders. *Journal of the American Academy of Child and Adolescent Psychiatry, 30,* 434–9.

Hewitt, L.E. & Jenkins, R.L. (1946). *Fundamental Patterns of Maladjustment, the Dynamics of Their Origin.* Springfield, Illinois.

Hinshaw, S.P., Lahey, B.B. & Hart, E.L. (1993). Issues of taxonomy and comorbidity in the development of conduct disorder. Special Issue: Toward a developmental perspective on conduct disorder. *Development and Psychopathology, 5,* 31–49.

Jensen, P.S., Martin, D. & Cantwell, D.P. (1997). Comorbidity in ADHD: implications for research practice, and DSM–V. *Journal of the American Academy of Child and Adolescent Psychiatry, 36,* 1065–79.

Johnston, C. & Pelham, W.E. (1986). Teacher ratings predict parent ratings of aggression at 3-year follow-up in boys with attention deficit disorder with hyperactivity. *Journal of Consulting and Clinical Psychology, 54,* 571–2.

Kandel, D.B., Davies, M., Karus, D. & Yamaguchi, K. (1986). The consequences in young adulthood of adolescent drug involvement. *Archives of General Psychiatry, 43,* 746–54.

Kaplan, H.J., Martin, S.S., Johnson, R.J. & Robbins, C.A. (1986). Escalation of marijuana use: Application of a general theory of deviant behavior. *Journal of Health and Social Behavior, 27,* 44–61.

Kashani, J.H., Beck, N.C., Hoeper, E.W., et al. (1987). Psychiatric disorders in a community sample of adolescents. *American Journal of Psychiatry, 144,* 584–9.

Kovacs, M., Paulauskas, S., Gatsonis, C. & Richards, C. (1988). Depressive disorders in childhood: III. A longitudinal study of comorbidity with and risk for conduct disorders. *Journal of Affective Disorders, 15,* 205–17.

Kuhne, M., Schaechar, R. & Tannock, R. (1997). Impact of comorbid oppositional or conduct problems on attention-deficit hyperactivity disorder. *Journal of the American Academy of Child and Adolescent Psychiatry*, 36, 1715–25.

Lahey, B., Loeber, R., Quay, H., et al. (1998). Validity of DSM–IV subtypes of Conduct Disorder based on age of onset. *Journal of the American Academy of Child and Adolescent Psychiatry*, 37, 435–42.

Lahey, B.B., Piacentini, J.C., McBurnett, K., et al. (1988). Psychopathology in the parents of children with conduct disorder and hyperactivity. *Journal of the American Academy of Child and Adolescent Psychiatry*, 27, 163–70.

Lahey, B.B., Schwab-Stone, M., Goodman, S.H., et al. (in press). Age and gender differences in oppositional behavior and conduct problems: a cross-sectional household study of middle childhood and adolescence. *Journal of Abnormal Psychology*.

Laucht, M. & Schmidt, M.H. (1987). Psychiatric disorders at the age of 13: results and problems of a long-term study. In B. Cooper (Ed.), *Psychiatric Epidemiology: Progress and Prospects* (pp. 212–24). London: Croom Helm.

Lavigne, J.V., Gibbons, R.D., Christoffel, K.K., et al. (1996). Prevalence rates and correlates of psychiatric disorders among preschool children. *Journal of the American Academy of Child and Adolescent Psychiatry*, 35, 204–14.

Le Blanc, M. & Fréchette, M. (1989). *Male Criminal Activity from Childhood through Youth: Multilevel and Developmental Perspectives*. New York: Springer-Verlag.

Lewinsohn, P.M., Hops, H., Roberts, R.E., Seeley, J.R. & Andrews, J.A. (1993). Adolescent psychopathology: I. Prevalence and incidence of depression and other DSM–III–R disorders in high school students. *Journal of Abnormal Psychology*, 102, 133–44.

Lewinsohn, P.M., Rohde, P. & Seeley, J.R. (1994). Psychosocial risk factors for future adolescent suicide attempts. *Journal of Consulting and Clinical Psychology*, 62, 297–305.

Loeber, R. (1988). Natural histories of conduct problems, delinquency, and associated substance use: evidence for developemental progressions. In B.B. Lahey & A.E. Kazdin (Eds.), *Advances in Clinical Child Psychology* (pp. 73–125). New York: Plenum Press.

Loeber, R. (1990). Development and risk factors of juvenile antisocial behavior and delinquency. *Clinical Psychology Review*, 10, 1–41.

Loeber, R., Farrington, D.P. & Waschbusch, D.A. (1998). Serious and violent juvenile offenders. In R. Loeber & D.P. Farrington (Eds.), *Serious & Violent Juvenile Offenders: Risk Factors and Successful Interventions* (pp. 13–29). Thousand Oaks: Sage Publications.

Loeber, R., Green, S., Keenan, K. & Lahey, B.B. (1995). Which boys will fare worse? Early predictors of the onset of conduct disorder in a six-year longitudinal study. *Journal of the American Academy of Child and Adolescent Psychiatry*, 34, 499–509.

Loeber, R., Green, S.M., Lahey, B.B., Christ, M.A.G & Frick, P.J. (1992). Developmental sequences in the age of onset of disruptive child behaviors. *Journal of Child and Family Studies*, 1, 21–41.

Loeber, R. & Hay, D.F. (1994). Developmental approaches to aggression and conduct problems. In M. Rutter & D.F. Hay (Eds.), *Development Through Life: A Handbook for Clinicians* (pp. 488–516). London: Blackwell Scientific Publications.

Loeber, R. & Keenan, K. (1994). Interaction between conduct disorder and its comorbid conditions: effects of age and gender. *Clinical Psychology Review, 14,* 497–523.

Loeber, R., Keenan, K., Lahey, B.B., Green, S.M. & Thomas, C. (1993). Evidence for developmentally based diagnoses of oppositional defiant disorder and conduct disorder. *Journal of Abnormal Child Psychology, 21,* 377–410.

Loeber, R., Lahey, B.B. & Thomas, C. (1991). Diagnostic conundrum of oppositional defiant disorder and conduct disorder. *Journal of Abnormal Psychology, 100,* 379–90.

Loeber, R. & Stouthamer-Loeber, M. (1997). The development of juvenile aggression and violence: some common misconceptions and controversies. *American Psychologist, 53,* 242–59.

Loney, J. (1988). *Adolescent Drug Abuse: Analyses of Treatment Research.* Rockville, MD: National Institute on Drug Abuse Office of Science.

Long, A. (1941). Parents' reports of undesirable behavior in children. *Child Development, 12,* 43–62.

Lyons, J., Serbin, L.A. & Marchessault, K. (1988). The social behavior of peer-identified aggressive, withdrawn, and aggressive/withdrawn children. *Journal of Abnormal Child Psychology, 16,* 539–52.

Macfarlane, J.W., Allen, L. & Honzik, M.P. (1954). *University of California Publications in Child Development.* Berkeley: University of California Press.

Marriage, K., Fine, S., Moretti, M. & Haley, G. (1986). Relationship between depression and conduct disorder in children and adolescents. *Journal of the American Academy of Child Psychiatry, 25,* 687–91.

Martunnen, M.J., Aro, H.M., Henriksson, M.M. & Lönnqvist, J.K. (1991). Mental disorders in adolescent suicide: DSM–III–R axes I and II diagnoses in suicides among 13 to 19 year-olds in Finland. *Archives of General Psychiatry, 48,* 834–9.

McBurnett, K., Lahey, B.B., Frick, P.J., et al. (1991). Anxiety, inhibition, and conduct disorder in children: II. Relation to salivary cortisol. *Journal of the American Academy of Child and Adolescent Psychiatry, 30,* 192–6.

McConaughy, S.H. & Achenbach, T.M. (1994). Comorbidity of empirically based syndromes in matched general population and clinical samples. *Journal of Child Psychology and Psychiatry, 35,* 1141–57.

McFie, B.S. (1934). Behavior and personality difficulties in school children. *British Journal of Educational Psychology, 4,* 34.

McGee, R., Feehan, M., Williams, S. & Anderson, J. (1992). DSM–III disorders from age 11 to age 15 years. *Journal of the American Academy of Child and Adolescent Psychiatry, 31,* 51–9.

McGee, R., Feehan, M., Williams, S., et al. (1990). DSM–III disorders in a large sample of adolescents. *Journal of the American Academy of Child and Adolescent Psychiatry, 29,* 611–19.

Milich, R. & Dodge, K.A. (1984). Social information processing in child psychiatric populations. *Journal of Abnormal Child Psychology, 12,* 471–90.

Mills, C.J. & Noyes, H.L. (1984). Patterns and correlates of initial and subsequent drug use among adolescents. *Journal of Consulting and Clinical Psychology, 52,* 231–43.

Moffitt, T.E. (1990). Juvenile delinquency and attention deficit disorder: boys' developmental trajectories from age 3 to age 15. *Child Development, 61,* 893–910.

Moffitt, T.E. (1993). The neuropsychology of conduct disorder. *Development and Psychopathology*, 5, 135–51.

Moffitt, T.E., Caspi, A., Dickson, N., Silva, P. & Stanton, W. (1996). Childhood-onset versus adolescent-onset antisocial conduct problems in males: natural history from ages 3 to 18 years. *Development and Psychopathology*, 8, 399–424.

Moffitt, T.E. & Lynam, Jr., D. (1992). The neuropsychology of conduct disorder and delinquency: Implications for understanding antisocial behavior. *Progress in Experimental Personality and Psychopathology Research*, 15, 233–62.

Munir, K., Biederman, J. & Knee, D. (1987). Psychiatric comorbidity in patients with attention deficit disorder: A controlled study. *Journal of the American Academy of Child and Adolescent Psychiatry*, 26, 844–8.

Noam, G.G., Paget, K., Valiant, G., Borst, S. & Bartok, J. (1994). Conduct and affective disorders in developmental perspective: a systematic study of adolescent psychopathology. *Development and Psychopathology*, 6, 519–32.

Offord, D.R., Sullivan, K., Allen, N. & Abrams, N. (1979). Delinquency and hyperactivity. *Journal of Nervous and Mental Disorders*, 167, 734–41.

Olson, W.C. (1930). *Problem Tendencies in Children*. Minneapolis: The University of Minnesota Press.

Quay, H.C. (1986). Conduct disorders. In H.C. Quay & J.S. Werry (Eds.), *Psychopathological Disorders of Childhood* (pp. 35–72). New York: John Wiley & Sons.

Quay, H.C. (1993). The psychobiology of undersocialized aggressive conduct disorder: A theoretical perspective. *Development and Psychopathology*, 5, 165–80.

Quiggle, N.L., Garber, J., Panak, W.F. & Dodge, K.A. (1992). Social information processing in aggressive and depressed children. *Child Development*, 63, 1305–20.

Reeves, J.C., Werry, J.S., Elkind, G.S. & Zametkin, A. (1987). Attention deficit, conduct, oppositional and anxiety disorders in children: II. Clinical characteristics. *Journal of the American Academy of Child and Adolescent Psychiatry*, 26, 144–55.

Renouf, A.G., Kovacs, M. & Mukerji, P. (1997). Relationship of depressive, conduct, and comorbid disorders and social functioning in childhood. *Journal of the American Academy of Child and Adolescent Psychiatry*, 36, 998–1004.

Rey, J.M., Bashir, M.R. & Schwartz, M. (1988). Oppositional disorder: fact or fiction? *Journal of the American Academy of Child and Adolescent Psychiatry*, 27, 157–62.

Rhode, P., Lewinsohn, P.M. & Seeley, J.R. (1991). Comorbidity of unipolar depression: II. Comorbidity with other mental disorders in adolescents and adults. *Journal of Abnormal Psychology*, 100, 214–22.

Robins, E. & Guze, S.B. (1970). Establishment of diagnostic validity in psychiatric illness: Its application to schizophrenia. *American Journal of Psychiatry*, 126, 107–11.

Robins, L. (1998). A 70-year history of conduct disorder: variations in definition, prevalence, and correlates. In P. Cohen, C. Slomkowski & L.N. Robins (Eds.), *Time, Place, and Psychopathology*. Mahwah, NJ: Lawrence Erlbaum.

Robins, L.N. (1974). *Deviant Children Grown Up*. Huntington, NY: Krieger.

Robins, L.N. (1978). Sturdy childhood predictors of adult antisocial behavior: Replications from longitudinal studies. *Psychological Medicine, 8*, 611–22.

Robins, L.N. & McEvoy, L. (1990). Conduct problems as predictors of substance abuse. In L.N. Robins & M. Rutter (Eds.), *Straight and Devious Pathways from Childhood to Adulthood* (pp. 182–204). Cambridge: Cambridge University Press.

Robins, L.N. & Murphy, G.E. (1967). Drug use in a normal population of young negro men. *American Journal of Public Health and the Nation's Health, 57*, 1580–96.

Robins, L.N. & Przybeck, T.R. (1985). *Age of Onset of Drug Use as a Factor in Drug and Other Disorders.* Rockville, MD: National Institute of Drug Abuse Research.

Robins, L.N. & Ratcliff, K.S. (1980). Childhood conduct disorders and later arrest. In L.N. Robins, P.J. Clayton & J.K. Wing (Eds.), *The Social Consequences of Psychiatric Illness* (pp. 248–63). New York: Brunner/Mazel.

Rohde, P., Lewinsohn, P.M. & Seeley, J.R. (1996). Psychiatric comorbidity in problematic alcohol use in high school students. *Journal of the American Academy of Child and Adolescent Psychiatry, 35*, 101–9.

Rudolph, K.D., Hammen, C. & Burge, D. (1994). Interpersonal functioning and depressive symptoms in childhood: addressing the issues of specificity and comorbidity. *Journal of Abnormal Child Psychology, 22*, 355–71.

Russo, M.F., Loeber, R., Lahey, B.B. & Keenan, K. (1994). Oppositional defiant and conduct disorders: validation of the DSM–III–R and an alternative diagnostic option. *Journal of Clinical Child Psychology, 23*, 56–68.

Rutter, M. (1978). Diagnostic validity in child psychiatry. *Advances in Biological Psychiatry, 2*, 2–22.

Rutter, M. (1997). Comorbidity: concepts, claims and choices. *Criminal Behavior and Mental Health, 7*, 265–85.

Rutter, M. & Graham, P. (1966). Psychiatric disorder in 10- and 11-year-old children. *Proceedings of the Royal Society of Medicine, 59*, 382–7.

Rutter, M., Tizard, J. & Whitmore, K. (1970). *Education, Health, and Behaviour.* London: Longman.

Rutter, M.L., Shaffer, D. & Sturge, C. (1979). *A Guide to a Multi-axial Classification Scheme for Psychiatric Disorders in Childhood and Adolescence.* London: Frowde & Co. (Printers) Ltd.

Satterfield, J.H. & Schell, A. (1997). A perspective study of hyperactive boys with conduct problems and normal boys: adolescent and adult criminality. *Journal of the American Academy of Child and Adolescent Psychiatry, 36*, 1726–35.

Schachar, R. & Logan, G.D. (1990). Impulsivity and inhibitory control in development and psychopathology. *Development and Psychopathology, 26*, 1–11.

Schachar, R. & Rannock, R. (1995). Test of four hypotheses for the comorbidity of attention-deficit hyperactivity disorder and conduct disorder. *Journal of the American Academy of Child and Adolescent Psychiatry, 34*, 639–48.

Schachar, R. & Wachsmuth, R. (1990). Hyperactivity and parental psychopathology. *Journal of Child Psychology and Psychiatry, 31*, 381–92.

Seidman, L.J., Biederman, J., Faraone, S.V., et al. (1995). Effects of family history and comorbidity on the neuropsychological performance of children with ADHD: preliminary findings. *Journal of the American Academy of Child and Adolescent Psychiatry*, 34, 1015–24.

Shaffer, D. (1993). Suicide: risk factors and the public health. *American Journal of Public Health*, 83, 171–2.

Shaffer, D. & Fisher, P.W. (1981). The epidemiology of suicide in children and young adolescents. *Journal of the American Academy of Child Psychiatry*, 20, 545–65.

Silberg, J., Meyer, J., Pickles, A., et al. (1996a). Heterogeneity among juvenile antisocial behaviours: findings from the Virginia Twin Study of Adolescent Behavioural Development (VTSABD). *Genetics of Criminal and Antisocial Behaviour: Ciba Foundation Symposium*, 194, 76–92.

Silberg, J.L., Rutter, M.L., Meyer, J.M., et al. (1996b). Genetic and environmental influences on the covariation between hyperactivity and conduct disturbances in juvenile twins. *Journal of Child Psychology and Psychiatry*, 37, 803–16.

Simonoff, E., Pickles, A., Meyer, J.M., et al. (1997). The Virginia twin study of adolescent behavioral development: influences of age, sex and impairment on rates of disorder. *Archives of General Psychiatry*, 54, 801–8.

Stein, J.A., Newcomb, M.D. & Bentler, P.M. (1987). An 8-year study of multiple influences on drug use and drug use consequences. *Journal of Personality and Social Psychology*, 53, 1094–105.

Steinhausen, H.-C. & Reitzle, M. (1996). The validity of mixed disorders of conduct and emotions in children and adolescents: a research note. *Journal of Child Psychology and Psychiatry and Allied Disciplines*, 37, 339–43.

Taylor, E. (1994). Similarities and differences in DSM–IV and ICD–10 diagnostic criteria. *Child and Adolescent Psychiatric Clinics of North America*, 3, 209–26.

Taylor, E., Chadwick, O., Heptinstall, E. & Danckaerts, M. (1996). Hyperactivity and conduct problems as risk factors for adolescent development. *Journal of the American Academy of Child and Adolescent Psychiatry*, 35, 1213–26.

Tolan, P.H. & Gorman-Smith, D. (1997). Development of serious and violent offending careers. In R. Loeber & D.P. Farrington (Eds.), *Never Too Early, Never Too Late: Risk Factors and Successful Interventions for Serious and Violent Juvenile Offenders*. Thousand Oaks, CA: Sage Publications.

Tubman, J.G., Vicary, J.R., von Eye, A. & Lerner, J.V. (1990). Longitudinal substance use and adult adjustment. *Journal of Substance Abuse*, 2, 317–34.

Van Kammen, W.B. & Loeber, R. (1994). Are fluctuations in delinquent activities related to the onset and offset in juvenile illegal drug use and drug dealing? *Journal of Drug Issues*, 24, 9–24.

Van Kammen, W.B., Loeber, R. & Stouthamer-Loeber, M. (1991). Substance use and its relationship to conduct problems and delinquency in young boys. *Journal of Youth and Adolescence*, 20, 399–413.

Velez, C.N., Johnson, J. & Cohen, P. (1989). A longitudinal analysis of selected risk factors of childhood psychopathology. *Journal of the American Academy of Child and Adolescent Psychiatry*, 28, 861–4.

Verhulst, F.C. (1995). A review of community studies. In F.C. Verhulst & H.M. Koot (Eds.), *The*

Epidemiology of Child and Adolescent Psychopathology (pp. 146–77). Oxford: Oxford University Press.

Verhulst, F.C. & Achenbach, T.M. (1995). Empirically based assessment and taxonomy of psychopathology: cross-cultural applications. A review. *European Child & Adolescent Psychiatry,* 4, 61–76.

Verhulst, F.C. & van der Ende, J. (1993). 'Comorbidity' in an epidemiological sample: a longitudinal perspective. *Journal of Child Psychology and Psychiatry,* 34, 767–83.

Verhulst, F.C., van der Ende, J., Ferdinand, R.F. & Kasius, M.C. (1997). The prevalence of DSM–III–R diagnoses in a national sample of Dutch adolescents. *Archives of General Psychiatry,* 54, 329–36.

Vikan, A. (1985). Psychiatric epidemiology in a sample of 1510 ten-year-old children: I. Prevalence. *Journal of Child Psychology and Psychiatry,* 26, 55–75.

Walker, J.L., Lahey, B.B., Hynd, G.W. & Frame, C.L. (1987). Comparison of specific patterns of antisocial behavior in children with conduct disorder with or without co-existing hyperactivity. *Journal of Consulting and Clinical Psychology,* 55, 910–13.

Walker, J.L., Lahey, B.B., Russo, M.F., et al. (1991). Anxiety, inhibition, and conduct disorder in children: I. Relations to social impairment. *Journal of the American Academy of Child and Adolescent Psychiatry,* 30, 187–91.

Welte, J.W. & Barnes, G.M. (1985). Alcohol: The gateway to other drug use among secondary-school students. *Journal of Youth and Adolescence,* 14, 487–98.

Wickman, E.K. (1928). *Children's Behavior and Teachers' Attitudes.* New York: The Commonwealth Fund.

Windle, M. (1990). A longitudinal study of antisocial behaviors in early adolescence as predictors of late adolescent substance use: gender and ethnic group differences. *Journal of Abnormal Psychology,* 99, 86–91.

Yamaguchi, K. & Kandel, D.B. (1984). Patterns of drug use from adolescence to young adulthood: II. Sequences of progression. *American Journal of Public Health,* 74, 668–72.

Young-Masten, I. (1938). Behavior problems of elementary school children: a descriptive and comparative study. *Genetic Psychology Monographs,* 20, 123–80.

Yourman, J. (1932). Children identified by their teachers as problems. *Journal of Educational Sociology,* 5, 334–43.

Zoccolillo, M. (1992). Co-occurrence of conduct disorder and its adult outcomes with depressive and anxiety disorders: A review. *Journal of the American Academy of Child and Adolescent Psychiatry,* 31, 547–56.

Zoccolillo, M. (1993). Gender and the development of conduct disorder. *Development and Psychopathology,* 5, 65–78.

Zoccolillo, M., Tremblay, R. & Vitaro, F. (1996). DSM–III–R and DSM–III criteria for conduct disorder in preadolescent girls: specific but insensitive. *Journal of the American Academy of Child and Adolescent Psychiatry,* 35, 461–99.

Zucker, R.A. & Gomberg, E.S.L. (1986). Etiology of alcoholism reconsidered: the case for biopsychosocial process. *American Psychologist,* 41, 783–93.

7

Conduct disorder in context

Barbara Maughan

Introduction

Of all child psychiatric disorders, conduct problems show perhaps the strongest associations with psychosocial adversity. Both within the family and beyond, decades of research has documented links between disruptive behaviour problems and adverse environments: poverty and social disadvantage, disorganized neighbourhoods, poor schools, family breakdown, parental psychopathology, harsh and ineffective parenting and inadequate supervision all occur at higher than expected rates in conduct-disordered samples (Earls, 1994; Loeber & Stouthamer-Loeber, 1986).

The consistency of these associations is in no doubt; interpreting their meaning has proved more challenging. First, especially in relation to family and peer-based correlates, there are quite basic questions of the direction of effects: children influence, as well as being influenced by, those around them (Lytton, 1990), so no simple assumptions can be made about the direction of the causal arrow. Second, behaviour genetic studies have shown that many ostensibly 'environmental' measures involve genetic mediation (Plomin & Bergeman, 1991), and that risks for conduct disorder are likely to involve a complex interplay between nature and nurture. Third, the environmental factors measured in many epidemiological studies – low SES, parental discord, harsh parenting, and so forth – are cast at too general a level to be more than broad brush indicators of the processes that are actually likely to put children at risk. To understand their effects, we need to 'unpack' their meaning. And finally, increasing awareness of the heterogeneity of antisocial behaviour (Rutter et al., 1997) suggests that different patterns of risk, both individual and environmental, may be important for different subgroups of conduct-disordered children.

Over time, each of these veins of theorizing promises to cast new light on the ways in which environmental adversities impact on the onset or persistence of conduct problems. At this stage, they are only beginning to be explored. This chapter examines recent progress in understanding contextual risks for conduct problems, focusing on three central contexts for children's development: the family, the neighbourhood and the school. Peer influences, a further key element in environmental risk, are considered by Vitaro and colleagues (chapter 13, this volume). We begin by discussing a number of general conceptual and methodological issues that have implications across a range of domains.

Correlates, causes and chains of risk

Though much early research on psychosocial risks assumed unidirectional effects of adverse environments on the child, several different lines of evidence have converged to demand more complex models. From infancy onwards, investigators have documented how children's own behaviour contributes to the regulation of their interactions with others (Gianino & Tronick, 1988). At older ages, both naturalistic and experimental studies have shown that disruptive behaviours elicit negative responses from both parent figures (Lytton, 1990) and peers (Parker & Asher, 1987). Indeed, in reviewing this literature Lytton (1990) concluded that 'child effects' may be especially important in relation to conduct problems. Patterson's detailed studies (Patterson, 1982, 1995) have elegantly charted the bidirectional processes involved, with hostility from each interactional partner fuelling increasingly coercive spirals of effects. Although less systematically documented, reciprocal processes of this kind almost certainly arise in other settings, such as classrooms and schools (Nichol et al., 1985).

In addition to these effects on immediate interaction patterns, children's behaviour may also function to shape and select environments in more wide-ranging ways (Scarr & McCartney, 1983). Robins' classic follow-up of child guidance patients provided striking examples of this kind: in adulthood, previously conduct-disordered children were more likely to be unemployed, to be sacked from their jobs, to face marital difficulties and breakdowns, and to be in debt (Robins, 1966). The long-term consequences of their problems led them into experiences that researchers in other traditions would regard as stressful life events. Subsequent findings have reinforced this view: in adolescence, disruptive and aggressive teenagers are more likely to affiliate with deviant peers (Fergusson & Horwood, 1996), to drop out of school or leave with few educational qualifications (Kessler et al., 1995), to begin sexual and intimate relationships earlier than their peers (Bardone et al., 1996), and take on the responsibilities of parenthood at young ages (Kessler et al., 1997a; Maughan & Lindelow, 1997). Behaviour at one developmental period can play a central role in selecting young people into life circumstances that restrict their opportunities, and increase their exposure to subsequent stress (Rutter et al., 1995).

Selection effects of this kind in no sense negate the possibility that later environments carry independent risk potential. As Robins (1978) pointed out many years ago, unemployment, debt and divorce are likely to carry similar connotations however they arise – and may even be especially deleterious for young people already vulnerable to antisocial behaviour (Farrington et al., 1986). What they do underscore, however, is the need for research designs capable of teasing these reciprocities and chains of risk apart. Time-ordered assessments, with putative risk factors measured before child outcomes, are a basic prerequisite for demonstrating the causal status of any risk factor (Kraemer et al., 1997). Cross-sectional studies are important in generating hypotheses, but longitudinal designs, with postulated risk factors measured before child outcomes, are essential if we are to move beyond correlational findings. As Farrington (1988) has argued, designs addressing risks for within-individual change – factors associated with the onset of conduct disorder, with increases in its severity, or with its offset – are especially valuable here. To examine more complex processes, repeated data-waves, along with appropriate measurements, are essential (Willett et al., 1998). Although designs of this kind are increasingly being employed in psychosocial risk research, many findings still rest on cross-sectional data, or on assessments from two-wave longitudinal designs. Insofar as this is the case, interpretations about causal direction must inevitably remain tentative.

Environmental lessons from genetic research

A second major influence on thinking about environmental risk has derived from behavioural genetic research. As Simonoff details (chapter 8, this volume), current twin study findings all point to nontrivial environmental influences on conduct problems, and some suggest that environmental effects are substantial. As estimated in twin studies, environmental influences seem as important for boys as for girls, but are likely to vary in their salience for different subgroups of conduct-disordered children. At this stage, evidence suggests that genetic influences are likely to predominate in relation to aggression (Edelbrock et al., 1995), conduct problems that persist to adulthood (Lyons et al., 1995) and those that overlap with hyperactivity (Silberg et al., 1996), but that environmental factors may carry greater weight in shaping adolescent delinquency and 'pure' conduct problems.

In addition to findings on specific disorders, behaviour genetic analyses have also highlighted a series of more general issues relevant to models of environmental influence. First, both twin and adoption studies have shown that apparently 'environmental' measures may involve genetic mediation (Plomin & Bergeman, 1991). Parental genes affect the environments parents provide for their children, and heritable child characteristics may evoke particular patterns of parental response. Gene–environment correlations of this kind may be of particular importance in relation to antisocial behaviour. Antisocial parents are well known to provide adverse rearing environments (Rutter et al., 1998), with increased rates of just those factors identified as risks for their children – harsh parenting, marital breakdown and negative parent–child relationships. Although it is unclear at this stage how far passive gene–environment correlations of this kind mediate effects of adverse parenting, they almost certainly play some part. In a parallel way, child effects on the environment are also likely to reflect some element of gene–environment correlation, this time of an active or evocative kind (Ge et al., 1996).

These findings clearly mark important advances in our appreciation of family-related risks. Their interpretation, however, is by no means straightforward. In particular, they do not – as is sometimes assumed – obviate the possibility that the risk *mechanisms* involved are predominantly environmental. As Rutter (1997) has argued, the origins of a risk factor carry no direct implications for its mode of operation: the pathogenic effects of harsh parenting, for example, may still lie in environmentally influenced risk processes even though their origins reflect effects of parental genes. Once again, the challenge is for research designs capable of teasing these differing interpretations apart. Genetically informative designs – twin and adoption studies, along with more complex 'blended family' designs (Reiss et al., 1994) – are clearly central here, but are by no means the only approaches of value. Rutter et al. (1998) provide an overview of other informative designs.

A further key issue concerns the nature of environmental influences. Genetic analyses suggest that for most aspects of personality and psychopathology, nonshared environmental factors – influences that function to make children in the same family different from one another, rather than more alike – are markedly more important than shared effects (Pike & Plomin, 1996). More recent findings suggest some modifications to this position (Rutter et al., 1999), and conduct disorder and delinquency have often been seen as exceptions to this 'rule'. Even so, some nonshared effects are typically documented. What does this imply for environmental risks? Some commentators have assumed that it casts doubt on the importance of many of the family-wide factors so consistently identified in correlational studies – social disadvantage, parental marital discord, and so forth – and suggests instead that the focus should turn to nonfamilial risks. In relation to conduct disorder, these clearly play a central role: peer influences are undoubtedly of key importance, and, as we discuss in later sections, school and community-level factors also warrant attention. But nonshared influences can also arise within the family, through processes such as scapegoating, the differential exposure of siblings to ostensibly 'family-wide' risks, or the differing perceptions that individual children hold of family-based experiences. To date, much risk research has studied just one child per family, so that processes of this kind have been difficult to identify. More complex designs involving siblings (Reiss et al., 1995) are already beginning to highlight the advantages of exploring both shared and nonshared risks.

Finally, although twin studies partition variance into separate genetic and environmental components, in many instances nature and nurture seem likely to combine to elevate risks for conduct problems (Rutter, 1997). One of the most consistent findings to emerge from studies of psychosocial risks is the marked individual variability in children's response: exposed to risk factor X, some go on to show disorder, while others do not. To date, we know very little about the bases for these variations in susceptibility. Hill (chapter 5, this volume) discusses evidence for biosocial interactions, while Simonoff (chapter 8, this volume) describes findings from adoption studies that suggest an interplay between genetic predisposition and environmental risk (Bohman, 1996; Cadoret et al., 1995). Here, adoptees at genetic risk seemed more sensitive to adverse environmental features than those whose biological parents showed no evidence of criminality or antisocial personality. Because adoptive homes are selected to have low risks of the problems so characteristic of conduct-disordered children's families, these findings are likely to provide very conservative estimates of the importance of gene–environment interactions. As well as increasing exposure to adverse environments, heritable factors may also increase children's sensitivity to their effects (Kendler, 1995).

Conceptualizing contexts

Charting the differing aspects of children's social worlds that may have implications for disorder is a complex enterprise. Bronfenbrenner (1979), Sameroff (1983) and Cicchetti & Richters (1997) are among key theorists who have proposed ecological models of environmental influence, whereby more proximal contexts – relationships with parents, siblings, teachers and peers – are seen as nested or embedded within wider systems of family and peer group, school, neighbourhood and culture. The implications of individual relationships for children's adjustment may vary with characteristics of other relationships, and of these wider systems, and influences at each of these levels, and at the interface between them, may be important for development. Taken alone, structural markers of children's 'social addresses' – single parent families, low social class and so forth – will usually require translation to more process-oriented variables to uncover their effects; processes may, however, vary systematically between social addresses, or differ in their implications depending on the context in which they occur.

As children develop, so their social worlds expand, and their understandings of them change. Potential sources of environmental risk are likely to vary widely between early childhood and adolescence, and exposure to objectively similar risks – marital discord between parents, or ineffective supervision – may differ in their effects at different developmental stages. Developmentally sensitive models of environmental risk (Costello & Angold, 1993) must be designed to take these changing contingencies into account. Time and place may also be important, with contextual influences varying in their impact for children growing up in different geographical locations (Farrington & Loeber, 1998), and born and passing through key phases of development in different historical eras (Elder, 1998).

Formulations of this kind now inform much research on normal development. In general, research on psychopathology has been slower to take them on board. Boyce et al. (1998), surveying the current state of research on social contexts in developmental psychopathology, concluded that – with some notable exceptions – coherent models of context influence are all too often missing from studies of psychopathology. Many focus on isolated aspects of children's environments, or include 'laundry lists' of environmental factors as covariates in their analyses, with little apparent rationale for their selection. Systematic explorations of the ways in which individual factors may be mediated or moderated by other influences (Baron & Kenny, 1986) are still quite limited, and despite extensive evidence that risks for conduct problems overlap, the implications of multiple risks remain relatively little explored.

Heterogeneity of conduct disorder and specificity of risk

It has long been recognized that conduct disorders are heterogeneous: current classifications almost certainly include distinctively different subgroups of children, varying in phenotypic presentation or etiology. Genetic studies, for example, now point to the distinctiveness of a subgroup comorbid with ADHD (Silberg et al., 1996), and a variety of investigators have proposed developmental typologies based on age at onset (DiLalla & Gottesman, 1989; Moffitt, 1993; Patterson & Yoerger, 1997). Environmental influences may differ in their relative importance in these different subgroups, and also in the types of risk that prove most salient. Moffitt (1993), for example, has argued that while adolescent onset conduct problems largely reflect status frustration and social mimicry of deviant peers, early onset disorder has quite different roots, depending more heavily on both individual vulnerabilities and exposure to family adversity. More differentiated, comparative models of this kind, examining risks in contrasting subgroups of antisocial and delinquent youth, are likely to be especially important in furthering our understanding of environmental risks.

Complementary issues arise in relation to specificity. Many of the family and social correlates of conduct problems also show links with other child psychiatric disorders, raising important questions about the ways in which they exert their effects. On the one hand, nonspecific associations might suggest that some types of adversity carry broadly pathogenic implications; where this is so, differences in child outcomes may owe as much to individual vulnerabilities as to the nature of the external risk. Alternatively, apparently nonspecific links may suggest that different mechanisms, at this stage little understood, are operating to elevate risks of different disorders. Medicine provides numerous examples of this kind: cigarette smoking, for instance, is associated with increased risks of lung cancer, coronary artery disease and osteoporosis, but each through distinct and different physiological pathways. Similar processes may well arise in the psychosocial domain. Once again, however, we are only in the beginning stages of teasing them apart.

Risk variables and risk processes

At a more general level, examples of this kind underscore the need to move beyond the study of risk variables to investigations of risk processes: which aspects of any identified risk factor carry the main potential for disorder, and how do their effects 'get under the skin' (Taylor et al., 1997)? As Rutter (1994) has argued, the central needs here are for clearly articulated hypotheses about competing risk mechanisms, combined with research designs capable of testing them out. Natural experiments often provide important leverage here. In exploring the links between 'broken homes' and conduct disorder, for example, investigators have used a variety of contrasts – between the effects of parental death and divorce, between levels of children's disturbance before and after parental separation, and between exposure to family change and family discord – to identify the particular aspects of marital breakdown that seem most pathogenic in their effects (Rodgers & Pryor, 1998).

Once these more proximal factors have been identified, a second series of questions concern the mechanisms through which adverse family and social factors function to compromise children's development. A variety of models are currently being explored here. The first concern children's perceptions of their experiences: like adults, children actively process experience, and there is ample evidence that they hold quite particular views, often different from those of other family members. These varying perceptions may prove key mediators of effects. Cummings et al. (1994), for example, found that boys' perceptions of marital discord tended to agree much more closely with those of their mothers than did girls'. These differing perceptions held important implications: boys' risks of externalizing behaviour were associated with their perceptions of the threat involved in parental discord, while for girls, the likelihood of internalizing difficulties was associated with perceptions of self-blame. Some of the sex differences in response to marital discord may thus run through the differing ways in which girls and boys perceive and respond to hostility between their parents. In a rather similar way, cultural variations in perceptions of the legitimacy of physical punishment appear to mediate its impact (Deater-Deckard et al., 1996). How children process and evaluate their experiences may hold important keys to understanding their effects.

In addition to these perceptual variations, the majority of the family and social risks identified for conduct problems might plausibly operate through a variety of psychological, and possibly some physiological, routes. Some of these – the impact of early parent–child relationships on attachment security, the role of social learning, and the effects of exposure to hostility on the development of biased information processing and attributions – are examined in detail in other chapters in this volume. We note others in the sections that follow. As we shall see, however, although some progress is being made in examining more specific risk processes, in most cases we are still only in the very beginning stages of understanding how environmental adversities impact on the child.

Individual differences and group levels

Contextual factors are likely to contribute to variations in antisocial behaviours in two rather different ways: in terms of individual differences in risk, and also in relation to variations in overall *levels* of antisocial behaviour in different settings and time periods. Rates of many childhood and adolescent disorders have risen over recent decades (Rutter & Smith, 1995). Juvenile crime statistics clearly mirror these trends (Rutter et al., 1998), and, as Angold & Costello note (chapter 6, this volume), although data on conduct disorder are less satisfactory, they too are consistent with the view that levels of antisocial behaviour have been rising over time. Secular trends of this kind almost certainly reflect environmental influences; some may overlap with risks for individual differences in disorder, but others may be quite distinct. In relation to changing rates of delinquency, for example, Rutter et al. (1998) suggest that changes in the meaning of adolescence, an increasing disparity between aspirations and opportunities, a rise in the use of alcohol and drugs, diminished surveillance and increased opportunities for crime, along with increased rates of family breakdown, may all play some part. While some of these may impact on individual differences in vulnerability to disorder, others may not. The present chapter focuses on risks for individual differences in conduct problems. Any comprehensive model of environmental influence, however, needs to take both sets of factors into account.

Sex differences

Finally, we turn briefly to the question of sex differences. From early childhood onwards, boys are more likely to show noncompliant and disruptive behaviours than girls (Campbell, 1995). At this stage, we know very little about the extent to which variations in either exposure or response to psychosocial adversities may contribute to these differences. Like much research on conduct problems, most early studies of environmental risks focused solely on boys, and a number of the more informative current programmes continue to do so. As a result, evidence on sex differences is still slim. Because of this, we make only brief reference to gender differences in the individual sections that follow, and attempt to draw the findings together in a separate section at the end of the chapter, highlighting the few general conclusions that can be drawn at this stage.

With these general issues in mind, we turn to evidence on the role of specific environmental factors as risks for conduct disorder, beginning with the most proximal context for young children's development: the family.

Family context

From the time of the first systematic studies of conduct disorder and delinquency, family structure and processes have emerged as central correlates of childhood conduct problems (McCord, 1979; Robins, 1966; Rutter et al., 1970). Many of the features identified in these early investigations – family poverty and disadvantage, large family size, parental psychopathology, harsh and inept parenting, conflicted relationships and family breakdown – have since shown robust links with conduct disorder in numerous other samples (see Coie & Dodge, 1998; Hawkins et al., 1998; Loeber & Stouthamer-Loeber, 1986; Rutter et al., 1998, for reviews). Especially in childhood, conduct problems seem most likely to arise in families facing high rates of external adversities, where parents are stressed and relationships strained, and where parenting strategies are less than optimal.

Parents, children and parenting

As early as the preschool years, noncompliant child behaviours are associated with particular patterns of parenting and parent–child relationships (see Campbell, 1995 for a review). Studies of the early emergence of disruptive, aggressive behaviours suggest that biological propensities in the child – as indexed, for example, by difficult temperament – interact with caregiving environments to contribute to more and less adaptive outcomes. The extensive literature on parenting (Bornstein, 1995; Maccoby & Martin, 1983) makes clear that parental behaviours that combine warmth, firm but fair control, and the use of explanation and reasoning are associated with the establishment of compliance and the internalization of controls in the toddler period. Parents of noncompliant preschoolers often show the polar opposites of this profile: they are arbitrary, inconsistent and negative in their interactions with their children. Observational studies report more parent–child confrontations, with mothers less likely to follow through on instructions until they achieve compliance. In addition, affective relationships also seem compromised: mothers of difficult preschoolers have lower rates of positive, harmonious interactions with their children, and are less likely to show mutual enjoyment in activities that they share.

These themes of negativity and hostility in parent–child relationships, along with inconsistent, inept strategies for control, emerge repeatedly as correlates of conduct problems throughout the childhood and adolescent years. Studies at different age-periods also agree that these patterns are most likely to arise in families that are stressed in other ways: by poverty and social disadvantage, adverse life events, parental psychopathology, marital discord and separation and divorce. Indeed, some evidence suggests that the combination of negative parenting, low social status, family instability and parental disagreements may be somewhat specific to antisocial outcomes, rather than to adjustment problems more generally (Henry et al., 1993).

As Campbell (1995) underlined, these findings might plausibly reflect either genetic or environmental influences, or their interplay. Antisocial children are disproportionately drawn from families where one or both parents also show antisocial tendencies (Cohen et al., 1990; Farrington et al., 1996; Frick et al., 1992), and antisocial parents are known to provide less than optimal rearing environments (Rutter et al., 1998). Some of the observed associations between parenting styles and child behaviours are thus likely to reflect passive gene–

environment correlations. At this stage, the extent of these influences is difficult to estimate, as no studies have yet examined parental characteristics and parenting styles within genetically informative designs. Current findings suggest that the most proximal risks lie in harsh, coercive parenting, and that antisocial traits in parents are largely influential through their effects on parenting styles (Bank et al., 1993). We must await further studies, however, to clarify these conclusions.

Evidence on the role of evocative and active correlations – whereby child behaviours evoke negative parenting – is slightly more extensive. Two adoption studies (Ge et al., 1996; O'Connor et al., 1998a) have now shown that adoptees at genetic risk of antisocial disorders are more likely than low risk children to receive negative parenting in their adoptive homes. Child characteristics clearly play some part in evoking particular styles of parental response. Longitudinal evidence, however, suggests that these processes form part of a reciprocal parent–child dynamic. Campbell et al. (1996), for example, found that negative control at age 4 predicted antisocial problems at age 9 after controlling for prior behaviour problems and the stability of these two sets of measures. Importantly, the cross-lagged correlation from early maternal control to later behaviour problems was stronger than the link from child behaviour to parental control. Cohen & Brook (1995) reported a similar pattern. Taking account of confounding variables, they found that punishment early in childhood was associated with later conduct problems with an odds ratio of over 3. Child behaviour also had significant effects on parental punishment, but only in the younger children in their sample, studied from early childhood to early adolescence. Moving later into adolescence, these effects dropped out. The effects of punishment were similar for boys and girls, but interacted with early conduct problems: severe punishment had the strongest impact on later behaviour problems for children who were already showing difficulties at the first assessment point.

These findings suggest that some of the effects of adverse parenting almost certainly involve environmental mediation. On that assumption, investigators have attempted to tease out the particular aspects of parenting that are most deleterious, and how they have their effects. Three main constructs have emerged across a range of studies: first, harsh, coercive parenting, including the use of physical punishment; second, hostile, critical parent–child relationships; and third, ineffective, inconsistent management styles, often involving poor monitoring and supervision. Other chapters in this volume examine some of the key psychological processes that are likely to underlie these links: compromised attachment security (DeKlyen & Speltz, chapter 12, this volume); social learning processes (Kiesner et al., chapter 10, this volume); and the effects of exposure to hostility and aggression on children's information processing and attributions (Pettit et al., chapter 11, this volume). We focus briefly here on one particular issue that has been the subject of much controversy: the effects of physical punishment.

How far does physical punishment per se, when it falls short of abuse, have negative effects on children's development? The question is a central one for parents, policy makers and researchers alike, and has generated continuing debate. Current evidence is not conclusive, but suggests that several rather different issues may be involved. Firstly, effects may vary with the meaning of punishment for the child. Deater-Deckard et al. (1996), for example, found that effects differed in different cultural groups: physical punishment showed clear links with behaviour problems in the white children in their US sample, but few if any effects in an African-American sample. These authors suggested that although in many cultures authoritarian parenting is seen as rejecting, in some it can be regarded as a marker of parental involvement and concern. Where it is viewed as acceptable and legitimate, the negative effects of physical punishment seem less marked. In a similar way, the underlying nature of parent–child relationships may also moderate effects, so that physical punishments administered in the context of generally warm parent–child bonds may also have less deleterious consequences than when relationships are strained.

Secondly, Deater-Deckard & Dodge (1997) proposed that associations with risks for problem behaviours may be nonlinear, varying with the severity, frequency and intensity of the punishment involved. A model of this kind would go some way to reconciling the inconsistent findings on the links between physical punishment and problems behaviours reported in clinical and nonclinical samples: correlations are often modest in community studies (Rothbaum & Weisz, 1994), but much stronger in referred or disordered groups. Parents of conduct-disordered children may use substantially higher levels of physical discipline than most other parents; markedly stronger correlations between harsh discipline and externalizing behaviours may thus arise in the extremes of the range. Finally, there may be important individual differences in children's susceptibility to adverse parenting, so that, for example, difficult temperament interacts with parenting variables to produce adverse outcomes. Once again, the few findings currently available support this view, but much more evidence is needed to determine which particular characteristics put children most at risk.

Returning to the more general question of parenting, it seems likely that different aspects of parenting styles are associated with risks for conduct problems at different developmental periods. As outlined earlier, patterns of hostile, coercive parenting seem especially characteristic of early onset conduct problems, beginning in the childhood years. Where onset is later, different constellations of influences are likely to be involved (Moffitt, 1993). In particular, individual vulnerabilities seem less marked, and environmental influences turn more centrally on affiliations with deviant peers than on family risks per se. In keeping with this view, Capaldi & Patterson (1994) found that families of adolescent onset delinquents tended to be intermediate between early onset and nondelinquent groups in terms of income, social disadvantage, rates of parental antisociality and frequency of family transitions. Discipline and monitoring were more positive than in childhood onset families, and showed no differences from nondelinquent groups. For later onset conduct problems, the key appears to lie in processes that promote, or fail to hinder, involvement with delinquent peers. Family processes may of course continue to be important here: stressed family relationships may contribute to a flight into peer involvements, and poor monitoring and supervision may fail to inhibit links with deviant peers. In addition, neighbourhood and school influences may also take on a more central role. We return to these possibilities in later sections.

Finally, although nonshared risks seem less central for conduct problems than other forms of child psychopathology, the effects of adverse parenting may of course vary in important ways for individual children within a family. Scapegoating and other forms of differential treatment have long been recognized as important in clinical practice. It is only recently, however, that researchers have begun to explore issues of this kind. Reiss et al. (1995), for example, examined effects of parental negativity in families with at least two same-sex adolescent siblings. Though negativity to siblings was significantly correlated, overlaps were by no means complete; importantly, parenting behaviours directed specifically towards each adolescent proved the strongest correlates of his or her problem levels, and there were suggestions that negativity towards the other sibling might in some instances offer protection against antisocial behaviour. O'Connor et al. (1998b) took these findings further, using clustering methods with measures of multiple family relationships to approximate a family systems perspective on developmental context. Differing relationship clusters clearly emerged, and reliably predicted variations in levels of antisocial behaviour. Variations in risk could not simply be captured by main effects models of individual relationships; the patterning of relationships between parents, between parents and children, and between siblings, each contributed to effects. Adverse family relationships, along with less than optimal parenting, clearly contribute in central ways to risks for conduct problems. As they become more widespread, these more complex research designs clearly promise important gains in our understanding of these effects.

Abuse and neglect

Though it is often difficult to draw clear distinctions between harsh parenting and more uncontrolled, abusive forms of punishment, a somewhat separate literature has explored how far maltreatment in childhood – including sexual abuse and neglect as well as physical abuse – is associated with increased risks of aggression, conduct problems and criminality.

Current evidence suggests that they do play a part, though more modest than once anticipated, and far from specific to antisocial outcomes. In early childhood, maltreatment is associated with a wide spectrum of difficulties, including externalizing and internalizing symptoms and low self-esteem (Cicchetti & Toth, 1995). At these ages it is physical abuse, rather than sexual abuse or neglect, that seems most clearly associated with externalizing problems (see Coie & Dodge, 1998, for a review). In adolescence, community surveys of both physical maltreatment (Fergusson & Lynskey, 1997) and sexual abuse (Fergusson et al., 1996) show links with increased risks of psychopathology; once again, conduct disorder is just one of a number of domains affected. There are of course both methodological and ethical problems in studying the effects of abuse. As a result, much current evidence is derived either from case-control comparisons of referred groups in childhood, or from retrospective reports of maltreatment collected later in life. In terms of risks for offending, Widom's prospective study of substantiated cases of abuse and neglect provides some of the most satisfactory evidence to date (Widom, 1989, 1997). In adolescence, 26% of abused and neglected young people were arrested, by contrast with 17% in a well-matched comparison group; comparable rates in adulthood were 29% and 21% respectively. As these figures suggest, although maltreatment was linked with some increased risk for offending, effects were relatively modest, and the majority of the maltreated sample did not go on to become offenders. Risks for specifically violent crime were also modestly increased, a pattern reported in other studies (Smith & Thornberry, 1995; Zingraff et al., 1993).

Widom (1997) also examined rates of antisocial personality disorder in her sample in adult life. Here, risks were more substantially elevated in maltreated young adult males (20.3% versus 10.1% in the comparison group), although contrasts for females failed to reach statistical significance. In the National Comorbidity Study, retrospective reports of aggression by fathers were also more strongly associated with antisocial personality disorder (OR = 4.4) than with childhood conduct disorder (OR = 2.5) (Kessler et al., 1997b). The prime

risks from physical abuse may apply to more wide-ranging personality problems rather than to conduct disorder or delinquency per se. The mechanisms
underlying these associations continue to be explored. At this stage, it seems
likely that they include both affective and cognitive components, with abusive
treatment compromising the development of secure attachments, affecting
emotion regulation, and contributing to the development of hostile attributional biases. Children reared in homes where they are exposed to threats and
physical abuse appear to develop a heightened arousal to conflict, anger and
distress. In addition, as Pettit and colleagues discuss in chapter 11 (this volume),
they may become hypervigilant to hostility, come to expect hostile intentions
from others, and be more likely to respond accordingly. Finally, some effects
may be mediated through the physiological effects of early stress (see Widom,
1997).

Marital discord and family breakdown

In addition to hostility directed towards the child, conduct disorder also shows
strong links with discord between parents. From the time of the first epidemiological studies in child psychiatry, 'broken homes' have been highlighted
as risks for conduct disorder (Rutter et al., 1970) and an extensive range of
evidence now links parental divorce with increased rates of aggressive behaviour, conduct problems, delinquency and adult crime (see Rodgers & Pryor,
1998, for a review). Typically, risks for externalizing behaviours are approximately doubled for children from divorced families; are most marked in the
immediately post-divorce period; and are stronger for boys than for girls. Once
again, these effects are far from specific: parental divorce is associated with a
wide range of adverse outcomes including emotional distress, poor educational
attainments and effects on physical health (Rodgers & Pryor, 1998).

As outlined earlier, a variety of hypotheses have been explored to identify
which aspects of poor marital relationships are central to these effects. Contrasts between parental death and divorce suggest that parental loss alone is not
the key element; although bereaved children clearly show distress, they are less
likely to show long-term difficulties than children whose parents divorce. In the
National Comorbidity Study, for example, odds ratios for childhood conduct
problems were not elevated for parental death, but were increased three-fold
by divorce (Kessler et al., 1997b). Next, there has been increasing appreciation
that divorce represents a process, rather than a single event. Relationships
between parents are often strained long before the eventual separation takes
place, and may continue to be so long afterwards. Prospective studies have
shown that many children have raised levels of behaviour problems before

divorce, suggesting that the conflict and discord that so frequently precede marital breakdown may be central components of risk (Cherlin et al., 1991).

After divorce, children often face a cascade of other difficulties: distressed parents, with reduced capacities to respond to their children's needs; family financial pressures; house and school moves; and, if parents remarry, relationships with new parent figures and stepsiblings. Each of these factors might plausibly contribute to risk for conduct problems. Current findings suggest that marital discord, together perhaps with the experience of repeated family transitions, are likely to constitute the most important mediators. The key role of parental conflict has emerged in a variety of studies. Outcomes are poorer, for example, for children in intact but conflictual families than for those in affectionate but broken homes, and family conflict predicts risks for antisocial behaviour controlling for separations, but the reverse is not the case (see Rutter et al., 1998). Repeated family transitions may also, however, have independent effects, perhaps through disrupting parenting (Patterson & Capaldi, 1991).

How do marital and family conflicts impact on the child? A variety of possibilities have been explored (Fincham et al., 1994; Rutter, 1994; Moffitt & Caspi, 1998). First, effects may arise through modelling of aggression and hostility observed within the family, or through effects on social information processing. Second, emotional stress on the child may impair capacities to regulate emotional responses and develop appropriate coping strategies. Third, discord may disrupt the quality of parenting. Here, commentators have suggested that marital conflict may affect the consistency and quality of discipline, increase the likelihood of harsh disciplinary methods, or lead to arguments over discipline between parents that directly involve the child. In a rather different way, the affective quality of parent–child relations may also be compromised. Marital quality predicts warmth and sensitivity to children, so marital discord, together with its related emotional stress on parents, may reduce their capacity to respond sensitively to their children's needs. Some effects on parent–child relationships may also emanate from what have been described as 'spillover' effects (Engfer, 1988), whereby deteriorating marital relationships directly affect the ways in which parents interact with their children. Finally, in this domain as in others, individual differences in response are marked. To date, relatively little is known about the factors that render some children especially vulnerable to parental discord. As Moffitt & Caspi (1998) note, however, some of the observed associations may reflect genetic mediation. As outlined earlier, Cadoret et al. (1995) reported gene–environment interactions in their adoption study of conduct problems, with adoptees at genetic risk being most susceptible to environmental adversities – including, in this instance, marital conflict between adoptive parents. Genetic vulnerabilities may render some children especially susceptible to exposure to discord and violence in the family.

Poverty and social disadvantage

Many families of conduct-disordered children face high levels of social as well as interpersonal stressors. Recent evidence suggests that the effects of poverty and social disadvantage are most strongly associated with children's cognitive skills and educational achievements (Duncan & Brooks-Gunn, 1997). Nonetheless, consistent links with behavioural outcomes have been reported. Effects on externalizing problems appear to be more marked for boys than for girls; intermittent hardship is associated with some increased risk for conduct problems, but effects are most marked for children in families facing persistent economic difficulties (Bolger et al., 1995). Farrington & Loeber (1998) reported odds ratios of 2.6 and 3.2 in London and Pittsburgh respectively for effects of low income on boys' delinquency, and in the Ontario Child Health Study, Lipman et al. (1996) calculated attributable risks associated with poverty for a range of child psychiatric disorders. Estimates of this kind depend heavily, of course, on the extent of poverty in the population under study. In the Ontario sample, 17.5% of children were assessed as living in low income families. Attributable risks were highest – at 36% – for conduct disorder among 6–11-year-olds, but were also elevated for emotional disorders (32%), and for general measures of social impairment at these ages. In general, effects were more modest in adolescence.

The processes underlying these links have been examined from two main perspectives: viewing individual family poverty in the context of community disadvantage, and looking within families to identify more proximal risks. As we discuss below, community-level factors do appear to contribute independent effects. Even with these controlled, however, individual family poverty is associated with increased risks of aggression and violent crime. Most current evidence suggests that these effects are indirect. McLoyd (1990), for example, argued that the more proximal influences lie in the quality of parenting. Poverty imposes stress on parents, and reduces the supports available to them. These in turn increase risks of harsh or coercive parenting, and reduce parents' emotional availability to children's needs. Findings broadly consistent with this model have now emerged in both urban and rural samples, and in early childhood and adolescence (Conger et al., 1994; Dodge et al., 1994). They also appear to show consistency over time. Sampson & Laub (1994), for example, reanalysed data from the Glueck's classic study of delinquency, begun in the

1930s depression in the US. They too found that proximal measures of harsh discipline, low supervision and weak parent–child attachments mediated the effects of poverty and structural background factors on delinquency. Across these various studies, between a half and two-thirds of the observed associations between low income, social disadvantage and childhood conduct problems can be 'explained' through family socialization mediators of this kind.

In many societies, minority ethnic groups are disproportionately exposed to severe economic hardship. A number of investigators have now reported, however, that effects seem less marked in minority groups. Guerra et al. (1995), for example, found that although African-American and Hispanic children in US cities were more likely than whites to come from families near the official poverty level, individual family poverty was only associated with aggression among white children. Bolger et al. (1995) documented a similar pattern. Costello et al. (1999) explored effects in the rural south of the US, where a quarter of white children, but almost two-thirds of American Indians, came from families with incomes below federal poverty guidelines. Once again, poverty increased prediction of childhood disorder in the white community, but not significantly for American Indians. As these authors suggest, where social mobility is checked by restricted employment opportunities and extremely low income levels, the social selection processes that link mental health problems with social status in many communities may not apply. Even here, however, relative poverty had some effects, suggesting that perceived status may contribute to risk even within severely disadvantaged groups.

Neighbourhood and community contexts

Many children in poor families also grow up in disadvantaged neighbourhoods, and rates of conduct problems, aggression and other externalizing behaviours vary systematically in different community contexts. In the UK, Rutter et al. (1975a) found that rates of disorder were roughly doubled in an inner city area, and similar effects of urbanization have been documented in Scandinavia (Wichström et al., 1996). In one of the few studies to examine neighbourhood effects in samples at genetic risk, Majumder et al. (1998) found that neighbourhood crime rates and social cohesion contributed to the prediction of disruptive behaviour problems in boys.

From an ecological perspective, the central question raised by these findings is the extent to which community-level predictors, independent of or additional to those deriving from individual and family risks, contribute to risk for disorder. A long tradition of criminological theory has posited that community level factors – in particular poverty, residential instability and the disruption of community social integration – mediate rates of violent crime (see Sampson & Lauritsen, 1994, for a review). Processes of this kind do now seem fairly robustly established in relation to adult crime. One important study, for example, has demonstrated that associations between violent crime, concentrated disadvantage and residential instability are considerably mediated by neighbourhood variations in social cohesion and informal social controls (Sampson et al., 1997).

For child and adolescent outcomes, effects may vary by developmental stage. In their studies of 10-year-olds, for example, Rutter et al. (1975b) argued that area differences in child disorder reflected parallel variations in rates of family and school-based risks: inner city stressors operated primarily via their impact on families and schools. More recent analyses suggest both direct and indirect effects. In relation to maltreatment, for example, rates of child abuse are known to be higher in communities marked by social disorganization and other forms of violence, suggesting that community-level factors influence rates of family-based risks. In addition, independent effects of exposure to community violence are beginning to be identified (Lynch & Cicchetti, 1998). In some cases, these risks seem quite direct and proximal to the child: in chronically disadvantaged neighbourhoods even very young children are reported to witness shootings, stabbings and other forms of street violence (Osofsky, 1995). Importantly, variations in exposure to community violence do not seem strongly associated with family relationships or parenting characteristics, so may reflect somewhat independent, neighbourhood-specific features (Gorman-Smith & Tolan, 1998).

For older children and adolescents, other neighbourhood-level processes may apply. Jencks & Mayer (1990) suggest a variety of possibilities here, including contagion mechanisms, whereby problem behaviours are spread via peer influences; collective socialization, whereby neighbourhood role models and levels of monitoring contribute to informal social controls; competition models, whereby individuals compete for scarce neighbourhood resources; and relative deprivation processes, whereby individuals evaluate their relative standing in the light of neighbourhood comparisons. Hawkins et al. (1998) provide an overview of findings relevant to these models in north American samples. Risks of youth violence were increased in neighbourhoods in which drugs were readily available, where adolescents were exposed to models of adult crime and racial prejudice, and where perceptions of community disorganization were high. Urban–rural differences in rates of conduct problems were also associated with variations in substance use and peer antisocial behaviours in the very different setting of a Norwegian city (Wichström et al., 1996). In small US communities, Simons et al. (1996) found indirect effects of community disadvantage on rates of conduct problems among boys, and effects associated with the proportions of single-parent household in the neighbourhood for girls; both seemed mediated through links with deviant peers. Contagion-related peer influences may thus contribute in important ways to neighbourhood effects in adolescence.

School context

The school constitutes a further important context for children's development. Criminological theories have long argued that academic failure, truancy and low bonding to school play a part in the genesis of delinquency (see Hawkins et al., 1999), and school experiences constitute one obvious source of nonshared environmental effects on behavioural development. To date, however, school influences have received only limited attention in relation to child psychiatric disorders (Maughan, 1994).

Prima facie evidence for links between school experiences and conduct-related difficulties is clear. Individual schools vary in their rates of delinquency, classroom disruptiveness and absenteeism even when variations in intakes are controlled (Mortimore, 1995; Rutter et al., 1979). Mortimore et al. (1988), for example, found that school membership accounted for approaching 10% of the variance in a composite measure of behaviour problems in urban junior schools, controlling for age, sex and social background. Kasen et al. (1990), in a longitudinal study of adolescents, found links between school climate and changes in rates of attention deficits, oppositional behaviours and conduct problems over a 2-year follow-up; and Maughan et al. (1990), in a longitudinal study of schools, reported marked reductions in levels of nonattendance in failing schools where new head teachers had been appointed. Although school differences in behavioural outcomes are generally more modest than those for cognitive attainments, variations between schools do nonetheless appear to be associated with consistent differences in risk for behaviour problems.

Several rather different processes, some direct and some indirect, seem likely to be involved here. The first relate to aspects of school climate and organization. Schools with more positive child outcomes are characterized by purposeful leadership, constructive classroom management techniques, an appropriate academic emphasis, and consistent but not over-severe sanctions (Mortimore, 1998). Some of the factors identified provide interesting echoes of family correlates of conduct problems: Kasen et al. (1990), for example, found that low levels of school conflict (indexed by items such as teachers often shouting at pupils), were associated with a decline in attentional and behavioural problems in adolescence, while Nichol et al. (1985), focusing on severely disruptive children, described escalating spirals of negative teacher–pupil interchanges strongly reminiscent of coercive relationships within families.

Less is known about how these variations in school climate come about. Naturalistic studies of school change (Ouston & Maughan, 1991), as well as the burgeoning literature on 'school improvement' (Mortimore, 1998), suggest that purposive strategies by school staff can do much to influence school ethos and organization. Equally clearly, school climate, like family climate, will reflect an interplay of both child and teacher effects. Child characteristics are known to affect teachers' approaches to behaviour management (Eder, 1982), and staff in some schools with high rates of disruption may retreat from attempts to manage difficult situations if problems rise above certain critical levels (Ouston & Maughan, 1991). Just as disruptive behaviours evoke negative responses from parents, so too they may contribute to the organizational climate in schools.

A second main route for school-related influences seems unequivocally child-based. Schools provide one obvious setting for the development of peer groups, and much of the 'school' influence demonstrated to date may be attributable to peer effects. As early as first grade, the composition of pupil groupings is associated with the development of both shy and aggressive behaviours (Werthamer-Larsson et al., 1991). Even with children randomly assigned to classrooms, Kellam et al. (1998) found that group differences in levels of aggression quickly developed. Importantly, these group characteristics predicted later outcomes: risks of aggression were markedly increased for individually aggressive boys in high aggressive classes, but not for those in low aggressive groups. Rutter et al. (1979) documented similar effects in adolescence: the overall ability balance in the schools they studied constituted an independent predictor of delinquency in boys, over and above risks associated with individual child characteristics. Caspi et al. (1993), examining girls' delinquency, found that affiliations with delinquent peers mediated both the initiation and persistence of behaviour problems. In this case, effects were especially marked in co-educational schools, where peer support for delinquency was presumably more widespread.

Other effects may arise indirectly. Many conduct-disordered children show poor educational attainments, and academic failure in its turn has consistently been found to predict delinquency (Maguin & Loeber, 1996). Once again, peer influences may be implicated here: Dishion et al. (1991), for example, found that academic failure and peer rejection in late childhood were key predictors of early adolescent involvement with delinquent peers. From a somewhat different perspective, social control theorists have argued that a positive attachment to school may function as a protective factor against delinquency and crime (Hirschi, 1969). In line with these predictions, Lynam et al. (1993) showed that the IQ–delinquency relationship was mediated by school achievement for black but not white youth in the early teens, suggesting that commitment to schooling may be especially important when other social bonds are weak.

These still scattered findings suggest that school-related experiences, however mediated, warrant continued attention in models of contextual risks for conduct problems. As in other risk domains, effects are likely to vary for different subgroups of children. Early onset, highly aggressive children, for example, show strong cross-setting consistency in behaviour as they begin school (Ramsey et al., 1990), and their school careers seem likely to be marked discipline problems, academic failure and peer rejection from an early age. Adolescent onset groups, by contrast, may show few difficulties in the early school years, but the school context may play an important contributory role, primarily perhaps via the medium of peer influences, in the development of disruptive behaviour in the teens.

Cumulations and configurations of risk

Taken together, these findings suggest that comprehensive models of contextual influences on conduct problems need to consider each of these varying types and levels of effects. For some children, they will of course covary. Early epidemiological findings (Rutter et al., 1975b) suggested that isolated single risks have relatively little impact on disorder, but that rates rise sharply when risk factors combine. More recently, investigators have begun to examine these effects in more detail, testing how far outcomes in multiply disadvantaged children reflect effects of a general cumulation of adversities, or whether specific configurations of risk show specific impacts. Deater-Deckard et al. (1998), for example, explored both the specific and the cumulative impact of child, sociocultural, parenting and peer-related risks on the development of behaviour problems from ages 5 to 10 years. Each risk domain added uniquely to prediction for both boys and girls; in addition, a cumulative model was also supported, with the total number of risks, regardless of which they were, explaining further variance in outcomes. Cluster analyses identified differing configurations of risks. Each predicted equally strongly to later externalizing behaviours; differing risk pathways, some involving child and parenting factors, others focusing on sociocultural risks and peer influences, were equally likely to contribute to poor subsequent outcomes. Gorman-Smith et al. (1998) also identified different clusters of risks predicting to serious chronic juvenile offending. If replicated, these findings are important in suggesting that conduct problems may flow from diverse developmental risk pathways, differing for different subgroups of children.

Sex differences

Finally, we return to the question of sex differences. As Rutter et al. (1998) note, psychosocial processes might be implicated in boys' and girls' differing risks for conduct problems in three rather different ways: through differential exposure to adverse environmental influences; differential susceptibility to them; or through variations in boys' and girls' typical modes of response to stress and adversity.

Because sex differences in rates of disruptive behaviours emerge most clearly in the late preschool years, that may be an especially fruitful period to begin examining effects. Keenan & Shaw (1997), reviewing evidence from a range of studies, put forward two main hypotheses. First, socialization experiences do appear to differ in some ways between the sexes in early childhood: mothers are more likely to encourage young girls to behave prosocially, and they respond more positively to shy rather than to moody or intense behaviours in girls. Girls may thus be encouraged to show over- rather than undercontrolled behaviour, so that when problems arise, they are channelled into 'internalizing' rather than 'externalizing' modes of expression. Second, girls' more rapid biological, cognitive and socio-emotional development in early childhood may foster adaptive skills that buffer against effects of environmental stressors, and allow for more adaptive modes of response. Though empirical support remains limited, both hypotheses seem worthy of further exploration.

Later in childhood, evidence of differential exposure to adverse family experiences is mixed. In the case of some risks, such as growing up in poverty or experiencing parental divorce, overall levels of exposure will of course be similar for boys and girls. It remains possible, however, that boys may be more likely to be scapegoated, or to become targets of criticism and hostility, when parents are under stress. In population samples, studies of family socialization processes suggest few systematic sex differences (Lytton & Romney, 1991), but these may not, of course, reflect the more extreme modes of treatment associated with conduct problems. Findings on harsh parenting are informative here. A number of investigations, focusing on children and adolescents of different ages, have now reported very similar risks of exposure for boys and girls. Cohen & Brook (1995), for example, found that girls were just as likely as boys to be exposed to power-assertive punishment in their community sample; in addition, links between punishment and risk for conduct problems were almost exactly the same. Findings on supervision are conflicting: some studies report that girls are more likely to be closely supervised than boys, while others find few variations (Rutter et al., 1998). Some protection for girls may nonetheless come via this route. Overall, however, although evidence on within-family variations is still at best limited, there are few indications of systematic differences between boys and girls in exposure to adverse family features. Where variations are more likely is in relation to peer influences. Variations in base rates of behaviour problems mean that male peer groups are inevitably likely to include more deviant models than do girls'; in adolescence in particular, this may prove an important source of differential influence and deviance-amplifying effects (see Giordano & Cernkovich, 1997, for a review).

Turning to vulnerability and response, the clear evidence that males are more vulnerable to physical hazards suggests that there may well be parallels in the psychosocial domain (Rutter, 1970). As we have seen, at least in the short term boys seem more vulnerable to the effects of parental divorce, and effects of poverty also seem stronger in boys. Few other consistent differences have been reported, however; boys and girls seem equally vulnerable to effects of institutional care (Rutter et al., 1990), and, as outlined earlier, physical punishment has shown closely comparable links with later outcomes in males and females in a number of studies. Deater-Deckard et al. (1998), exploring a more extensive array of risk factors, reached similar conclusions. Though base rates of early childhood behaviour problems were higher among boys, predictions from individual, socio-cultural, family and peer-based factors were similar for both sexes, suggesting that at this developmental period at least, vulnerability to contextual risks was very similar for boys and girls. If sex differences in vulnerability do occur, the limited evidence currently available thus suggests that they are restricted to particular domains.

Conclusions

Risk research in childhood conduct problems has a long and illustrious past. Many key contextual risks were identified decades ago, and have since been confirmed with striking regularity in different samples, settings and eras. As this chapter has underscored, however, we are in many ways still at the beginning rather than the end of the journey in understanding their effects. New perspectives have brought new challenges, and cast new light on well-established associations. Questions of process remain little understood, and the complex links between biology and social risks are only now beginning to be explored. Research designs have lagged behind conceptual models of contextual influence; here too, as we have seen, more complex models are beginning to be introduced. The next generation of research, building on these various advances, should bring us closer to appreciating the contextual difficulties that represent the reality of many children's lives.

REFERENCES

Bank, L., Forgatch, M.S., Patterson, G.R. & Fetrow, R.A. (1993). Parenting practices of single mothers: mediators of negative contextual effects. *Journal of Marriage and the Family, 55,* 371–84.

Bardone, A.M., Moffitt, T.E., Caspi, A., Dickson, N. & Silva, P.A. (1996). Adult mental health and social outcomes of adolescent girls with depression and conduct disorder. *Development and Psychopathology, 8,* 811–29.

Baron, R. & Kenny, D. (1986). The moderator–mediator variable distinction in social psychological research: conceptual, strategic, and statistical considerations. *Journal of Personality and Social Psychology, 51,* 1173–82.

Bohman, M. (1996). Predisposition to criminality: Swedish adoption studies in retrospect. CIBA Foundation Symposium 194. *1995 Genetics of Criminal and Antisocial Behaviour,* pp. 99–194.

Bolger, K.E., Patterson, C.J., Thompson, W.W. & Kupersmidt. J.B. (1995). Psychosocial adjustment among children experiencing persistent and intermittent family economic hardship. *Child Development, 66,* 1107–29.

Bornstein, M.H. (Ed.) (1995). *Handbook of Parenting.* Mahwah, NJ: Lawrence Erlbaum.

Boyce, W.T., Frank, E., Jensen, P.S., et al. (1998). Social context in developmental psychopathology: Recommendations for future research from the MacArthur Network on Psychopathology and Development. *Development and Psychopathology, 10,* 143–64.

Bronfenbrenner, U. (1979). *The Ecology of Human Development: Experiments by Nature and Design.* Cambridge, MA: Harvard University Press.

Cadoret, R.J., Yates, W.R., Troughton, E., Woodworth, G. & Stewart, M.A. (1995). Genetic–environmental interaction in the genesis of aggressivity and conduct disorders. *Archives of General Psychiatry, 52,* 916–24.

Campbell, S.B. (1995). Behavior problems in prechool children: a review of recent research. *Journal of Child Psychology and Psychiatry, 36,* 113–49.

Campbell, S.B., Pierce, E.W., Moore, G., Marakovitz, S. & Newby, K. (1996). Boys' externalizing problems at elementary school age: pathways from early behavior problems, maternal control, and family stress. *Development and Psychopathology, 8,* 701–19.

Capaldi, D. & Patterson, G.R. (1994). Interrelated influences of contextual factors on antisocial behavior in childhood and adolescence for males. In D. Fowles, P. Sutker & S. Goodman (Eds.), *Psychopathy and Social Personality: a developmental perspective* (pp. 165–98). New York: Springer.

Caspi A., Lynam D., Moffitt T.E. & Silva P.A. (1993). Unraveling girls' delinquency: biological, dispositional, and contextual contributions to adolescent misbehavior. *Developmental Psychology*, 29, 19–30.

Cherlin, A.J., Furstenberg, F.F., Chase-Lansdale, P.L., et al. (1991). Longitudinal studies of effects of divorce on children in Great Britain and the United States. *Science*, 252, 1386–9.

Cicchetti, D. & Richters, J.E. (1997). Examining the conceptual and scientific underpinnings of research in developmental psychopathology. *Development and Psychopathology*, 9, 189–91.

Cicchetti, D. & Toth, S.L. (1995). A developmental psychopathology perspective on child abuse and neglect. *Journal of the American Academy of Child & Adolescent Psychiatry*, 34, 541–65.

Cohen, P. & Brook, J. (1995). The reciprocal influence of punishment and child behavior disorder. In J. McCord (Ed.), *Coercion and Punishment in Long-term Perspectives* (pp. 154–64). Cambridge: Cambridge University Press.

Cohen, P., Brook, J.S., Cohen, J., Velez, C.N. & Garcia, M. (1990). Common and uncommon pathways to adolescent psychopathology and problem behavior. In L.N. Robins & M. Rutter (Eds.), *Straight and Devious Pathways from Childhood to Adulthood* (pp. 242–58). New York: Cambridge University Press.

Coie, J.D. & Dodge, K.A. (1998). Aggression and antisocial behavior. In N. Eisenberg (Vol. Ed.), *Handbook of Child Psychology. Vol 3: Social, Emotional and Personality Development*, pp. 779–862.

Conger, R.D., Ge, X., Elder, G.H., Lorenz, F.O. & Simons, R.L. (1994). Economic stress, coercive family process, and developmental problems of adolescents. *Child Development*, 65, 541–61.

Costello, E.J. & Angold, A. (1993). Toward a developmental epidemiology of the disruptive behavior disorders. *Development and Psychopathology*, 5, 91–101.

Costello, E.J., Farmer, E.M.Z. & Angold, A. (1999). Same place, different children: White and American Indian children in the Appalachian mountains. In P. Cohen, C. Slomkowski & L.N. Robins (Eds). *Historical and Geographical Aspects of Psychopathology*, pp. 279–98. Mahwah, NJ: Lawrence Erlbaum.

Cummings, E.M., Davies, P.T. & Simpson, K.S. (1994). Marital conflict, gender, and children's appraisals and coping efficacy as mediators of child adjustment. *Journal of Family Psychology*, 8, 141–9.

Deater-Deckard, K. & Dodge, K.A. (1997). Externalizing behavior problems and discipline revisited: nonlinear effects and variation by culture, context and gender. *Psychological Inquiry*, 8, 161–75.

Deater-Deckard, K., Dodge, K.A., Bates, J.E. & Pettit, G.S. (1996). Physical discipline among African American and European American mothers: links to children's externalizing behaviours. *Developmental Psychology*, 32, 1065–72.

Deater-Deckard, K., Dodge, K.A., Bates, J.E. & Pettit, G.S. (1998). Multiple risk factors in the development of externalizing behavior problems: group and individual differences. *Development and Psychopathology*, 10, 469–93.

DiLalla, L.F. & Gottesman, I.I. (1989). Heterogeneity of causes for delinquency and criminality: lifespan perspectives. *Development and Psychopathology, 1,* 339–49.

Dishion T.J., Patterson G.R., Stoolmiller, M. & Skinner M.L. (1991). Family, school, and behavioral antecedents to early adolescent involvement with antisocial peers. *Developmental Psychology, 27,* 172–80.

Dodge, K.A., Pettit, G.S. & Bates, J.E. (1994). Socialization mediators of the relation between socioeconomic status and child conduct problems. *Child Development, 65,* 649–65.

Duncan, G.J. & Brooks-Gunn, J. (Eds.) (1997). *Consequences of Growing Up Poor.* New York: Russell Sage.

Earls, F. (1994). Oppositional-defiant and conduct disorders. In M. Rutter, E. Taylor & L. Hersov (Eds.), *Child and Adolescent Psychiatry: Modern Approaches* (3rd edn, pp. 308–29). Oxford: Blackwell Scientific Publications.

Edelbrock, C., Rende, R., Plomin, R. & Thompson, L.A. (1995). A twin study of competence and problem behavior in childhood and early adolescence. *Journal of Child Psychology and Psychiatry, 39,* 775–85.

Eder, D. (1982). Differences in communicative styles across ability groups. In L.C. Wilkinson (Ed.), *Communicating in the Classroom* (pp. 245–65). New York: Academic Press.

Elder, G.H.J. (1998). The life course and human development. In R.M. Lerner (Ed.), *Handbook of Child Psychology Vol 1: Theoretical Models of Human Development* (pp. 939–91). New York: John Wiley & Sons.

Engfer, A. (1988). The interrelatedness of marriage and the mother–child relationship. In R.A. Hinde & J. Stevenson-Hinde (Eds.), *Relationships within Families* (pp. 104–18). Oxford: Clarendon Press.

Farrington, D.P. (1988). Studying changes within individuals: the causes of offending. In M. Rutter (Ed.), *Studies of Psychosocial Risk: The Power of Longitudinal Data* (pp. 158–83). Cambridge: Cambridge University Press.

Farrington, D.P., Barnes, G. & Lambert, S. (1996). The concentration of offending in families. *Legal and Criminological Psychology, 1,* 47–63.

Farrington, D.P., Gallagher, B., Morley, L., St Ledger, R.J. & West, D.J. (1986). Unemployment, school leaving and crime. *British Journal of Criminology, 26,* 335–56.

Farrington, D.P. & Loeber, R. (1998). Transatlantic replicability of risk factors in the development of delinquency. In P. Cohen, C. Slomkowski & L.N. Robins (Eds.), *Where and When: The Influence of History and Geography on Aspects of Psychopathology,* (pp. 299–329). Mahwah, NJ: Lawrence Erlbaum.

Fergusson, D.M. & Horwood, L.J. (1996). The role of adolescent peer affiliations in the continuity between childhood behavioral adjustment and juvenile offending. *Journal of Abnormal Child Psychology, 24,* 205–21.

Fergusson, D.M., Horwood, L.J. & Lynskey, M.T. (1996). Childhood sexual abuse and psychiatric disorder in young adulthood: II. Psychiatric outcomes of childhood sexual abuse. *Journal of the American Academy of Child and Adolescent Psychiatry, 35,* 1365–74.

Fergusson, D.M. & Lynskey, M.T. (1997). Physical punishment/maltreatment during childhood and adjustment in young adulthood. *Child Abuse and Neglect, 21,* 617–30.

Fincham, F.D., Grych, J.H. & Osborne, L.N. (1994). Does marital conflict cause child maladjust-ment? Directions and challenges for longitudinal research. *Journal of Family Psychology, 8,* 128–40.

Frick, P.J., Lahey, B.B., Loeber, R., Stouthamer-Loeber, M., Christ, M.A.G. & Hanson, K. (1992). Familial risk factors to oppositional defiant disorder and conduct disorder: parental psycho-pathology and maternal parenting. *Journal of Consulting and Clinical Psychology, 60,* 49–55.

Ge, X., Conger, R., Cadoret, R.J. et al. (1996). The developmental interface between nature and nurture: a mutual influence model of child antisocial behavior and parent behaviors. *Develop-mental Psychology, 32,* 574–89.

Gianino, A. & Tronick, E.Z. (1988). The mutual regulation model: The infant's self and interactive regulation and coping and defensive capacities. In T.M. Field, P.M. McCabe & N. Schneiderman (Eds.), *Stress and Coping across Development,* (p. 264). Hillsdale, NJ: Lawrence Erlbaum.

Giordano, P.C. & Cernkovich, S.A. (1997). Gender and antisocial behavior. In D.M. Stoff, J. Breiling & J.D. Maser (Eds.), *Handbook of Antisocial Behavior* (pp. 496–510). New York: John Wiley & Sons.

Gorman-Smith, D. & Tolan, P. (1998). The role of exposure to community violence and developmental problems among inner-city youth. *Development and Psychopathology, 10,* 101–16.

Gorman-Smith, D., Tolan, P., Loeber, R. & Henry, D.B. (1998). Relation of family problems to patterns of delinquent involvement among urban youth. *Journal of Abnormal Child Psychology, 26,* 319–34.

Guerra, N.G., Huesmann, L.R., Tolan, P.H., Acker, R.V. & Eron, L.D. (1995). Stressful events and individual beliefs as correlates of economic disadvantage and aggression among urban children. *Journal of Consulting and Clinical Psychology, 63,* 518–28.

Hawkins, J.D., Herrenkohl, T. Farrington, D.P., et al. (1998). A review of predictors of youth violence. In R. Loeber & D.P. Farrington (Eds.), *Serious and Violent Juvenile Offenders: Risk Factors and Successful Interventions.* Thousand Oaks: Sage.

Hawkins, J.D., Farrington, D.P. & Catalano, R.F. (1999). Reducing violence through the schools. In D.S. Elliott, B.A. Hamburg & K.R. Williams (Eds.), *Youth Violence: New Perspectives for Schools and Communities* (pp. 188–216). Cambridge: Cambridge University Press.

Henry, B., Moffitt, T.E., Robins, L., Earls, F. & Silva, P. (1993). Early family predictors of child and adolescent antisocial behavior: who are the mothers of delinquents? *Criminal Behaviour and Mental Health, 3,* 97–118.

Hirschi, T. (1969). *Causes of Delinquency.* Berkeley: University of California Press.

Jencks, C. & Mayer, S.E. (1990). The social consequences of growing up in a poor neighbour-hood. In L.E. Lynn & M.G.H. McGeary (Eds.), *Inner-City Poverty in the United States.* Washing-ton DC: National Academy Press.

Kasen, S., Johnson, J. & Cohen, P. (1990). The impact of school emotional climate on student psychopathology. *Journal of Abnormal Child Psychology, 18,* 165–77.

Keenan, K. & Shaw, D. (1997). Developmental and social influences on young girls' early problem behavior. *Psychological Bulletin, 121,* 95–113.

Kellam, S.G., Ling, X., Merisca, R., Brown, C.H. & Ialongo, N. (1998). The effect of the level of aggression in the first grade classroom on the course and malleability of aggressive behavior into middle school. *Development and Psychopathology, 10,* 165–85.

Kendler, K.S. (1995). Genetic epidemiology in psychiatry: taking both genes and environment seriously. *Archives of General Psychiatry, 52,* 895–9.

Kessler, R.C., Foster, C.L., Saunders, W.B. & Stang, P.E. (1995). Social consequences of psychiatric disorder: I. Educational attainment. *American Journal of Psychiatry, 52,* 1026–32.

Kessler, R.C., Berglund, P.A., Foster, C.L., et al. (1997a). Social consequences of psychiatric disorders, II: Teenage parenthood. *American Journal of Psychiatry, 154,* 1405–11.

Kessler, R.C., David, C.G. & Kendler, K.S. (1997b). Childhood adversity and adult psychiatric disorder in the US National Comorbidity Survey. *Psychological Medicine, 27,* 1101–19.

Kraemer, H.C., Kazdin, A.E., Offord, D.R., et al. (1997). Coming to terms with the terms of risk. *Archives of General Psychiatry, 54,* 337–43.

Lipman, E.L., Offord, D.R. & Boyle, M.H. (1996). What if we could eliminate child poverty? The theoretical effect on child psychosocial morbidity. *Social Psychiatry Epidemiology, 31,* 303–7.

Loeber, R. & Stouthamer-Loeber, M. (1986). Family factors as correlates and predictors of juvenile conduct problems and delinquency. In N. Morris & M. Tonry (Eds.), *Crime and Justice: An Annual Review of Research,* Vol. 7 (pp. 29–149). Chicago: University of Chicago Press.

Lynam, D., Moffitt, T. & Stouthamer-Loeber, M. (1993). Explaining the relation between IQ and delinquency: class, race, test motivation, school failure or self control? *Journal of Abnormal Psychology, 102,* 187–96.

Lynch, L. & Cicchetti, D. (1998). An ecological–transactional analysis of children and contexts: the longitudinal interplay among child maltreatment, community violence, and children's symptomatology. *Development and Psychopathology, 10,* 235–57.

Lyons, M.J., True, W.R., Eisen, S.A., et al. (1995). Differential heritability of adult and juvenile antisocial traits. *Archives of General Psychiatry, 52,* 906–15.

Lytton, H. (1990). Child and parent effects in boys' conduct disorder: A reinterpretation. *Developmental Psychology, 5,* 101–32.

Lytton, H. & Romney, D.M. (1991). Parents' differential socialization of boys and girls: a meta-analysis. *Psychological Bulletin, 109,* 267–96.

McCord, J. (1979). Some child-rearing antecedents of criminal behavior in adult men. *Journal of Personality and Social Psychology, 37,* 1477–86.

McLoyd, V.C. (1990). The impact of economic hardship on Black families and children: psychological distress, parenting, and socioemotional development. *Child Development, 61,* 311–46.

Maccoby, E.E. & Martin, J.A. (1983). Socialization in the context of the family: parent–child interaction. In P.H. Mussen & M.E. Hetherington (Eds.), *Handbook of Child Psychology: Vol. 4. Socialization, Personality and Social Development* (pp. 1–101). New York: John Wiley & Sons.

Maguin, E. & Loeber, R. (1996). Academic performance and delinquency. *Crime and Justice, 20,* 145–264.

Majumder, P.P., Moss, H.B. & Murrelle, L. (1998). Familial and nonfamilial factors in the prediction of disruptive behaviors in boys at risk for substance abuse. *Journal of Child Psychology and Psychiatry, 39,* 203–13.

Maughan, B. (1994). School influences. In M. Rutter & D.F. Hay (Eds.), *Development Through Life: A Handbook for Clinicians* (pp. 134–58). Oxford: Blackwell Scientific Publications.

Maughan, B.M. & Lindelow, M. (1997). Secular change in psychosocial risks: the case of teenage motherhood. *Psychological Medicine, 27,* 1129–44.

Maughan, B., Ouston, J., Pickles, A. & Rutter, M. (1990). Can schools change? I. Outcomes at six London secondary schools. *School Effectiveness and School Improvement, 1,* 188–210.

Moffitt, T.E. (1993). Adolescence-limited and life-course-persistent antisocial behaviour: a developmental taxonomy. *Psychological Review, 100,* 674–701.

Moffitt, T.E. & Caspi, A. (1998). Annotation: implications of violence between intimate partners for child psychologists and psychiatrists. *Journal of Child Psychology & Psychiatry, 39,* 137–44.

Mortimore, P. (1995). The positive effects of schooling. In M. Rutter (Ed.), *Psychosocial Disturbances in Young People: Challenges for Prevention* (pp. 333–63). Cambridge: Cambridge University Press.

Mortimore, P. (1998). *The Road to School Improvement: Reflections on School Effectiveness.* Lisse: Swets & Zeitlinger.

Mortimore, P., Sammons, P., Stoll, L., Lewis, D. & Ecob, R. (1988). *School Matters.* London: Open Books.

Nichol, A.R., Wilcox, C. & Hibbert, K. (1985). What sort of children are suspended from school and what can we do for them? In A.R. Nichol (Ed.), *Longitudinal Studies on Child Psychology and Psychiatry* (pp. 33–49). Chichester: John Wiley & Sons.

O'Connor, T.G., Deater-Deckard, K., Fulker, D., Rutter, M. & Plomin, R. (1998a). Genotype–environment correlations in late childhood and early adolescence: antisocial behavioral problems and coercive parenting. *Development Psychology, 34,* 970–81.

O'Connor, T.G., Hetherington, E.M. & Reiss, D. (1998b). Family systems and adolescent development: shared and nonshared risk and protective factors in nondivorced and remarried families. *Development and Psychopathology, 10,* 353–75.

Osofsky, J.D. (1995). The effects of exposure to violence on young children. *American Psychologist, 50,* 782–8.

Ouston, J. & Maughan, B. (1991). Can schools change? II: Practice in six London secondary schools. *School Effectiveness and School Improvement, 2,* 3–13.

Parker, J.G. & Asher, S.R. (1987). Peer relations and later personal adjustment: are low-accepted children at risk? *Psychological Bulletin, 102,* 357–89.

Patterson, G.R. (1982). *Coercive Family Interactions.* Eugene, OR: Castalia Press.

Patterson, G.R. (1995). Coercion as a basis for early age of onset for arrest. In J. McCord (Ed.), *Coercion and Punishment in Long-term Perspectives* (pp. 81–105). Cambridge: Cambridge University Press.

Patterson, G.R. & Capaldi, D.M. (1991). Antisocial parents: unskilled and vulnerable. In P.A. Cowan & E.M. Hetherington (Eds.), *Family Transitions* (pp. 195–218). Hillsdale NJ: Lawrence Erlbaum.

Patterson, G.R. & Yoerger, K. (1997). A developmental model for late-onset delinquency. In R. Dienstbier (Series Ed.) & D.W. Osgood (Vol. Ed.), *Nebraska Symposium on Motivation: Vol. 44. Motivation and Delinquency* (pp. 119–77). Lincoln, NE: University of Nebraska Press.

Pike, A. & Plomin, R. (1996). Importance of nonshared environmental factors for childhood and adolescent psychopathology. *Journal of the American Academy of Child and Adolescent Psychiatry, 35, 56–570.*

Pike, A., McGuire, S., Hetherington, E.M., Reiss, D. & Plomin, R. (1996). Family environment and adolescent depressive symptoms and antisocial behavior: a multivariate genetic analysis. *Developmental Psychology, 32, 590–603.*

Plomin, R. & Bergeman, C.S. (1991). The nature of nurture. Genetic influences on 'environmental' measures. *Behavioral and Brain Sciences, 14, 373–86.*

Ramsey, E., Patterson, G.R. & Walker, H.M. (1990). Generalization of the antisocial trait from home to school settings. *Journal of Applied Developmental Psychology, 11, 209–33.*

Reiss, D. Plomin, R., Hetherington, E.M., et al. (1994). The separate worlds of teenage siblings: an introduction to the study of the nonshared environment and adolescent development. In E.M. Hetherington, D. Reiss & R. Plomin (Eds.), *Separate Social Worlds of Siblings: Importance of Nonshared Environment on Development.* Hillsdale, NJ: Lawrence Erlbaum.

Reiss, D., Hetherington, E.M., Plomin, R., et al. (1995). Genetic questions for environmental studies: differential parenting and psychopathology in adolescence. *Archives of General Psychiatry, 52, 925–36.*

Robins, L.N. (1966). *Deviant Children Grown Up: A Sociological and Psychiatric Study of Sociopathic Personality.* Baltimore, MD: Williams & Wilkins.

Robins, L.N. (1978). Sturdy childhood predictors of adult antisocial behavior: Replications from longitudinal studies. *Psychological Medicine, 8, 611–22.*

Rodgers, B. & Pryor, J. (1998). *Divorce and Separation: The Outcomes for Children.* York: Joseph Rowntree Foundation.

Rothbaum, F. & Weisz, J. (1994). Parental caregiving and child externalizing behavior in non-clinical samples: A meta-analysis. *Psychological Bulletin, 116, 55–74.*

Rutter, M. (1970). Sex differences in children's responses to family stress. In E.J. Anthony & C. Koupernik (Eds.), *The Child in his Family* (pp. 165–96). New York: John Wiley & Sons.

Rutter, M. (1994). Family discord and conduct disorder: cause, consequence or correlate? *Journal of Family Psychology, 8, 170–86.*

Rutter, M.L. (1997). Nature-nurture integration: the example of antisocial behavior. *American Psychologist, 52, 390–8.*

Rutter, M., Cox, A., Tupling, C., Berger, M. & Yule, W. (1975a). Attainment and adjustment in two geographical areas: I. The prevalence of psychiatric disorder. *British Journal of Psychiatry, 17, 35–56.*

Rutter, M., Champion, L., Quinton, D., Maughan, B. & Pickles, A. (1995). Understanding individual differences in environmental risk exposure. In P. Moen, G.H.J. Elder & K. Luscher (Eds.), *Examining Lives in Context: Perspectives on the Ecology of Human Development* (pp. 61–93). Washington, DC: American Psychological Association.

Rutter, M., Giller, H. & Hagell, A. (1998). *Antisocial Behavior by Young People.* New York: Cambridge University Press.

Rutter, M.R., Maughan, B., Meyer, J., et al. (1997). Heterogeneity of antisocial behaviour: Causes, continuities and consequences. In R. Dienstbier (Series Ed.) & D.W. Osgood (Vol.

Ed.), *Nebraska Symposium on Motivation: Vol. 44. Motivation and Delinquency* (pp. 45–118). Lincoln, NE: University of Nebraska Press.

Rutter, M., Maughan, B., Mortimore, P. & Ouston, J., with Smith, A. (1979). *Fifteen Thousand Hours: Secondary Schools and their Effects on Children*. London: Open Books.

Rutter, M., Quinton, D. & Hill, J. (1990). Adult outcome of institution-reared children: males and females compared. In L. Robins & M. Rutter (Eds.), *Straight and Devious Pathways from Childhood to Adulthood* (pp. 135–57). New York: Cambridge University Press.

Rutter, M.R., Silberg, J., O'Connor, T. & Simonoff, E. (1999). Genetics and child psychiatry: I Advances in quantitative and molecular genetics. *Journal of Child Psychology and Psychiatry, 40,* 3–18.

Rutter, M. & Smith, D.J. (1995). *Psychosocial Disorder in Young People: Times, Trends and their Causes*. Chichester: John Wiley & Sons.

Rutter, M., Tizard, J. & Whitmore, K. (1970). *Education, Health and Behaviour*. London: Longmans (Reprinted, 1981, Krieger, Melbourne, FL).

Rutter, M., Yule, B., Quinton, D., et al. (1975b). Attainment and adjustment in two geographical areas: III. Some factors accounting for area differences. *British Journal of Psychiatry, 126,* 520–33.

Sameroff, A.J. (1983). Developmental systems: Contexts and evolution. In W. Kessen (Ed.), *History, Theory, and Methods,* (4th edn, Vol. 1, pp. 237–94). New York: John Wiley & Sons.

Sampson, R.J. & Laub, J.H. (1994). Urban poverty and the family context of delinquency: A new look at structure and process in a classic study. *Child Development, 65,* 523–40.

Sampson, R.J. & Lauritsen, J. (1994). Violent victimization and offending: individual-, situational-, and community-level risk factors. In A.J. Reiss & J.A. Rough (Eds.), *Understanding and Preventing Violence: Vol. 3: Social influences* (pp. 1–115). Washington DC: National Academy Press.

Sampson, R.J., Raudenbush, S.W. & Earls, F. (1997). Neighborhoods and violent crime: A multilevel study of collective efficacy. *Science, 277,* 918–24.

Scarr, S. & McCartney, K. (1983). How people make their own environments: A theory of genotype → environment effects. *Child Development, 54,* 424–35.

Silberg, J., Meyer, J., Pickles, A., et al. (1996). Heterogeneity among juvenile antisocial behaviours: Findings from the Virginia Twin Study of Adolescent Behavioural Development. In G.R. Bock & J.A. Goode (Eds.), *Genetics of Criminal and Antisocial Behaviour: CIBA Foundation Symposium, 194* (pp. 76–92). Chichester: John Wiley & Sons.

Simons, R.L., Johnson, C., Beaman, J., Conger, R.D., et al. (1996). Parents and peer group as mediators of the effects of community structure on adolescent problem behavior. *American Journal of Community Psychology, 24,* 145–71.

Smith, C. & Thornberry, T.P. (1995). The relationship between childhood maltreatment and involvement in delinquency. *Criminology, 33,* 451–81.

Taylor, S.E., Repetti, R.L. & Seeman, T. (1997). What is an unhealthy environment and how does it get under the skin? *Annual Review of Psychology 1997, 48,* 411–47.

Werthamer-Larsson, L., Kellam, S.G. & Wheeler, L. (1991). Effect of classroom environment on shy behavior, aggressive behavior and concentration problems. *American Journal of Community Psychology, 19,* 585–602.

Wichström, L., Skogen, K. & Oia, T. (1996). Increased rate of conduct problems in urban areas: What is the mechanism? *Journal of the American Academy of Child & Adolescent Psychiatry, 35*, 471–9.

Widom, C.S. (1989). Child abuse, neglect and adult behavior: research design and findings on criminality, violence, and child abuse. *American Journal of Orthopsychiatry, 59*, 355–67.

Widom, C.S. (1997). Child abuse, neglect, and witnessing violence. In D. Stoff, J. Breiling & J.D. Maser (Eds.), *Handbook of Antisocial Behavior* (pp. 159–70). New York: John Wiley & Sons.

Willett, J.B., Singer, J.D. & Martin, N.C. (1998). The design and analysis of longitudinal studies of development and psychopathology in context: Statistical models and methodological recommendations. *Development and Psychopathology, 10*, 395–426.

Zingraff, M.T., Leiter, J., Myers, K.A. & Johnson, M. (1993). Child maltreatment and youthful problem behavior. *Criminology, 31*, 173–202.

8

Genetic influences on conduct disorder

Emily Simonoff

Introduction

In the last decade, there has been an increasing appreciation of the role of genetic influences on many child behavioural traits and disorders (Rutter et al., 1999a,b). Although there has been a growing acceptance of the importance of genetic factors for many behaviours and psychiatric problems, there has been a tendency to view conduct disorder as the exception. The reasons for this point of view are varied. They include the fact that rates of conduct disorder and juvenile delinquency vary considerably from one population to another (Rutter et al., 1998) and that much of this variation can be explained by environmental adversity (Rutter et al., 1975). Rates of both juvenile and adult crime have also changed enormously over time (Rutter et al., 1998), a phenomenon that cannot be explained by genetic effects (because the genetic makeup of a population takes many generations to change). Family-based influences have included a number of risk factors for which a direct effect on disruptive behaviour has seemed likely such as inconsistent discipline and poor supervision (Rutter, 1978). For all these reasons, it has only been in very recent years that the possibility of significant genetic influences has been entertained seriously.

Risk factors for conduct disorder include behavioural problems such as hyperactivity (Stewart et al., 1979; Taylor et al., 1986a, b), a variety of family factors (Frick et al., 1992; Hamdan-Allen et al., 1989) and cognitive deficits that include misinterpretation of social interactions (Dodge et al., 1994) and discrepancies in verbal and performance intellectual abilities (Moffitt, 1993), as well as reading problems (Maughan & Hagell, 1996). In addition to hyperactivity, conduct disorder is comorbid with most other common child psychiatric disorders (Simonoff et al., 1997) and the reasons for this comorbidity are uncertain (Caron & Rutter, 1991). It seems likely that different risk factors, or combinations of risk factors, will operate in different individuals, and that conduct disorders will be etiologically heterogeneous. This heterogeneity is also likely to apply to genetic risk factors, and is likely to be a cause of variability in the findings from both behavioural and molecular genetic studies.

Although this chapter emphasizes genetic influences, in part because many of the other chapters deal with the effects of specific environmental risk factors, this emphasis should not lead the reader to assume that those exploring genetic risk factors are uninterested in the effects of the environment. Genetic designs, both behavioural and molecular, are one of the most powerful means of disentangling the mechanisms by which observed risk factors exert their effects. Genetically informative studies can specify the nature of gene–environment interplay, in particular, gene–environment correlations and interactions, through examining the impact of environmental risk in different genotypes.

Clinical heterogeneity does not necessarily reflect genetic heterogeneity. On the one hand, it is quite possible for clinically indistinguishable conditions to have different genetic abnormalities; this has been demonstrated for tuberose sclerosis, retinitis pigmentosa and red blood cell elliptocytosis, as well as many other disorders in which multiple genetic mutations have been identified. On the other hand, it is also possible for individuals with the same susceptibility genes to show very different features. Disorders such as Noonan syndrome, Marfan syndrome and neurofibromatosis are all single gene disorders with widely varying characteristics. There is an enormous range of phenotypic abnormalities between identical twins with autism, in which some are affected with classical autism and others only with relatively mild social and cognitive impairments, and where the IQ difference between co-twins may be as great as 60 points (Le Couteur et al., 1996). The implication for conduct disorder is that current clinical subtypes, such as early- versus late-onset, socialized versus unsocialized, aggressive versus nonaggressive, may not index genetic risk factors.

Animal models of genetic influences on aggression highlight in a different way that our clinical classification schemes may not be meaningful with respect to the genetic architecture of conduct disorder symptoms. For example, Popova & Kalikov (1986) have shown that the components of aggression in mice may be separately inherited. Using methods of selective in-breeding, they demonstrated that the inheritance of the probability of a male mouse ever attacking another male was distinct from that for either the number of attacks or the accumulated attack time. This highlights that aggression has separate components which may only be distinguishable with experimental designs that allow manipulation of influences on these components. In humans, there have been no designs that allow decomposition of individual behaviours into genetically meaningful entities. There is even very little evidence clarifying the extent to which traits such as impulsivity, sensation-seeking, and hostility index the genetic risk in conduct disorder. Further developments in behaviour genetic research need to include studies aimed at identifying which of the risk factors for conduct disorder are highly heritable, and the extent to which genetic influences are shared or distinct for different risk factors. This will provide a first step in identifying genetic heterogeneity.

A further question is the extent to which risk factors, both genetic and environmental, act across the dimension of aggressive, antisocial behaviour or alternatively only influence the extremes of behaviour. There is considerable evidence to suggest much of conduct disorder can be considered dimensionally (Robins, 1991) and this would be compatible with multiple susceptibility genes whose presence increases the probability of conduct disorder behaviour. On the other hand, this does not exclude the possibility of extremes that are influenced by different genetic (and environmental) risk factors. Height provides such an example; height within the normal range appears to be influenced by a number of genetic and environmental factors acting dimensionally. However extremes of stature are often influenced by distinct pathological (and often genetic) disorders such as achondroplasia causing short stature and Marfan syndrome being associated with extreme height. The findings with respect to the monoamine oxidase gene (see below) suggest that certain forms of aggressive behaviour may be influenced by single gene mutations. In this chapter, the term 'conduct disorder' refers to the diagnostic categories of conduct disorder and oppositional defiant disorder. Conduct disorder symptoms, aggression and antisocial behaviour will refer to the dimension of such behaviour.

The chapter starts with a brief review of the key methodologies and their strengths and weaknesses; the description is only brief as this has been dealt with in detail elsewhere (Rutter et al., 1990a, 1999a; Simonoff et al., 1994). It then discusses the current knowledge and, finally, highlights the key research questions for the future.

Genetic strategies

Behaviour genetic designs

Most psychiatric disorders are considered genetically complex and conduct disorder is no exception. The term 'complex disorders' is used to refer to ones in which there is evidence that family members of an affected individual (or proband) are at increased risk for having the disorder, but where the mode of inheritance does not follow the Mendelian rules that are found in disorders due to a single abnormal gene. Disorders may be complex because multiple genes are involved, each conferring a degree of risk or susceptibility, but each in itself being insufficient to produce the disorder. Such disorders are referred to as oligogenic when it is thought that only a few genes are involved, or polygenic when many genes are implicated. Alternatively, inheritance may be complex because both susceptibility genes and environmental risk factors are required for disease expression; such disorders are referred to as multifactorial. It is generally assumed that many psychiatric disorders may have multifactorial inheritance. Behaviour genetic studies can estimate the extent to which the phenotypic variation is due to genetic and environmental factors, by decomposing the total phenotypic variance into that due to genetic influences, termed the 'heritability' and that due to environmental effects. Environmental variation can be further decomposed into family-wide versus individual-specific effects (Plomin, 1995).

Twin studies

The most common behaviour genetic design currently in use is the twin design. Although there are a number of variants (see Rutter et al., 1990a and Simonoff et al., 1994 for a fuller discussion), the most widely used method is the comparison of monozygotic (MZ) and dizygotic (DZ) twin pairs. The design is based on the principles firstly, that MZ twin pairs share all their genes while DZ pairs share on average only half their genes and, secondly, that both types of twins share their environment to the same extent. The latter 'equal environments' assumption has been questioned in a number of studies (for example Hopper & Culross, 1983; Kaprio et al., 1990) and greater similarity of intra-pair environment has been found for MZ compared to DZ twins. However, it has been argued that the increased environmental similarity represents increased genetic similarity (a form of gene–environment correlation, see below – Kendler et al., 1993b). While this may be true, it will be important to consider whether the greater environmental similarity for MZ twins then leads to increased phenotypic similarity (Rutter et al., 1999a).

The comparison of MZ and DZ twins allows three components of variance to be estimated and usually these are additive genetic, shared or common environmental and nonshared or unique environmental effects. Shared environmental effects are family-wide effects that make both MZ and DZ twin pairs more similar to each other; nonshared effects are individual-specific and make both twin types different from each other. It is usually the case that the genetic and environmental variance components are comprised of latent, or unobserved, measures. Thus, just as the actual genes involved are not specified, nor are the individual environmental influences that affect the trait. Individual measured environmental risk factors can be included, but typically to date they have accounted for only a small proportion of the total environmental effect (Kendler et al., 1991; Meyer et al., in press). A frequent misconception is that shared environment is a measure of the importance of family-wide factors, such as marital discord or home environment. However, shared environment is rather a measure of family-wide factors that affect both twins in a similar manner. Similarly nonshared environmental influences are not necessarily ones that occur outside the family; they may include ones within the family which affect siblings differently.

Most twin models assume that genes and environment act in an additive, or independent, fashion. However, there are many examples of gene–environment correlations and gene–environment interactions. Both concepts are discussed in detail elsewhere (Rutter et al., 1999a; Simonoff et al., 1994). Gene–environment (GE) correlation refers to covariation between genetic predisposition and environmental exposure. In children raised by biological parents, passive GE correlation occurs because parents provide both genes and environment. In relation to conduct disorder, this might be expressed by antisocial parents (who may then pass on genetic susceptibility for antisocial behaviour) also providing suboptimal parenting and exposure to aggression and criminality. As children develop, both evocative (eliciting a response from others based on behaviour which is genetically influenced) and active (selecting environments through one's behaviour) GE correlation may become more important. In relation to evocative GE correlation, children with genetic susceptibility to conduct disorder, possibly indexed by a challenging, defiant style, may elicit more coercive and inconsistent responses from their parents and others (Patterson & Fleischman, 1979). For active GE correlation, genetic susceptibility mediated through traits such as sensation-seeking behaviour, could influence children to search out peers and situations likely to lead to antisocial behaviour. GE interaction occurs when individuals of differing genetic predisposition vary in the effect resulting from exposure to a particular environment. For example, children with a genetic susceptibility to conduct disorder (possibly indexed for example by impulsivity or challenging behaviour) may only be at greater risk of developing conduct disorder than those without genetic susceptibility where there is suboptimal parenting. Both GE correlation and interaction are difficult to measure in behaviour genetic designs, especially twin studies, and there is currently very little knowledge of their importance. The degree and nature of these effects will be more easily measured once susceptibility genes have been identified. Where they are not measured, GE correlation and interaction will be included in the additive genetic component (leading to a possible overestimate of heritability, although other inaccuracies in measurement may have the effect of under-estimating heritability).

Assortative, or nonrandom, mating of parents is an important consideration in behaviour genetic studies of conduct disorder or antisocial behaviour. Assortative mating for antisocial behaviour is well recognized (Rutter et al., 1998). Assortative mating can have important effects on heritability estimates, when not accounted for. In twin studies, the effect is to inflate the DZ correlation (because parents will share some of their genes and therefore DZ genetic similarity will be greater then 0.5) and to underestimate heritability while overestimating shared environment. In adoption designs (see below), genetic effects will be overestimated because the component of biological parent–adopted offspring similarity that is due to parental assortment (and therefore similarity with the other biological parent) will not be taken into account.

The statistical method of structural equation modelling revolutionized the use and interpretation of twin data (Heath et al., 1989). Prior to its implementation, heritabilities were estimated from twin correlations or concordances. Structural equation modelling allowed two advances: first, it allowed more complex models to be explored and, second, it provided a means of testing how well any given model explained the data. The power of these two features had marked effects on the use and misuse of structural equation modelling. One potential misuse has been the selection of the most parsimonious model fitting the data, without due consideration of the implications. Studies of individual rather than group variation require much larger sample sizes to obtain precise estimates and even large sample sizes may produce broad confidence intervals, as witnessed in the study of retrospectively recalled conduct disorder by Slutske et al. (1997). Thus, the usual practice of publishing parameter estimates, i.e. estimates of genetic and environmental influence, for the most parsimonious model has often led to rejection of a role for shared environment, when the 95% confidence intervals often may include estimates well above 0, because it is the parameter that twin studies have least power to detect.

The use of structural equation modelling has also led to certain types of more complex models being asserted without reference to alternative pathways of effect. One area has involved exploring shared genetic and environmental risk as an explanation for association among correlated phenotypes. When the data involve closely linked concepts, such as items contributing to a scale of conduct disorder symptoms, it may be reasonable to assume the covariance between variables is due to shared genetic and environmental risk factors. However, when dealing with less closely integrated phenotypes, such as conduct disorder and hyperactivity, the possibility of other mechanisms such as one phenotype causing the other (e.g. hyperactivity causing conduct disorder) requires consideration (Simonoff, 2000).

Despite these drawbacks, twin studies provide an excellent tool for estimating the relative importance of genetic and environmental effects and for exploring more complex models of effect. Extended twin designs, including twins reared apart, twin-family designs and the offspring of twins can further delineate causes of variation, including intergenerational transmission (Eaves, 1982; Kendler, 1993).

Twins are relatively common (about 1 in 40 individuals is a twin), making it possible to ascertain the large samples required for powerful analyses. For many of the traits in which psychiatry is interested, twins appear to be broadly representative of the general population (Rutter & Redshaw, 1991), making it possible to generalize from findings. There have been some suggestions that conduct disorder could be more common in twins (Simonoff, 1992), and that the phenomenon of a co-twin providing a 'partner in crime' might lead to twin-specific interactions (Carey, 1992), but current general population data have not suggested an increased rate in twins (Gjone & Novik, 1995; Van Den Oord et al., 1995) and systematic exploration of twin interaction effects has not revealed any for conduct disorder (Eaves et al., 1997).

Adoption studies

There are several adoption paradigms in use; most involve the comparison between adopted relatives who share environmental influences but no genes and biological relatives who may share environmental influences (such as biological siblings) or may not (for example, the biological parents of adopted-away offspring). Differences in similarity allow estimation of the strength of genetic and environmental effects. Adoption designs are also potentially more powerful than twin studies in demonstrating gene–environment correlations and interactions, because of the separate origins of genetic and environmental influences. However, an important limiting step in adoption designs using biological parents is the lack of detailed information on parents. Scandinavian adoption studies have made use of register data, including those from psychiatric care and criminal records. In some of the US studies, assessments of biological parents at the time of placement for adoption have been made, including psychiatric and intellectual evaluations. However, the quality of information is usually very limited, and information on biological fathers may be particularly lacking.

Adoption designs using biological parents are probably least helpful in examining genetic and environmental influences on children's behaviour, because information about parental behaviour during childhood is particularly likely to be lacking. Designs comparing biological and adoptive sibs overcome this. Because adoption designs involve comparisons between groups of individuals less strongly related than in twin studies, the power of such designs to detect genetic effects is lower.

A major concern about modern adoption studies must be the generalizability to the population at large. In Western countries where the birth of a child out of wedlock is no longer a taboo, the group of parents who give up their children for adoption differ systematically with respect to demographic and psychiatric factors (Rutter et al., 1999a). There is also little information on the impact of the pre-adoption environment including the intra-uterine environment of the child, for example in relation to prenatal alcohol exposure (Cadoret, 1986). Other methodological problems may include selective placement and time in institutional care.

Family studies

Conventional family studies fall into two groups: those comparing familial aggregation for a disorder or trait in the relatives of probands versus controls, and those making use of family members who are differentially related. In the former case, a key design issue is the selection of the control group, where the concern is often to take into account 'nonspecific' risk factors that might distort the conclusions. Particularly with patient populations, biases influencing whether individuals come to clinical attention may relate to extent and type of family aggregation (Leckman et al., 1987). Like adoption studies, family studies may suffer from the difficulty of obtaining accurate data on the child psychiatric phenotypes of adult family members. Unless family studies include individuals of different degrees of relatedness, familiarity cannot be decomposed to genetic and environmental effects. Even when different relatives are used, degree of relatedness will covary with sharing of the environment, making extrapolation difficult.

More recently, family studies have looked at youngsters of different degrees of relatedness living in the same home. The Nonshared Environment in Adolescent Development (NEAD) project has used biological families with adolescent twins and siblings and reconstituted stepfamilies with full, half and unrelated siblings (McGuire et al., 1994; O'Connor et al., 1995). The innovative design has primarily focused on similarity among children and thereby by-passed the difficulties of parental data. However, it is unknown whether aspects of relationships in stepfamilies affect their behaviour (or ratings of behaviour) in ways that are different from biological families. There is some suggestion from the NEAD data that such effects may occur, as evidenced by differences in the full sibling correlations for biological and stepfamilies and the variance differences among different pairs of siblings (Pike et al., 1996). Furthermore, the assumption that relevant aspects of the environment are equally shared across all types of sib pairs may be incorrect.

Molecular genetic strategies

The astonishing rapidity of advances in molecular genetics are now being applied to child psychiatry. Early molecular genetic studies of adult psychiatric disorders used strategies designed to detect single genes whose individual effects accounted for a very substantial proportion of the phenotypic variance. Not surprisingly, the successes from this approach were very limited and occurred primarily in those disorders in which patterns of familial segregation suggested a single major gene. However, the combination of awareness that such strategies were inappropriate for neuropsychiatric disorders of complex inheritance and of laboratory and statistical advances have led to the use of methods that are likely to be more appropriate for psychiatric disorders such as conduct disorder. Because the findings to date have limited implications for conduct disorder, the current discussion will be brief, and the reader is directed to other sources (Rutter et al., 1999a).

Two main strategies are used: linkage and association; in both cases it is possible to take either a candidate gene or genome screen approach. In the candidate gene approach, a specific gene of known location is postulated to be involved. This usually occurs when there is already an understanding of the pathophysiology of the disorder, such as in diabetes. When there are no strong hypotheses about which genes might be involved in a disorder, scientists may elect to undertake a genome scan, in which biological markers are examined at regular intervals across all the chromosomes. Such a strategy can run foul of both false positives and false negatives. False positives occur because a relatively low significance level is used to indicate areas of interest and there is multiple testing; this can be resolved with the use of a finer genetic map of markers and replication in other samples. False negatives may occur for several reasons. The markers used in scanning may be too far from the disease gene, the susceptibility gene may account for too small a proportion of variance, and the disorder may be too heterogeneous. All of these can be reduced, at least in theory, but extremely large sample sizes may be required to do so (Risch & Merikangas, 1996).

Linkage studies are aimed at detecting a relationship between allelic variation (differences within individual genes) and disease status within families. The design requires families with multiple affected members in at least two generations, because the strategy examines transmission of genes. Early psychiatric genetic studies used few pedigrees that were heavily loaded with affected individuals over several generations, a strategy that had proved highly successful for Mendelian disorders of dominant inheritance, such as Huntington's disease (The Huntington's Disease Collaborative Research Group, 1993), and early-onset Alzheimer's disease (St George-Hyslop et al., 1989), but gave unreplicable findings for schizophrenia, bipolar disorder and Tourette syndrome. Concerns were also expressed about the appropriateness of the design for complex psychiatric disorders where usually only 2–3 people are affected in multiplex families (Watt & Edwards, 1991), and where the phenotypic classification (diagnosis) of key individuals can have major effects on the significance of the linkage (measured by the lod – logarithm of the odds ratio – score) (Baron et al., 1990). More recently, psychiatric geneticists have made use of affected-sib or affected-relative pair designs, in which families with pairs of relatives who are both affected are studied. The advantages are that these families show more typical patterns of familial segregation and there is no need to classify those in whom diagnosis is uncertain. However, large numbers of families are required for many disorders; current power calculations estimate that over 200 relative pairs may be required (Risch & Merikangas, 1996).

In association studies, affected individuals are compared with controls with the goal of detecting particular genotypes that are associated with the disorder. Association strategies are aimed at detecting susceptibility genes that are neither necessary nor sufficient for the disorder and, as such, the design is suited to complex disorders. Association studies require the biological test marker to be very close to the susceptibility gene. Therefore, until recently, only candidate gene association strategies were practical. Genome-wide association studies have recently been considered although their utility remains to be seen. A major drawback to association studies has been the need for appropriate control groups. The method depends on linkage disequilibrium between the susceptibility gene and the marker, which occurs when the two are in close proximity and therefore are unlikely to recombine during cell division. However, if the case and control groups come from genetically different populations, false positive results can occur because of population stratification. The methods of haplotype relative risk (HRR – Falk & Rubinstein, 1987) and the transmission disequilibrium test (TDT – Spielman & Ewens, 1996) have aided greatly in this problem by using parents, who have the same genetic origin as their offspring, as controls for gene frequency. Although this may be difficult for adult psychiatric disorders (because parents may be dead or unavailable), this is relatively easy for childhood disorders and provides a good control for possible stratification.

Cytogenetics

The detection of chromosomal anomalies has been used primarily to identify syndromes, such as Down syndrome and Turner syndrome, but also to localize single genes causing well-defined disorders. Generally, the former occurs in the case of gross chromosomal abnormalities, where the phenotypic effects are widespread and often involve moderate to severe mental retardation. Other behavioural phenomena may include aggression, but it is likely that this aggression is secondary to the broader abnormalities, and the genetic defect is unlikely to provide useful information about conduct disorder more broadly. On the other hand, small chromosomal deletions and duplications have provided useful clues as to the location of individual genes causing disorder, although its utility is likely to be greatest in disorders of Mendelian inheritance. Submicroscopic deletions detected with molecular genetic techniques, termed microdeletions, have been associated with mental retardation (although their causative role has not been resolved) and could prove to be associated with other behavioural problems in the future (Flint et al., 1995).

Genetic and environmental influences

Twin studies

The generally accepted wisdom from twin studies has been that childhood traits associated with conduct disorder such as delinquency are strongly influenced by shared environmental components, differentiating them from adult antisocial behaviour, which is much more highly genetic (DiLalla & Gottesman, 1991; Rutter et al., 1990b). The key recent twin studies are summarized in Table 8.1. Increasing evidence in the 1990s has emerged to suggest that the picture is more complex. Some studies continue to support this earlier view. Lyons et al. (1995) studied a large cohort of male twin pairs ascertained through the Vietnam Era Twin Register, where enrolment depended upon both twins having been inducted into the US Armed Forces. DSM–III–R conduct disorder (retrospectively) and adult antisocial personality disorder were determined by telephone interviews based on the Diagnostic Interview Schedule (DIS). Structural equation modelling revealed that shared environment (31% of the variance) was more important than genetic influences (7%) for conduct disorder. This contrasted with antisocial personality, for which shared environmental influences accounted for only 5% of the variance while genetic influences accounted for 43%. The influences responsible for continuity over time were roughly equally divided among genetic, shared environmental and nonshared environmental effects. A similar trend over the life span was reported by Simonoff et al. (submitted) from the Maudsley Follow-Up Twin Register, based on a clinic sample of systematically ascertained twins referred to child psychiatric services for conduct and/or emotional problems. In this sample, proband concordances for conduct disorder in MZ and DZ same-sex pairs were identical (64%), highlighting the importance of shared environment. However, there were larger differences in the concordances for both antisocial personality (67% versus 60%) and pervasive personality dysfunction (50% versus 21%). The latter category required poor functioning in most areas of psychosocial functioning, including intimate relationships, work, friendships, other relationships and general coping, and has been strongly associated with childhood conduct disorder (Zoccolillo et al., 1992).

Other recent twin studies of childhood antisocial behaviour suggest that the picture is less consistent than these two studies might suggest. Findings from two recent large-scale general population twin studies have found little support for an important role for shared environment. The Virginia Twin Study of Adolescent Behavioral Development (VTSABD), based on over 1400 8–16-year-old twin pairs systematically ascertained through the school system, reported heritability estimates for a variety of measures of antisocial behaviour (Eaves et al., 1997). These included mother, father and child reports of oppositional and conduct disorder clinical symptoms on the Child and Adolescent Psychiatric Assessment (CAPA) psychiatric interview; and a variety of antisocial acts recorded on a modified version of the questionnaire developed by Olweus (1989). There were also mother, father and teacher reports based on the Rutter A and B scales (Rutter et al., 1970). The findings highlight several features. First, there was considerable variability in the heritability estimates across informants; in particular, children's self-reports showed smaller genetic effects and larger nonshared environmental effects than did reports from their parents. The reason for this is unclear, but it cannot be explained by lower reliability in children's reports because the longitudinal stability (18 month re-assessment) was roughly the same for child and parent reports. Second, for interview measures of oppositional and conduct disorder, there was relatively little evidence for a role for shared environment, with only 2 of the 12 ratings reporting a shared environmental component. However, the picture was different for questionnaire measures and particularly for the Olweus questionnaire; in the latter case, 10 of the 12 ratings showed a shared environmental

Table 8.1. Twin studies of childhood antisocial behaviour

Study	Sample	N	Measure	Informant	Correlations			Variance estimates		
					MZ	DZ-SS	DZ-OS	h^2	c^2	e^2
Eaves et al. (1997)	General population sample 8–16 years	1400 pairs	CAPA conduct	Mother	0.66	0.38	0.32	0.69	—	0.31
					0.59	0.27	—	0.69	—	0.31
				Father	0.62	0.49	0.44	0.27	0.37	0.36
					0.64	0.26	—	0.58	0.09	0.33
			Rutter – conduct	Mother	0.73	0.35	0.44	0.74	—	0.26
					0.70	0.49	—	0.72	—	0.28
				Father	0.64	0.40	0.39	0.55	0.11	0.24
					0.60	0.32	—	0.25	0.37	0.28
				Teacher	0.52	0.25	0.31	0.53	—	0.47
					0.53	0.13	—	0.54	—	0.46
			Olweus – conduct	Mother	0.77	0.42	0.46	0.61	0.14	0.25
					0.75	0.59	—	0.31	0.44	0.25
				Father	0.73	0.54	0.46	0.36	0.38	0.26
					0.76	0.56	—	0.64	0.14	0.23
				Child	0.46	0.35	0.27	0.24	0.24	0.52
					0.48	0.43	—	0.05	0.42	0.53
			CAPA oppositional	Mother	0.46	0.40	0.22	0.53	—	0.47
					0.50	0.21	—	0.51	—	0.49
				Father	0.66	0.21	0.39	0.69	—	0.36
					0.50	0.14	—	0.49	—	0.51
				Child	0.20	0.13	0.08	0.21	—	0.79
					0.26	0.00	—	0.23	—	0.77
			Olweus – oppositional	Mother	0.72	0.56	0.56	0.35	0.38	0.27
					0.72	0.53	—	0.36	0.37	0.28
				Father	0.79	0.64	0.63	0.39	0.42	0.19
					0.77	0.68	—	0.14	0.63	0.24
				Child	0.42	0.20	0.15	0.45	—	0.55
					0.41	0.34	—	0.41	—	0.59
Slutske et al. (1997)	General population volunteers; sample adult twins	2882 pairs	SSAGA via telephone interview, retrospective reports	DSM–III–R diagnosis	0.70	0.37	0.34	0.71	—	0.29
								(0.32–0.79)	(0.32)	(0.21–0.41)
					0.68	0.48	—	0.71	—	0.29
								(0.32–0.79)	(0–0.32)	(0.21–0.41)

Study	Population	N	Measure	Informant						
(continued)				DSM-III-R symptoms	0.59	0.29	0.31	0.53 (0.32–0.59)	– (0.0–0.15)	0.47 (0.41–0.56)
Gjone & Stevenson (1997)	General population 5–9, 12–15 years	905 pairs same sex	CBC-L externalizing	Mother 5–9	0.63	0.41	–	0.53 (0.32–0.59)	0.12 (0.05–0.29)	0.35 (0.31–0.41)
				12–15	0.94	0.67	–	0.46	0.47	0.07
Thapar & McGuffin (1996)	General population 8–16 years	197 pairs same sex	Rutter questionnaires	Mother	0.88	0.68	–	0.38	0.50	0.12
					0.89	0.63	–	0.57	0.33	0.10
					0.87	0.57	–	0.65	0.23	0.12
McGuffin & Thapar (1997)	General population 12–16 years	81 same sex pairs	Olweus questionnaire	Self-report	0.62	0.60	–	0.28	0.40	0.32
					0.62	0.60	–	0.81	–	–
Lyons et al. (1995)	General population, Armed Forces Register, adult	3226 male–male pairs	DIS telephone interview	Self-report retrospective	0.81	0.29	–	0.07	0.31	0.19
				current (ASP symptoms)	0.39	0.33	–	0.43	0.05	0.62
Edelbrock et al. (1995)	General population volunteer sample 7–15 years	181 same sex pairs	CBC-L externalizing	Mother	0.47	0.27	–	0.51 (±0.22)	0.28 (±0.20)	0.52
			delinquency		0.79	0.53	–	0.35 (±0.22)	0.37 (±0.18)	0.21
			aggression		0.72	0.55	–	0.60 (±0.22)	0.15 (±0.20)	–
Stevenson & Graham (1988)	General population volunteer sample 13 years	285 pairs	Rutter A scale	Mother	0.75	0.45	–	–	–	0.28
					0.61	0.40	0.42	–	–	–
					0.29	0.49	–	–	0.28	0.25
Rowe (1983)	General population volunteer sample 13–17 years	265 pairs	Antisocial scale	Self-report	0.62	0.52	–	0.39	–	–
					0.66	0.46	–	–	0.30	–
Zahn-Waxler et al. (1996)	General population volunteer sample 5 years	~300 same sex pairs	CBC-L externalizing	Mother	0.87	0.59	–	0.57	0.35	0.33
				Father	0.85	0.60	–	0.48	–	–
Schmitz et al. (1994)	General population + B7 2–4 years	232 pairs	Pre-school behaviour questionnaire	Teacher	0.76	0.28	–	0.70	–	–
			CBC-L externalizing	Mother	0.55	0.46	0.45	0.03	0.49	0.48
					0.71	0.39	–	0.18	0.39	0.44

component. Although 95% confidence intervals were not given, and the degree of overlap in parameter estimates is therefore unclear, the findings suggested consistent differences. Whether these represent etiological heterogeneity with respect to the behaviours being measured, i.e. trait variance, or an effect of the form of measurement, i.e. method variance, remains unclear.

The findings from the VTSABD also highlight how little the proportions of variance differed according to sex. In only one of the 15 measures (fathers' interview ratings of oppositional-defiant behaviour) was the parameter estimate significantly different for males and females. This indicates that the differences in the rates of conduct disorder for boys and girls cannot be explained by different proportions of genetic and environmental variance. Furthermore, the fact that the DZ opposite sex correlations were not much smaller than those for the DZ same sex pairs makes it unlikely that the type of genetic and environmental influences on conduct disorder vary according to sex.

The Australian Twin Register comprises a large adult volunteer register of whom over 2600 pairs participated in a telephone interview study that included lifetime DSM–III–R conduct disorder symptoms recalled retrospectively (Slutske et al., 1997). Models were fitted both to the diagnosis of conduct disorder (reported as having a lifetime prevalence of 17–20% in males and 2–3% in females) and to conduct disorder symptoms. For conduct disorder, the best fitting model gave a heritability estimate of 71% with no shared environment, although the 95% confidence intervals ranged from 0–32%, and no difference in the estimates for males and females. For conduct disorder symptoms, 53% of the variance in males was due to genetic influences and 0% to shared environment (95% confidence intervals 0–15%); for females, heritability was also 53% but there was evidence for a small shared environmental component of 12%. The range of the 95% confidence intervals highlights the large sample sizes required to obtain precise estimates in studies of individual differences and the danger in smaller studies of accepting more parsimonious models, where parameters have been set to 0. While in general, researchers should be encouraged to publish 95% confidence intervals for their parameter estimates, there are greater problems of interpretation in complex, multivariate models.

The findings of Gjone & Stevenson (1997) are quite different from those in Virginia and Australia. The sample of 905 pairs of same-sex Norwegian twins returned maternal reports on the Child Behavior Checklist (CBC-L – Achenbach & Edelbrock, 1985). They found not only substantial genetic but also shared environmental influences for the externalizing behaviour scale. The reasons for these differences are unclear; they could represent true difference in the populations or an effect of the scale. It seems unlikely to be entirely an effect of using mailed questionnaires, as other studies doing this (Edelbrock et al., 1995; McGuffin & Thapar, 1997), did not show similarly high correlations.

These findings highlight that not only population differences but also rater and measurement differences can lead to wide variation in heritability estimates. In an attempt to deal with these issues, Simonoff et al. (1995) used a multi-method (interview and questionnaire measures), multi-trait (mother, father and child ratings) latent variable model in which genetic and environmental influences were estimated for the latent variable of conduct disorder symptoms. The model took systematic differences among raters into account and gave a heritability of 81%, with only 2% of the variance being due to shared environment. The findings should be interpreted with caution because of the only moderate agreement among raters, which meant that only a proportion of each informant's rating was included in the latent variable, raising the question as to what aspect of conduct disorder is being evaluated. On the other hand, this approach to reducing measurement error indicates that the presence of measurement error may lead to spurious increases in both shared environmental estimates (through parental rating biases) and nonshared environment (through unreliability). Other strategies of using multiple measures to reduce measurement error have also increased heritability estimates (Kendler et al., 1993a).

Twin studies have suggested that there may be a difference between the relative importance of genetic and environmental influences on different components of conduct disorder behaviour. Edelbrock et al. (1995) used the aggression and delinquency subscales from the CBC-L in a relatively small twin study. For aggression, the genetic and shared environmental estimates were 60% and 15%, respectively; for delinquency, these estimates were 35% and 37%, suggesting that aggression was more heritable. Eley et al. (1999) reported similar differences on the CBC-L with aggression showing heritability estimates of 50–70% and delinquency 0–47%. The findings are of interest because of the suggestion that aggression is one predictor of continuing antisocial problems (Farrington et al., 1990; Loeber, 1982; Loeber et al., 1995; Olweus, 1989). If aggression is strongly genetic, this could provide part of the explanation for increased genetic effects on antisocial behaviour in adult life. Simonoff et al. (1998) used the Frick et al. (1993) typology of property violations, status violations, aggression and oppositional behaviour to examine genetic and environmental influences on these symptom subtypes using ratings from both mothers and boys. While these findings agreed with Edelbrock et al. (1995) and Eley et al. (1999) in showing a higher heritability for aggression (57%), the heritability was also relatively high for property violations (47%), which might be considered part of delinquency. In addition, this analysis again raised the question of informant differences, as the pattern of results was somewhat different for boys and their mothers.

Twin studies have explored the causes of comorbidity between conduct disorder and hyperactivity. Silberg et al. (1996) showed that the correlation between the hyperactivity and conduct disorder subscales of the Rutter A Scale in the Virginia Twin Study could be explained on the basis of common genetic risk factors for both disorders. Common environmental risk factors (whether for shared or nonshared environment) were not required. Furthermore, for this measure of conduct disorder symptomatology, the genetic influences were entirely shared with those for hyperactivity. A strong interpretation of the finding would be that conduct disorder that is comorbid with hyperactivity represents a genetically distinct subtype and, furthermore, that other forms of conduct disorder, i.e. those that are not comorbid with hyperactivity, are under little if any genetic influence. However, further work is needed and, in particular, the model of phenotypic causation (hyperactivity causing conduct disorder) needs to be considered as an alternative.

The extent to which genetic influences on conduct disorder are distinct from those for problem behaviour more generally has been examined by Gjone & Stevenson (1997), with the externalizing and internalizing subscales of the CBC-L from the Norwegian Twin Register. The results suggested that shared environmental influences were common to both traits with no evidence of common environment influencing one but not the other, while there were genetic factors common to both areas of psychopathology but also others that were specific to each area. Here, a strong interpretation would suggest that family-wide influences have a nonspecific effect on the presence of psychopathology, while genetic factors influence the type of problem behaviour. Replication is required.

For the most part, the large twin studies fail to find large sex differences in the proportions of variance accounted for by genetic and environmental influences. There is also relatively little evidence to suggest large differences in the individual genes or environments influencing conduct disorder, because the opposite-sex DZ twin correlations are similar to the same-sex correlations. However, differences in numbers of symptoms and rates of disorder can be explained by differential impact of genes and/or environment, when such risk factors are present. Measures of susceptibility genes and environments will help to clarify the mechanisms influencing sex differences.

Adoption studies

As highlighted earlier, a limiting feature of adoption studies has been the absence of information with respect to conduct disorder in biological (and adoptive) parents. Most adoption studies have used criminal records to index antisocial behaviour. Although there is a strong association between the two, not all youngsters with conduct disorder have problems in adult life, and when they do, they do not always involve criminality. Furthermore, criminality, particularly violent crime, can be associated with different types of psychopathology, including psychotic illness. In the Swedish (Bohman, 1995; Cloninger et al., 1982), and Danish (Brennan et al., 1995; Mednick et al., 1984) adoption studies, criminal registration data only have been used to index antisocial outcomes in adoptees and their biological and adoptive parents. The Iowa adoption study has more systematic psychiatric data on adoptees and their adoptive parents but data are more limited on biological parents (Cadoret et al., 1990, 1995b).

The Swedish and Danish adoption registers have focused on crime in adoptees, in comparison to biological and adoptive parents, but with somewhat different areas of emphasis. The Swedish study has examined criminality in relation to alcohol abuse. In the Swedish adoption data, the overall rate of criminality in adoptees was the same as that for the general population, although the rate was raised 2 to 3-fold in biological parents; a similar pattern was seen with respect to alcohol abuse (Bohman, 1995). Both adoptive and biological parental criminality significantly raised the rate of criminality in the offspring from 2.9% when both parental backgrounds were classified as low risk, to 6.7% when only adoptive parental background was high risk and to 12.1% when only biological parental background was high risk. An interaction was suggested, but not formally tested, by the criminality rate of 40.0% in the adoptees when both backgrounds were high risk. With respect to environmental factors, prolonged institutional rearing was a risk factor for female criminality only, while multiple placements and socioeconomically disadvantaged adoptive homes constituted risk factors for boys but not girls. The Swedish data further suggested that the types of criminality were genetically distinct, with petty, recidivist criminality showing stronger genetic effects. The finding that criminality in a biological mother increased the risk of adoptee criminality more than that of biological father criminality is consistent with a multiple threshold model suggesting that criminal women represent a more severe group than criminal men. In a multiple threshold model, this increased severity is associated with greater genetic liability, and therefore an increased probability that offspring will inherit genetic susceptibility.

The Danish adoption study also found a relationship between biological father and adoptive offspring risk of criminality (Brennan et al., 1995). They further showed increasing concordance in criminality rates among related adoptees, depending on the degree of relationship, from 8.5% for unrelated adoptees reared in separate homes, to 12.9% for half sibs reared apart, to 20.0% for full sibs, a finding supported by the Swedish study. The parent–offspring relationship was markedly attenuated for violent crime. Their findings are intriguing in showing a relationship between biological fathers' violence and schizophrenia in the offspring, that could not be explained by factors such as socioeconomic status, time to adoptive placement, or the presence of either schizophrenia or other mental illness in either of the biological parents. Replication and careful multivariate analysis is required to ensure that a combination of factors does not explain the findings. Furthermore, violent crime may be more heterogeneous in its origins, although it is generally associated with high rates of recidivism. The findings raise questions about a possible shared genetic basis for violent crime and psychotic illness.

Cadoret et al. (1995a, b, 1996) have used the Iowa adoption sample to select 197 individuals in whom biological parent data were sufficient to determine the presence of antisocial personality disorder. Structured psychiatric interviews using the DIS obtained on the adoptees included childhood aggression, conduct disorder, substance abuse and adult antisocial personality, and information about psychiatric illness in the adoptive parents was also collected. For childhood and adolescent aggression and conduct disorder before age 15, interactions were found between the presence of antisocial personality in the biological parent and psychiatric disorder in the adoptive parents. For adult antisocial personality, the genetic and environmental factors showed main, independent effects, with the interaction term falling just short of significance. For adult antisocial personality, adverse rearing environment had an impact in the absence of a deleterious biological background.

The findings for drug abuse in males suggest two biological pathways. The first is through biological parent alcohol abuse, with a direct effect on drug abuse. The second was via biological parent antisocial personality. In the latter case, drug abuse was mediated through antisocial behaviour, which increased risk for aggression, which in turn mediated conduct disorder and then drug abuse. In both, there were interactions with an adverse rearing environment. In females, they were unable to find evidence for a pathway from biological parent alcohol abuse, and the impact of biological parent antisocial personality was directly on conduct disorder, rather than via aggression (Cadoret et al., 1996). As with the males, adverse rearing environment had a direct effect on aggression, which subsequently increased the risk of drug abuse/dependency. These different pathways to drug abuse/dependency are broadly in line with the findings from the Swedish adoption data in highlighting different patterns of risk leading to substance abuse.

It is interesting to note that two of the three major adoption studies indicate a role for gene–environment interactions, a phenomenon more easily detectable in adoption than twin studies. In general, the genetic effects reported in adoption studies are somewhat weaker than those for twin studies; one explanation of this would be that undetected gene–environment interactions (and correlations) in twin studies are included in the heritability estimate (Carey, 1994). This possibility highlights the need for studies that include direct measures of nature–nurture interplay.

Family risk factors

Family studies of conduct disorder and antisocial behaviour in the past have documented the increased rate of family-based adversity (Emery, 1982; Fergusson et al., 1992; Haapasalo & Hamalainen, 1996; Hamdan-Allen et al., 1989; Olweus, 1980). There is no doubt about the relationship between antisocial behaviour and a number of aspects of family adversity. However, much less is understood about the specificity of these relationships and their mechanism of action. To what extent does family adversity have an independent effect, mediated through environmental exposure, on the development of conduct disorder and to what extent is it only indexing genetic susceptibility? Szatmari et al. (1993) compared the extent to which various family factors had differential impact on familial aggregation of conduct, emotional and hyperactivity problems in the Ontario Child Health Study. There were few factors having a clear-cut differential impact on conduct disorder, with the presence of a sibling with conduct disorder and all male sibships being among the few factors. In general, the factors measured (sibship size, sex and age composition of siblings) showed a stronger relationship to conduct and emotional problems than to hyperactivity, and the differentiation in the first two categories was weak. These findings are in line with those of the Gjone & Stevenson (1997) twin study showing shared environmental effects were not specific for externalizing or internalizing behaviour problems.

Frick et al. (1992) compared the role of parental psychopathology and parenting practices in clinically referred families with conduct disorder, oppositional defiant disorder, and psychiatric controls. The rates of paternal antisocial personality disorder and substance abuse/dependency were increased in conduct disorder, as were poor maternal supervision and inconsistent discipline.

However, in a multivariate analysis, the parenting practices no longer discriminated among the groups when paternal psychopathology was taken into account. Similar analyses, using a smaller but overlapping sample, suggested that parental antisocial personality but not divorce influenced the diagnosis of clinic attenders (Lahey et al., 1988). A strong interpretation would be that poor parenting in this group was a marker of assortative mating with an antisocial spouse, where genetic liability was the underlying mediator. However, methodological limitations, in particular the use of a clinically referred group, means that further research on general population groups and with independently obtained measures of parental psychopathology and environmental risk is needed (Meyer et al., in press). Lytton (1990) reviewed the literature on child and parent effects on conduct disorder and concluded that parental behaviour was at least as likely to reflect as to be the cause of child antisocial behaviour. A small adoption study showed an association between a history of antisocial behaviour and substance abuse in biological parents and both aggression in the adoptee and the disciplinary practices of the adoptive parent (Ge et al., 1996). While the study is small, it raises several interesting points about gene–environment correlation. First, the association between adoptive parents' discipline and biological parents' psychiatric history suggested an evocative or active gene–environment correlation, where children's behaviour was influencing their experiences of parenting. However, the strength of the associations further suggested that maternal behaviour towards their adopted children has further reciprocal effects on their antisocial behaviour. Finally, there was an independent effect of maternal hostility toward the child (which was associated with marital discord) on the child's antisocial behaviour, suggesting that there can also be important pure environmental influences. The findings require replication in a larger sample.

Findings from the Nonshared Environment and Adolescent Development (NEAD) study support the impact of child behaviour on parents. Aggressive, explosive and inconsistent parenting predicted nearly 60% of adolescent antisocial behaviour (Reiss et al., 1995). In comparing remarried families with half versus unrelated sibs, within-family differences in both parenting and problem behaviour were greater in the unrelated sib families (Mekos et al., 1996). In rating observational data from the entire sample, O'Connor et al. (1995) reported greater genetic correlations for adolescent conduct disorder than for parental style. The findings are consistent with the idea of child effects on parental behaviour, or evocative or active GE correlation, as they suggest that an underlying parental style may be influenced by the behaviour of different children (where behaviour may be genetically mediated).

Chromosomal influences

There is interest in the role of the Y chromosome with respect to aggression, because of the higher rate of aggression in males and the fact that Y chromosome genes are responsible for testosterone production. Males with an abnormal sex chromosome complement have provided one model, with the particular suggestion that XYY males (Klinefelter's syndrome) may be more aggressive because of their slightly increased prevalence in prisons. Despite the prevalence of the anomaly, affecting 1 in 1000 males, there has been little in the way of objective work on systematically ascertained samples. Possible confounds with respect to the increased rate in prisons include the lower IQ and tall stature in men with Klinefelter's syndrome. In addition, it may be difficult to disentangle direct effects of the chromosomal anomaly from those due to the individuals' knowledge of the abnormality. However, the available findings suggest both that XYY males may have greater behavioural adjustment difficulties and also that these are not specifically aggressive in nature (Robinson & de la Chapelle, 1997). In childhood, clinical descriptions have suggested XYY boys are hyperactive, distractible and prone to temper tantrums. However, about 50% have learning and developmental problems, although most have an IQ in the normal range, and it is unclear whether the behavioural abnormalities cosegregate with and are possibly caused by the intellectual difficulties. There is a suggestion of emotional immaturity and lack of emotional control in adult life, but it is unclear how pervasive this is. XYY individuals may be more susceptible to stress, as indicated by the observation that those raised in dysfunctional families fare worse than their unaffected siblings.

Molecular genetic studies

Molecular genetic studies have relevance to conduct disorder both through the study of phenotypes in which aggression is a prominent feature and also through other psychiatric disorders such as hyperactivity and alcohol and drug abuse, which are frequently comorbid with conduct disorder or antisocial personality. There have to date been no molecular genetic studies taking conduct disorder as the phenotype of interest. A point mutation (a single DNA base pair change) in the monoamine oxidase A (MAOA) gene has been described in one family with borderline mental retardation and intermittent, explosive aggression (Brunner et al., 1993). Both MAOA and MAOB are enzymes involved in the breakdown of several neurotransmitters, including dopamine, norepinephrine and serotonin. The pharmacological effect of MAO, and MAOA in particular, is demonstrated by the use of MAO inhibitors in depression. However, attempts to correlate MAOB levels (which can be measured from platelets, but whose role in the central nervous system remains to be established) with impulsive, sensation-seeking behaviour have led to variable results (Hsu et al., 1989). To date, the abnormality has not been replicated in other families and therefore the observed relationship cannot be accepted as causative. Furthermore, the findings by themselves give very little information about the pathophysiology of aggression, because of the wide-ranging impact of the mutation on a variety of neurotransmitter systems. In the affected family members, the plasma neurotransmitter levels were higher than normal, while aggression in other samples has been linked to low cerebrospinal fluid (CSF) levels of serotonin metabolites. Although these findings are apparently contradictory, the regulation of neurotransmitter systems is highly complex and the impact of congenital effects through mutations may be very different from those of altered function later in life.

Several reports in the last few years have suggested a relationship between genes associated with dopamine function and hyperactivity. Positive findings have focused on two genes: the D4 dopamine receptor (DRD4) and the dopamine transporter (DAT1) (Thapar et al., 1999). Genes associated with dopamine neurotransmission are obvious candidate genes for several reasons, including drug response to amphetamines and related substances, which stimulate release of dopamine and other neuroamines in the brain. Animal models and neuroimaging studies also suggest a role for dopamine neurotransmission in hyperactivity. However, it is equally likely that disturbances in other neurotransmitters play an important role in the mediation of hyperactivity. The studies reporting an association to DRD4 include both studies of youngsters diagnosed with attention deficit hyperactivity disorder (ADHD) and studies of individual differences in sensation seeking. An association between ADHD and a variant of the DRD4 allele has been reported (Lahoste et al., 1996; Swanson et al., 1998), although there are also currently unpublished reports of other nonreplications. The same DRD4 allelic variant have also been associated with the dimensional trait of novelty seeking (Benjamin et al., 1996; Ebstein et al., 1996, 1997; Ono et al., 1997) although there have also been reports failing to find the association (Benjamin et al., 1998; Sander et al., 1997). The 7-repeat DRD4 allele is thought to mediate a blunted intracellular response to dopamine, which has been postulated as the physiological mechanism underlying the behavioural differences (Van Tol et al., 1992).

An association between DAT1 and ADHD has also been reported by two groups (Cook et al., 1995; Gill et al., 1997). While, for both dopamine genes, the methods used make population differences between cases and controls an unlikely confound in the findings, there are still uncertainties about the generalizability of the findings. It is uncertain how widely replicable the positive results are because of the difficulty in publishing negative findings. It will also be crucial to clarify what aspects of behaviour are most closely linked to these susceptibility genes. At this point, the relationship to conduct disorder may become clearer.

Resistance to thyroid hormone has been associated with hyperactivity (Brucker-Davis et al., 1995). The exact prevalence of thyroid hormone resistance is unknown but it is thought to be rare. Rates of ADHD are significantly higher (73%) amongst those family members with thyroid resistance than amongst those without (27%), suggesting that the genetic effects of thyroid resistance may confer an increased risk for hyperactivity. The relationship between hyperactivity and thyroid resistance requires replication; even if findings are consistent, it is likely to be a rare cause of hyperactivity and its relationship to conduct disorder is uncertain.

Genetic studies of alcohol abuse are of some relevance to conduct disorder, because a proportion of those with adult alcohol problems will have had childhood conduct disorder. Although findings related to the alcohol dehydrogenase (ADH) and aldehyde dehydrogenase (ALDH) genes are currently the most promising, these are unlikely to relate to conduct disorder, as the pathophysiological susceptibility is probably only through alcohol metabolism. The dopamine D2 receptor (DRD2) gene has also been implicated in alcohol abuse/dependency through a number of association studies, with both positive (Blum et al., 1990; Parsian et al., 1991) and negative (Bolos et al., 1990; Cook et al., 1992; Gelernter et al., 1991; Suarez et al., 1994; Turner et al., 1992) findings, so that the current status is unclear. Further molecular genetic research on alcohol abuse may shed light on the genetic liability to conduct disorder, particularly if characteristics of abuse and related features are more closely defined.

A number of studies have linked impulsive, aggressive behaviour, to low levels of plasma serotonin (5-HT) and CSF 5HIAA (a serotonin metabolite) (Asberg & Traskmanbendz, 1987; Linnoila et al., 1983) and therefore genes involved in its regulation become candidate genes for aggressive behaviour. While increased aggression has been reported in mice lacking the 5-HT1B receptor (Saudou et al., 1994), there are as yet no relevant human studies. This will be an area of interest in the future.

Conclusions

It is clear that conduct disorders are influenced in important ways by genetic factors, although environmental factors also have a considerable role. It is likely that some of the family factors associated with conduct disorder either have their impact partly through genetic routes, or are primarily an index of other factors which are genetically influenced. The very mixed results with respect to the importance of genetic influences are difficult to interpret with confidence at this point. The variability in findings for conduct disorder are similar to those for other child psychiatric phenotypes (Eaves et al., 1997; Thapar & McGuffin, 1994). The exception is hyperactivity, which has shown very stable heritability estimates of 60–90%. A crucial question with respect to conduct disorder is whether the substantial differences reflect true genetic heterogeneity in the qualities of aggressive and antisocial behaviour, whether they derive from testing different populations, or whether they are artefacts of an assessment method. More work is needed to establish whether there are links between clinically meaningful subtypes and the extent and type of genetic influences. The example of comorbidity with hyperactivity highlights the possibility of one clinically meaningful genetically distinct subtype, but this will need replication.

The lack of evidence for sex differences in the extent and type of genetic and environmental influences, demonstrated in the twin and adoption studies, is interesting given the different prevalence rates. The implication of these findings is that there are influences independent from those determining conduct disorder that affect the rates. It may be as important to understand these influences, which may act at a group rather than individual level, in terms of developing effective interventions.

Although behaviour genetic studies are a useful tool in outlining the potential mechanisms for the development and maintenance of psychopathology, they frequently are limited to latent measures and do not specify the actual influences involved. Behaviour genetic studies in the future can be more productive if they link closely to current knowledge of psychopathology and include observed measures such as environmental risk, parental and comorbid psychopathology and, when possible, molecular genetic susceptibility. It is also important that future studies are designed to explore the interplay between genes and environment.

To date, molecular genetics has suggested some interesting routes for further study. However, the current findings both need replication and are likely to apply only to a small subset of those with conduct disorder. As with other neuropsychiatric disorders, the candidate gene approach is limited, because of our lack of understanding of the pathophysiology of conduct disorder. While it is hoped that the discovery of genes for conduct disorder may help to delineate this process, it should be recognized that this will need to be a boot-strapping operation in which genetic and other research strategies will need to inform each other. With respect to genetic studies, such information will come not only from biological but also from environmental studies, that alert us to important influences. There is disagreement in the field as to whether the time is ripe for large-scale genome-wide searches for genes of small to moderate effect size. While some will argue this is the most effective strategy for common disorders, others will say that more knowledge is needed about which aspects of the phenotype are inherited and what are the indices of genetic heterogeneity. Once again, there is an argument for a boot-strapping approach.

We should expect genetic studies in the future to tell us as much about the environment as they do about genes. Thus, genetic studies should help us to understand why some children are vulnerable to environmental adversity and not others, why some children have long-term difficulties, and why some respond to particular interventions, to highlight just a few questions. Genetic strategies should also help us to understand which aspects of conduct disorder behaviour are core, or cause, and which are consequence. This applies not only to questions such as comorbidity with hyperactivity, but also to issues such as the relationship to social cognitive deficits. A long-term goal of genetic research must be to aid in prevention and treatment of conduct disorder. Prevention can be enhanced by the detection at an early stage of individuals at risk for the development of problems. Genetic research should also improve treatment by contributing to our knowledge of meaningful subgroups and by helping to define the mechanisms involved in persistence, thereby clarifying the points at which intervention may be useful.

REFERENCES

Achenbach, T.M. & Edelbrock, C. (1985). *Manual for the Child Behavior Checklist and the Revised Child Behavior Profile*. Burlington, VT: University of Vermont.

Asberg, A.U. & Traskmanbendz, L. (1987). Is CSF 5-HIA a suicide predictor. *International Journal of Neuroscience*, 31, 253–4.

Baron, M., Hamburger, R., Sandkuyl, L.A., et al. (1990). The impact of phenotypic variation on genetic analysis: application to X-linkage in manic-depressive illness. *Acta Psychiatrica Scandinavica*, 82, 196–203.

Benjamin, J., Lin, L., Patterson, C., et al. (1996). Population and familial association between the D4 dopamine receptor gene and measures of novelty seeking. *Nature Genetics*, 12, 81–4.

Benjamin, J., Osher, Y., Belmaker, R.H. & Ebstein, R. (1998). No significant associations between two dopamine receptor polymorphisms and normal temperament. *Human Psychopharmacology – Clinical and Experimental*, 13, 11–15.

Blum, K., Noble, E.P., Sheridan, P.J., et al. (1990). Allelic association of human dopamine D2 receptor gene in alcoholism. *Journal of the American Medical Association, 263*, 2055–60.

Bohman, M. (1995). Predisposition to criminality: Swedish adoption studies in retrospect. In G.R. Bock & J.A. Goode (Eds.), *Genetics of Criminal and Antisocial Behaviour (Ciba Foundation Symposium 194)* (pp. 99–114). Chichester: John Wiley & Sons.

Bolos, A.M., Dean, M., Lucas-Derse, S., et al. (1990). Population and pedigree studies reveal a lack of association between the dopamine D2 receptor gene and alcoholism. *Journal of the American Medical Association, 264*, 3156–60.

Brennan, P.A., Mednick, S.A. & Jacobsen, B. (1995). Assessing the role of genetics in crime using adoption cohorts. In G.R. Bock & J.A. Goode (Eds.), *Genetics of Criminal and Antisocial Behaviour (Ciba Foundation Symposium 194)* (pp. 115–28). Chichester: John Wiley & Sons.

Brucker-Davis, F., Skarulis, M.C., Grace, M.B., et al. (1995). Genetic and clinical features of 42 kindreds with resistance to thyroid hormone. *Annals of Internal Medicine, 123*, 572–83.

Brunner, H.G., Nelen, M.R., van Zandvoort, P., et al. (1993). X-linked borderline mental retardation with prominent behavioral disturbance: Phenotype, genetic localization, and evidence for disturbed monoamine metabolism. *American Journal of Human Genetics, 52*, 1032–9.

Cadoret, R. (1986). Adoption studies: historical and methodological critique. *Psychiatric Developments, 1*, 45–64.

Cadoret, R.J., Troughton, E., Bagford, J. & Woodworth, G. (1990). Genetic and environmental factors in adoptee antisocial personality. *European Archives of Psychiatric Neurological Science, 239*, 231–40.

Cadoret, R.J., Yates, W.R., Troughton, E., Woodworth, G. & Stewart, M.A. (1995a). Adoption study demonstrating two genetic pathways to drug abuse. *Archive of General Psychiatry, 52*, 42–52.

Cadoret, R.J., Yates, W.R., Troughton, E., Woodworth, G. & Stewart, M.A. (1995b). Genetic–environmental interaction in the genesis of aggressivity and conduct disorders. *Archives of General Psychiatry, 52*, 916–24.

Cadoret, R.J., Yates, W.R., Troughton, E., Woodworth, G. & Stewart, M.A. (1996). An adoption study of drug abuse/dependency in females. *Comprehensive Psychiatry, 37*, 88–94.

Carey, G. (1992). Twin imitation for antisocial behavior: Implications for genetic and family environment research. *Journal of Abnormal Psychology, 101*, 18–25.

Carey, G. (1994). *Genetics and Violence*. Washington: National Academy Press.

Caron, C. & Rutter, M. (1991). Comorbidity in child psychopathology: concepts, issues and research strategies. *Journal of Child Psychology and Psychiatry, 32*, 1063–81.

Cloninger, C.R., Sigvardsson, S., Bohman, M. & von Knorring, A.L. (1982). Predisposition to petty criminality in Swedish adoptees: II. Cross-fostering analysis of gene–environment interaction. *Archives of General Psychiatry, 39*, 1242–7.

Cook, B.L., Wang, Z.W., Crowe, R.R., Hauser, R. & Friemer, M. (1992). Alcoholism and the D2 receptor gene. *Alcoholism: Clinical and Experimental Research, 16*, 806–9.

Cook, E.H., Stein, M.A., Krasowski, M.D., et al. (1995). Association of attention-deficit disorder and the dopamine transporter gene. *American Journal of Human Genetics, 56*, 993–8.

DiLalla, L.F. & Gottesman, I.I. (1991). Biological and genetic contributors to violence – Widom's untold tale. *Psychological Bulletin, 109*, 125–9.

Dodge, K.A., Pettit, G.S. & Bates, J.E. (1994). Socialization mediators of the relation between socioeconomic status and child conduct problems. *Child Development, 65,* 649–65.

Eaves, L.J. (1982). The utility of twins. In V.E. Anderson, W.A. Hausner, J.K. Penry & C.F. Sing (Eds.), *Genetic Basis of the Epilepsies* (pp. 249–75). New York: Raven Press.

Eaves, L.J., Silberg, J.L., Meyer, J.M., et al. (1997). Genetics and developmental psychopathology: 2. The main effects of genes and environment on behavioral problems in the Virginia Twin Study of Adolescent Behavioral Development. *Journal of Child Psychology and Psychiatry, 38,* 965–80.

Ebstein, R.P., Nemanov, L., Klotz, I., Gritsenko, I. & Belmaker, R.H. (1997). Additional evidence for an association between the dopamine D4 receptor (D4DR) exon III repeat polymorphism and the human personality trait of novelty seeking. *Molecular Psychiatry, 2,* 472–7.

Ebstein, R.P., Novick, O., Umansky, R., et al. (1996). Dopamine D4 receptor (D4DR) exon III polymorphism associated with the human personality trait of novelty seeking. *Nature Genetics, 12,* 78–80.

Edelbrock, C., Rende, R., Plomin, R. & Thompson, L.A. (1995). A twin study of competence and problem behaviour in childhood and early adolescence. *Journal of Child Psychology and Psychiatry, 36,* 775–85.

Eley, T.C., Lichtenstein, P. & Stevenson, J. (1999). Sex differences in the aetiology of aggressive and non-aggressive antisocial behavior: Results from two twin studies. *Child Development, 8,* 155–68.

Emery, R.E. (1982). Interparental conflict and the children of discord and divorce. *Psychopharmacology Bulletin, 92,* 310–20.

Falk, C.T. & Rubinstein, P. (1987). Haplotype relative risks: an easy reliable way to construct a proper control sample for risk calculations. *Annals of Human Genetics, 51,* 227–33.

Farrington, D., Loeber, R. & Van Kammen, W.B. (1990). Long-term criminal outcomes of hyperactivity-impulsivity-attention deficit and conduct problems in childhood. In L.N. Robins & M. Rutter (Eds.), *Straight and Devious Pathways from Childhood to Adulthood* (pp. 62–81). Cambridge: Cambridge University Press.

Fergusson, D.M., Horwood, L.J. & Lynsky, M.T. (1992). Family change, parental discord and early offending. *Journal of Child Psychology and Psychiatry, 33,* 1059–75.

Flint, J., Wilkie, A.O.M., Buckle, V.J., et al. (1995). The detection of subtelomeric chromosomal rearrangements in idiopathic mental retardation. *Nature Genetics, 9,* 132–40.

Frick, P.J., Lahey, B.B., Loeber, R., et al. (1992). Familial risk factors to oppositional defiant disorder and conduct disorder: Parental psychopathology and maternal parenting. *Journal of Consulting and Clinical Psychology, 60,* 49–55.

Frick, P.J., Van Horn, Y., Lahey, B.B., et al. (1993). Oppositional defiant disorder and conduct disorder: a meta-analytic review of factor analyses and cross-validation in a clinic sample. *Clinical Psychology Review, 13,* 319–40.

Ge, X.J., Conger, R.D., Cadoret, R.J., et al. (1996). The developmental interface between nature and nurture: A mutual influence model of child antisocial behavior and parent behaviors. *Developmental Psychology, 32,* 574–89.

Gelernter, J., O'Malley, S., Risch, N., et al. (1991). No association between an allele at the D2 dopamine receptor gene (DRD2) and alcoholism. *Journal of the American Medical Association*, *266*, 1801–7.

Gill, M., Daly, G., Heron, S., Hawi, Z. & Fitzgerald, M. (1997). Confirmation of association between attention deficit hyperactivity disorder and a dopamine transporter polymorphism. *Molecular Psychiatry*, *2*, 311–13.

Gjone, H. & Novik, T.S. (1995). Parental ratings of behaviour problems: a twin and general population comparison. *Journal of Child Psychology and Psychiatry*, *36*, 1213–24.

Gjone, H. & Stevenson, J. (1997). The association between internalizing and externalizing behaviour in childhood and early adolescence: genetic or environmental common influences? *Journal of Abnormal Child Psychology*, *25*, 277–86.

Haapasalo, J. & Hamalainen, T. (1996). Childhood family problems and current psychiatric problems among young violent and property offenders. *Journal of the American Academy of Child and Adolescent Psychiatry*, *34*, 1394–401.

Hamdan-Allen, G., Stewart, M.A. & Beeghly, J.H. (1989). Subgrouping conduct disorder by psychiatric family history. *Journal of Child Psychology and Psychiatry*, *30*, 889–97.

Heath, A.C., Neale, M.C., Hewitt, J.L., Eaves, L.J. & Fuilker, D.W. (1989). Testing structural equation models for twin data using LISREL. *Behavior Genetics*, *19*, 9–35.

Hopper, J.L. & Culross, P. (1983). Covariation between family members as a function of cohabitation history. *Behavior Genetics*, *13*, 439–71.

Hsu, Y.-P., Powell, J.F., Sims, K.B. & Breakefield, X.O. (1989). Short review – Molecular genetics of the monoamine oxidases. *Journal of Neurochemistry*, *53*, 12–18.

Kaprio, J., Koskenvuo, M. & Rose, R.J. (1990). Change in cohabitation and intrapair similarity of monozygotic (MZ) co-twins for alcohol use, extraversion and neuroticism. *Behavior Genetics*, *20*, 265–76.

Kendler, K.S. (1993). Twin studies of psychiatric illness: current status and future directions. *Archives of General Psychiatry*, *50*, 905–15.

Kendler, K.S., Neale, M.C., Kessler, R.C., et al. (1993*a*). The lifetime history of major depression in women. *Archives of General Psychiatry*, *50*, 863–70.

Kendler, K.S., Neale, M.C., Heath, A.C., Kessler, R.C. & Eaves, L.J. (Eds.). (1991). *Life Events and Depressive Symptoms: A Twin Study Perspective*. Oxford: Butterworth-Heineman.

Kendler, K.S., Neale, M.C., Kessler, R.C., Heath, A.C. & Eaves, L.J. (1993*b*). A test of the equal-environment assumption in twin studies of psychiatric illness. *Behavior Genetics*, *23*, 21–7.

Lahey, B.B., Hartdagen, S.E., Frick, P.J., et al. (1988). Conduct disorder: parsing the confounded relation to parental divorce and antisocial personality. *Journal of Abnormal Psychology*, *97*, 334–7.

Lahoste, G.J., Swanson, J.M., Wigal, S.B., et al. (1996). Dopamine D4 receptor gene polymorphism is associated with attention deficit hyperactivity disorder. *Molecular Psychiatry*, *1*, 121–4.

Le Couteur, A., Bailey, A., Goode, S., et al. (1996). A broader phenotype of autism: the clinical spectrum in twins. *Journal of Child Psychology and Psychiatry*, *37*, 785–801.

Leckman, J.F., Weissman, M.M., Pauls, D.L. & Kidd, K.K. (1987). Family-genetic studies and identification of valid diagnostic categories in adult and child psychiatry. *British Journal of Psychiatry*, *151*, 39–44.

Linnoila, M., Virkkunen, M., Scheinin, M., et al. (1983). Low cerebrospinal-fluid 5 hydroxyindoleacetic acid concentration differentiates impulsive from nonimpulsive violent behavior. *Life Sciences*, *33*, 2609–14.

Loeber, R. (1982). The stability of antisocial and delinquent child behavior: a review. *Child Development*, 1431–46.

Loeber, R., Green, S.M., Keenan, K. & Lahey, B.B. (1995). Which boys will fare worse? Early predictors of the onset of conduct disorder in a six-year longitudinal study. *Journal of the American Academy of Child and Adolescent Psychiatry*, *34*, 499–509.

Lyons, M.J., True, W.R., Elsen, S.A., et al. (1995). Differential heritability of adult and juvenile antisocial traits. *Archives of General Psychiatry*, *52*, 905–15.

Lytton, H. (1990). Child effects – still unwelcome? Response to Dodge and Wahler. *Developmental Psychology*, *26*, 705–9.

Maughan, B. & Hagell, A. (1996). Poor readers in adulthood: psychosocial functioning. *Development and Psychopathology*, *8*, 457–76.

McGuffin, P. & Thapar, A. (1997). Genetic basis of bad behaviour in adolescents. *Lancet*, *350*, 411–12.

McGuire, S., Neiderhiser, J.M., Reiss, D., Hetherington, E.M. & Plomin, R. (1994). Genetic and environmental influences on perceptions of self-worth and competence in adolescence: a study of twins, full siblings, and step-siblings. *Child Development*, *65*, 785–99.

Mednick, S.A., Gabrielli, W.F. & Hutchings, B. (1984). Genetic influences in criminal convictions: Evidence from an adoption court. *Science*, *224*, 891–3.

Mekos, D., Hetherington, E. & Reiss, D. (1996). Sibling differences in problem behavior and parental treatment in nondivorced and remarried families. *Child Development*, *67*, 2148–65.

Meyer, J.M., Rutter, M., Silberg, J., et al. (in press). Familial aggregation for conduct disorder symptomatology: the role of gender, marital discord and family adaptability. *Psychological Medicine*, in press.

Moffitt, T.E. (1993). The neuropsychology of conduct disorder. *Development and Psychopathology*, *5*, 135–51.

O'Connor, T.G., Hetherington, E.M., Reiss, D. & Plomin, R. (1995). A twin-sibling study of observed parent–adolescent interactions. *Child Development*, *66*, 812–29.

Olweus, D. (1980). Familial and temperamental determinants of aggressive behavior in adolescent boys: a causal analysis. *Development Psychology*, *16*, 644–60.

Olweus, D. (1989). Persistence and prevalence in the study of antisocial behavior: definitions and management. In M.W. Klein (Eds.), *Cross-national Research in Self-reported Crime and Delinquency*. Dordrecht, The Netherlands: Kluwer.

Ono, Y., Manki, H., Yoshimura, K., et al. (1997). Association between dopamine D4 receptor (D4DR) exon III polymorphism and novelty seeking in Japanese subjects. *American Journal of Medical Genetics*, *74*, 501–3.

Parsian, A., Todd, R.D., Devor, E.J., et al. (1991). Alcoholism and alleles of the human D2 dopamine receptor locus. *Archives of General Psychiatry*, *48*, 655–63.

Patterson, G. & Fleischman, M.J. (1979). Maintenance of treatment effects. Some considerations concerning family systems and follow-up data. *Behavior Therapy*, *10*, 168–85.

Pike, A., Reiss, D., Hetherington, E.M. & Plomin, R. (1996). Using MZ differences in the search for nonshared environmental effects. *Journal of Child Psychology and Psychiatry, 37*, 695–704.

Plomin, R. (1995). Genetics and children's experiences in the family. *Journal of Child Psychology and Psychiatry, 36*, 33–68.

Popova, N. & Kalikov, A.V. (1986). Genetic analysis of spontaneous internal aggression in mice. *Aggressive Behaviour, 12*, 425–31.

Reiss, D., Hetherington, M., Plomin, R., et al. (1995). Genetic questions for environmental studies. *Archives of General Psychiatry, 52*, 925–36.

Risch, N. & Merikangas, K. (1996). The future of genetic studies of complex human disease. *Science, 275*, 1516–17.

Robins, L.N. (1991). Conduct disorder. *Journal of Child Psychiatry and Psychology, 32*, 193–212.

Robinson, A. & de la Chapelle, A. (1997). Sex chromosome anomalies. In D. Rimoin, J.M. Connor & R.E. Pyeritz (Eds.), *Principles and Practice of Medical Genetics* (pp. 973–99). New York: Churchill Livingstone.

Rowe, D.C. (1983). Biometrical genetic models of self-reported delinquent behavior: a twin study. *Behavior Genetics, 13*, 473–89.

Rutter, M. (Ed.) (1978). *Family, Area and School Influences in the Genesis of Conduct Disorders.* Oxford: Pergamon Press.

Rutter, M., Bolton, P., Harrington, R. et al. (1990a). Genetic factors in child psychiatric disorders – I. A review of research strategies. *Journal of Child Psychology and Psychiatry, 31*, 3–37.

Rutter, M., Giller, H. & Hagell, A. (1998). *Antisocial Behavior by Young People.* Cambridge: Cambridge University Press.

Rutter, M., Macdonald, H., Le Couteur, A., et al. (1990b). Genetic factors in child psychiatric disorders – II. Empirical findings. *Journal of Child Psychology and Psychiatry, 31*, 39–83.

Rutter, M. & Redshaw, J. (1991). Growing up as a twin: twin singleton differences in psychological development. *Journal of Child Psychology and Psychiatry, 32*, 885–95.

Rutter, M., Silberg, J., O'Connor, T.J. & Simonoff, E. (1999a). Genetics and child psychiatry. I: Advances in quantitative and molecular genetics. *Journal of Child Psychology and Psychiatry. 40*, 3–18.

Rutter, M., Silberg, J., O'Connor, T. & Simonoff, E. (1999b). Genetics and child psychiatry. II: Empirical research findings. *Journal of Child Psychology and Psychiatry, 40*, 19–56.

Rutter, M., Tizard, J. & Whitmore, K. (1970). *Education, Health and Behaviour.* London: Longman.

Rutter, M., Yule, B., Quinton, D., et al. (1975). Attainment and adjustment in two geographical areas: III – Some factors accounting for area differences. *British Journal of Psychiatry, 125*, 520–33.

Sander, T., Harms, H., Dufeu, P., et al. (1997). Dopamine D4 receptor exon III alleles and variation of novelty seeking, exploratory excitability. *American Journal of Medical Genetics, 74*, 483–7.

Saudou, F., Amara, D.A., Dierich, A., et al. (1994). Enhanced aggressive behavior in mice lacking 5-HT$_{1B}$ receptor. *Science, 265*, 1875–8.

Schmitz, S., Cherny, S.S., Fulker, D.W. & Mrazek, D.A. (1994). Genetic and environmental influences on early childhood behavior. *Behavior Genetics, 24*, 25–34.

Silberg, J., Rutter, M., Meyer, J., et al. (1996). Genetic and environmental influences on the covariation between hyperactivity and conduct disturbance in juvenile twins. *Journal of Child Psychology and Psychiatry, 37*, 803–16.

Simonoff, E. (1992). A comparison of twins and singletons with child psychiatric disorders: an item sheet analysis. *Journal of Child Psychology and Psychiatry, 33*, 1319–32.

Simonoff, E. (2000). Extracting meaning from comorbidity: genetic analyses that make sense. *Journal of Child Psychology and Psychiatry, 41*, 667–74.

Simonoff, E., Elander, J., Holmshaw, J., Murray, R. & Rutter, M. (submitted). The genetics of antisocial behaviour: evidence for increasing genetic effects from childhood to adult life.

Simonoff, E., McGuffin, P. & Gottesman, I.I. (1994). Genetic influences on normal and abnormal development. In M. Rutter, E.A. Taylor & L. Hersov (Eds.), *Child and Adolescent Psychiatry: Modern Approaches* (pp. 129–51). Oxford: Blackwell Scientific Publications.

Simonoff, E., Pickles, A., Hewitt, J., et al. (1995). Multiple raters of disruptive child behavior: using a genetic strategy to examine shared views and bias. *Behavior Genetics, 25*, 311–26.

Simonoff, E., Pickles, E., Meyer, J., Silberg, J. & Maes, H. (1998). Genetic and environmental influences on subtypes of conduct disorder. *Journal of Abnormal Child Psychology, 27*, 497–511.

Simonoff, E., Pickles, A., Meyr, J.M., et al. (1997). The Virginia Twin Study of Adolescent Behavioral Development: influences of age, gender and impairment on rates of disorder. *Archives of General Psychiatry, 54*, 801–8.

Slutske, W.S., Heath, A.C., Dinwiddie, S.H., et al. (1997). Modeling genetic and environmental influences in the etiology of conduct disorder: A study of 2682 adult twin pairs. *Journal of Abnormal Psychology, 106*, 269–79.

Spielman, R.S. & Ewens, W.J. (1996). Invited editorial: The TDT and other family-based tests for linkage disequilibrium and association. *American Journal of Human Genetics, 59*, 983–9.

St. George-Hyslop, P.H., Myers, R.H., Haines, J.L., et al. (1989). Familial Alzheimer's disease: progress and problems. *Neurobiology of Aging, 10*, 417–25.

Stevenson, J. & Graham, P. (1988). Behavioral deviance in 13-year old twins: An item analysis. *Journal of the American Academy of Child and Adolescent Psychiatry, 27*, 791–7.

Stewart, M.A., Cummings, C., Singer, S. & DeBlois, C.S. (1979). The overlap between hyperactive and unsocialized aggressive children. *Journal of Child Psychology and Psychiatry, 22*, 35–45.

Suarez, B.K., Parsian, A., Hampe, C.L., et al. (1994). Linkage disequilibria at the D2 dopamine receptor locus (DRD2) in alcoholics and controls. *Genomics, 19*, 12–20.

Swanson, J.M., Sunohara, G.A., Kennedy, J.L., et al. (1998). Association of the dopamine receptor D4 (DRD4) gene with a refined phenotype of attention deficit hyperactivity disorder (ADHD); A family-based approach. *Molecular Psychiatry, 3*, 38–41.

Szatmari, P., Boyle, M. & Offord, D. (1993). Familial aggregation of emotional and behavioral problems in adulthood in the general population. *American Journal of Psychiatry, 150*, 1398–1405.

Taylor, E., Everitt, B., Thorley, G., et al. (1986a). Conduct disorder and hyperactivity: II. A cluster analytic approach to the identification of a behavioural syndrome. *British Journal of Psychiatry, 149*, 768–77.

Taylor, E., Schachar, R., Thorley, G. & Wiselberg, M. (1986b). Conduct disorder and hyperactivity:

I. Separation of hyperactivity and antisocial conduct in British child psychiatric patients. *British Journal of Psychiatry*, 149, 760–77.

Thapar, A., Holmes, J., Poulton, K. & Harrington, R. (1999). Genetic basis of attention deficit and hyperactivity. *British Journal of Psychiatry*, 174, 105–11.

Thapar, A. & McGuffin, P. (1994). A twin study of depressive symptoms in childhood. *British Journal of Psychiatry*, 165, 259–65.

Thapar, A. & McGuffin, P. (1996). A twin study of antisocial and neurotic symptoms in childhood. *Psychological Medicine*, 26, 1111–18.

The Huntington's Disease Collaborative Research Group (1993). A novel gene containing a trinucleotide repeat that is expanded and unstable on Huntington's disease chromosomes. *Cell*, 72, 971–83.

Turner, E., Ewing, J., Shilling, P., et al. (1992). Lack of association between an RFLP near the D2 dopamine receptor gene and severe alcoholism. *Biological Psychiatry*, 31, 285–90.

Van Den Oord, E.J., Koot, H.M., Boomsma, D.I., Verhulst, F.C. & Orlebeke, J.F. (1995). A twin–singleton comparison of problem behaviour in 2–3-year-olds. *Journal of Child Psychology and Psychiatry*, 36, 449–58.

Van Tol, H.H., Wu, C.M., Guan, H.C., et al. (1992). Multiple dopamine D4 receptor variants in the human population. *Nature*, 358, 149–52.

Watt, D.C. & Edwards, J.H. (1991). Doubt about evidence for a schizophrenia gene on chromosome 5. *Psychological Medicine*, 21, 279–85.

Zahn-Waxler, C., Schmitz, S., Fulker, D., Robinson, J. & Emde, R. (1996). Behavior problems in 5-year-old monozygotic and dizygotic twins: genetic and environmental influences, patterns of regulation, and internalization of control. *Development and Psychopathology*, 8, 103–22.

Zoccolillo, M., Pickles, A., Quinton, D. & Rutter, M. (1992). The outcome of childhood conduct disorder: implications for defining adult personality disorder and conduct disorder. *Psychological Medicine*, 22, 971–88.

9

The role of neuropsychological deficits in conduct disorders

Donald R. Lynam and Bill Henry

Introduction

The idea of a link between the physical health of an individual's brain and his or her level of antisocial behaviour has been in the literature for centuries. Benjamin Rush (1812, cited in Elliott, 1978, p. 147) referred to the 'total perversion of the moral faculties' in people who displayed 'innate preternatural moral depravity'. Rush further suggested that 'there is probably an original defective organization in those parts of the body which are occupied by the moral faculties of the mind'. Since Rush's day, there have been numerous advances in our understanding of the human brain and in our ability to measure its functioning. Using this new information and technologies, scientists have worked to put more specific accounts of the 'neuropsychological hypothesis' to the scientific test.

In what is to follow, we examine the accumulated evidence for the relation between neuropsychology and conduct problems in children and adolescents. Specifically, we will demonstrate that antisocial behaviour is related to impairments in two specific domains of functioning: language-based verbal skills and 'executive' or self-control functions. Next, we will also examine several proximal and distal accounts that attempt to make sense of these relations. We will present in some detail a comprehensive, developmental theory that draws from research in neuropsychology, criminology, personality and development and that offers one of the most satisfying explanations. Finally, we will end with a discussion of the methodological and theoretical shortcomings of the present research and an outline for the future.

In what follows, we provide evidence for a link between neuropsychological health and conduct disorder. Before beginning our review, however, three caveats are in order. First, we conceive of conduct disorder as an extreme variant of antisocial behaviour. Thus, studies examining antisocial, aggressive, and delinquent children and adolescents are considered relevant. This is important because very few studies have dealt specifically with conduct disorder.

Therefore, we refer primarily to the syndrome of conduct problems throughout.

Second, it is difficult to unequivocally demonstrate causality in most areas of psychology; the area of conduct problems is no exception. To say that neuropsychological problems cause antisocial behaviour, three conditions must be met: (1) neuropsychological problems must be positively related to antisocial behaviour; (2) neuropsychological problems must precede the antisocial behaviour; and (3) it must be possible to rule out plausible alternative explanations of the relation (Rosenthal & Rosnow, 1991). Although no single study has successfully met all three conditions, it is our contention that, taken together, studies on the relation between neuropsychological health and antisocial behaviour suggest that neuropsychological deficits cause serious antisocial behaviour. All of the evidence to be reviewed in the pages that follow suggests that poorer neuropsychological health is associated with more severe antisocial behaviour; importantly, the effect sizes are in the moderate range and survive frequent, conservative controls for other variables. Additionally, several observational studies suggest that poor neuropsychological health is present before the onset of serious antisocial behaviour (Denno, 1990; Moffitt, 1993), and there are no studies that demonstrate the reverse sequence. Natural experiments in which individuals have sustained severe head injury also suggest that changes in neuropsychological status are associated with changes in antisocial status with the case of Phineas Gage being the best known. Finally, several studies have tested and ruled out viable third variable explanations of the relation (Lynam et al., 1993).

The third caveat concerns the heterogeneity of the samples. Most studies have used heterogeneous samples of mid-adolescent male delinquents as research subjects with little effort to distinguish late- from early-starters. Thus, subjects from one study may not be directly comparable to subjects from another study. Rather than invalidate our conclusions, however, we believe that this heterogeneity actually strengthens them; we agree with Robins (1978) that 'the more the populations studied differ, the wider the historical eras they span, the more the details of the methods vary, the more convincing becomes that replication' (p. 611). Nonetheless, whenever possible, we have attempted to identify from within this heterogeneous mix the most disordered individuals. The literature reveals clearly that the most consequential offenders begin earlier, commit a greater variety of offences, commit more serious offences, and are more likely to have co-occurring symptoms of hyperactivity, impulsivity and attention problems. The concept of hyperactivity (a pattern of restless, inattentive, and impulsive behaviour in childhood) has been in the medical literature since the early 1900s. Across the years, however, terminology and diagnostic criteria have changed greatly, because of these changes we will avoid specific diagnostic labels in our general discussion. Instead, we will refer to the syndrome of hyperactivity (i.e. hyperactivity, impulsivity and attention deficits) as HIA (Hyperactivity-Impulsivity-Attention).

Empirical evidence for a verbal deficit

One of the most robust correlates of severe conduct problems is impaired verbal ability. Verbal deficits have been found in conduct-disordered children, serious adolescent delinquents and adult criminals. Since Wechsler (1944) first remarked on the diagnostic utility of a Performance IQ score greater than a Verbal IQ score to identify delinquents, a multitude of studies has been published on the deficient verbal intelligence of antisocials. Prentice & Kelly (1963), West & Farrington (1973), Moffitt (1990a), and Moffitt & Lynam (1994) have all provided comprehensive literature reviews with increasing numbers of studies in each review and with few disconfirming reports. In fact, the finding of decreased verbal ability in antisocials continues to find support (Fergusson et al., 1996; Lahey et al., 1995; Lynam et al., 1993; Moffitt et al., 1994; Walsh et al., 1987; Werry et al., 1987). It is important to note that the differences between antisocials and nonantisocials remain even after controlling for potential confounds, such as race (Lynam et al., 1993; Short & Strodtbeck, 1965; Wolfgang et al., 1972), socioeconomic status (Lynam et al., 1993, Moffitt et al., 1981; Reiss & Rhodes, 1961; Wolfgang et al., 1972), academic attainment (Denno, 1989; Lynam et al., 1993), test motivation (Lynam et al., 1993) and the differential detection of low-IQ delinquents (Moffitt & Silva, 1988a). The robustness of delinquents' deficient VIQs (especially relative to their near-normal PIQs), has been taken as strongly supporting a specific deficit in language manipulation. Because language functions are subserved by the left cerebral hemisphere in almost all individuals, these findings have also been interpreted as evidence for dysfunction of the left cerebral hemisphere.

In addition to studies utilizing IQ tests, studies using more standard neuropsychological tests have also provided evidence for specific verbal deficits in antisocials. For example, Karniski et al. (1982) tested 54 teenaged incarcerated boys using 29 tasks that were collapsed on a rational basis into six composite measures of 'neuromaturation, gross motor function, temporal-sequential organization, visual processing, and auditory-language function'. A comparison group consisted of 51 boys from schools in a predominantly blue-collar community. Notable group differences were obtained for two of the composite measures: visual processing and auditory language function, but differences were greatest for the auditory language area. When the tails of the distribution were examined, 29.6% of the delinquents, but only 2% of the comparison boys, scored two or more standard deviations below the comparison group's mean score on language skills. Other studies have provided similar results (Berman & Siegal, 1976; Sobotowicz et al., 1987; Wolff et al., 1982).

The strongest support for a specific language deficit in conduct disorder, however, comes from the series of reports from a longitudinal project in New Zealand. The New Zealand sample consists of a birth cohort of over 1000 subjects who have been studied extensively from birth to age 21 through comprehensive, bi-annual assessments. Importantly, when the subjects were 13 years old, they were administered a comprehensive neuropsychological assessment battery. This battery yielded five theoretically meaningful factors (Moffitt & Henry, 1989): (1) verbal, (2) visual-spatial, (3) verbal memory, (4) visual-motor integration, and (5) mental flexibility. This study is an important one for the field because it was designed to correct many of the flaws of previous research, and to provide an 'acid test' for the neuropsychological hypothesis (see Moffitt, 1988). The neuropsychological findings from this study have been reported in several articles to date (Frost et al., 1989; Moffitt, 1990a, b; Moffitt & Henry, 1989; Moffitt et al., 1994; Moffitt & Silva, 1988a, b, c; White et al., 1989, 1990). Because of the importance of this study, several of the most important findings will be reviewed here.

One of the major findings from this study has been that boys with severe conduct problems, particularly those with comorbid HIA, are the most neuropsychologically impaired (Moffitt & Silva, 1988c). These impairments occur primarily on the verbal, and verbal memory factors. (The combination of conduct problems and HIA predicts an especially poor outcome. Boys with both types of problems tend to be more antisocial in terms of variety, seriousness and frequency of antisocial actions, are more likely to persist in their antisocial behaviour through adolescence and into adulthood, and are more likely to receive diagnoses of antisocial personality disorder. See Lynam (1996) for a complete review.) When Moffitt (1990b) examined the developmental trajectories of these boys and boys with only conduct problems or only HIA from age 3 to age 15, the comorbid cases were found to have histories of extreme antisocial behaviour that remained stable across this period. Their neuropsychological problems were as long-standing as their antisocial behaviour. At ages 3 and 5, these boys had scored more than a standard deviation below the age-norm for boys on the Bayley and McCarthy tests of motor coordination; at each age (5, 7, 9, 11 and 13), these boys scored a more than 3/4 of a standard deviation below the age-norm for boys on verbal IQ.

Moffitt et al. (1994) demonstrated the ability of deficits in neuropsychological functioning at 13 to predict antisocial behaviour in later adolescence. (Late adolescence (15–18) represents the peak prevalence of involvement in anti-social behaviour. Given the large number of individuals involved in antisocial acts at this time, the ability of neuropsychological variables to predict involvement is especially noteworthy.) Whether antisocial behaviour was measured with self-reports, police reports, or court reports, the poorer a boy's neuropsychological functioning at age 13, the more likely he was to have committed crimes at age 18. Neuropsychological status also related to the ages of first police contact and first conviction. The strongest relations were obtained on the verbal and verbal memory factors of the test battery, and the results held despite controlling for socioeconomic status; zero-order correlations ranged from 0.13 to 0.38. Particularly interesting in this study was the effect that neuropsychological status had on the persistence of offending across time. Not only did scores on verbal and verbal memory factors relate to the early onset of offending, they also related to the persistence of offending across time. Boys who were delinquent at 13 and who scored poorly on the neuropsychological battery were the most delinquent at ages 15 and 18. For example, the 45 boys who had 'high' delinquency and 'poor' neuropsychological status at age 13 self-reported significantly more offenses that their peers at age 18, 0.70 S.D. more than the male average. Although those 45 boys constituted only 12% of the 375 males in the age-13 sample, they accounted for 46% of the 251 juvenile offenses on record and for 59% of the 255 convictions in juvenile and adult court.

The relation between poor verbal ability and the persistence of antisocial behaviour has also been found among children with diagnoses of conduct disorder. Lahey et al. (1995) examined factors related to the persistence of conduct disorder across four years in a relatively large, prospective study of clinic-referred boys. As expected, low verbal IQ was related to conduct disorder at Time 1. More importantly, low verbal IQ was related to the persistence of CD over time, particularly when VIQ was considered in conjunction with a parental history of Antisocial Personality Disorder; only boys with above average VIQ and without a parental history of APD improved across time. Similarly, Farrington & Hawkins (1991) found that low VIQ at age 8–10 predicted persistence in crime after the 21st birthday (phi = 0.23) even after controlling for several other predictors (see also Fergusson et al., 1996).

In the end, poor verbal ability, as indexed by low VIQ and other more specific neuropsychological measures, is associated with relatively severe and persistent conduct problems in childhood and adolescence. There is also evidence that poor verbal ability may be especially related to the comorbidity of conduct problems and HIA – a combination with a particularly poor prognosis (see Lynam, 1996).

Empirical evidence for executive dysfunctions

Verbal deficits are not the only neuropsychological correlates of antisocial behaviour. Antisocial behaviour has also been found to be associated with deficiencies in the brain's self-control or 'executive' functions which include operations such as sustaining attention and concentration, abstract reasoning and concept formation, formulating goals, anticipating and planning, programming and initiating purposive sequences of behaviour, and inhibiting unsuccessful, inappropriate, or impulsive behaviours. Evidence of the relation between executive deficits and conduct problems has been found among incarcerated subjects, among non-conduct-disordered subjects in laboratory situations, and among general-population samples. This relationship holds when controlling for IQ, and, as will be described later, appears to be especially strong for a subgroup of offenders characterized by both antisocial behaviour and symptoms of HIA.

Several studies that have applied batteries of formal tests of executive functions to delinquent subjects have now shown that the test scores can discriminate between antisocial and nonantisocial adolescents (see Henry & Moffitt, 1997; Moffitt, 1990a; Moffitt & Henry, 1991, for reviews). In addition, there is some evidence that the persistent and impulsive behaviours characteristic of conduct-disordered children and adults with antisocial personality disorder may be associated with executive deficits, particularly in attention modulation (Newman, 1987; Newman & Kosson, 1986; Raine, 1988; Shapiro et al., 1988).

Several studies have applied frontal lobe batteries to delinquent subjects. For example, Skoff & Libon (1987) compared the scores of 22 incarcerated delinquents to published test norms for the Wisconsin Card Sort Test (WCST), Porteus Mazes, Trails B, Verbal Fluency, and four additional executive tasks. One-third of their subjects scored in the impaired range on the battery as a whole. Similarly, the WCST, Verbal Fluency, Trails B, Mazes, and the Rey Osterreith Complex Figure Test were administered to a general-population sample in New Zealand (Moffitt & Henry, 1989). Multivariate analysis of variance demonstrated that a linear combination of these executive test scores significantly discriminated self-reported early delinquents from nondelinquents. This effect was most robust among the subgroup of delinquents who exhibited co-occurring HIA; differences between this comorbid group and nondisordered controls ranged from two-thirds to over one standard deviation. Furthermore, the effects remained even after controlling statistically for overall IQ (see also Lynam, 1998).

Other studies, while not focusing specifically upon executive functions, have reported data from individual measures typically included in frontal lobe batteries. Berman & Siegal (1976) found that delinquents scored poorly on the Category Test and Trails B. Wolff et al. (1982) reported delinquency-related impairments on tests of selective attention and on the Stroop Color Word Test. Five studies have shown delinquents to score poorly on various tests requiring sequencing of motor behaviour (Brickman et al., 1984; Hurwitz et al., 1972; Karniski et al., 1982; Lueger & Gill, 1990; Miller et al., 1980).

Recently, several investigators have employed more sophisticated measures, such as the Self-Ordered Pointing (SOP; Petrides & Milner, 1982) task and the Conditional Association Task (CAT; Petrides, 1985), to investigate the relation between aggression and frontal lobe functions. The SOP presents subjects with different arrangements of the same set of stimuli and forces the subject to choose a different stimulus on each trial until all stimuli have been selected; the SOP requires subjects to actively consider previous selections as they prepare their next response. On the CAT, subjects must learn associations between two sets of stimuli. Positron emission topography studies have found that the SOP is specifically associated with the mid dorsolateral frontal region, whereas the CAT is specifically associated with the posterior dorsolateral frontal region (Petrides et al., 1993). Lau et al. (1995) found that poor performance on these two measures was associated with aggression in a laboratory setting. However, Giancola & Zeichner (1994) reported that only performance on the CAT was associated with intensity of shocks administered to a fictitious opponent in a laboratory setting. This suggests that only deficits in the posterior dorsolateral region are associated with aggression. Lau & Pihl (1994) also found that performance on the SOP did not predict aggression above and beyond the CAT.

As was the case for verbal deficits, the evidence suggests that poor executive functioning may be especially characteristic of the most antisocial group – boys with symptoms of conduct problems and HIA. In the New Zealand study, adolescent boys who exhibited symptoms of both conduct disorder and HIA scored more poorly on neuropsychological tests of executive functions than their peers who had either CD or HIA alone (Moffitt & Henry, 1989; Moffitt & Silva, 1988c). In a companion study of executive functions and conduct problems in the Pittsburgh Youth Study (White et al., 1994), data were gathered on 'self-control and impulsivity' using multiple tests and measures for 430 12-year-old boys. The impulsivity measures were strongly related to delinquency at two ages even after controlling for IQ and SES (s = 0.38 and 0.43); additionally, these measures were related to the 3-year longevity of antisocial behaviour, even after controlling for initial levels of delinquency (s = 0.15). In a separate study, Aronowitz et al. (1994) reported that adolescents with both CD and HIA performed more poorly on measures of executive function than did CD-only adolescents.

In addition to these documented cross-sectional relations, recent longitudinal studies have demonstrated that executive function deficits are associated with the stability and continuity of conduct problems. Seguin et al. (1995) found that boys who exhibited a stable pattern of aggression between the ages of 6 and 12 performed significantly more poorly on measures of executive functions than did unstable aggressive or nonaggressive boys.

Taken together, these studies suggest that neuropsychological dysfunctions that manifest themselves as poor scores on tests of self-control are linked with the early onset of conduct disorder, and with its subsequent persistence. Additionally, the findings in regard to the group comorbid for HIA and conduct problems are of considerable interest in light of Lynam's (1996) suggestion that the co-occurrence of CD and hyperactivity/inattention may represent a distinct subtype of conduct disorder which is particularly severe and persistent, and which places the child at risk for serious antisocial behaviour in adolescence and adulthood.

An emerging area of research using neuroimaging techniques to examine patterns of brain functioning associated with antisocial behaviour deserves brief mention. Researchers have employed methods that assess both the structural (e.g. computerized tomography, magnetic resonance imaging) and functional (e.g. positron emission tomography, single photon emission computed tomography) characteristics of the brains of antisocial individuals (for a full review, see Henry & Moffitt, 1997). Results varied across studies, but where significant findings did emerge, they generally involved dysfunction in the temporal and frontal regions among offenders, a pattern supportive of results found in studies using performance tests. Interestingly, studies using measures of brain structure and brain function have yielded a different pattern of results. Studies of brain structure (Hucker et al., 1986, 1988; Langevin et al., 1987, 1988, 1989a, b; Tonkonogy, 1991; Wright et al., 1990) tend to find a relationship between temporal lobe abnormalities and antisocial behaviour; studies of brain function (Goyer et al., 1994; Hendricks et al., 1988; Raine et al., 1994b; Volkow et al., 1995) tend to highlight the role of the frontal region. However, this literature is far from complete. Reliance on small sample sizes, failure to consistently use noncriminal control groups, and use of a wide variety of types of offenders precludes the drawing of any firm conclusions. The very tentative suggestion is that the results of neuroimaging studies are consistent with results from performance tests of neuropsychological function. However, the two literatures are not integrated, and much future research is needed to more fully explore these issues.

Theoretical accounts of the relations between neuropsychological dysfunction and antisocial behaviour

Although much research has been directed at documenting the nature and strength of the relation, less research has been done towards understanding how neuropsychological deficits exert their effects. It seems most likely that there are both direct and indirect effects, as well as proximal and distal effects.

Several theories have been advanced to account for the relation between poor verbal ability and antisocial behaviour. For example, A.R. Luria (1961; Luria & Homskaya, 1964) outlined a comprehensive theory of the importance of normal language for the self-control of behaviour. According to Luria, normal auditory verbal memory and verbal abstract reasoning are essential abilities in the development of self-control, and they influence the success of socialization beginning with the earliest parent–child interactions. Language-based mechanisms of self-control range from virtually automatic motor programming for inhibiting simple childhood behaviours ('No!') to 'thinking things through' before embarking on a course of complex adult behaviour. Similarly, Wilson & Herrnstein (1985) suggest that low verbal intelligence contributes to a present-oriented cognitive style which, in turn, fosters irresponsible and exploitative behaviour. In his autonomic conditioning theory of antisocial behaviour, Eysenck (1977) speculates that stimulus generalization should be enhanced when parents verbally label their children's various misbehaviours as 'naughty', 'bad', or 'wicked'. But children with verbal deficits might not profit from the labelling of a class of behaviours as punishment-attracting; rather, they may have to learn by trial and error that each individual act is wrong. Normal language development is thus an essential ingredient in prosocial processes such as delaying gratification, anticipating consequences, and linking belated punishments with earlier transgressions.

In yet another account, Savitsky & Czyzewski (1978) speculate that a deficit in verbal skills may preclude children's ability to label their perceptions of the emotions expressed by others (victims or adversaries). Such deficiencies might also limit children's response options in threatening or ambiguous social situations, predisposing them to quick physical reactions rather than to more laborious verbal ones. As such, children who feel uncomfortable with verbal modes of communication may be more likely to strike out than to talk their way out of difficulties with others. This discussion is in line with work by Dodge and his colleagues. These researchers found that not only do aggressive children have a tendency to make hostile attributions in the face of ambiguous cues (Dodge et al., 1986), but these children also tend to generate fewer verbal solutions and more direct, action-oriented solutions in response to social problems (Lochman et al., 1989).

Sociological accounts emphasize the potentially indirect effects of poor verbal ability on antisocial behaviour through school achievement. For example, Hirschi's (1969) version of social control theory suggests that differences in intellectual capacity will have implications for how children experience school, a crucial agent in deterring children and adolescents from delinquency. Cognitively able students are likely to experience school as rewarding and valuable and will be more likely to develop bonds to the school and therefore will be more likely to refrain from delinquency. On the other hand, less able students will experience school as frustrating and unimportant. These less able students who do not care what their teachers think of them, who do not care about getting good grades, who do not spend much time on homework, who do not have high aspirations for the future, and who do not want to be in school will, by virtue of their weak attachment to school, be more likely to deviate. Similarly, strain theory (Cloward & Ohlin, 1960) also predicts that unpleasant school experiences and school failure, which are made more likely by poor verbal ability, are important precursors to antisocial behaviour.

Multiple theorists have also speculated on the processes by which executive deficits contribute to antisocial behaviour. In fact, one historical rationale for neuropsychological research with delinquents was the apparent resemblance between criminal behaviour and the disinhibited, antisocial symptoms of patients with injury to the frontal lobes of the brain (Elliott, 1978; see also Elliott, 1992). Several authors (Gorenstein, 1982; Pontius, 1972; Yeudall, 1980) have developed theories based on the observed similarity between the behaviour of delinquents and 'pseudopsychopathic' patients with frontal lobe brain injuries. The major features of the 'pseudopsychopathic syndrome' seen following trauma to the orbital frontal lobes include: facetiousness, sexual and personal hedonism, disinhibition, lack of judgement, impulsivity, irritability and absence of concern for others (Blumer & Benson, 1975). Gorenstein & Newman (1980) described functional similarities between disinhibited antisocial human behaviour and experimental animal models of damage to the structures of the frontal lobes and limbic system of the brain. More recently, Newman and colleagues (Newman & Wallace, 1993; Patterson & Newman, 1993) have extended this model, further clarifying the nature of 'disinhibitory psychopathology' (see also Quay, 1993). Newman & Wallace (1993) argued that disinhibitory psychopathology is based in deficiencies in 'response modulation' and 'self regulation'. Response modulation is described as an automatic process involving the suspension of an ongoing behavioural response in order to assimilate feedback. In contrast, self-regulation is viewed as a controlled process, and is described as the 'controlled examination of one's behaviour'. In sum, Newman and colleagues suggest that deficiencies in response modulation curtail an individual's capacity to pause in response to cues for punishment, and thus make self-regulation impossible. This process ultimately results in the failure of avoidance learning – learning to avoid behaviours which result in punishment.

Finally Lau et al. (1995) advanced a model of the mechanisms linking executive deficits and aggression. According to this model, frontal lobe deficits may interfere with the linkage between specific stimulus characteristics and pre-established rules for responding. In the absence of this linkage, the individual is unable to bring these response rules to bear on the regulation of behaviour. Instead, behaviour is governed by the immediate stimulus. Thus, under conditions of provocation or perceived threat, the rules that would normally act to inhibit aggressive responding are ineffective, and impulsive/ aggressive responses will emerge.

Many of the above perspectives are extremely proximal, nondevelopmental accounts. They emphasize the influence of poor neuropsychological health on antisocial behaviour in the very moment of its occurrence. For example, the child with verbal deficits will rely more heavily on physical modes for resolving conflict and getting his needs met. Similarly, the child with deficits in executive functioning, upon seeing something that he wants, will rashly grab it without reflecting on the possible consequences. These accounts apply equally well to the 6-year-old who beats up a peer on the playground as to the 25-year-old who shoots a peer in a bar. Additionally, these explanations fail to account for the increase in the severity of antisocial behaviour across time (Loeber, 1988). To take account of the increase in severity, these explanations would have to suggest that the neuropsychological deficit worsens across time; in fact, the temporal progression of neuropsychological problems is often one of amelioration. Some other process must be at work.

Moffitt (1993) has written extensively about the more distal and developmental effects of neuropsychological deficits. In her developmental taxonomy,

she differentiated between adolescent-limited offenders, whose antisocial behaviour is relatively late onset, and who are likely to desist offending upon
entering adulthood; and life-course persistent offenders, whose antisocial tendencies become apparent early in childhood, who account for a disproportionately large percentage of all criminal activity, and who are likely to continue
offending throughout adulthood. The key difference between these two groups
is thought to lie in the distinct developmental trajectories leading to each type
of antisocial outcome. Life-course persistent offenders are thought to be
characterized by early emerging neuropsychological deficits which set in
motion a series of social and academic failures. The cumulative effect of the
neuropsychological deficits and the consequent social and academic failures
results in a pattern of undercontrolled, explosive behaviour which persists
across the life course.

In Moffitt's theory, the development of LCP antisocial behaviour begins
with some prenatal, postnatal, or inherited factor capable of producing individual differences in the neuropsychological health of the infant nervous system.
Although we believe the most important neuropsychological functions to be
the verbal and executive functions, few of the developmental studies that we
discuss have made distinctions between different kinds of neuropsychological
problems. The studies have examined low birth weight children, children with
nonspecific neurological 'soft signs', children with 'minimal brain dysfunction',
and children with focal deficits. Thus, it is impossible to make statements about
'executive functioning' and early development; instead we speak more generally of 'poor neuropsychological health'. Whatever the genesis of poor
neuropsychological health, its presence is likely to be associated with a variety
of consequences for cognitive, motor, affective and personality development.
Commonly reported behavioural consequences of poor neuropsychological
health include poor motor coordination, attention problems, hyperactivity,
impulsivity, language problems and learning disabilities (Rutter, 1983; Thomas
& Chess, 1977). For example, Hertzig (1983) examined the neurological health
of 66 low birth weight infants from intact middle class families, some with focal
deficits and others with diffuse soft signs. Neurological impairments were
related to an index of difficult temperament taken at ages 1, 2 and 3. Thus, the
earliest manifestation of poor neuropsychological health may be a difficult
temperament.

This difficult temperament is translated into undercontrolled and more
overtly antisocial behaviour through interactions with the social environment,
primarily through a series of failed parent–child encounters. To explain this,
Moffitt draws on the notion of evocative person–environment interactions

(Caspi & Bem, 1990) which are evident when an individual's behaviour evokes characteristic reactions from the environment that may serve to reinforce the original behaviour. Difficult-to-manage children evoke typical reactions from parents that include harsh and erratic parental discipline (Lytton, 1990), reduction of parental efforts at socialization (Buss, 1981; Maccoby & Jacklin, 1983), and increases in permissiveness for later aggression (Olweus, 1980). All of these reactions are more likely to exacerbate than ameliorate the child's existing tendencies. For example, Henry et al. (1996) found that difficult temperament in infancy interacted with inconsistent parenting to produce convictions in young adulthood.

Work by Patterson and his colleagues (e.g. Patterson, 1982; Patterson et al., 1991) has explicitly demonstrated the potential reinforcing effects of evoked parental behaviour on child misbehaviour. In micro-analyses of interactional behaviour, these investigators have shown that children's oppositional behaviours (e.g. temper tantrums) often provoke and force adult family members to counter with highly punitive and angry responses. As the child, in turn, escalates his/her own aversive behaviour, parents eventually withdraw from these interactions, ceding to the child's demands and reinforcing evermore aversive behaviour. Moffitt suggests that this coercive style of interacting with parents may generalize; that is, this aversive interactional style, learned through interactions with the parent, may become a dominant mode of response outside the family as well. Patterson (1986) has provided evidence that children who coerce one family member are likely to be coercive with other family members as well.

These difficult children would pose challenges to the most capable and resourceful parents. Unfortunately, these children are not randomly assigned to home environments; some of the possible sources of the original neuropsychological difficulties are linked to parental actions, behaviour and characteristics (e.g. drug abuse, poor pre- and postnatal nutrition, lack of stimulation/affection, physical abuse and neglect; and the genetic transmission of impulsivity or irritability). Thus, the most difficult children are born to parents that are the least capable of resisting evocative pressures and adequately socializing the children.

Once a child begins his antisocial journey, he is kept to his path by two types of 'life-course consequences': contemporary consequences and cumulative consequences. Contemporary continuity arises when an individual carries with him into his later life-phases the same traits that got him into trouble earlier. An undercontrolled child may exhibit angry outbursts and aggression toward his peers, resulting in peer rejection and generally hostile relationships with peers.

These same angry outbursts as an adult may alienate employers, coworkers, and intimate others, resulting in the inability to maintain a job or relationship. Similarly, acting on the spur of the moment or without thinking things through will result in difficulties throughout life. Cumulative continuity operates when early behaviour structures future outcomes and opportunities and sets in motion a snowball effect that keeps the individual to this ill-started path. For example, the undercontrolled child who drops out of school may be limited to high-stress, frustrating, low-wage jobs; the resultant frustration and stress may then contribute to the individual's continued participation in criminal behaviour (Caspi et al., 1987). Moffitt identifies two particular sources of cumulative continuity: (1) the development of a restricted behavioural repertoire and (2) the ensnarement by consequences of antisocial behaviour. Antisocial and undercontrolled children miss out on opportunities to learn about and practice prosocial alternatives. Similarly, these children are more likely to make poor decisions that diminish the probability of later success; for example, teenaged parenthood, drug addiction, a criminal record, and spotty work history close the doors of legitimate opportunity.

Although Moffitt's theory focuses on large-scale mechanisms of development operating at the behavioural level, we would note that the development of particular brain systems must also be considered. Schore (1996) described the ways in which the regulatory systems of the orbital prefrontal cortex mature over the first two years of life. Most importantly, Schore argues that this maturation is experience dependent. Specifically, periods of intense stress during the first two years of life are thought to result in structural and functional deficits in the affect-regulating systems of the frontal lobes. This hypothesis is particularly interesting in light of the earlier evidence reviewed regarding the role of frontal deficits in the etiology of antisocial behaviour. If an infant is reared in a disorganized home, in which the caregiver is insensitive to the child's stressful experiences, that child may emerge from the first two years of life with self-regulatory deficits which place him/her at risk for antisocial outcomes. In this case, the risk may be two-fold: The risk represented by frontal deficits will be superimposed over the risk represented by being reared in a disorganized home environment.

There is accumulating evidence for Moffitt's taxonomy and her developmental system. Jeglum-Bartusch et al. (1997) identified two latent factors underlying antisocial behaviour from childhood to late adolescence. The first factor, related to early antisocial behaviour (ages 5, 7, 9 and 11), was most strongly correlated with low verbal ability, hyperactivity and negative/impulsive personality. On the other hand, the second factor, related to adolescent delinquency (ages 13 and 15), was most strongly correlated with peer delinquency. These findings were replicated across parent-, self- and teacher-ratings.

Moffitt et al. (1996) also provided support for the developmental theory. Using parent-, teacher- and self-reports of antisocial behaviour from ages 5 to 18, these authors formed and examined the developmental correlates of five groups of boys: Life-course Persistents (LCP), Adolescent-Limiteds (AL), Abstainers, Recoverers and Unclassifieds. LCP and AL boys differed from other groups on a variety of indices. Importantly, however, LCP and AL boys differed from each other on several theoretically meaningful measures. For example, at ages 3 and 5, relative to AL boys, LCP boys were rated by observers as more emotionally labile, restless, negative, wilful, rougher in play, and as having shorter attention spans; in short, LCP boys were more likely to demonstrate difficult temperaments in early childhood. In accord with Moffitt's theorizing, although AL and LCP boys did not differ in general delinquency during adolescence, LCP boys were much more likely to have been convicted of a violent offence by age 18; 25% of the LCP boys had been convicted of a violent offence compared to only 8% of AL boys. LCP boys also self-reported 'psychopathic' personalities; they described themselves as unconventional, impulsive, willing to take advantage of others, suspicious and callous. Finally, LCP boys tended to have experienced more 'snares' than other boys; they were more likely to report feeling distant from their families and were more likely to have dropped out of school.

Gender differences

Any account of conduct disorder must address the issue of gender differences. The DSM–IV (American Psychiatric Association, 1994) reports that the prevalence of conduct disorder is 2–3 times higher in males than it is in females. If one considers only cases of early onset conduct disorder, this discrepancy is even higher, and higher still if one considers the antisocial group comorbid with HIA. Gender differences extend to delinquency as well (Farrington, 1987); whether measured by official court and police records or self-report inventories, the prevalence and incidence of delinquent behaviour is higher among males than among females. Additionally these gender differences are found in both white and black populations, and are greatest for more serious offences.

The developmental theory outlined above offers a straightforward account of the gender difference in conduct disorder. This account suggests that neuropsychological problems contribute to antisocial behaviour in the same way for males as for females, but further suggests that males are at greater risk of conduct disorder because they are at greater risk of neuropsychological problems. Although we could identify no studies that specifically report on executive functioning, there is substantial evidence that males are at increased risk for birth complications and a host of neurodevelopmental disorders, including mental retardation, autism and learning disabilities (Raz et al., 1994). There is also evidence that females show more plasticity in development and are more capable than males of recovering from brain insult in general (Witelson, 1977). Raz et al. (1995) examined the cognitive development of a group of children who had experienced intracranial haemorrhage in association with premature birth. At age 4, girls performed significantly better than boys on measures of intelligence. Working with adult populations following neuro-surgical procedures, Lansdell (1989) reported that females showed greater recovery of cognitive ability than did males. These results suggest that males are at greater risk for persistent, neuropsychological difficulties which may lead to increased rates of conduct disorder. Unfortunately, direct tests of this account have not been conducted, in part, because studies of the relation between neuropsychological problems and antisocial behaviour in females are virtually nonexistent.

A second account of gender differences, not unique to the developmental account, emphasizes the differential socialization of males and females. For example, power-control theory (Hagan et al., 1985) attempts to account for gender differences in delinquency by arguing that greater pressure to conform to social norms is brought to bear on females than on males. According to this perspective, males have the 'freedom to deviate' – that is, undercontrolled behaviour exhibited by males is more likely to be tolerated than the same behaviour exhibited by females. Thus, when males begin to engage in delin-quent behaviour, less social pressure is exerted by parents and teachers to inhibit that behaviour. However, undercontrolled behaviour exhibited by females is likely to elicit a strenuous response directed toward modifying that behaviour. Similarly, Keenan & Shaw (1997) have recently argued that social influences and developmental differences between boys and girls (in biological, language and social-emotional development) work together to influence the course of early behaviour problems. These authors suggest that there is little difference between boys and girls in early behaviour problems; as time goes by, however, developmental differences and social influence serve to either ameli-orate or shape girls' behaviour problems into less aggressive forms.

Future directions

Research from a variety of perspectives has yielded a coherent picture of the relation between neuropsychological functioning and conduct problems.

Theoretical groundwork has been laid to allow understanding of these relations. However, the field is not without its complexities, and there are clear
directions for the field. Some of these future directions involve overcoming
existing shortcomings in the empirical literature. Other directions require
extending current theoretical and empirical work in new directions. We will
discuss both types of directions, beginning with how to address existing
methodological shortcomings.

Samples

First, a major difficulty in interpreting research on conduct problems lies in
attaining homogeneous samples. Individuals likely to receive a diagnosis of
conduct disorder represent a very heterogeneous group, and many previous
studies have used samples of convenience with unknown characteristics. Previous studies have lumped together different kinds of children with conduct
problems; this is especially true in studies of adolescent offenders. Samples of
adolescents will include children who began offending early in childhood and
children who did not offend until adolescence; these two types of offenders are
not easily discriminable in adolescence (see Moffitt et al., 1996). However,
these two types of adolescent offenders have different developmental trajectories and different psychological profiles; neuropsychological deficits are likely
more characteristic of the early starters than of the late starters. Lumping these
two types of offenders together will make a large difference (between early
starters and controls) seem small (the difference between adolescent offenders
and controls).

In addition to neglecting the distinction between early and late starters,
much previous research has failed to distinguish between boys with conduct
problems and comorbid HIA and boys without HIA. HIA and CP have been
found to co-occur in 30–50% of cases in both epidemiological (Anderson et al.,
1987; Szatmari et al., 1989) and clinical samples (Biederman et al., 1987; Loney,
1987). Failure to assess HIA symptomatology may be a particularly problematic
oversight for several reasons. First, given that several clinical studies have
found that children with HIA have deficits on a range of executive neuropsychological measures (Carte et al., 1996), it is possible that the relation
between CP and neuropsychological problems is spurious. The existing studies,
however, are not sufficient to demonstrate this possibility, because almost
without exception, these studies of children with HIA have failed to control for
comorbid conduct problems. Thus, it is equally likely that the relation between
neuropsychological problems and HIA is spurious.

A few studies have included children with HIA, CP and both types of
problems. These studies point to the second problem with the failure to

consider the overlap of HIA and CP: the group with both types of problems is the most neuropsychologically impaired. In fact, two studies suggest that neuropsychological deficits are unique to the comorbid group. As discussed earlier, Moffitt & Henry (1989) examined the frontal lobe functioning of four groups of children in the New Zealand cohort: HIA/CP, CP-only, HIA-only, and non-HIA-CP comparison subjects. They found that executive deficits were unique to the group comorbid for HIA and CP. More recently, Lynam (1998) examined the performance of four groups of children from the Pittsburgh Youth Study; he also found that the comorbid group, relative to CP-only, HIA-only and non-HIA-CP groups, was uniquely impaired on four measures of executive functioning. It may be that the deficits reportedly linked to HIA and CP are actually linked to the comorbid group. Because the comorbid group is clearly the most antisocial (see Lynam, 1996), failure to consider the comorbidity of HIA and CP may actually underestimate the true relation between neuropsychological problems and serious antisocial behaviour.

Control variables and control groups

A second set of methodological limitations in this area revolve around the issues of equating comparison groups on one or more variables and the nature of the comparison groups used. Some studies have not consistently matched the control and experimental groups on variables which are known to influence performance on neuropsychological tasks, i.e. race, age and previous substance use. On the other hand, some studies control for variables that may not be necessary. For example, some authors have included education in their lists of relevant control variables (Hare, 1984; Hart et al., 1990). Excluding subjects who failed to achieve a certain level of education can lead to two problems: firstly, such designs may exclude neuropsychologically impaired subjects, thus throwing the baby out with the bathwater. Secondly, such designs may create a select and unrepresentative sample of prisoners, thus compromising generalization. Requiring that subjects meet a minimum level of reading ability may have the same confounding effects as requiring a minimum level of education.

Finally, many studies have failed to include informative control groups. Some studies compared offenders with nonoffenders, while others compared one type of offender (e.g. sex offenders) with a different type of offender (e.g. property offenders). While a case may be made for either of these control groups depending on the hypotheses of the study, inclusion of both control groups will advance most quickly our knowledge of the relation between neuropsychological functioning and antisocial behaviour.

Tasks

A third methodological limitation has to do with the nature of the tasks used to assess neuropsychological deficit. Although performance measures of neuro-psychological functioning are sensitive to gross deficits, many lack the sensitivity necessary to more precisely identify the nature of that deficit. There are some promising exceptions, however; both the Self-Ordered Pointing (SOP) task and the Conditional Association Task (CAT) represent sophisticated advances in performance measures. Additionally, the recent emergence of imaging technologies has provided the opportunity to synthesize findings from these studies with findings from studies using neuropsychological performance measures. Such efforts can contribute to the construct validation of these performance measures, and assist in the localization of test scores to specific brain regions and systems. It is clear that speaking of antisocial behaviour being related to 'frontal lobe deficits' is at best a crude description. Utilizing both performance measures and imaging techniques may assist in developing a much more precise, fine-grained understanding of this relationship.

Additionally, many studies have administered large batteries of neuro-psychological tests to small numbers of subjects and then gone on to compare the groups on many of the individual tests. This procedure is problematic in several ways. Firstly, the large number of comparisons will lead to a large increase in the likelihood of making at least one Type I error – wrongly rejecting the null hypothesis of no difference. Secondly, the small number of subjects reduces the power of individual comparisons and increases the likelihood of making a Type II error – failing to reject the null hypothesis of no difference between groups when there is a difference. Finally, because many neuropsychological tests were designed as clinical 'sign tests' to distinguish cases of severe brain trauma or injury from normals, the sensitivity of these instruments may be limited; that is, they may be unreliable measures of the full range of individual differences in neuropsychological functioning. This insensitivity will reduce the power to detect subtle effects. These problems can be overcome by including more subjects, employing more reliable and sensitive measures, and by aggregating data from several indices into theoretical or empirical composites.

Prospective studies

Finally, the majority of the studies reviewed here have been cross-sectional and focused on either adolescents or adults. Prospective studies of children with conduct disorder or HIA would help to further clarify the role of these deficits in the onset of antisocial behaviour. In addition, recent research has highlighted the relation between antisocial outcomes and infant characteristics such as perinatal problems (Kandel & Mednick, 1991; Raine et al., 1994*a*) and difficult toddler temperament (Henry et al., 1996; Tremblay et al., 1994). Prospective studies will also provide information that is lacking about the specific infant characteristics that are linked to specific neuropsychological deficits. Studies of young children will contribute to an understanding of the neuropsychological correlates of temperament, thus possibly allowing these disparate fields to be linked.

Theory development

There are also theoretical directions that need to be pursued. These directions include moving toward more directed theory testing, increased theorizing on the specific brain mechanisms involved, and examination of some open issues. There seems little doubt that there exists a correlation between poor neuro-psychological health and antisocial behaviour; it also seems likely that the causal relation runs from poor neuropsychological health to antisocial behav-iour. Although theories abound, what is less well demonstrated is how these neuropsychological deficits exert their effects. Do they do so directly via deficient self-control and/or indirectly via school failure? What is the nature of the proximal and distal relations? We urge researchers to move beyond merely documenting the relation and onto testing theoretical formulations. This theory testing should involve testing both proximal and distal mechanisms. Ideally, to move us most quickly, this research will employ the method of strong inference and test various formulations against one another.

Additionally, more specific theories regarding the effects of the neuro-psychological deficits on behaviour are needed. That is, researchers on conduct problems should attend to research being conducted in basic neuropsychology. For example, Petrides (1995) has put forth a two-level model of the involve-ment of the mid-lateral frontal cortex in memory. Specifically, he argues that mid-dorsolateral frontal cortex is responsible for the active monitoring in working memory; this process involves monitoring and manipulating several pieces of information on the basis of task requirements or the person's current plans. On the other hand, the ventrolateral frontal cortex is critical for strategic encoding and retrieval of specific information held in long-term memory; it is thus important for selecting, comparing, or deciding on information held in short-term and long-term memory. Perhaps what happens for antisocial per-sons with neuropsychological difficulties is that they have difficulty retaining (or calling forth) long-term goals in working memory; thus they may be less able to compare current actions to long-term goals – a process necessary for adequate self-regulation. By understanding the nature of specific deficits and their influence on cognition and behaviour, we are in a better position to understand and prevent antisocial behaviour. The theory outlined by Lau et al. (1995) represents a good start in this direction.

Towards the above end, we briefly mention Barkley's (1997) recent presentation of a model of inhibition and executive functioning. Offered as a means of understanding the underlying deficit of children with HIA, Barkley's model is a hybrid of Bronowski's (1977) theory on the uniqueness of human language and Fuster's (1989) theory of prefrontal functions. The theory links behavioural inhibition to the performance of four executive functions that brings motor control, fluency, and syntax under the control of internally represented information. That is, the theory attempts to account for how the control of behaviour can move from control exclusively by the external environment to control by internal representations. Behavioural inhibition refers to inhibiting a prepotent response, stopping an ongoing response to allow a delay in the decision to respond, and/or interference control. Once behavioural inhibition occurs, the stage is set for the performance of any of the four executive functions. These four executive functions include working memory (e.g. holding events in mind and manipulating the information); self-regulation of affect, motivation and arousal; internalization of speech (e.g. description and reflection and problem solving); and reconstitution (e.g. analysis and synthesis). Barkley has outlined the potential problems arising from deficits at each stage of his model. Although he specifically attempts to apply the model to children with HIA, it is a fairly general model and may be applied to a broad variety of problems. We discuss the theory because we believe it represents an important theoretical advance and might be used to organize research on the relation between neuropsychological deficits and antisocial behaviour.

It may also be necessary to think critically about the relations between specific deficits and specific types of antisocial behaviour. For example, after reviewing several brain imaging studies, Raine (1993) suggested that frontal dysfunction may characterize violent offenders, whereas temporal dysfunction may characterize sexual offenders. There may even be important distinctions to be made within the same brain region. Raine & Venables (1992) highlighted the need for careful consideration of the nature of frontal deficits that may be linked to antisocial behaviour. Rather than referring to a general frontal dysfunction, these authors argued that the location of the frontal deficit determined the nature of psychopathology exhibited. Psychopathic behaviour was hypothesized to be associated with deficits in the orbitofrontal region; deficits in the dorsolateral region, on the other hand, were hypothesized to be associated with schizotypal behaviour. Individuals unfortunate enough to have deficits in both areas were expected to exhibit both types of psychopathology, and would thus appear as schizotypal psychopaths. Although in need of replication, the findings that aggression is specifically related to a task (the CAT) that taps functioning of the posterior dorsolateral region of the frontal lobes and not related to a task (the SOP) that taps functioning in the mid-dorsolateral area (Giancola & Zeichner, 1994; Lau & Pihl, 1994) is extremely provocative.

In summary, we have reviewed evidence that suggests poor verbal and/or executive functioning is linked to serious conduct problems. The relations between poor neuropsychological functioning and conduct problems were robust across diverse samples, particularly strong for severely antisocial sub-groups, and survived conservative controls for possible third variables. Although we believe that the evidence suggests the causal direction runs from poor neuropsychological functioning to serious conduct problems, this conclusion cannot be drawn unequivocally. Future prospective studies are clearly needed to address this point. We have also explored various theoretical accounts of this relation. Moffitt's (1993) developmental account was examined in particular detail because we believe the theory has much to recommend it and that it may serve as a theoretical basis for further research. The theory is developmental in nature and recognizes that neuropsychological deficits may exert their effects not only directly, but also indirectly by disrupting socialization, impairing attachments, narrowing opportunities for change, and accruing to the individual harmful labels. The theory has only begun to be tested, however, and much work remains. Importantly, the theory points us not only in new research directions, but provides some suggestions for prevention and intervention. One important implication of this theory is that prevention and intervention involve not just reducing the incidence of neuropsychological problems, but also acting to reduce some of its social and interpersonal consequences.

REFERENCES

American Psychiatric Association (1994). *Diagnostic and Statistical Manual of Mental Disorders* (4th edn) (DSM–IV). Washington, DC: American Psychiatric Association.

Anderson, J.C., Williams, S., McGee, R. & Silva, P.A. (1987). DSM–III disorders in preadolescent children: prevalence in a large sample from the general population. *Archives of General Psychiatry*, 44, 69–76.

Aronowitz, B., Liebowitz, M.R., Hollander, E., Fazzini, E., et al. (1994). Neuropsychiatric and neuropsychological findings in conduct disorder and attention-deficit hyperactivity disorder. *Journal of Neuropsychiatry & Clinical Neurosciences, 6,* 245–9.

Barkley, R.A. (1997). Behavioral inhibition, sustained attention, and executive functions: constructing a unifying theory of ADHD. *Psychological Bulletin, 121,* 65–94.

Berman, A. & Siegal, A.W. (1976). Adaptive and learning skills in juvenile delinquents: a neuropsychological analysis. *Journal of Learning Disabilities, 9,* 51–8.

Biederman, J., Munir, K. & Knee, D. (1987). Conduct and oppositional disorder in clinically referred children with attention deficit disorder: a controlled family study. *Journal of the American Academy of Child and Adolescent Psychiatry, 26,* 724–7.

Blumer, D. & Benson, D.F. (1975). Personality changes with frontal and temporal lobe lesions. In D.F. Benson & D. Blumer (Eds.), *Psychiatric Aspects of Neurologic Disease* (pp. 151–70). New York: Grune and Stratton.

Brickman, A.S., McManus, M.M., Grapentine, W.L. & Alessi, N. (1984). Neuropsychological assessment of seriously delinquent adolescents, *Journal of the American Academy of Child Psychiatry, 23,* 453–7.

Bronowski, J. (1977). Human and animal languages. In J. Bronowski (Ed.), *A Sense of the Future* (pp. 104–131). Cambridge, MA: MIT Press.

Buss, D.M. (1981). Predicting parent–child interactions from children's activity level. *Developmental Psychology, 17,* 59–65.

Carte, E.C., Nigg, J.T. & Hinshaw, S.P. (1996). Neuropsychological functioning, motor speed, and language processing in boys with and without ADHD. *Journal of Abnormal Child Psychology, 24,* 481–98.

Caspi, A. & Bem, D. (1990). Personality continuity and change across the life course. In L. Pervin (Ed.), *Handbook of Personality: Theory and Research* (pp. 549–75). New York: Guilford Press.

Caspi, A., Elder, G.H. & Bem, D.J. (1987). Moving against the world: life-course patterns of explosive children. *Developmental Psychology, 23,* 308–13.

Cloward, R.A. & Ohlin, L.E. (1960). *Delinquency and Opportunity: A Theory of Delinquent Gangs.* New York: Free Press.

Denno, D.J. (1989). *Biology, Crime and Violence: New Evidence.* Cambridge: Cambridge University Press.

Denno, D.W. (1990). *Biology and Violence: From Birth to Adulthood.* Cambridge: Cambridge University Press.

Dodge, K.A., Petit, G.S., McClaskey, C.L. & Brown, M.M. (1986). Social competence in children. *Monographs of the Society for Research in Child Development, 51* (2, Serial 213).

Elliott, F.A. (1978). Neurological aspects of antisocial behavior. In W.H. Reid (Ed.), *The Psychopath* (pp. 146–89). New York: Bruner/Mazel.

Elliott, F.A. (1992). Violence: The neurologic contribution. *Archives of Neurology, 49,* 595–603.

Eysenck, H.J. (1977). *Crime and Personality.* London: Routledge & Kegan Paul.

Farrington, D.P. (1987). Epidemiology. In H.C. Quay (Ed.), *Handbook of Juvenile Delinquency* (pp. 33–61). New York: John Wiley & Sons.

Farrington, D.P. & Hawkins (1991). Predicting participation, early onset, and later persistence in officially recorded offending. *Criminal Behavior and Mental Health, 1,* 1–33.

Fergusson, D., Lynskey & Horwood (1996). Factors associated with continuity and changes in disruptive behavior patterns between childhood and adolescence. *Journal of Abnormal Child Psychology, 24*, 533–53.

Frost, L.A., Moffitt, T.E. & McGee, R. (1989). Neuropsychological function and psychopathology in an unselected cohort of young adolescents. *Journal of Abnormal Psychology, 98*, 307–13.

Fuster, J.M. (1989). *The Prefrontal Cortex*. New York: Raven Press.

Giancola, P. & Zeichner, A. (1994). Neuropsychological performance on tests of frontal-lobe functioning and aggressive behavior in men. *Journal of Abnormal Psychology, 103*, 832–5.

Gorenstein, E.E. (1982). Frontal lobe functions in psychopaths. *Journal of Abnormal Psychology, 91*, 368–79.

Gorenstein, E.E. & Newman, J.P. (1980). Disinhibitory psychopathology: a new perspective and a model for research. *Psychological Review, 87*, 301–15.

Goyer, P., Andreasen, P., Semple, W., et al. (1994). Positron-emission tomography and personality disorders. *Neuropsychopharmacology, 10*, 21–8.

Hagan, J., Gillis, A.R. & Simpson, J. (1985). The class structure of gender and delinquency: toward a power-control theory of common delinquent behavior. *American Journal of Sociology, 90*, 1151–78.

Hare, R.D. (1984). Performance of psychopaths on cognitive tasks related to frontal lobe function. *Journal of Abnormal Psychology, 93*, 133–40.

Hart, S.D., Forth, A.H. & Hare, R.D. (1990). Performance of criminal psychopaths on selected neuropsychological tests. *Journal of Abnormal Psychology, 99*, 374–9.

Hendricks, S., Fitzpatrick, D., Hartman, K., et al. (1988). Brain structure and function in sexual molesters of children and adolescents. *Journal of Clinical Psychiatry, 49*, 108–12.

Henry, B., Caspi, A., Moffitt, T.E. & Silva, P.A. (1996). Temperamental and familial predictors of violent and nonviolent criminal convictions: from age 3 to age 18. *Developmental Psychology, 32*, 614–23.

Henry, B. & Moffitt, T.E. (1997). Neuropsychological and neuroimaging studies of juvenile delinquency and adult criminal behavior. In D. Stoff, J. Breiling & J.D. Maser (Eds.), *Handbook of Antisocial Behavior* (pp. 280–8). New York: John Wiley & Sons.

Hertzig, M. (1983). Temperament and neurological status. In M. Rutter (Ed.) *Developmental Neuropsychiatry* (pp. 164–80). New York: Guilford Press.

Hirschi, T. (1969). *Causes of Delinquency*. Berkeley, CA: University of California Press.

Hucker, S., Langevin, R., Wortzman, G., et al. (1986). Neuropsychological impairment in pedophiles. *Canadian Journal of Behavioral Science, 18*, 440–8.

Hucker, S., Langevin, R., Wortzman, G., et al. (1988). Cerebral damage and dysfunction in sexually aggressive men. *Annals of Sex Research, 1*, 33–47.

Hurwitz, I., Bibace, R.M.A., Wolff, P.H. & Rowbotham, B.M. (1972). Neurological function of normal boys, delinquent boys, and boys with learning problems. *Perceptual and Motor Skills, 35*, 387–94.

Jeglum-Bartusch, D., Lynam, D.R., Moffitt, T.E. & Silva, P.A. (1997). Is age important: testing general versus developmental theories of antisocial behavior. *Criminology, 35*, 13–48.

Kandel, E. & Mednick, S.A. (1991). Perinatal complications predict violent offending. *Criminology, 29*, 519–30.

Karniski, W.M., Levine, M.D., Clarke, S., Palfrey, J.S. & Meltzer, L.J. (1982). A study of neurodevelopmental findings in early adolescent delinquents. *Journal of Adolescent Health Care*, *3*, 151–9.

Keenan, K. & Shaw, D. (1997). Developmental and social influences on young girls' early problem behavior. *Psychological Bulletin*, *121*, 95–113.

Lahey, B.B., Loeber, R., Hart, E.L., et al. (1995). Four-year longitudinal study of conduct disorder in boys: patterns and predictors of persistence. *Journal of Abnormal Psychology*, *104*, 83–93.

Langevin, R., Ben-Aron, M., Wortzman, G., Dickey, R. & Handy, L. (1987). Brain damage, diagnosis, and substance abuse among violent offenders. *Behavioral Sciences and the Law*, *5*, 77–94.

Langevin, R., Lang, R., Wortzman, G., Frenzel, R. & Wright, P. (1989a). An examination of brain damage and dysfunction in genital exhibitionists. *Annals of Sex Research*, *2*, 77–87.

Langevin, R., Wortzman, G., Dickey, R., Wright, P. & Handy, L. (1988). Neuropsychological impairment in incest offenders. *Annals of Sex Research*, *1*, 401–15.

Langevin, R., Wortzman, G., Wright, P. & Handy, L. (1989b). Studies of brain damage and dysfunction in sex offenders. *Annals of Sex Research*, *2*, 163–79.

Lansdell, H. (1989). Sex differences in brain and personality correlates of the ability to identify popular word associations. *Behavioral Neuroscience*, *103*, 893–7.

Lau, M.A. & Pihl, R.O. (1994). Alcohol and the Taylor aggression paradigm: a repeated measures study. *Journal of Studies on Alcohol*, *55*, 701–6.

Lau, M.A., Pihl, R.O. & Peterson, J.B. (1995). Provocation, acute alcohol intoxication, cognitive performance and aggression. *Journal of Abnormal Psychology*, *104*, 150–5.

Lochman, J.E., Lampron, L.B. & Rabiner, D.L. (1989). Format and salience effects in the social problem-solving of aggressive and nonaggressive boys. *Journal of Consulting and Clinical Psychology*, *18*, 230–6.

Loeber, R. (1988). Natural histories of conduct problems, delinquency, and associated substance use: evidence for developmental progressions. In B.B. Lahey & A.E. Kazdin (Eds.), *Advances in Clinical Child Psychology*, (Vol. 11, pp. 73–124). New York: Plenum Press.

Loney, J. (1987). Hyperactivity and aggression in the diagnosis of attention deficit disorder. In B.B. Lahey & A.E. Kazdin (Eds.), *Advances in Clinical Child Psychology* (Vol. 10, pp. 99–135). New York: Plenum Press.

Lueger, R. & Gill, K. (1990). Frontal-lobe cognitive dysfunction in conduct disorder adolescents. *Journal of Clinical Psychology*, *46*, 696–706.

Luria, A.R. (1961). *The Role of Speech in the Regulation of Normal and Abnormal Behavior*. New York: Basic Books.

Luria, A.R. & Homskaya, E.D. (1964). Disturbance in the regulative role of speech with frontal lobe lesions. In J.M. Warren & K. Akert (Eds.), *The Frontal Granular Cortex and Behavior* (pp. 353–71). New York: McGraw Hill.

Lynam, D.R. (1996). The early identification of chronic offenders: Who is the fledgling psycho-path? *Psychological Bulletin*, *120*, 209–34.

Lynam, D.R. (1998). Early identification of the fledgling psychopath: locating the psychopathic child in the current nomenclature. *Journal of Abnormal Psychology*, *107*, 566–75.

Lynam, D., Moffitt, T. & Stouthamer-Loeber, M. (1993). Explaining the relation between IQ and delinquency: class, race, test motivation, school failure, or self-control? *Journal of Abnormal Psychology, 102,* 187–96.

Lytton, H. (1990). Child and parent effects in boys' conduct disorder. *Developmental Psychology, 26,* 683–97.

Maccoby, E.E. & Jacklin, C.N. (1983). The 'person' characteristics of children and the family as environment. In D. Magnusson & V.L. Allen (Eds.), *Human Development: An Interactional Perspective* (pp. 75–92). San Diego, CA: Academic Press.

Miller, L.J., Burdg, N.B. & Carpenter, D. (1980). Application of recategorized WISC-R scores of adjudicated adolescents. *Perceptual and Motor Skills, 51,* 187–91.

Moffitt, T.E. (1988). Neuropsychology and self-reported early delinquency in an unselected birth cohort: a preliminary report from New Zealand. In T.E. Moffitt & S.A. Mednick (Eds.), *Biological Contributions to Crime Causation* (pp. 93–120). Boston: Martinus Nijhoff Publishers.

Moffitt, T.E. (1990a). The neuropsychology of delinquency: a critical review of theory and research. In N. Morris & M. Tonry (Eds.), *Crime and Justice: An Annual Review of Research* (Vol. 12) (pp. 99–169). Chicago: University of Chicago Press.

Moffitt, T.E. (1990b). Juvenile delinquency and attention deficit disorder: Boys' developmental trajectories from age 3 to age 15. *Child Development, 61,* 893–910.

Moffitt, T.E. (1993). Adolescence-limited and life-course persistent antisocial behavior: a developmental taxonomy. *Psychological Review, 100,* 674–701.

Moffitt, T.E., Caspi, A., Dickson, N., Silva, P. & Stanton, W. (1996). Childhood-onset versus adolescent-onset antisocial conduct problems in males: Natural histories from ages 3 to 18 years. *Development and Psychopathology, 8,* 399–424.

Moffitt, T.E., Gabrielli, W.F. & Mednick, S.A. (1981). Socioeconomic status, IQ, and delinquency. *Journal of Abnormal Psychology, 90,* 152–6.

Moffitt, T.E. & Henry, B. (1989). Neuropsychological assessment of executive functions in self-reported delinquents. *Development and Psychopathology, 1,* 105–18.

Moffitt, T.E. & Henry, B. (1991). Neuropsychological studies of juvenile delinquency and violence: a review. In J. Milner (Ed.), *The Neuropsychology of Aggression* (pp. 67–91). Norwell, MA: Kluwer Academic Publishers.

Moffitt, T.E. & Lynam, D.R. (1994). The neuropsychology of conduct disorder and delinquency: implications for understanding antisocial behavior. In D. Fowles, P. Sutker & S. Goodman (Eds.), *Psychopathy and Antisocial Personality: A Developmental Perspective* (pp. 233–62). Vol. 18 in the series, Progress in Experimental Personality and Psychopathology Research. New York: Springer.

Moffitt, T.E., Lynam, D.R. & Silva, P.A. (1994). Neuropsychological tests predicting persistent male delinquency. *Criminology, 32,* 277–300.

Moffitt, T.E. & Silva, P.A. (1988a). IQ and delinquency: A direct test of the differential detection hypothesis. *Journal of Abnormal Psychology, 97,* 330–3.

Moffitt, T.E. & Silva, P.A. (1988b). Neuropsychological deficit and self-reported delinquency in an unselected birth cohort. *Journal of the American Academy of Child and Adolescent Psychiatry, 27,* 233–40.

Moffitt, T.E. & Silva, P.A. (1988c). Self-reported delinquency, neuropsychological deficit, and history of attention deficit disorder. *Journal of Abnormal Child Psychology, 16,* 553–69.

Newman, J.P. (1987). Reaction to punishment in extroverts and psychopaths: Implications for the impulsive behavior of disinhibited individuals. *Journal of Research in Personality, 21,* 464–80.

Newman, J.P. & Kosson, D.S. (1986). Passive avoidance learning in psychopathic and non-psychopathic offenders. *Journal of Abnormal Psychology, 95,* 257–63.

Newman, J.P. & Wallace, J.F. (1993). Divergent pathways to deficient self-regulation: implications for disinhibitory psychopathology in children. *Clinical Psychology Review, 13,* 699–720.

Olweus, D. (1980). Familial and temperamental determinants of aggressive-behavior in adolescent boys: a causal analysis. *Developmental Psychology, 16,* 644–60.

Patterson, G.R. (1982). *Coercive Family Process.* Eugene, OR: Castalia.

Patterson, G.R. (1986). Performance models for antisocial boys. *American Psychologist, 41,* 432–44.

Patterson, G.R., Capaldi, D. & Bank, L. (1991). An early starter model for predicting delinquency. In D. Pepler & K.H. Rubin (Eds.), *The Development and Treatment of Childhood Aggression* (pp. 139–68). Hillsdale, NJ: Lawrence Erlbaum.

Patterson, M.C. & Newman, J.P. (1993). Reflectivity and learning from aversive events: toward a psychological mechanism for the syndromes of disinhibition. *Psychological Review, 100,* 76–736.

Petrides, M. (1985). Deficits on conditional associative-learning tasks after frontal- and temporal-lobe lesions in man. *Neuropsychologia, 23,* 601–14.

Petrides, M. (1995). Functional organization of the human frontal cortex for mnemonic processing: evidence from neuroimaging studies. *Annals of the New York Academy of Sciences, 769,* 85–96.

Petrides, M., Alivisatos, B., Evans, A. & Meyer, E. (1993). Dissociation of human mid-dorsolateral frontal cortex in memory processing. *Proceedings of the National Academy of Sciences, USA, 90,* 873–7.

Petrides, M. & Milner, B. (1982). Deficits on subject-ordered tasks after frontal- and temporal-lobe lesions in man. *Neuropsychologia, 20,* 249–62.

Pontius, A.A. (1972). Neurological aspects in some type of delinquency, especially among juveniles: toward a neurological model of ethical action. *Adolescence, 7,* 289–308.

Prentice, N.M. & Kelly, F.J. (1963). Intelligence and delinquency: a reconsideration. *Journal of Social Psychology, 60,* 327–37.

Quay, H.C. (1993). The psychobiology of undersocialized aggressive conduct disorder: a theoretical perspective. *Development and Psychopathology, 5,* 165–80.

Raine, A. (1988). Evoked potentials and antisocial behavior. In T. Moffitt & S. Mednick (Eds.), *Biological Contributions to Crime Causation* (pp. 14–39). Dordrecht: Martinus Nijhoff Publishers.

Raine, A. (1993). *The Psychopathology of Crime: Criminal Behavior as a Clinical Disorder.* San Diego, CA: Academic Press.

Raine, A., Brennan, P. & Mednick, S.A. (1994a). Birth complications combined with early maternal rejection at age 1 year predispose to violent crime at age 18 years. *Archives of General Psychiatry, 51,* 984–8.

Raine, A., Buschbaum, M., Stanley, J., Lottenberg, S., Abel, L. & Stoddard, J. (1994b). Selective reductions in prefrontal glucose metabolism in murderers. *Biological Psychiatry, 36,* 365–73.

Raine, A. & Venables, P. (1992). Antisocial behavior: Evolution, genetics, neuropsychology, and psychophysiology. In A. Gale & M. Eysenck (Eds.), *Handbook of Individual Differences: Biological Perspectives* (pp. 287–321). London: John Wiley & Sons.

Raz, S., Goldstein, R., Hopkins, T.L., Lauterbach, M.D., et al. (1994). Sex differences in early vulnerability to cerebral injury and their neurodevelopmental implications. *Psychobiology, 22,* 244–53.

Raz, S., Lauterbach, M.D., Hopkins, T.L., Glogowski, B.K., et al. (1995). A female advantage in cognitive recovery from early cerebral insult. *Developmental Psychology, 31,* 958–66.

Reiss, A.J. & Rhodes, A.L. (1961). The distribution of juvenile delinquency in the social class structure. *American Sociological Review, 26,* 720–32.

Robins, L. (1978). Sturdy childhood predictors of adult antisocial behavior: replications from longitudinal studies. *Psychological Medicine, 8,* 611–22.

Rosenthal, R. & Rosnow, R.L. (1991). *Essentials of Behavioral Research: Methods and Data Analysis* (2nd edn). New York: McGraw-Hill.

Rutter, M. (Ed.) (1983). *Developmental Neuropsychiatry.* New York, NY: Guilford Press.

Savitsky, J.C. & Czyzewski, D. (1978). The reaction of adolescent offenders and nonoffenders to nonverbal emotional displays. *Journal of Abnormal Child Psychology, 6,* 89–96.

Schore, A.N. (1996). The experience-dependent maturation of a regulatory system in the orbital prefrontal cortex and the origin of developmental psychopathology. *Development and Psychopathology, 8,* 59–87.

Seguin, J.R., Pihl, R.O., Harden, P.W., Tremblay, R.E. & Boulerice, B. (1995). Cognitive and neuropsychological characteristics of physically aggressive boys. *Journal of Abnormal Psychology, 104,* 614–24.

Shapiro, S., Quay, H., Hogan, A. & Schwartz, K. (1988). Response perseveration and delayed responding in undersocialized aggressive conduct disorder. *Journal of Abnormal Psychology, 97,* 371–3.

Short, J.F. & Strodtbeck, F.L. (1965). *Group Process and Gang Delinquency.* Chicago: University of Chicago Press.

Skoff, B.F. & Libon, J. (1987). Impaired executive functions in a sample of male juvenile delinquents. *Journal of Clinical and Experimental Neuropsychology, 9,* 60.

Sobotowicz, W., Evans, J. R. & Laughlin, J. (1987). Neuropsychological function and social support in delinquency and learning disability. *International Journal of Clinical Neuropsychology, 9,* 178–86.

Szatmari, P., Offord, D.R. & Boyle, M. (1989). Ontario Child Health Study: prevalence of attention deficit disorder with hyperactivity. *Journal of Child Psychology and Psychiatry, 30,* 219–30.

Thomas, A. & Chess, S. (1977). *Temperament and Development.* New York: Brunner/Mazel.

Tonkonogy, J. (1991). Violence and temporal lobe lesion: head CT and MRI data. *Journal of Neuropsychiatry and Clinical Neurosciences, 3,* 189–96.

Tremblay, R.E., Pihl, R.O., Vitaro, F. & Dobkin, P.L. (1994). Predicting early onset of male antisocial behavior from preschool behavior. *Archives of General Psychiatry, 51,* 732–9.

Volkow, N.D., Tancredi, L.R., Grant, C., Gillespie, H., et al. (1995). Brain glucose metabolism in violent psychiatric patients: a preliminary study. *Psychiatry Research: Neuroimaging, 61,* 243–53.

Walsh, A., Petee, T.A. & Beyer, J.A. (1987). Intellectual imbalance and delinquency: comparing high verbal and high performance IQ delinquents. *Criminal Justice and Behavior*, 14, 370–9.

Wechsler, D. (1944). *The Measurement of Adult Intelligence*, 3rd edn. Baltimore: Williams and Wilkins.

Werry, J.S., Elkind, G.S. & Reeves, J.C. (1987). Attention deficit, conduct, oppositional, and anxiety disorders in children: III. Laboratory differences. *Journal of Abnormal Child Psychology*, 15, 409–28.

West, D.J. & Farrington, D.P. (1973). *Who Becomes Delinquent?* London: Heineman Educational Books.

White, J., Moffitt, T.E., Caspi, A., et al. (1994). Measuring impulsivity and examining its relation to delinquency. *Journal of Abnormal Psychology*, 103, 192–205.

White, J.L., Moffitt, T.E., Earls, F., Robins, L. & Silva, P.A. (1990). How early can we tell? Predictors of childhood conduct disorder and adolescent delinquency. *Criminology*, 28, 507–33.

White, J.L., Moffitt, T.E. & Silva, P.A. (1989). A prospective replication of the protective effects of IQ in subjects at high risk for juvenile delinquency. *Journal of Consulting and Clinical Psychology*, 57, 719–24.

Wilson, J.Q. & Herrnstein, R.J. (1985). *Crime and Human Nature*. New York: Simon & Schuster.

Witelson, S.F. (1977). Neural and cognitive correlates of developmental dyslexia: age and sex differences. In C. Shagass, S. Gershan & A.J. Friedhoff (Eds.), *Psychopathology and Brain Dysfunction* (pp. 121–53). New York: Raven Press.

Wolff, P.H., Waber, D., Bauermeister, M., Cohen, C. & Ferber, R. (1982). The neuropsychological status of adolescent delinquent boys. *Journal of Child Psychology and Psychiatry*, 23, 267–79.

Wolfgang, M.E., Figlio, R.M. & Sellin, T. (1972). *Delinquency in a Birth Cohort*. Chicago: The University of Chicago Press.

Wright, P., Nobrega, J., Langevin, R. & Wortzman, G. (1990). Brain density and symmetry in pedophilic and sexually aggressive offenders. *Annals of Sex Research*, 3, 319–28.

Yeudall, L.T. (1980). A neuropsychological perspective of persistent juvenile delinquency and criminal behavior. *Annals of the New York Academy of Science*, 347, 349–55.

10

A reinforcement model of conduct problems in children and adolescents: advances in theory and intervention

Jeff Kiesner, Thomas J. Dishion and François Poulin

Introduction

In the history of clinical psychology and psychiatry, troublesome children have been referred to with a variety of labels. The Diagnostic and Statistical Manual of Mental Disorders (DSM) and ICD systems of classification concur on the basic features and behaviours of this clinical syndrome, including behaviours considered to be oppositional by adults and conduct disordered by mental health professionals. The behaviours represented with these domains are quite heterogeneous and include: (a) noncompliance to adult requests; (b) verbal and physical aggressivity to siblings, peers, and adults; (c) behaviours such as lying, stealing and destruction of property.

From a syndrome perspective, the heterogeneity in the behavioural and social profile of troublesome children presents a theoretical dilemma. Theorists of the past have provided some organization to children's clinical presentation by posing subtypes of troublesome behaviour. For example, a distinction has been made between socialized and unsocialized conduct problems (Quay, 1964), or covert and overt behaviour (Loeber, 1988), or of late, proactive and reactive aggression (Dodge & Coie, 1987; Poulin & Boivin, 2000).

As we shall see, the distinctions are important to explore for model building and for understanding the functional mechanisms underlying various forms of conduct problems in children and adolescents (Dishion & Patterson, 1997). From a reinforcement perspective, however, we often use the term 'antisocial behaviour' to describe the wide array of behaviours falling within the ICD and DSM classification systems. Antisocial behaviour is defined simply as behaviour experienced as aversive by other social interactants (see also Patterson et al., 1992). Although the child's alleged intentions are certainly important for parents, teachers and peers when reacting to aversive behaviour, we have de-emphasized this component of the behaviour in our definition.

An unfortunate aspect of child antisocial behaviour is that it tends to be consistent across settings and informants (Achenbach et al., 1987; Bernal et al., 1976; Charlesbois et al., 1989; Loeber & Dishion, 1984; Patterson, 1986; Patterson et al., 1984), as well as stable over time (Loeber, 1982; Loeber & Dishion, 1983; Moore et al., 1979; Olweus, 1979; Patterson et al., 1991; Robins, 1966). Although most studies have focused on boys, recent research has also demonstrated temporal continuity of antisocial behaviour for girls. Bardone et al. (1996) showed that girls with conduct disorder at age 15 demonstrated significantly higher levels of adjustment problems at age 21, as compared to girls without a mental health disorder.

Research has indicated that children who become involved in antisocial behaviour at a very early age have the worst prognosis for adult involvement in antisocial and criminal behaviour. Studies of criminal conviction patterns suggest that antisocial behaviour beginning in childhood is persistent throughout life, and that the earliest offenders are those who are the most likely to have the highest levels of recidivism (Farrington & West, 1993; Gendreau et al., 1979; Koller & Gosden, 1984; Mandelzys, 1979).

The relation between age of onset and both stability and severity of antisocial behaviour has led to the conceptualization of two developmental pathways to adolescent antisocial behaviour (Patterson, 1995; Patterson et al., 1991; Patterson & Yoerger, 1997; Moffitt, 1993). There is a general consensus that youth who start early show the most pervasive developmental difficulties with respect to the continuance of antisocial behaviour, as well as the disruption of social, academic and other competencies necessary for adult adjustment (Patterson, 1982; Moffitt, 1993).

Relationship contingencies and development

Patterson et al. (1992) propose a theory based on social reinforcement, specifying that early starters begin training for antisocial behaviour as young children, as a result of a coercive family process (Dishion & Patterson, 1997; Patterson, 1996; Patterson et al., 1991). The coercive training the young child receives in the home results in massive social-skills and academic deficits. Confluence with a delinquent peer group is the next step and involves positive reinforcement from similar antisocial peers for increasingly high-risk behaviours. On the other hand, late starters begin around age 15, after a breakdown in effective family management and parental supervision. Affiliation with a delinquent peer group provides opportunities and reinforcement for antisocial acts. However, by the age of 15, these late starters have already developed sufficient prosocial and academic skills to facilitate desistence from antisocial behaviour (Simons et al.,

1996). Although early and late starters are on different developmental pathways with different probable outcomes, reinforcement plays a crucial role for both groups. The present chapter focuses on the role of reinforcement in both the early- and late-starter pathways.

According to reinforcement theory, antisocial behaviour is learned and practiced within the child's social environment. Relationships with parents, siblings, peers and teachers provide children with opportunities to learn and practice prosocial and antisocial behaviour, although the specific relationships that play dominant roles in socialization are believed to change throughout an individual's life. Presumably, what is learned within one relationship at a particular developmental period will affect social relationships in subsequent developmental periods. The developmental course of antisocial behaviour represents an individual's adaptation to these evolving relationships.

From both a clinical and developmental standpoint, parents are at centre stage when considering the development of antisocial behaviour. Parents begin the socialization process early in the child's life, and their role in managing the child's later social relationships continues to be important in determining adult outcomes. For this reason, parent–child interactions, as well as parenting practices in general, have been studied a great deal (Patterson et al., 1992). Also, our understanding of how peers and siblings affect the developmental course of antisocial behaviour is continuously expanding.

The reinforcement model presented here focuses on the functional action–reaction sequences of social interactions (Patterson & Reid, 1984). At the core of this model is the idea that antisocial behaviours resulting in benefits to the child by controlling unpleasant interactions (e.g. work demands) or promoting pleasant interactions (e.g. laughter with friends) are more likely to occur in the future (Dishion & Patterson, 1997). A child's antisocial behaviour, therefore, is seen as a social adaptation within the immediate microsocial environment. The child learns certain social responses through reinforcement, which sets the child on a course for either social adaptation or maladaptation.

Parenting practices and coercion

For many years, parenting practices have been recognized to be among the most powerful predictors of antisocial behaviour (Loeber & Dishion, 1983). These findings have been published in both psychology and criminology literature. For example, using structural equation modelling procedures, Patterson (1986) found a strong correlation between harsh, abrasive and inconsistent parental discipline and child antisocial behaviour. Forgatch (1991) replicated this model across the two cohorts of the Oregon Youth Study (OYS) with a single-parent sample and a clinical sample. Similarly, Patterson and colleagues (Patterson & Dishion, 1985; Patterson & Stouthamer-Loeber, 1984) found an association between inept parental discipline practices, parental monitoring and child antisocial behaviour in mid-adolescence. Recently, Fagot & Leve (1998) found that early harsh parenting was associated with the early emergence of antisocial behaviour in elementary school, as rated by teachers. In addition, Conger et al. (1995) found that the model replicates when using diverse measures and samples.

Moreover, these relationships have also been found using longitudinal data. For example, Patterson & Bank (1989) and Vuchinich et al. (1992) used structural equation modelling to demonstrate that parental discipline practices were associated with child antisocial behaviour during middle childhood and early adolescence. Importantly, the relation between parental discipline and antisocial behaviour in early adolescence held even after controlling for the stability of antisocial behaviour from ages 9 to 12. Researchers in criminology have also predicted adolescent antisocial behaviour from comprehensive measures of family functioning (including measures of parenting behaviours) during middle childhood (Farrington, 1978; McCord, 1979; McCord et al., 1961; Wadsworth, 1979; West & Farrington, 1977).

Although these studies, and many others, have established that parenting practices play an important role in the development of antisocial behaviour, a detailed model of the causal chain is needed to fully understand the socialization process of antisocial behaviour. Patterson's (1982) coercion model has provided such a detailed model, focusing specifically on the contributions of parent–child interactions to child antisocial behaviour (see Fig. 10.1).

A coercive act is defined as an aversive behaviour that results in a positive outcome. Initially, the child learns to avoid parental demands through the process of negative reinforcement. During one exchange, for example, the parent may make an unpleasant demand of the child, to which the child responds with some aversive behaviour. If the parent drops the demand in response to the aversive behaviour, the child will have been negatively reinforced for the aversive response.

Clearly, coercive interactions occur at some level in all families. Long-term exposure to a high rate of these exchanges, however, 'trains' the child in an antisocial pattern of social interaction. Gardner (1989) examined this problem by focusing on the outcome of parent–child conflicts. This is an important step because the end of a conflict determines whether the child has been negatively reinforced. Using a measure of parental consistency based on the final outcome

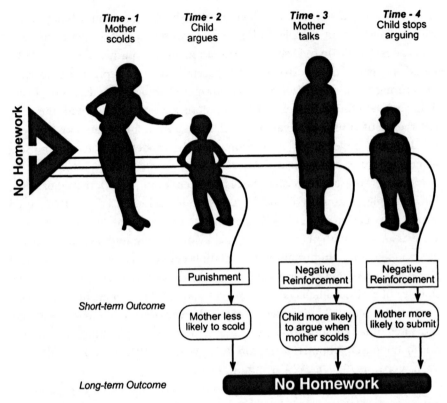

Fig. 10.1. A four-step escape-conditioning sequence. From *Antisocial Boys* by G.R. Patterson, J.B. Reid & T.J. Dishion, 1992 (p. 41). © 1992, Castalia Publishing Company; used with permission.

of a conflict, Gardner found that mothers of conduct problem children were eight times more likely to relinquish demands than their normal counterparts. Within the reinforcement model, the relinquishment of a demand following conflict results in negative reinforcement. Also, mothers of conduct problem children handled 43% of the conflict episodes inconsistently, compared with 5% for mothers of children without conduct problems. These data support the hypothesis that negative reinforcement is involved in the development of antisocial behaviour.

Snyder & Patterson (1995) applied a matching law analysis to children's and mothers' selection of specific responses. According to the matching law, the effect of reinforcement on behaviour is not a simple linear equation. One cannot go into an environment, count the reinforcing sequences, and correlate them with an individual's rate of responding, as the correlation would be negligible. What is necessary is to examine the relative utility of a particular response, compared with all the other responses in a person's repertoire

(McDowell, 1988). Specifically, the matching law predicts that the proportion of a target behaviour to all possible behaviours (target/target + nontarget) will 'match' or equal the proportion of the rate of reinforcement for the target behaviour to the rate of reinforcement for all behaviours (rate of reinforcement for targets/rate of reinforcement for targets + nontargets). Rather than hypothesizing simply that reinforcement for a response results in an increased rate of responding, one hypothesizes that as the rate of reinforcement for that response – relative to the rate of reinforcement for all responses – increases, the rate of the target response will increase proportionately to all other responses. According to coercion theory, negative reinforcement (escape conditioning) is the learning mechanism that accounts for the development of antisocial behaviour. The matching law would then predict that the rate of a particular coercive response will be determined, not just by the frequency of negative reinforcement, but the relative rate of negative reinforcement for that response with respect to the rate of negative reinforcement for all possible responses.

Using the matching law framework, Snyder & Patterson (1995) accounted for individual, as well as intra-individual differences in preschool children's aggressive responding. Using a sample of 10 aggressive and 10 nonaggressive mother–child dyads, they found that during 5 hours of direct observation, the functional utility of a child's response was associated with the relative occurrence of that response in a second 5-hour observation period. That is to say, the rate with which the child used a particular response (relative to all possible responses) in the second 5 hours of observation matched the payoff (relative rate of negative reinforcement by the mother) of that response during the first 5 hours ($r = 0.64$). The same was found for the mother's choice of responses ($r = 0.59$). Because this relationship was found for both child and mother responding it was concluded that negative reinforcement of aversive behaviour is bidirectional. Moreover, these correlations are based on both constructive/positive and aggressive tactics for conflict termination. Thus, the findings suggest that the matching law applies to both aversive and prosocial behaviours. In addition, they found individual differences in aggressive and non-aggressive children: for the former group, lag sequential analyses revealed a contingent connection between aggressive behaviour and conflict termination. In the nonaggressive group, conflict termination was not associated with the child's aversive reaction, but rather, with the more functional 'No Response' by the mother.

Recent work by Snyder et al. (1997b) further examined the role of negative reinforcement in the development of antisocial behaviour. Using a sample of 57 boys (6 to 13 years old) referred to a clinic for conduct problems, these researchers found a positive relation between parent negative reinforcement of child aggressive behaviour during conflict and child antisocial behaviour two years later. Moreover, this research revealed a positive relationship between a composite score representing a child's tendency to initiate and reciprocate conflict and the probability that the parent would negatively reinforce the child's aggressive (relative to nonaggressive) behaviour during a conflict ($r = 0.48$). This means that boys who tended to initiate and reciprocate conflict were also more likely to be negatively reinforced for their aggressive behaviour.

Central to the coercion process is the parents' inconsistent, harsh or erratic efforts to set limits on their young child (Loeber & Dishion, 1983). However, the exact process is not clear. One possibility is that these harsh and erratic efforts to discipline represent the parent's attempt to regain control of the family. The child, in response, escalates the aversive behaviour until eventually the parent backs off, reinforcing intra-episodic escalation of coercive behaviour, as well. This intermittent type of reinforcement schedule results in a learned behaviour that is particularly resistant to change.

Intra-episodic escalation of aversive behaviour has, in fact, been noted in the literature. Snyder et al. (1994) found that families with an antisocial child were more likely to react to conflict with an escalation of aversive behaviour, whereas other families were more likely to de-escalate. Similarly, other research has found that nondistressed families tended to disengage within a conflict bout rather than escalate (Dishion et al., 1983).

Despite these problems, parents frequently believe that they use good parenting practices and blame the child for not responding. In fact, data indicate that aversive parent–child interactions, even in the most disruptive families, represent only about 10% of the total interactions (Patterson et al., 1992). While these parents may be using a variety of positive parenting practices, the 10% of aversive interactions appear to strongly impact the child's trajectory toward antisocial development. Although positive interactions between the parent and child are plentiful, they do not discriminate between clinical and normative families (see Patterson et al., 1992). Moreover, this low base rate of aversive exchange, even in clinical samples, makes the recognition of the problem difficult for both parents and clinicians, resulting in judgements biased toward blaming the child rather than the process.

These microsocial studies have been critical for researchers to get a sense of the moment-by-moment interactions that may seem trivial to the participants, but actually, over time, may lead to chronic antisocial behaviour. As described by Dishion & Patterson (1997), positive and negative reinforcement in close relationships is largely unnoticed by the untrained participants, as such interactions are not consciously driven and tend to proceed as if on 'automatic pilot'.

Intervention trials

The reinforcement theory has also been tested in the context of intervention trials. The effectiveness of such interventions is reviewed by Kazdin (chapter 15, this volume). Here we focus on their value for increasing contingent reinforcement for prosocial behaviour and reducing coercive exchanges in order to reduce problem behaviours. Dishion & Andrews (1995) randomly assigned families of 158 at-risk adolescent boys and girls to either the Adolescent Transitions Program (ATP) or to a nontreatment quasi-experimental control group. The ATP comprises four versions of intervention: parent-focused training, teen-focused training, a joint focus on parent and teen, and a self-directed group. Involvement in either the parent or teen focus groups was associated with a decrease in observed parent–child negative engagement. More importantly, parent-focused training was also related to reductions in smoking and teacher ratings of antisocial behaviour in school. These data suggest that family management skills can decrease negative engagement, and in turn, antisocial behaviour, thus providing experimental evidence to support the reinforcement model, as well as reinforcement-based interventions.

More recently, Dishion & Kavanagh (in press) have studied the impact of parenting interventions on changes in antisocial behaviour. In these analyses (see Fig. 10.2 for summary), we looked at families with high-risk young adolescents, videotaping their interactions between parent and child while discussing hot family topics. Overall, parenting interventions were associated with a reduction in conflict between the parent and child during these discussions of hot topics. Moreover, reductions in negative interactions were associated with reductions in teacher reports of externalizing problems in the children's schools. This final link is critical for theory testing and has practical value, as well. When working with parents of troubled children, it is vitally important to find and support their use of family management skills that reduce the level of coercion between the parent and child. Success in this area appears to have real-life benefits to the adolescent in settings outside the home.

It is important to acknowledge that the parent is not solely responsible for their child's behaviour. Children who are temperamental or who have learned to respond coercively are more difficult to manage and will likely strain their parents' already tenuous parenting abilities (Dishion et al., 1995b). Past research has demonstrated that parents' negative emotions (anger, depression,

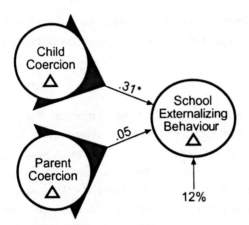

Fig. 10.2. Predicting change in teacher ratings of externalizing behaviour at school from changes in parent–child coercion.

irritability) undermine their attempts to set limits and problem-solve (Forgatch, 1984). The more difficult a child becomes, the more likely the parent will experience negative emotions that further jeopardize family management.

Changing contexts and evolving problems

The coercion model predicts that, as a child grows, a coercive style of social interaction learned in the family will be taken outside the home, disrupting social relationships and academic learning. For example, the effects of poor parenting skills on peer rejection in the school setting should be mediated by the child's antisocial behaviour and skills deficits, which have resulted from the coercive family process. Dishion (1990) demonstrated that, for 206 boys in middle childhood, the effects of parent discipline on peer rejection were mediated through child antisocial behaviour and low academic achievement (together explaining 60% of the variance in the peer relations score). Parenting practices were implicated in poor peer relations, not directly, but indirectly, through a more general pattern of antisocial behaviour, which was associated with parent discipline practices.

A second study by Dishion et al. (1994) examined the unique contribution of coercive exchanges of both parents and peers to antisocial behaviour. Using a sample of 374 first and fifth graders (52% girls), these researchers found that both child-to-parent and child-to-peer coercion accounted for unique variance in antisocial behaviour. Together, coercive exchanges with parents and peers accounted for 21% and 19% of the variance in antisocial behaviour, for girls and boys, respectively. Surprisingly, child-to-parent and child-to-peer coercion were only modestly correlated ($r = 0.19$). This low correlation is likely to be an underestimate, resulting from the brief laboratory task used to measure child-to-parent coercion. This measure might be unable to capture the coercive interactions that may normally take place in the family. Although gender differences were observed for absolute levels of coercion and antisocial behaviour, the same model fitted equally well for both genders.

As children move into adolescence, the social world outside the family takes on an increasingly important role in the development of antisocial behaviour. However, parenting practices, such as monitoring youth activities, continue to play an important role. Research has demonstrated a strong correlation between parental monitoring practices, adolescent delinquent behaviour and deviant peer association (French et al., 1991; Patterson & Dishion, 1985). Similarly, Dishion et al. (1995a) found that parental monitoring was negatively related to deviant peer association, and that deviant peer association was positively related to drug use. Thus, the effects of poor parental monitoring on drug use appears to be mediated through association with deviant peers. This research points out that, although new social relationships begin to contribute to the socialization of antisocial behaviour, parents remain important players.

Contribution of peers: deviancy training

Children with conduct problems are more likely to associate with deviant peers, to have discordant peer relationships, and to be rejected by peers. Current models linking deviant friends to the development of antisocial problems are reviewed by Vitaro et al. (chapter 13, this volume). Here we focus on the coercion model of Patterson et al. (1992) which hypothesizes that the aversive interactional style learned in the family will be generalized to the peer system, resulting in rejection and reinforcement of deviant behaviour by peers. As early as preschool, there is evidence that antisocial children experience rejection by their peers (Wasik, 1987). In elementary and middle school (ages 5 to 14), antisocial behaviour has emerged as the most consistent correlate of peer rejection in children (Coie & Dodge, 1988; Coie et al., 1988; French & Waas, 1987). Moreover, playgroup studies aggregating previously unacquainted children provided evidence of a causal relationship between antisocial behaviour and peer rejection (Coie & Kupersmidt, 1983; Dodge, 1983).

Antisocial behaviour is not, however, consistently associated with peer disapproval. According to Wright et al. (1986), the relation between antisocial behaviour (or aggression) and peer status is moderated by the group composition. More specifically, aggression is likely to be related to peer rejection when a child is dissimilar from his peers, but not when he is behaving in a way that is normative for his group. This model received empirical support in studies conducted in a summer camp (Wright et al., 1986) and with the playgroups procedure (Boivin et al., 1995).

In their naturalistic environment, antisocial children apparently tend to seek out social settings in which their antisocial behaviour will be normative and receive the maximum level of social reinforcement for the minimum social energy (Dishion et al., 1994). As early as preschool, aggressive children tend to form social networks with similar peers, the nuclear members of which are the most aggressive individuals (Farver, 1996). Recent work by Snyder et al. (1997a) applied the matching law to peer relations. These researchers hypothesized that children would allocate their 'associational time with and indicate verbal preference for each peer in proportion to the probability at which the child received positive social consequences during interaction with that peer relative to other peers' (Snyder et al., 1996, p. 218). In fact, results demonstrated that, for a sample of 74 preschoolers (36 boys, 38 girls), the relative rate of positive consequences received from peers predicted peer affiliation. Of more interest, partial correlations demonstrated that for same- and mixed-gender peer affiliations the relative probability of positive consequences from peers predicted changes in affiliation after earlier peer affiliation was accounted for (partial rs from 0.68 to 0.79). These findings held for both girls and boys.

In a study using 72 preschool-age, high-risk, African-American boys and girls, Snyder et al. (1997a) observed that aggressive children made as many attempts as nonaggressive children to establish associations, but their efforts were less likely to be reciprocated by their peers. The successful mutual relationships that aggressive children did establish tended to be with similar aggressive peers and were associated with a subsequent increase in their negative behaviour. Snyder et al. (1996) suggest that both negative reinforcement (as conceptualized in Patterson's model) or positive reinforcement (i.e. access to desired resources) can explain these findings. These data suggest that reinforcement for mutually approved aggressive behaviour may contribute to group formation. In childhood, antisocial children pursue and crystallize their tendency to associate together (Cairns et al., 1988; Kupersmidt et al., 1995; Poulin et al., 1997).

Recently, Poulin & Boivin (2000) argued that this affiliative tendency in antisocial children might be a function of the proactive aggressive behaviour displayed by the child. This hypothesis is based on the work of Dodge & Coie (1987), who proposed a distinction between proactive aggression (a non-provoked aversive means of influencing another) and reactive aggression (an impulsive and hostile act displayed in response to a perceived threat or provocation). The former is acquired by social learning processes and maintained by reinforcement (especially in the context of the peer group), as opposed to the latter, that comes from a history of physical abuse and harsh discipline (Dodge et al., 1997). Poulin & Boivin (2000) observed that, in elementary classrooms, proactively aggressive boys tended to select each other as friends, which was not the case for reactively aggressive boys. In other words, proactive aggressive behaviour appears instrumental in shaping the social context in which this class of behaviour is reinforced.

What are the immediate and long-term consequences of being associated with other antisocial children? There is sufficient evidence that mutual affiliation of aggressive preschool children is associated with increases in aggression over the course of the year (Snyder et al., 1997a). Studies by Patterson et al. (1967), as well as subsequent researchers (Strayer & Noel, 1986), suggest that the overall pattern of action–reaction among children on the playground, as well as coalitions, account for a sizable percentage of the variance in overall aggressive behaviour among preschool children. In childhood, Boivin & Vitaro (1995) reported that aggressive boys who were not involved in a friendship clique were more likely to decrease their aggressive behaviour over time than aggressive boys who were members of a clique, suggesting that the clique plays a role in the maintenance of aggressive behaviour. Antisocial cliques in childhood are also seen as a developmental pathway leading to gang involvement in late adolescence (Cairns et al., 1997). For instance, criminal acts are often committed by groups of antisocial adolescents (Aultman, 1980; Gold, 1970).

The role of deviant peers in the etiology of adolescent delinquent behaviour and substance use is illustrated in a longitudinal study using a national probability sample reported by Elliott et al. (1985). They found that self-reported involvement in a deviant peer group accounted for substantial variance in subsequent levels of self-reported delinquency and substance use in middle and late adolescence, even after accounting for previous levels of delinquency. The role of the deviant peer group in the development of various forms of problem behaviour has also been put forward by several other longitudinal investigations (Biglan et al., 1995; Fergusson & Horwood, 1996; Keena et al., 1995; Patterson & Dishion, 1985).

These longitudinal studies suggest a causal relationship between involvement in a deviant peer group and later escalation in problem behaviour. However, conclusions about causality are stronger when they are based on studies using an experimental design, as is the case in clinical research with random assignment. Iatrogenic effects observed when at-risk youth are aggregated in groups for intervention purposes provide such empirical support. In their evaluation of the ATP, Dishion & Andrews (1995) reported iatrogenic effects resulting from the teen focus component. Specifically, youth aggregated into treatment groups designed to improve their social and problem-solving skills escalated in terms of self-reported smoking and teacher-reported delinquent behaviour, compared with the control condition. Unfortunately, this effect persisted for 3 years after the intervention. It is important to note that only the postpubertal adolescents (i.e. ages 13 and 14) exhibited the iatrogenic effects. This age effect is consistent with the developmental literature, suggesting that as they reach adolescence, individuals are at an increasing risk of escalation if exposed to other high-risk youth.

Other empirical evidence of the unfortunate consequences of aggregating high-risk youth comes from a re-examination of the long-term effects of the Cambridge–Sommerville Youth Study (McCord, 1992). This prevention study revealed that youth who participated in a 5-year multilevel intervention (family consultation, mentoring, counselling, etc.) showed more adjustment problems 30 years later than their control counterparts. A more recent series of analyses has revealed that it was specifically those youth who had participated in a summer camp programme who demonstrated the poorest long-term outcomes (Dishion et al., 1999).

These studies have serious implications. Theoretically, the data support the hypothesis that association with other at-risk peers plays a role in the escalation of antisocial behaviour. These effects appear to exist even in highly controlled treatment settings. Clinically, these data provide a strong criticism against treatments that place at-risk adolescents in close proximity with one another.

Longitudinal and prevention studies with random assignment provide empirical support for the hypothesis that association with deviant peers is causally related to subsequent behaviour problems. Early formulations of social learning theory placed the reinforcements provided by peers as a critical part of the learning process (Akers, 1973; Burgess & Akers, 1966). In his social learning theory of aggression, Bandura (1973, 1989) also underlined the role of peers as a source of reinforcement. More direct empirical support for the role of peers in the reinforcement process comes from the work of Dishion et al. (1996).

To study the mechanisms through which friends impact behavioural adjustment, the OYS boys (13 to 14 years old) and their closest friends participated in a 25-minute videotaped problem-solving discussion. These videotapes were analysed using a coding system that focuses on verbal content and affective reactions. Two topics were defined: rule-breaking talk and normative talk. The possible reactions were 'laugh' and 'pause'. Rule-breaking talk occurred four times more frequently in antisocial dyads. Also, sequential analyses revealed a statistically reliable difference between groups in reciprocal response patterns. Whereas nonantisocial and mixed dyads responded to normative talk with a laugh, antisocial dyads were found to respond to rule-breaking talk with a laugh.

The most important issue concerns the impact of these dyadic processes on developmental trajectories. Friendship dyads that provided contingent positive reinforcement for rule-breaking talk were found to escalate in self-reported delinquent behaviour during the following 2 years, even controlling for prior levels (Dishion et al., 1996). Dishion et al. (1995a) found that a tendency for the dyad to react positively to rule-breaking topics was associated with increased probability of escalating from abstinence to patterned alcohol, tobacco and marijuana use over the ensuing 2 years. Dishion et al. (1997) also found that both self-reported violence and police contacts for violence was associated with deviancy training during adolescence, as assessed over three time points (ages 13–14, 15–16, 17–18).

In summary, the data linking deviant peer association with the development and escalation of antisocial behaviour is overwhelming. Moreover, recent research has provided rich information regarding the specific mechanisms through which deviant peers reinforce one another's deviant behaviour. These findings also suggest that interventions grouping together at-risk youth should be approached with great caution.

Contributions of siblings

It makes sense that both the coercion and deviancy training reinforcement mechanisms would apply to sibling interaction and the possible influence of siblings on social development. The study of siblings, however, is just beginning.

At the most basic level, we are faced with data indicating that siblings are behaviourally similar. For example, based on direct observation conducted in the home, Patterson (1986) reported a correlation of 0.61 among boys referred for conduct problems and their nonreferred brothers. These data, however, are confounded by the fact that the brothers were observed while at home, frequently interacting with each other.

Other research (Lewin et al., 1993) found that siblings are similar on measures of negative peer nominations ($r = 0.65$), teacher ratings of aggression ($r = 0.26$), likability ($r = 0.55$), behaviour adjustment ($r = 0.48$), and observed positive peer behaviour in the classroom ($r = 0.47$). Of note, these observations were conducted in different classrooms and with different teachers. This research has revealed a correlation of 0.72 among siblings on direct observation measures of teacher disapproval. The most important implication here is that these siblings are not only behaviourally similar, but they elicit similar responses from their individual social environments.

From a reinforcement perspective, it is hypothesized that these behavioural similarities result, at least in part, from similar reinforcement backgrounds. In fact, support for this hypothesis has been provided by Arnold et al. (1975), who found that all siblings in a family decreased observed aversive behaviour following a parent training intervention, even though only one child was targeted in the treatment.

However, we also should expect siblings within a family to be treated differently in relation to differences in age and family circumstances as each child grows (Conger & Conger, 1994). Such differential parenting has been one way of examining the effects of a nonshared family environment (Anderson et al., 1994). Recent longitudinal studies have shown that differential discipline (McGuire et al., 1995) and differential parent hostility from both mothers and fathers (Conger & Conger, 1994) are related to different levels of problem behaviour at a later time.

However, it is possible that differential treatment of siblings would account for no additional variance in child adjustment after accounting for the effects of direct parenting to the child (McGuire et al., 1995). In response to this concern, McGuire et al. included measures both of differential and direct parenting. Differential parenting was defined as the treatment of one child relative to the treatment of the other child. That is, the difference in treatment between the siblings, ignoring the individual parenting directed to each. Thus, differential parenting was similar to nonshared parenting. Direct parenting was defined as the parenting directed towards the individual child, ignoring the difference or similarity with the sibling. Since this measure ignores the difference or similarity between parenting towards the siblings, it corresponds neither to shared nor nonshared parenting. Including both measures allows one to ask whether the presence of differential parenting (e.g. one child receiving more severe punishment than a sibling) has a unique effect beyond the direct parenting (e.g. amount of punishment) given to that child. Surprisingly, preliminary analyses of time 1 direct parenting revealed no significant correlations with outcome measures at time 2, so the direct-parenting measures were dropped. Therefore, no strong conclusions regarding the unique effects of differential treatment toward siblings can be drawn from these studies.

Other research has taken a different approach to examining the effects of shared and nonshared parenting received by siblings. Anderson et al. (1994)

examined three components of parenting: (a) nonshared parenting to child, (b) nonshared parenting to sibling and (c) shared parenting (shared variance in the two direct-parenting measures). Using a cross-sectional design with 720 same-sex sibling pairs, these researchers attempted to examine the unique effects of shared parenting and nonshared parenting to a target child and to a sibling on social adjustment. They found that shared parenting and nonshared parenting directed toward the target child were related to measures of social competence and cognitive agency (explaining 13% to 28% of the variance in 10 of 24 analyses), whereas nonshared parenting directed toward the sibling never explained more than 2% of the variance in social adjustment directed toward the target child. No differences were found with respect to gender.

It is important to note that this study only focused on social competence. However, further analyses of the same data set (Reiss et al., 1995), focusing only on nonshared parenting to each child and sibling in relation to antisocial behaviour, further demonstrated that parenting specifically directed toward a sibling is not related to child outcomes. Again, no gender differences were found. Together, these findings are consistent with the reinforcement model, which would predict that the direct microsocial interactions between the parent and child should have the greatest effects within the family.

Finally, we must also understand how siblings affect each other's social development. Dishion (1987) addressed this question by examining the correlation between children's aversive behaviour with their siblings and peer acceptance and antisocial behaviour at school. Results indicated that the correlation between sibling interactions and peer relations were primarily nonexistent, suggesting that the influence of peers and siblings are somewhat unique. Other research failed to support the hypothesis that there is a direct transfer of interactions with siblings to those with peers (Abramovitch et al., 1986).

However, research by Snyder et al. (1997b) is relevant to this point. These researchers reported a positive relationship between a composite score representing a target child's tendency to initiate and reciprocate conflict and the probability that a sibling would negatively reinforce the target child's aggressive, relative to nonaggressive, behaviour during a conflict ($r = 0.52$). Apparently, coercion is also used with and reinforced by siblings.

In summary, although siblings show a great deal of behavioural similarity, the evidence examining how siblings affect one another's antisocial development remains unclear. This area of research, however, is relatively new and undeveloped. The effect of peer relations on the development of antisocial behaviour is much more developed and may help us understand the effects of siblings, as well.

Contextual factors

From a reinforcement point of view, contextual factors, such as family stress and neighbourhood, all affect the microsocial interactions within relationships. Thus, the effects of the larger context on antisocial behaviour are hypothesized, at least in part, to be mediated through the microsocial interactions.

In support of this hypothesis, McLeod & Shanahan (1996) have studied the effects of family stress on the development of antisocial behaviour. They found that the number of years of childhood poverty was significantly related to changes in antisocial behaviour over a 4-year period. More specifically, Patterson (1983) showed that parenting practices covaried on a day-by-day basis with daily ratings of stress, as did the child's display of aversive behaviour in the home. These findings link stress to child antisocial behaviour via parenting practices. Similarly, Forgatch et al. (1985) found that parental discipline mediated the relation between maternal stress and child antisocial behaviour. Finally, Conger et al. (1993) found support for a model that economic stress leads to depression and demoralization, which in time disrupts skilful parenting. Most importantly, disrupted parenting then plays a mediating role from economic hardship to adolescent adjustment.

Neighbourhood settings have been implicated in the development of antisocial behaviour, as well. For example, Crane (1991) used census data to look at the rate of high school dropouts as a function of neighbourhood risk status. In the largest US metropolitan areas, results showed that as the percentage of high-status workers fell below 3.5%, the probability of adolescent dropout doubled from 11% to 22% (see Fig. 10.3). Boys from the highest risk neighbourhoods demonstrated a dramatic nonlinear increase in dropping out, whereas girls demonstrated a linear trend.

Again, it is likely that the effects of the neighbourhood are mediated through microsocial variables, such as parenting practices. Rutter (1981) found that the association between context and antisocial behaviour was, in part, mediated through the disruption of families as indexed by a family adversity scale. However, more research is needed to demonstrate the role of reinforcement as a mediator of sociological factors, such as neighbourhood settings.

Niche-building

Environment selection is an emergent but central issue in understanding children's development. Behaviour genetics has pointed out that the selection of settings and relationships is influenced considerably by the genetic constitu-

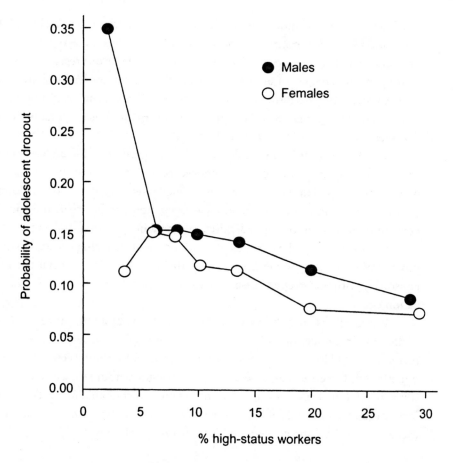

Fig. 10.3. Estimated dropout probability as a function of the percentage of high-status workers in the neighbourhood for black males and black females in the largest cities. From 'The Epidemic Theory of Ghettos and Neighborhood Effects on Dropping Out and Teenage Childbearing' by J. Crane (1991), *American Journal of Sociology*, 100, p. 1240. © 1991, University of Chicago; used with permission.

tion of the individual. Scarr & McCartney (1983) suggested that the differences in changing correlations between monozygotic twins, dizygotic twins and nonrelated adopted siblings provide support for a genetic-based niche-building model. These authors argue that during early and middle childhood, all siblings share a great deal of environment, regardless of genetic similarity. However, as these siblings get older and start selecting their own environment (friends, sports, intellectual pursuits), they will either remain similar or diverge and become more dissimilar, depending on shared genetic endowment. Specifically, the correlation between monozygotic twins remains high from childhood to adolescence, correlations between dizygotic twins drop moderately and the correlation between nonrelated adopted siblings drops to zero. The most dramatic evidence in support of this model is provided from research demonstrating the high degree of similarity between identical twins reared apart (Scarr & McCartney, 1983). They maintain that the high level of similarity among the monozygotic twins reared apart is the result of similar choices about activities and social relations, primarily in adolescence.

An important contribution of the niche-building model is the understanding that the overall environment is composed of a selected (e.g. friends) and a nonselected (e.g. family) environment (Elicker et al., 1992). By including measures of an individual's unchosen environment, rather than the specific environments chosen by the individual, we may be watering down the environment construct, adding irrelevant variance and reducing its explanatory power. We endorse the perspective that the act of finding a social network consonant with one's repertoire and personality has the most powerful socialization effect.

One hypothesis that draws from both the niche-building model and the reinforcement model of antisocial behaviour suggests that self-selected social relations should have a relatively stronger potential for reinforcement. Consequently, reinforcement may be relatively stronger within self-selected friendships than familial relationships. A reinforcement niche-building model, therefore, would be supported if data were to demonstrate that deviancy training is more powerful among chosen friends than among siblings.

Conclusion

We have examined the literature relating the social world of antisocial youth to their specific developmental course. The richness of the research findings presented in this chapter is not found in the general conclusion that parents and peers are important in the socialization of a child. Rather, the richness lies in the specification of the process through which the family and peers affect the development of an enduring antisocial behavioural trait.

For example, findings demonstrating the powerful and long-term effects of microsocial coercive exchanges between parents and children, in combination with the coercion model proposed by Patterson et al. (1992), illuminate the step-by-step life-course progression of antisocial behaviour. Moreover, the observed differences between antisocial and nonantisocial adolescent boys in microsocial interactions with friends have given us a deeper understanding of the processes involved in escalation of and the changing contingencies for antisocial behaviour across the life span. Evidence suggests that, although the process starts with negative reinforcement of coercive escape behaviours, adolescents are positively reinforcing each other's rule-breaking talk and anti-social behaviour.

The reinforcement model and the demonstrated functional utility of these antisocial acts suggest promise for intervention. By changing contingencies within the parent–child relationship, we should be able to positively affect the developmental trajectory of the child. Moreover, both theory and research have helped specify which parenting behaviours and contingencies are most important at different ages. With younger children, it is critical that parents set clear contingencies for positive and negative behaviours, and consistently adhere to those contingencies. During adolescence, parents should pay special attention to monitoring peer activities, ensuring that their adolescent associates with prosocial peers and has limited time with peers unsupervised by an adult. From microsocial analyses, we are able to break down parenting behaviours and describe in detail how they can improve their skills.

Although the reinforcement model provides clear direction and promise for reducing antisocial behaviour, barriers still exist. First, individual characteristics of the child may make parenting particularly difficult. For example, Moffitt et al. (1996) demonstrated differences in temperament between childhood-onset and adolescent-onset cases of antisocial behaviour as early as age 3. Given a child with a difficult temperament, parenting behaviours may be especially difficult to change. Also, larger social contexts, such as economic and marital difficulties, unstable employment, parent psychopathology, and the effects of bad neighbourhoods, all present forces that maintain poor family management practices.

Although barriers exist, research has already demonstrated that clinical change is possible (Dishion & Andrews, 1995). One approach now being tested to curb the development of antisocial behaviour is based on motivational interviewing, originally developed to be used with problem drinkers (Miller et al., 1993). Dishion et al. (in press a) proposed a multiple gating approach to motivate parents to utilize appropriate levels of intervention. At one level, the parents and child complete a broad-based assessment of personal and family adjustment, termed the Family Check-Up. The parents are then presented with the results of the assessment. Emphasis is placed on how parents may positively change the present situation. One particular strength of this approach is that it helps place family difficulties into a larger picture. For example, some families may be experiencing an abundance of extrafamilial stress, which bleeds into their daily family life. Others may discover that their family interactions are highly coercive. Relationships between microsocial interactions and larger contextual factors can be emphasized. Parents are then able to identify which area of difficulty they want to address. This procedure (Dishion et al., in press *b*) has been found to result in reductions in parent-reported behaviour problems (Rao, 1998).

A final note regarding gender differences is needed. Although the studies, including both boys and girls typically found no differences in the role of reinforcement in the development of antisocial behaviour, it is too early to draw strong conclusions. Results demonstrating that teachers rated the aggressiveness of rejected boys and girls quite differently, and that boys' antisocial behaviour was more strongly correlated with academic difficulties than the girls' (Dishion et al., 1994), suggest that differences likely exist. Further research is clearly needed to understand gender differences in the socialization and expression of antisocial behaviour.

Popular solutions that have not considered the developmental etiology and microsocial processes of antisocial behaviour are highly risky. For example, placing antisocial youth in a 'boot camp' type of institution allows these youth to push each other further down the path of antisocial development. Escalation of problem behaviour is likely to occur, even while the youth are within the institution. Moreover, once the children or adolescents return to the same neighbourhood, friends and family, they are likely to respond to that environment in the same manner as before. Instead, intervention and prevention efforts should be directed at changing the children's environment and immediate social contingencies. A reinforcement model offers a strong tool with which we can address the problems of antisocial behaviour.

Acknowledgements

This project was supported by grant DA 07031 from the National Institute on Drug Abuse at the National Institutes of Health to the second author, by grant MH 46690 from the National Institute of Mental Health to Gerald R. Patterson, PhD, and by grant MH 37940 from the National Institute of Mental Health to John B. Reid, PhD. Our thanks to the NIDA, OYS and PIRC families and staff for their participation in this project and to Ann Simas for her editorial and graphic assistance.

REFERENCES

Abramovitch, P., Carter, C., Pepler, D.J. & Stanhope, L. (1986). Sibling and peer interaction: a final follow-up and a comparison. *Child Development, 57*, 217–29.

Achenbach, T.M., McConaughy, S.H. & Howell, C.T. (1987). Child/adolescent behavioral and emotional problems: implications of cross-information correlations for situational specificity. *Psychological Bulletin, 101*, 213–32.

Akers, R.L. (1973). *Deviant Behavior: A Social Learning Perspective.* Belmont, CA: Wadsworth Publishing Company.

Anderson, E.R., Hetherington, E.M., Reiss, D. & Howe, G. (1994). Parents' nonshared treatment of siblings and the development of social competence during adolescence. *Journal of Family Psychology, 8*, 303–20.

Arnold, J.E., Levine, A.G. & Patterson, G.R. (1975). Changes in sibling behavior following family intervention. *Journal of Consulting and Clinical Psychology, 43*, 683–8.

Aultman, M.G. (1980). Group involvement in delinquent acts: a study of offense types and male–female participation. *Criminal Justice and Behavior, 7*, 185–92.

Bandura, A. (1973). Social learning theory of aggression. In J.F. Knutson (Ed.), *The Control of Aggression* (pp. 201–50). Chicago: Aldine.

Bandura, A. (1989). Social cognitive theory. In R. Vasta (Ed.), *Annals of Child Development,* (Vol. 6, pp. 1–60). Greenwich, CT: JAI Press.

Bardone, A.M., Moffitt, T., Caspi, A. & Dickson, N. (1996). Adult mental health and social outcomes of adolescent girls with depression and conduct disorder. *Development and Psychopathology, 8*, 811–29.

Bernal, M.E., Delfini, L.F., North, J.A. & Kreutzer, S.L. (1976). Comparison of boys' behaviors in homes and classrooms. In E.J. Mash, L.A. Hamerlynck & L.C. Hardy (Eds.), *Behavior Modification and Families* (pp. 125–39). New York: Brunner/Mazel.

Biglan, A., Duncan, T.E., Ary, D. & Smolkowski, P. (1995). Peer and parental influences on adolescent tobacco use. *Journal of Behavioral Medicine, 18*, 315–30.

Boivin, M., Dodge, K.A. & Coie, J.D. (1995). Individual-group behavioral similarity and peer status in experimental playgroups of boys: the social misfit revisited. *Journal of Personality and Social Psychology, 69*, 269–79.

Boivin, M. & Vitaro, F. (1995). The impact of peer relationships on aggression in childhood: inhibition through coercion or promotion through peer support. In J. McCord (Ed.), *Coercion and Punishment in Long-term Perspectives* (pp. 183–97). New York: Cambridge University Press.

Burgess, R.L. & Akers, R.L. (1966). A differential association reinforcement theory of criminal behavior. *Social Problems, 14*, 128–47.

Cairns, R.B., Cadwallader, T.W., Estell, D. & Neckerman, H. (1997). Groups to gangs: developmental and criminological perspectives and relevance for prevention. In D.M. Stoff, J. Breiling & J.D. Maser (Eds.), *Handbook of Antisocial Behavior* (pp. 194–204). New York: John Wiley & Sons.

Cairns, R.B., Cairns, B.D., Neckerman, H.J., Gest, S.D. & Gariepy, J. (1988). Social networks and aggressive behavior: Peer support or peer rejection. *Developmental Psychology, 24*, 815–23.

Charlebois, P., Tremblay, R.E., Gagnon, C., Larivee, S. & Laurent, D. (1989). Situational consistency in behavioral patterns of aggressive boys: methodological considerations on observational measures. *Journal of Psychopathology and Behavioral Assessment*, *11*, 15–27.

Coie, J.D., Belding, M. & Underwood, M. (1988). Aggression and peer rejection in childhood. In B.B. Lahey & A. Kazdin (Eds.), *Advances in Clinical Psychology*, (Vol. 11, pp. 38–57). New York: Plenum Press.

Coie, J.D. & Dodge, K.A. (1988). Multiple sources of data on social behavior and social status in the school: across-age comparison. *Child Development*, *59*, 815–29.

Coie, J.D. & Kupersmidt, J.B. (1983). A behavioral analysis of emerging social status in boys groups. *Child Development*, *54*, 1400–16.

Conger, K.J. & Conger, R.D. (1994). Differential parenting and change in sibling differences in delinquency. *Journal of Family Psychology*, *8*, 287–302.

Conger, R.D., Conger, K.J., Elder, G.H., Jr., et al. (1993). Family economic stress and adjustment of early adolescent girls. *Developmental Psychology*, *29*, 206–19.

Conger, R.D., Patterson, G.R. & Ge, X. (1995). It takes two to replicate: a mediational model for the impact of parents' stress on adolescent adjustment. *Child Development*, *66*, 80–97.

Crane, J. (1991). The epidemic theory of ghettos and neighborhood effects on dropping out and teenage childbearing. *American Journal of Sociology*, *100*, 1226–59.

Dishion, T.J. (1987). *A developmental model for peer relations: Middle childhood correlates and one-year sequelae*. PhD dissertation, University of Oregon, Eugene, OR.

Dishion, T.J. (1990). The family ecology of boys' peer relations in middle childhood. *Child Development*, *61*, 874–92.

Dishion, T.J. & Andrews, D.W. (1995). Preventing escalation in problem behaviors with high risk young adolescents: immediate and 1-year outcomes. *Journal of Consulting and Clinical Psychology*, *63*, 538–48.

Dishion, T.J., Capaldi, D., Spracklen, K.M. & Li, F. (1995a). Peer ecology of male adolescent drug use. *Development and Psychopathology*, *7*, 803–24.

Dishion, T.J., Eddy, J.M., Haas, E., Li, F. & Spracklen, K.M. (1997). Friendships and violent behavior during adolescence. *Social Development*, *6*, 207–25.

Dishion, T.J., French, D.C. & Patterson, G.R. (1995b). The development and ecology of antisocial behavior. In D. Cicchetti & D.J. Cohen (Eds.), *Developmental Psychopathology. Vol. 2: Risk, Disorder, and Adaptation* (pp. 421–71). New York, NY: John Wiley & Sons.

Dishion, T.J., Gardner, K., Patterson, G.R., Reid, J.R., Spyrou, S. & Thibodeaux, S. (1983). *The Family Process Code: A Multidimensional System for Observing Family Interaction*. Unpublished technical report. (Available from Oregon Social Learning Center, 160 East 4th Avenue, Eugene, OR 97401-2426.)

Dishion, T.J. & Kavanagh, K. (in press). *Adolescent Problem Behavior: An Intervention and Assessment Sourcebook for Working with Families in Schools*. New York, NY: Guilford Press.

Dishion, T.J., Kavanagh, K. & Kiesner, J. (in press a). Prevention of early adolescent substance use among high-risk youth: A multiple gating approach to parent intervention. In R.S. Ashery (Ed.), *Research meeting on drug abuse prevention through family interventions*. NIDA Research Monograph.

Dishion, T.J., Kavanagh, K. & Rao, S. (in press b). A selected intervention for family change. In T.J. Dishion & K. Kavanagh (Eds.), *Adolescent Problem Behavior: A Family-Centered Intervention and Assessment Sourcebook*. New York, NY: Guilford Press.

Dishion, T.J., McCord, J. & Poulin, F. (1999). When interventions harm: peer groups and problem behavior. *American Psychologist*, *54*, 755–64.

Dishion, T.J. & Patterson, G.R. (1997). The timing and severity of antisocial behavior: Three hypotheses within an ecological framework. In D. Stoff, J. Breiling & J. Maser (Eds.), *Handbook of Antisocial Behavior* (pp. 205–17). New York: John Wiley & Sons.

Dishion, T.J., Patterson, G.R. & Griesler, P.C. (1994). Peer adaptation in the development of antisocial behavior: A confluence model. In L.R. Huesmann (Ed.), *Aggressive Behavior: Current Perspectives* (pp. 61–95). New York, NY: Plenum Press.

Dishion, T.J., Spracklen, K.M., Andrews, D.W. & Patterson, G.R. (1996). Deviancy training in male adolescent friendships. *Behavior Therapy*, *27*, 373–90.

Dodge, K.A. (1983). Behavioral antecedents: a peer social status. *Child Development*, *54*, 1386–99.

Dodge, K.A. & Coie, J.D. (1987). Social information-processing factors in reactive and proactive aggression in children's peer groups. *Journal of Personality and Social Psychology*, *53*, 1146–57.

Dodge, K.A., Lochman, J.E., Harnish, J.D. & Bates, J.E. (1997). Reactive and proactive aggression in school children and psychiatrically impaired chronically assaultive youth. *Journal of Abnormal Psychology*, *106*, 37–51.

Elicker, J., Englund, M. & Sroufe, L.A. (1992). Predicting peer competence and peer relationships in childhood from early parent–child relationships. In R.D. Parke & G.W. Ladd (Eds.), *Family–Peer Relationships: Modes of Linkage* (pp. 77–106). Hillsdale, NJ: Lawrence Erlbaum.

Elliott, D., Huizinga, D. & Ageton, S. (1985). *Explaining Delinquency and Drug Use*. Beverly Hills, CA: Sage Publications.

Fagot, B.I. & Leve, L.D. (1998). Teacher ratings of externalizing behavior at school entry for boys and girls: similar early predictors and different correlates. *Journal of Child Psychology and Psychiatry*, *39*, 555–66.

Farrington, D.P. (1978). The family backgrounds of aggressive youths. In L.A. Herson, M. Berger & D. Shaffer (Eds.), *Aggression and Antisocial Behavior in Childhood and Adolescence* (pp. 73–93). Oxford: Pergamon Press.

Farrington, D.P. & West, D.J. (1993). Criminal, penal and life histories of chronic offenders: risk and protective factors and early identification. *Criminal Behaviour and Mental Health*, *3*, 492–523.

Farver, J.M. (1996). Aggressive behavior in preschoolers' social networks: do birds of a feather flock together? *Early Childhood Research Quarterly*, *11*, 333–50.

Fergusson, D.M. & Horwood, L.J. (1996). The role of adolescent peer affiliations in the continuity between childhood behavioral adjustment and juvenile offending. *Journal of Abnormal Child Psychology*, *24*, 205–21.

Forgatch, M.S. (1984). *A two-stage analysis of family problem-solving: global and microsocial*. PhD dissertation, University of Oregon, Eugene, OR.

Forgatch, M.S. (1991). The clinical science vortex: Developing a theory for antisocial behavior. In D.J. Pepler & K.H. Rubin (Eds.), *The Development and Treatment of Childhood Aggression* (pp. 291–315). Hillsdale, NJ: Lawrence Erlbaum.

Forgatch, M.S., Patterson, G.R. & Skinner, M.L. (1985). A mediational model for the effect of divorce on antisocial behavior in boys. In E.M. Hetherington & J.D. Arasteh (Eds.), *Impact of Divorce, Single Parenting and Step-parenting on Children* (pp. 135–54). Hillsdale, NJ: Lawrence Erlbaum.

French, D.C. & Waas, G.A. (1987). Social-cognitive and behavioral characteristics of peer-rejected boys. *Professional School Psychology, 2,* 103–12.

French, D.C., Conrad, J. & Neill, S. (1991, April). *Social adjustment of antisocial and nonantisocial early adolescents.* Paper presented at the biennial meeting of the Society for Research in Child Development, Seattle, WA.

Gardner, F.E.M. (1989). Inconsistent parenting: Is there evidence for a link with children's conduct problems? *Journal of Abnormal Child Psychology, 17,* 223–33.

Gendreau, P., Madden, P. & Leipciger, M. (1979). Norms and recidivism for first incarcerates: implications for programming. *Canadian Journal of Criminology, 21,* 416–41.

Gold, M. (1970). *Delinquent Behavior in an American city.* San Francisco: Brooks and Coleman.

Keenan, K. Loeber, R., Zhang, Q., Stouthamer-Loeber, M. & Van Kammen, W.B. (1995). The influence of deviant peers on the development of boys' disruptive and delinquent behavior: a temporal analysis. *Development and Psychopathology, 7,* 715–26.

Koller, K. & Gosden, S. (1984). On living alone, social isolation and psychological disorder. *Australian and New Zealand Journal of Sociology, 20,* 81–92.

Kupersmidt, J.B., DeRosier, M.E. & Patterson, C.P. (1995). Similarity as the basis for children's friendships: the roles of sociometric status, aggressive and withdrawn behavior, academic achievement and demographic characteristics. *Journal of Social and Personal Relationships, 12,* 439–52.

Lewin, L.N., Hops, H., Davis, B. & Dishion, T.J. (1993). Multimethod comparison of similarity in school adjustment of siblings in unrelated children. *Developmental Psychology, 29,* 963–9.

Loeber, R. (1982). The stability of antisocial and delinquent child behavior: a review. *Child Development, 53,* 1431–46.

Loeber, R. (1988). Behavioral precursors and accelerators of delinquency. In W. Buikhuisen et al. (Eds.), *Explaining Criminal Behaviour: Interdisciplinary Approaches* (pp. 51–67). Leiden, Netherlands: E.J. Brill.

Loeber, R. & Dishion, T.J. (1983). Early predictors of male delinquency: a review. *Psychological Bulletin, 94,* 68–98.

Loeber, R. & Dishion, T.J. (1984). Boys who fight at home and school: family conditions influencing cross-setting consistency. *Journal of Consulting and Clinical Psychology, 52,* 759–68.

Mandelzys, N. (1979). Correlates of offense severity and recidivism probability in a Canadian sample. *Journal of Clinical Psychology, 35,* 897–907.

McCord, J. (1979). Some child-rearing antecedents of criminal behavior in adult men. *Journal of Personality and Social Psychology, 37,* 1477–86.

McCord, J. (1992). The Cambridge-Sommerville Study: a pioneering longitudinal-experimental study of delinquency prevention. In J. McCord & R. Tremblay (Eds.), *Preventing Antisocial Behavior: Interventions from Birth to Adolescence* (pp. 196–209). New York: Guilford Press.

McCord, W., McCord, J. & Howard, A. (1961). Familial correlates of aggression in nondelinquent male children. *Journal of Abnormal and Social Psychology, 62,* 79–93.

McDowell, J.J. (1988). Matching theory in natural human environments. *Behavior Analyst, 11*, 95–109.

McGuire, S., Dunn, J. & Plomin, R. (1995). Maternal differential treatment of siblings and children's behavioral problems: a longitudinal study. *Development and Psychopathology, 7*, 515–28.

McLeod, J.D. & Shanahan, M.J. (1996). Trajectories of poverty and children's mental health. *Journal of Health and Social Behavior, 37*, 207–20.

Miller, W.R., Benefield, R.G. & Tonigan, J.S. (1993). Enhancing motivation for change in problem drinking: a controlled comparison of two therapist styles. *Journal of Consulting & Clinical Psychology, 61*, 455–61.

Moffitt, T.E. (1993). Adolescence-limited and life course persistent antisocial behavior: developmental taxonomy. *Psychological Review, 100*, 674–701.

Moffitt, T.E., Caspi, A., Dickson, N. & Silva, P. (1996). Childhood-onset versus adolescent-onset antisocial conduct problems in males: natural history from ages 3 to 18 years. *Development and Psychopathology, 8*, 399–424.

Moore, D., Chamberlain, P. & Mukai, L. (1979). Children at risk for delinquency: a follow-up comparison of aggressive children and children who steal. *Journal of Abnormal Child Psychology, 7*, 345–55.

Olweus, D. (1979). Stability of aggressive reaction patterns in males: a review. *Psychological Bulletin, 86*, 852–75.

Patterson, G.R. (1982). *Coercive Family Process*. Eugene, OR: Castalia Publishing Company.

Patterson, G.R. (1983). Stress: a change agent for family process. In N. Garmezy & M. Rutter (Eds.), *Stress, Coping, and Development in Children* (pp. 235–64). New York: McGraw-Hill.

Patterson, G.R. (1986). Performance models for antisocial boys. *American Psychologist, 41*, 432–44.

Patterson, G.R. (1995). Coercion as a basis for early age of onset for arrest. In J. McCord (Ed.), *Coercion and Punishment in Long-term Perspectives* (pp. 81–105). New York: Cambridge University Press.

Patterson, G.R. (1996). Some characteristics of a developmental theory for early onset delinquency. In M.F. Lenzenweger & J.J. Haugaard (Eds.), *Frontiers of Developmental Psychopathology* (pp. 81–124). New York: Oxford University Press.

Patterson, G.R. & Bank, L. (1989). Some amplifying mechanisms for pathologic processes in families. In M.R. Gunnar & E. Thelen (Eds.), *Systems and Development: The Minnesota Symposia on Child Psychology*, (Vol. 22, pp. 167–209). Hillsdale, NJ: Lawrence Erlbaum Associates.

Patterson, G.R., Capaldi, D.M. & Bank, L. (1991). An early starter model predicting delinquency. In D.J. Pepler & K.H. Rubin (Eds.), *The Development and Treatment of Childhood Aggression* (pp. 139–68). Hillsdale, NJ: Lawrence Erlbaum Associates.

Patterson, G.R. & Dishion, T.J. (1985). Contributions of families and peers to delinquency. *Criminology, 23*, 63–79.

Patterson, G.R., Dishion, T.J. & Bank, L. (1984). Family interaction: a process model of deviancy training. *Aggressive Behavior, 10*, 253–67.

Patterson, G.R., Littman, R.A. & Bricker, W. (1967). Assertive behavior in children: a step toward a theory of aggression. *Monographs of the Society for Research in Child Development, 32*(5).

Patterson, G.R. & Reid, J.B. (1984). Social interactional processes within the family: the study of moment-by-moment family transactions in which human social development is embedded. *Journal of Applied Developmental Psychology, 5*, 237–62.

Patterson, G.R., Reid, J.B. & Dishion, T.J. (1992). *A Social Learning Approach. IV. Antisocial Boys.* Eugene, OR: Castalia Publishing Company.

Patterson, G.R. & Stouthamer-Loeber, M. (1984). The correlation of family management practices and delinquency. *Child Development, 55*, 1299–1307.

Patterson, G.R. & Yoerger, K. (1997). A developmental model for late-onset delinquency. In W.D. Osgood (Ed.), *Motivation and Delinquency* (pp. 119–77). Lincoln, NE: University of Nebraska Press.

Poulin, F. & Boivin, M. (2000). The formation and development of friendship in childhood: the role of proactive and reactive aggression. *Developmental Psychology*, in press.

Poulin, F., Cillessen, A.H.N., Hubbard, J.A. & Coie, J.D. (1997). Children's friends and behavioral similarity in two social contexts. *Social Development, 6*, 224–36.

Quay, H.C. (1964). Dimensions of personality in delinquent boys as inferred from the factor analysis of case history data. *Child Development, 35*, 479–84.

Rao, S. (1998). *An evaluation of the Family Check-Up with high risk young adolescents.* PhD dissertation, University of Oregon, Eugene, OR.

Reiss, D., Hetherington, M., Plomin, R., et al. (1995). Genetic questions for environmental studies: differential parenting and psychopathology in adolescence. *Archives of General Psychiatry, 52*, 925–36.

Robins, L.N. (1966). *Deviant Children Grow Up: A Sociological and Psychiatric Study of Sociopathic Personality.* Baltimore, MD: Williams & Wilkins Company.

Rutter, M. (1981). The city and the child. *American Journal of Orthopsychiatry, 51*, 610–25.

Scarr, S. & McCartney, K. (1983). How people make their own environments: a theory of genotype to environment effects. *Child Development, 54*, 424–35.

Simons, R.L., Wu, C., Conger, R.D. & Lorenz, F.O. (1996). Two routes to delinquency: Differences between early and late starters in the impact of parenting and deviant peers. *Criminology, 32*, 247–74.

Snyder, J., Edwards, P., McGraw, K., Kilgore, K. & Holton, A. (1994). Escalation and reinforcement in mother–child conflict: Social processes associated with the development of physical aggression. *Development and Psychopathology, 6*, 305–21.

Snyder, J., Horsch, E. & Childs, J. (1997a). Peer relationships of young children: affiliative choices and the shaping of aggressive behavior. *Journal of Child Clinical Psychology, 26*, 145–56.

Snyder, J.J. & Patterson, G.R. (1995). Individual differences in social aggression: a test of a reinforcement model of socialization in the natural environment. *Behavior Therapy, 26*, 371–91.

Snyder, J., Schrepferman, L. & St. Peter, C. (1997b). Origins of antisocial behavior: negative reinforcement and affect dysregulation of behavior as socialization mechanisms in family interaction. *Behavior Modification, 21*, 187–215.

Snyder, J., West, L., Stockemer, V., Givens, S. & Almquist-Parks, L. (1996). A social learning model of peer choice in the natural environment. *Journal of Applied Developmental Psychology, 17*, 215–37.

Strayer, F.F. & Noel, J.M. (1986). The prosocial and antisocial functions of preschool aggression:

an ethological study of triadic conflict among young children. In C. Zahn-Waxler, E.M. Cummings & R. Iannotti (Eds.), *Altruism and Aggression: Biological and Social Origins* (pp. 107–131). Cambridge: Cambridge University Press.

Vuchinich, S., Bank, L. & Patterson, G.R. (1992). Parenting, peers and the stability of antisocial behavior in preadolescent males. *Developmental Psychology, 28*, 510–21.

Wadsworth, M.E.J. (1979). *Roots of Delinquency: Infancy, Adolescence, and Crime*. Oxford: Robertson.

Wasik, B.H. (1987). Sociometric measures and peer descriptors of kindergarten children: a study of reliability and validity. *Journal of Clinical Child Psychology, 16*, 218–24.

West, D. & Farrington, D. (1977). *The Delinquent Way of Life*. London: Heinemann.

Wright, J.C., Giammarino, M. & Parad, H.W. (1986). Social status in small groups: individual-group similarity and the social 'misfit'. *Journal of Personality and Social Psychology, 50*, 523–36.

11

Perceptual and attributional processes in aggression and conduct problems

Gregory S. Pettit, Jodi A. Polaha and Jacquelyn Mize

Processing and the development of conduct problems

Aspects of social cognition and social information-processing have been studied intensively in recent years, as researchers and clinicians search for the underlying perceptual and mental processes that give rise to aggressive behaviour and conduct problems. What sets this period of inquiry apart from earlier research is the systematic effort now being made to integrate and synthesize the various pieces of the perceptual–attributional puzzle into coherent models depicting the interface of cognition, affect and behaviour. Our goal in writing the present chapter is not to fashion yet another synthetic model, but rather to scrutinize recent research in terms of its fit with current models, and the extent to which emerging findings amplify, contradict or are mute with respect to the prevailing theories. We will rely heavily on Dodge's social information-processing model (Crick & Dodge, 1994; Dodge et al., 1986), as it has provided perhaps the best known integrative perspective.

Dodge's model depicts a sequential series of steps in the processing of information in a specific social situation. It is a heuristic for summarizing distinctive perceptual, problem-solving and evaluative components thought to lead to the activation of a particular response or set of responses. Variations in these social cue-elicited patterns of activation are presumed to explain within-individual responding across differing situations and cross-individual responding within similar situations (Dodge, 1993). Early in the sequence of information-processing steps are components that characterize the perceptual encoding of social information and the assignment of meaning to the encoded cues, including judgements and attributions about the motives and intentions of social partners. It is these two components – perception and attribution – that are the focus of the current chapter. Because detailed summaries of the research literature bearing on these issues were published in the early 1990s (e.g. Crick & Dodge, 1994; Dodge & Feldman, 1990), we concern ourselves here primarily with research conducted in the latter part of the decade. We do, however, comment on earlier research that is most central to understanding the link between social perception, attributions, and aggression and related conduct problems.

Overview of models of social information-processing and social cognition

The decade of the 1980s witnessed the formulation of integrative models and theories of social information-processing that yielded an array of testable hypotheses regarding the role of conscious and nonconscious mental operations in children's maladaptive social behaviour (Dodge et al., 1986; Huesmann, 1988; Rubin & Krasnor, 1986). These theories sought to describe the mental processes that are proximally responsible for the display of maladaptive behaviour. The theories were integrative in the sense that more than a single cognitive domain was represented. The theories were synthetic in that they pulled together ideas and concepts from a variety of social-psychological and information-processing perspectives. Each stipulated a series of steps in the processing of external and internal sources of information, beginning with some form of information intake (perception of social cues), progressing through a judgement phase (making attributions regarding the intent of others), and culminating with some form of decision making and action. According to these models, to understand why a child responds to a particular situation (being teased) with a particular response (hitting), one would seek to identify how the child perceived the situation, the kinds of attributions the child made about the situation, and how these perceptions and attributions directed the child toward a particular kind of behavioural response. Behavioural responses that are considered to be ineffective, aggressive or otherwise problematic are hypothesized to be the result of deficits or biases encountered in one or more steps in the sequence of social information processing.

The first step in Dodge's (Crick & Dodge, 1994; Dodge et al., 1986) information-processing model is encoding, which describes the perceptual task of scanning the environment and attending to relevant social cues, and storage of cue information into short-term memory. Because the stimulus array typically is complex and potentially overwhelming, the individual learns to attend selectively to certain features, at the expense of other features, in order to respond more effectively. For example, in a situation in which a child has been provoked by a peer whose intentions are unclear, both deficits (failure to encode mitigating cues) and biases (selective attention to hostile cues) in encoding could lead the child to respond aggressively.

The next step is to mentally represent the encoded cues and assign meaning to them, particularly as regards others' intentions and potential threats to the self. The individual stores in memory a meaningful interpretation of the stimulus rather than a literal and specific (i.e. iconic) representation of the stimulus (Dodge, 1993). The meanings that are applied necessarily relate the stimulus array to the individual's emotional needs and goals (Crick & Dodge, 1994). Interpretation has been shown to be strongly linked to how an individual responds to an event (e.g. aggressive retaliation is more likely to follow if the individual interprets cues as threatening rather than as benign; Dodge, 1980). This means that both hostile attributional biases (a term coined by Nasby et al., 1979) and errors (such as misinterpreting a clearly benign teasing cue as malicious) could increase the likelihood of aggressive responding.

Subsequent steps (not a focus of this chapter) follow, including those in which the individual mentally generates one or more potential behavioural responses to the interpreted cues, evaluates its likely effects and the extent to which he or she feels capable of enacting it, then implements the behaviour, monitors its effects, and makes adjustments accordingly. As noted, variations in processing at these steps are thought to be correlated with the patterns of encoding and interpretation occurring earlier in the sequential model (e.g. perceived threat elicits aggressive retaliation as a viable response option). The magnitude of these relations typically is not large, however. In fact, the processing steps appear to be somewhat independent of each other, as has been documented in studies where assessments of differing steps of the processing model provide significant incremental prediction of aggressive behaviour (Dodge et al., 1986; Slaby & Guerra, 1988; Waldman, 1996).

Issues in conceptualization and measurement of perceptual and attributional processes

Latent structures versus on-line processing

Social information-processing models are thought to reflect the more proximal mental operations that are associated with behavioural responding. As such, these models describe how a particular behaviour comes to be displayed, rather than why a particular behaviour is displayed (Dodge, 1993). The 'why' issue is best addressed by considering how past experiences influence the construction of enduring mental structures (sometimes called latent knowledge structures) that, in turn, influence the processing of future social cues. These latent structures are presumed to be more distally removed from actual behavioural responding, but serve to guide on-line processing, which is the more proximal cause of behavioural responding. Although many theoretical accounts of perceptual and attributional processes in social behaviour and adjustment hypothesize the existence of enduring latent structures, there is considerable variation in how these structures are described or conceptualized.

Attachment theory provides one view of the nature of these enduring latent structures. In attachment theory, dynamic mental representations of relationships – known as internal working models – are thought to derive initially from early social relationships with caregivers. (Evidence of empirical relations between attachment history and perceptual-attributional processes is discussed in a later section.) Attachment theorists suggest that working models 'provide rules . . . that permit or limit the individual's access to certain forms of knowledge' (Main et al., 1985; p. 77) and thus influence on-line processing in ways that engender consistency between perceptions and attributions and one's working model. That is, persons with 'secure' models of the self and others are thought to perceive and remember more positive events and characteristics of others during social interaction and are likely to make benign attributions, whereas individuals with 'insecure' models see and remember more negative characteristics and events and are more likely to make hostile attributions (Belsky et al., 1996; Suess et al., 1992).

Cognitive social psychology offers alternative views and alternative nomenclature for describing latent structures that constrain processing. In contrast to work in the attachment tradition, social psychological literature offers greater specificity of mechanisms and an abundance of empirical evidence about how latent structures guide information processing. Generalized mental representations of previous experiences, often referred to as scripts (Shank & Abelson, 1977), relationship schema (Baldwin, 1992), or constructs of social concepts (Higgins & Bargh, 1987) are seen as facilitating understanding of events and guiding perceptions, attributions and behaviour. People differ in the types and accessibility of their social constructs, and in some individuals, constructs associated with aggression and hostility are rich and easily accessed. Cognitions (e.g. attributions of hostility) and behaviours consistent with a schema or construct are called into play when the particular schema is triggered or 'primed'. A child may, for instance, have a schema for 'friendly roughhousing' and a schema for hostile encounters with peers. Whether the roughhousing or the hostile schema is accessed when a peer tackles the child from behind depends, in part, on recent environmental and internal cues or events, such that an individual is more likely to access a schema that is consistent with the recent event or the affect that accompanied the event. Thus, children who have just been teased by a peer, or are in an angry mood because of conflict with a parent, or who have recently observed a violent television episode may be more likely to access a construct of hostility. Subsequent perceptions and attributions are likely to be consistent with the accessed schema. Experimental studies suggest that it is possible to prime access to schema by previously presenting, in a different context, words or ideas consistent with the primed schema (Bargh et al., 1988; Higgins & Bargh, 1987).

Although all individuals are subject to temporary priming effects (e.g. recent criticism by a boss or a bad mood make hostile or angry schemes more accessible, whereas hearing about a kind act makes a construct of kindness more easily accessible), constructs also can become chronically primed or accessible. Constructs become chronically accessible because of repeated experience with specific domains of social behaviour (e.g. hostility, selfishness, kindness). Children may develop a chronically accessible construct for hostility from living in a family in which blame routinely is assigned to others when negative events occur (Graham & Hudley, 1994), in which parents often attribute hostile intent to the child (Pettit et al., 1988), or in which violence and anger are prevalent (Coie & Dodge, 1998). That is, chronically accessible constructs are highly likely to be used to interpret social behaviour even in the absence of recent priming, so the construct is, in effect, perpetually at the 'top of the heap' when a situation in which it is potentially relevant arises. Application of chronically accessible constructs is automatic, unintentional, and uncontrollable (Bargh et al., 1988). Therefore, for aggressive children, hostile schemas may be the most easily and routinely accessed schemas in situations of potential threat.

Evidence that aggressive children acquire chronically accessible constructs of hostility (and that these are not easily countered by priming more benign constructs) comes from an experimental study by Graham & Hudley (1994). Nonaggressive children became as likely as their aggressive peers to attribute hostility in an ambiguous provocation story when they were 'primed' beforehand with stories of characters who were to blame for negative events. Aggressive children were not less likely to attribute hostile intent when primed with stories in which the characters had not been responsible for the negative events, however. These data are consistent with the idea that environmental events can prime access to constructs of hostility even for nonaggressive children, but that aggressive children may live in a state in which hostile constructs are perpetually primed, easily accessible and not easily preempted by exposure to more benign constructs.

Both attachment views and social cognitive views of latent structures offer insights into processes by which children come to be aggressive. However, social cognitive models credit a broader range of experiences as potential determinants of the structures (e.g. exposure to violence, parental treatment), and also provide greater insights into when and how latent structures affect on-line processing (Coie & Dodge, 1998).

The role of emotion

Social information-processing models of adjustment have been criticized for paying too little attention to emotion and its role in social cognition and social behaviour (Gottman, 1986). Partly as a response to these criticisms, more recent perspectives on social information-processing have been more explicit in incorporating affective elements as key ingredients. According to Crick & Dodge (1994), emotion is integral to each processing step. This includes perception, where emotional arousal (e.g. an increase in heart rate) may serve as an internal cue that must be encoded, and attribution, where emotions may influence the child's interpretation of a particular situation. For example, a child who feels anger or anxiety in an initial meeting with a peer may experience very strong affective reactions in subsequent encounters with that peer, reactions that may colour how the child interprets the peer's behaviour. When physiologically aroused owing to intensely experienced emotion (e.g. heart rate acceleration accompanying a fear reaction), it is difficult to maintain attention and engage in efficient processing (Thompson, 1994). Other kinds of arousal (e.g. such as that induced by drugs) can alter an individual's skill in making accurate attributions. Moreover, attributions themselves may induce certain emotions, such as when the interpretation of a peer's behaviour as hostile induces feelings of anger or wariness (Crick & Dodge, 1994).

To date, few investigators have examined both emotion and cognitive processing within the same study. In one study that did attempt to do so (Dodge & Somberg, 1987) induced emotional arousal was found to lead to decrements in information processing efficiency (i.e. a heightened tendency to make biased attributions), especially among aggressive children. However, the arousal induction paradigm used does not easily map onto current technologies for assessing emotion regulation and knowledge (e.g. Eisenberg et al., 1997). What are needed are investigations that use carefully designed and methodologically independent measures of emotional regulation and reactivity, underlying physiological concomitants and social cognition.

Contextual factors

Relations between processing biases and deficits and maladaptive behaviour are constrained by contextual factors, including type of situation. Situation refers to the setting or context within which children may experience social difficulties.

For example, some children may find it difficult to gain access to a group of peers already at play. Other children may have problems in situations in which they have been bothered or irritated by a peer. These two kinds of situation, referred to as peer group entry and response to provocation, respectively, appear to be especially challenging for rejected aggressive children (Dodge & Feldman, 1990). Assessments of children's social information-processing in peer group-entry situations have been found to be significantly related to children's actual behaviour in analogous situations but not in provocation-type situations. Correspondingly, processing about provocation situations has been found to predict children's actual behaviour in those situations in which a provocation occurs, but not in group entry situations (Dodge et al., 1986). This suggests that situational factors may be important determinants of the processing-behaviour linkage.

Characteristics of the target child recently have been examined as a possible situational factor in social information-processing. The standard assessment approach is to use hypothetical, generalized peers (e.g. 'imagine that a kid in your class . . .') as targets so as to allow children to use their own past experiences and expectations as a basis for responding. But when characteristics of the target are systematically modified (e.g. the target selected is a real classroom peer known to be aggressive) there are predictable changes in processing (e.g. the aggressive peer's behaviour is interpreted in a more negative light) (Dodge & Frame, 1982). Target characteristics do not appear to interact with maladjustment level, however, so it is not clear whether the specification of target information improves understanding of the relation between processing and social and behavioural adjustment (Crick & Dodge, 1994).

Heterogeneity of outcome groups

Advances in the study of links between perceptual-attributional processes and social and behavioural maladjustment have been hampered by ambiguity with respect to the types of outcome being predicted. Most research on social information-processing has been concerned with differences between normal-typical children and fairly extreme groups of problematic children. These latter groups have consisted of sociometrically rejected children, physically abused children, aggressive children, conduct-problem children, and incarcerated children and adolescents (Coie & Dodge, 1998). Comparatively little research has been conducted on nonclinical (or nondeviant) samples, so that normative-developmental variations in patterns of social information-processing across the childhood years are not clear. At least one study, however, has shown that individual differences in processing are predictive of social behaviour in an unselected sample of school-aged boys and girls (Dodge & Price, 1994).

By contrasting the processing patterns of children showing different kinds of maladjustment, researchers hope to be able to identify which aspects of processing are characteristic of deviance in general (e.g. poor encoding skills might heighten the likelihood of a range of antisocial outcomes) and which are specific to particular disorders (e.g. hypervigilance to perceived threats to self might lead to a tendency to display angry, reactive aggression but not proactive, instrumental aggression). In general, however, there has as yet been little empirical work devoted to using perceptual-attributional assessments to distinguish among children showing differing problem-behaviour profiles. In a later section, we offer a detailed critique of the empirical evidence of processing-outcome relations, with reference to the specificity of such relations. Here we would like to address briefly some issues bearing on comorbidity and age-of-onset.

With respect to comorbidity, conduct problems frequently have been found to covary with other kinds of behavioural problems, and particularly with internalizing problems (Bates et al., 1995) and with hyperactivity/attention deficit disorders (Hinshaw, 1987). The extent to which the perceptual-attributional patterns exhibited by aggressive children are unique versus characteristic of a general syndrome of behavioural dysfunction cannot be determined from existing literature. Quiggle et al. (1992) found that depressed children showed a depressogenic attributional style (i.e. they attributed negative events to internal, stable and global causes), whereas aggressive children did not. However, both depressed and aggressive children exhibited a hostile attributional bias. It may be, as Quiggle et al. (1992) speculate, that biased perceptions and attributions are typical of both aggressive and depressed children, but aggressive children are more likely to view the cause of the event as being external to themselves whereas the depressed children may be more likely to view the event as being caused by internal factors. Interestingly, children in a comorbid group showed processing patterns characteristic of both aggressive children and depressed children. Studies in this vein are clearly needed to sort out the specificity and overlap in processing in children with 'pure' versus comorbid types of behavioural maladjustment.

Processing patterns as related to age-of-onset of conduct problems have been studied even less frequently. In fact, no study could be located that explicitly contrasted the perceptual and attributional patterns of children showing differing profiles of the emergence and continuance of conduct problems. It might be expected, however, that early-onset problems would converge more strongly with hostile, reactive forms of aggression, whereas adolescent-limited problems might converge more strongly with proactive forms of aggression. This seems a reasonable possibility because early-onset problems are known to be more developmentally persistent, to be more closely linked with early socialization traumas, and to be associated with a broader array of concurrent and subsequent adjustment difficulties, compared to adolescent-limited conduct problems (Coie & Dodge, 1998). Comparable patterns have been reported for reactively and proactively aggressive children, respectively (Dodge et al., 1997). Insofar as reactive aggression has been linked to early-stage social information processing problems (e.g. biased attributions), whereas proactive aggression has been linked with later-stage processing problems (e.g. positively evaluating the likely outcome of being aggressive), it would seem possible that children showing the early-onset pattern of conduct problems might have deficits in perceptual and attributional processes, whereas adolescent-limited children might show processing patterns in decision-making and problem-solving facets – especially as they concern adult authority figures – of social information processing.

Aggregation across behaviours as a factor in prediction

Dodge (1993) has argued that, at the level of the single event, processing patterns should in theory account for all of the variance in behaviour (because processing describes how a behaviour comes about), measurement error notwithstanding. But at the level of patterns of processing and patterns of responding, the correlation necessarily will be weaker, because of contextual factors that are present to varying degrees across situations. Dodge (1993) illustrates this measurement problem in terms of the relative accuracy of prediction when the outcome is a categorical psychiatric diagnosis and when the outcome is a dimensional score indicating presence of a clinical problem. A range of problem behaviours are reflected in the typical dimensional score. For example, the broad-band externalizing behaviour problems score (Achenbach, 1985) includes aggression as well as noncompliance, covert antisocial behaviour and sexual perversion. Given the varied constituents of the score, it is unlikely that processing will correlate very highly with the composite scale. That is, whereas processing might strongly predict some of the individual behaviours that, together, contribute to a child being rated high on externalizing, the prediction of externalizing in general necessarily will be weaker.

At the categorical level of psychopathology, the goal is to identify constellations of behaviours that show some cross-time and cross-situational stability. As noted earlier, there is some evidence that processing–behaviour linkages show a fairly high degree of situation specificity, i.e. that processing patterns in one situation predict behaviours in the same kind of situation, but not in other kinds of situations (Dodge et al., 1986). This runs counter to the categorical psychopathology requirement of cross-situational consistency in behaviour. Aggregating across situations probably will reduce the psychometric reliability of the processing measures, thus attenuating the correlation between processing and categorical outcome. The point is that the strongest relations are likely to be found when processing patterns are used to predict discrete behavioural acts in specific kinds of situations (Dodge & Price, 1994).

Summary of research findings

We now turn our attention to an examination of research that has been concerned with perceptual and attributional processes as related to behavioural maladjustment, including aggression and conduct problems. We focus more on research published in the past five years; earlier work in this area has been amply summarized in a number of publications (Crick & Dodge, 1994; Dodge, 1993; Dodge & Feldman, 1990).

Perceptual processes: the encoding of social cues

Little research has been concerned directly with the examination of encoding-relevant variables, in contrast to the fairly extensive body of research on interpretation and attribution. In their review of the extant research published as of the early 1990s, Crick & Dodge (1994) identified only four studies that examined the relation between social adjustment and children's encoding and use of social cues. The general paradigm employed in these studies was to present children with hypothetical provocation situations and information about the intent of the peer in each situation. For example, Dodge & Tomlin (1987) found that aggressive children, compared to nonaggressive children, made use of significantly fewer benign cues, relied more on cues present late in the social interaction, rather than early in the interaction (a recency effect), and more often based their interpretation on information that was not a part of the presented scene, i.e. they appeared to rely more on preexisting schemas for interpreting peer-provocation situations. Other research also suggests that aggressive children are deficient in their use of social cues, either because they are overly attentive to hostile cues (Gouze, 1987) or because they make use of fewer cues of any type (Dodge & Newman, 1981).

On the basis of these early reports, Crick & Dodge (1994) hypothesize that, compared to their better adjusted peers, aggressive and socially maladjusted children's encoding of social cues is limited because of (a) memory deficits that do not allow them to store or recall the full range of presented cues, (b) selective attention to particular types of social cues (i.e. hostile cues) and (c) entrenched schemas for social situations (i.e. chronically primed for interpreting ambiguous situations as threatening) that interfere with the ability (or inclination) to process and use available social information. In the years subsequent to the Crick & Dodge (1994) review, only a handful of new studies have been published that address one or more of these hypothesized encoding limitations. One reason for the paucity of new data is that the most common paradigm for assessing encoding deficits relies on global assessments of the accuracy or 'relevance' of children's encoding. Much of the recent research by Dodge, Pettit, and their colleagues (e.g. Dodge et al., 1995) entails the presentation to the child of specially prepared videotapes depicting differing kinds of problematic social situation. The situations vary with respect to the 'goal' (e.g. dealing with a peer who has acted in a provocative way, responding to the demands of an adult authority figure) and the apparent intentions of the principal actors. Intentions typically are manipulated to depict clearly hostile behaviour, clearly benign or accidental behaviour, or behaviour that is ambiguous with respect to intention. The task of the child subject is to view the scene on tape and then to describe as fully as possible all details that can be recollected. From these descriptions, the child is assigned a score indicating the extent to which he or she encoded relevant or irrelevant details of the portrayed scene. In a series of studies, Dodge et al. have shown that aggressive children are less skilled than nonaggressive children in identifying relevant details of the depicted presentations (Dodge et al., 1990, 1995; Harrist et al., 1997). An advantage of this technique is that it allows for the modelling of real-life, complex social situations (i.e. where there are multiple actors in naturalistic settings with verbal and nonverbal cues present). A disadvantage is that little is learned about on-line encoding processes (e.g. the selective deployment of attention) that may underlie 'irrelevant' cognitions. The possibility also exists that when a 'recall' task is used to measure encoding, responses – including putative relevance of descriptions – may be biased by interpretations that occur subsequent to the presentation of the hypothetical vignette or may reflect general cognitive skill.

Attributional processes: the interpretation of social cues

A considerable amount of research has been devoted to the study of attributional processes. Such processes may be described broadly in terms of attributions of causality and attributions of intent (Crick & Dodge, 1994). The way in which children explain why events occur may have an effect on their eventual response to that event. These kinds of explanations are known as causal reasoning or causal attributions (Weiner & Graham, 1994). Most research on children's causal attributions has centred on children's explanations of events in achievement situations (e.g. explanations for success or failure), with a much smaller body of research examining children's causal reasoning in social situations. In the realm of aggression and conduct problems, the study of causal attributions is important because such attributions may explain how children come to make judgements about the behaviour of others, as well as children's appraisals of their own successes and failures in social situations.

Children who are rejected by their peers have been found to make external attributions (e.g. 'I am not responsible for this') for positive social outcomes, in comparison to their more accepted peers, who tend to make internal attributions for the same sorts of outcomes (Aydin & Markova, 1979). The kinds of attributions made by rejected children about positive events are thus more likely to contribute to negative self-evaluations. Evidence is less clear with respect to differences in attributions of negative social outcomes, with some research suggesting that low-status children, compared to high-status children, tend to blame themselves for undesirable social outcomes (Goetz & Dweck, 1980), and other research suggesting that low-status children blame external circumstances for undesirable outcomes (Crick & Ladd, 1993).

The Quiggle et al. (1992) study discussed earlier is one of the very few studies to examine children's aggression as related to their causal attributions. Whereas depressed children demonstrated a clear pattern of making internal and stable attributions for failure, aggressive children's responses were not significantly different from those of nonaggressive children. One explanation for why aggressive or rejected children do not differ consistently from their nonaggressive, nonrejected peers in attributions of social failure is that the former's use of an external attributional style serves a self-protection function. That is, it is possible that aggressive children, like their nonaggressive peers, explain failure in terms of external factors to protect themselves from experiencing distress or depressive symptoms.

The kinds of attributions made by aggressive children about others' intentions in social situations have been studied extensively. Nasby et al. (1979) were the first to describe empirical findings of a link between aggressive behaviour and biased attributions. The tendency of aggressive children to judge peers' intentions as hostile in ambiguous provocation situations subsequently has been demonstrated in a large number of studies by Dodge (Dodge, 1980; Dodge & Frame, 1982; Dodge et al. 1986) and others (Guerra & Slaby, 1989;

Waas, 1988). There is some recent evidence that this relation may be specific to children displaying a reactive, retaliatory style of aggressive behaviour. Crick & Dodge (1996) tested the hypothesis that hostile attribution bias is characteristic of reactively aggressive children but not proactively aggressive children. A standard hypothetical-stories procedure was used to assess attributions. As predicted, the reactive group had higher hostile attribution scores than did the nonaggressive group, although this difference was apparent only among older children (fifth and sixth graders). The proactive group did not differ from the nonaggressive group in terms of hostile attributions. These findings generally are consistent with the premise that children who engage in high rates of angry, retaliatory forms of aggression tend to show a bias toward interpreting ambiguous peer provocations as hostile acts. However, Dodge et al. (1997) found no evidence of hostile attributional tendencies among reactively aggressive children, compared to control children, although the reactively aggressive groups did show more encoding deficits (i.e. lower 'relevance' scores) than did contrast groups. The lack of consistent findings across studies may be due in part to the use of the hypothetical stories format for assessing intent attributions. Because this requires that the child consider the provocation scene in a deliberate sort of way, it may be that the kind of impulsive, preemptive processing that is thought to co-occur with reactive-aggressive tendencies is not 'pulled' from the child. If this were the case, then current methods may be insensitive to important variations in the kinds of automatic, scripted processing that is presumed to be a distinguishing characteristic of highly reactive youth (Crick & Dodge, 1996).

The role of impulsivity in encoding and interpretation was studied in greater detail by Waldman (1996). Socially maladjusted (aggressive, isolate and aggressive-isolate) and adjusted school-aged boys were compared on several standard measures of processing. Controlling for inattention/impulsivity, there still was a significant difference between aggressive and nonaggressive boys on hostile misidentifications of intentions (analogous to the hostile attribution bias studied by Dodge and others) and on hostile versus nonhostile discriminations of intentions. These latter two measures were conceptualized as indicators of hostile perceptual bias. There were no differences in what Waldman (1996) refers to as general social perceptual deficit, that is, discrimination among nonhostile (i.e. accidental, prosocial, ambiguous and 'merely present') intention cues. From these data it would appear that aggressive boys are characterized by a hostile social perceptual bias rather than a general social perceptual deficit. This bias could not be explained by individual differences in impulsivity and distractibility.

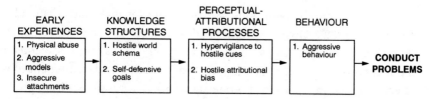

Fig. 11.1. Model of the development of aggression and conduct problems.

Do early family experiences predict individual differences in processing?

Increasingly in recent years researchers have sought to describe the etiology of social and behavioural maladjustment in terms of early experience, latent knowledge structures and social information-processing biases and deficits (Belsky et al., 1996; Cassidy et al., 1996; Dodge et al., 1990; Pettit et al., 1988). One version of such a model (adapted from Dodge, 1993) is depicted in Fig.11.1. In this model, early life experiences interact with biologically based limits in memory and neural functioning to produce generalized knowledge structures. These structures consist of beliefs and expectations for social relationships, and broad schemes for social interaction based on past experience. When the individual encounters a problematic social situation, the knowledge structures serve to guide how cues are encoded and interpreted in that situation. Deficits and biases in processing can lead to deviant behaviour; chronically deviant behaviour can lead to the psychiatric diagnosis of conduct disorder.

The model suggests that processing patterns will mediate the relation between early experience (and accompanying knowledge structures) and subsequent psychopathology. In a later section we evaluate the extent to which the empirical literature provides evidence consistent with this premise. Before addressing the issue of statistical mediation we examine research that has been concerned with the early experience antecedents and correlates of perceptual and attributional processes. Much of this research has been aimed at describing the role of maltreatment (Dodge et al., 1990), exposure to aggressive models (Bandura, 1973), and insecure attachments (Belsky et al., 1996) in the development of distinct social information processing styles. A smaller literature also has examined links between caregiver and child processing patterns (MacKinnon-Lewis et al., 1994; Pettit et al., 1988).

The role of maltreatment and physical abuse

It has been proposed that the experience of maltreatment leads to a tendency to be hypervigilant to hostile cues and to interpret ambiguous provocation stimuli as threatening and the intentions of provocateurs as malicious (Crittendon & Ainsworth, 1989). Given that the maltreated child is being reared in an environment that typically is characterized by high levels of stress, inconsistent and indiscriminate parenting, and threats to the self, the development of such defensive processing patterns is understandable. Several studies have provided evidence that maltreated youngsters, compared to their nonmaltreated peers, display a variety of social information-processing biases and deficits. For example, Dodge et al. (1990) found that maltreated children differed from their peers in both encoding of cues (i.e. lower 'relevance' ratings) and attributions about those cues (i.e. more hostile interpretations of ambiguous peer provocation behaviour). These findings subsequently were replicated with a second cohort of participants who were administered the same assessment battery (Dodge et al., 1995). Possible child confounds (e.g. temperament) were controlled in this latter study.

Aggressive models

There is some emerging evidence that social information processing biases and deficits are associated with power-assertive family interaction styles (Hart et al., 1990; MacKinnon-Lewis et al., 1994) and with parental aggressiveness and endorsement of aggression as a viable strategy for resolving conflicts (Pettit et al., 1988). Such findings are consistent with the cognitive social learning perspective (Bandura, 1973) that children acquire aggressive behavioural orientations – including the perceptual and attributional processes that support aggression – in part by being exposed to aggressive models, by being directly reinforced for behaving aggressively (and by observing aggressive models being reinforced), and by having parents who condone, or even encourage, the use of aggressive problem-solving strategies.

Insecure attachments

Central to formulations of the role of attachment security in interpersonal adjustment is the notion of the internal working model (Bretherton et al., 1990; Main et al., 1985). As noted earlier, the internal working model may be construed as a latent knowledge structure that derives from patterns of caregiver responsiveness and sensitivity. The working model is presumed to provide a filter through which social information must pass. Information is filtered selectively as a function of individual attachment history. In spite of its ubiquity as an explanation for obtained relations between attachment security/ insecurity and important developmental outcomes (including behavioural adjustment), scant empirical evidence exists that documents the actual operation of working models of peer relationships. Recent studies by Belsky et al. (1996) and Cassidy et al. (1996) bear directly on this issue, however.

Belsky et al. (1996) tested the hypothesis that young boys' attention toward and memory of affectively laden information would vary as a function of attachment history. A puppet technique was used to present positive and negative events embedded within a series of stories. A distracting stimulus (hand clicker) accompanied the presentation of each affective cue. The boys proved more distractible during negative cues than positive cues, irrespective of attachment history. Securely attached boys remembered significantly more positive cues, whereas insecurely attached children remembered significantly more negative cues. According to Belsky et al., insofar as attachment security and insecurity are anteceded by differing caregiving styles (pleasurable/positive in the case of security; unpleasurable/negative for insecurity), children's subsequent memories for affective cues should be expected to be concordant with their earlier experiences. This is because schema-consistent information appears to be attended to more and remembered better than schema-inconsistent information. The findings of Belsky et al. (1996) appear to be consistent with this premise, at least for boys' recall of affective cues.

Cassidy et al. (1996) report three loosely connected studies that seek to link attachment-relevant variables to aspects of children's social information-processing. In the first study, preschool-aged children with known attachment histories were orally administered a standard social information-processing interview (taken from Dodge & Frame, 1982). No differences were found between secure and insecure groups on attributions of intent, but some differences were found for behavioural responses to the event (e.g. children in the insecure groups were more likely to state that the peer should be punished). In a second study of somewhat older (kindergarten and first grade) children, attachment security and peer 'representations' (again, based on the Dodge & Frame (1982) interview) were assessed. Securely attached children, compared to insecurely attached children, made more spontaneous positive attributions of the protagonist's behaviour (i.e. interpreted the act as accidental rather than intentional). As in the first study, differences also were found for responses to the provocation (i.e. less negative/aggressive responding by securely attached children). A third study with preadolescent children focused on associations between perceptions of parenting and perceived intent of peers in hypothetical provocation situations. Perceived rejection by parents, which was considered to be an attachment-related component of the child's relationship with parents, was significantly correlated with perceived hostile peer intent. The Cassidy et al. (1996) research therefore does provide some support for a statistical link between children's attachment history and perceptual and attributional processes. What is less clear, however, is whether the findings of either Cassidy et al. or Belsky et al. support the theoretical connection between internal working models – the latent knowledge structure that derives from the attachment relationships – and subsequent social information-processing patterns. It has been challenging for researchers to develop methods for assessing latent structures that are distinct from those typically used to assess social information-processing components. It might be argued that instead of measuring separate constructs, researchers simply have developed alternative ways of assessing proximal processing patterns.

Caregiver–child commonalities in processing

An intriguing question – but one that has as yet received virtually no research attention – is whether parents' processing styles are mirrored in their children's social information-processing. It is possible that parents' ways of mentally representing and responding to social situations is only indirectly related to children's processing, with parents' coaching and instruction in how to respond in social contexts serving as a connecting link (Mize & Pettit, 1997). However, it also may be that by observing and listening to what their parents do in social situations, children are imbued with a distinct social information-processing orientation. MacKinnon-Lewis et al. (1994) assessed school-aged boys' attributions about their mothers' intentions and mothers' attributions about their sons' intentions in hypothetical ambiguous provocation situations. Children's and mothers' attributions were not significantly correlated, but boys' aggressiveness with their mothers was predicted by the hostility of the children's attributions about their mothers, and mothers' aggressiveness with their sons likewise was predicted by the hostility of mothers' attributions about their sons.

Keane et al. (1990) also examined associations between children's and mothers' intent attributions. A variant of the Dodge et al. (1986) intention-cue detection procedure was administered to sociometrically popular and rejected first-grade children and their mothers. The prediction that rejected children (and their mothers) would evince a hostile bias, compared to popular children (and their mothers), was not supported for either the children or their mothers. Descriptive statistics indicated fairly high levels of convergence in children's and mothers' intention-cue interpretations, but mainly for interpretations of hostile cues. Taken together, the findings of MacKinnon-Lewis et al. (1994) and Keane et al. (1990) provide only very modest support for the hypothesis that children and their parents share a common social information-processing style, at least in terms of attributions for others' behaviour.

Do perceptual and attributional processes mediate the link between early socialization experiences and later conduct problems?

Because social information-processing has been conceived as a proximal factor in the display of aggression and conduct problems, researchers increasingly have become interested in whether perceptual and attributional processes may help to account for the association between early family and social experiences and children's behavioural maladjustment. That is, it has been proposed that processing styles serve as a mechanism by which early experiences become linked with later aggression and conduct problems (Dodge et al., 1990).

An early demonstration of the utility of processing-relevant constructs as possible mediators of the relation between children's experience in the family and individual differences in preschool-aged children's aggression was provided by Pettit et al. (1988). In this cross-sectional study, family experience was assessed via an interview with the mother, children's social problem-solving skills were assessed with videotaped vignettes and hypothetical stories, and children's social behaviour (including aggressiveness) was indexed through teacher and peer ratings. Children's aggressiveness was associated with deviant problem solving patterns (higher likelihood of generating aggressive responses and lower likelihood of generating relevant or prosocial responses) and with mothers' reported use of harsh discipline. In regression analyses it was found that harsh discipline no longer predicted behaviour when social problem solving was controlled. Follow-up studies by Dodge and Pettit and their colleagues have yielded qualified support for the mediational model. Dodge et al. (1990) assessed 5-year-old children's processing using standard methods and multiple measures were derived to index each of the first four steps in Dodge's social information-processing model (i.e. encoding accuracy, hostile attributional bias, response generation and quality, and response evaluation). Family experience information was obtained from mothers. Results indicated that children identified as physically maltreated, compared to the nonmaltreated children, had significantly higher aggression scores in kindergarten. Moreover, maltreated children (relative to nonharmed children) were less attentive to relevant social cues, more biased toward attributing hostile intent, and less likely to generate competent solutions to hypothetical social problems. These processing patterns also were significantly related to the children's aggressiveness at school. When the social information-processing scores were controlled in a regression analysis, maltreatment was no longer significantly associated with aggressive behavioural outcomes. These findings are consistent with the hypothesis that harsh and abusive early family experience has its effects on a child's development of aggressive behaviour largely by altering the ways in which the child processes social information.

Although compelling as an explanatory device, the processing-as-mediator notion is in need of further testing and refinement. Some studies have failed to find evidence that the impact of family experience on child adjustment is mediated by social-cognitive factors (Downey & Walker, 1989) and even among those finding supportive evidence (Dodge et al., 1990, 1995; Pettit et al., 1988) there is an absence of precision and specificity with respect to the presumed causal relations among early experience, processing patterns, and outcome.

The rather equivocal support for the mediation hypothesis can be illustrated by careful examination of two studies, drawing on different data sets, that often are cited as providing evidence of mediation (Dodge et al., 1990; Pettit et al., 1988). The Pettit et al. (1988) study had a small number of participants ($N = 46$ for the principal analyses) with six family predictors, five processing measures and three outcomes. This resulted in a total of 90 possible mediational tests. The minimal requirements for a test of mediation (Baron & Kenny, 1986) are that the predictor be significantly correlated with the mediator and outcome, and that the mediator be significantly correlated with the outcome. Only seven of the 90 possible tests met these requirements, none of which was specified a priori as a probable linkage.

Dodge et al. (1990) had a fairly large number of participants (about 300 for the main analyses), with a single early experience predictor (maltreatment), seven social information-processing measures and three outcomes. This resulted in 21 possible mediational links. Four links were significant, involving three different types of processing, including encoding relevance and hostile attributional bias. An omnibus mediational test was conducted, in which all seven processing variables were used as covariates, regardless of whether they had a significant bivariate relation with either the predictor (maltreated versus not maltreated) or the aggression outcomes. The results showed that maltreatment groups no longer differed in aggression once the processing measures were controlled, but the amount of the effect (i.e. per cent of variance in the abuse–aggression relation) that was accounted for was not reported, nor were separate statistics (e.g. betas) presented for individual processing scores. Interestingly, in a later follow-up with a second cohort of participants (Dodge et al., 1995), the only processing variable not to contribute to the mediation of the maltreatment–aggression relation was hostile bias.

From these two studies it seems fair to conclude that processing – at least as measured to date – accounts for a modest portion of the effect of early experience on later aggression outcomes. Moreover, there is considerable variation across studies in the aspects of processing contributing to the mediational effect. Even though empirical demonstrations of the experience → processing → outcome linkage thus far have not been very strong, the mediational model remains an exciting and potentially useful explanatory mechanism. Refinements in the technology of information processing assessment, coupled with more sophisticated theoretical formulations of the complex, transactional nature of conduct problem development, may yield models that provide a more solid foundation for future empirical inquiry (Mize et al., in press).

Future directions in the study of perceptual and attributional processes

Understanding gender and developmental effects

Gender effects

There is reason to expect sex differences on both sides of the processing-outcome relation. The longstanding assumption that boys are more aggressive than girls and more likely to display conduct problems than girls is giving way to newer perspectives that emphasize the differing topological and functional features of boys' and girls' aggression (Crick & Grotpeter, 1995). It has become increasingly clear that whereas boys display more overt, physical forms of aggression than girls, girls engage in more relationally oriented forms of aggression than boys. The social information-processing correlates of the two forms appear to be somewhat different, with processing about physical acts of aggression predicting overt aggression most strongly, and processing about relational acts of aggression predicting relational aggression most strongly (Crick, 1995).

These patterns of outcome distinctiveness notwithstanding, there still is evidence that individual differences in processing predict boys' behavioural adjustment more strongly than they predict girls' adjustment. For example, Rabiner et al. (1990) found differences in boys' controlled and automatic processing as a function of sociometric status and aggression level, but no differences in girls' processing. Perhaps it is premature to attempt to draw strong conclusions about sex differences in patterns of processing, because many studies of links between processing and maladjustment only include boys as participants (Waldman, 1996). Also, because many studies of behavioural adjustment have focused on overt forms of aggression (known to occur more commonly among boys), the magnitude of the relation between processing and outcome may be underestimated for girls.

Developmental issues

Remarkably little research has been devoted to the study of stability and change in social information-processing. Consequently, it is necessary to rely on theory and data on children's cognitive development more generally, and nonsocial information processing more specifically, to address issues of development. Although information processing accounts of 'what develops' vary (see Meadows, 1993, for a comprehensive review of research on developmental changes in information processing), two domains in particular would seem to serve as good candidates for explaining developmental changes in perceptual and attributional processes: (a) enhanced basic capacities, especially greater attentional skills and perhaps increased processing speed or working memory capacity, and (b) a larger base of knowledge and experience.

Encoding is fundamentally about the perception of cues in a given social situation. And what children perceive, of course, depends in large degree on how well and to what they direct their attention. Developmentally, attention comes increasingly under effortful control so that by middle childhood normally developing children are quite proficient at deploying attention in the service of a goal. Children become faster at encoding information, and they become more systematic and exhaustive in scanning for cues, which may mean that they spend more time examining a stimulus array. In fact, older children, compared to younger children, have been found to utilize social cues in a more deliberate and planned fashion in peer-provocation situations (Dodge & Newman, 1981).

Hypothesized developmental change in a related basic process – working memory capacity – may have implications for attributional processes. With development, children are able to hold in memory and perform operations on more 'bits' of information at once. For example, most 6-year-olds can perform the mental operation of adding single digits, but are unable to hold enough bits of information in memory to compute double-digit sums. This limit in capacity also may apply to social information-processing and may explain why young children tend to assume that a harmful act was intentional: weighing simultaneously the effects of an act and the motivations of the actor may exceed the cognitive competence of most young thinkers.

The second component thought to be responsible for developmental change, a growing knowledge or experience base, also has obvious implications for attributional processes. Memory stores, perhaps in the form of generalized or specific event representations, are thought to provide the data base for social perception and interpretation. Knowledge and experience appear to play a critical role in influencing perceptual learning – the largely unconscious process of learning to selectively 'see' and interpret (and ultimately recall) relevant cues from an almost infinite array of possibilities. Individual differences in experience, therefore, will affect which cues are salient and available to interpretation. In this light, the tendency to see and recall more negative (Belsky et al., 1996) or aggressive (Gouze, 1987) cues may be thought of as a natural developmental consequence of perceptual learning for children with aggressogenic early experiences.

Another developmental issue concerns the salience of differing social information processes as children grow older. There is some suggestion that, among preschool-aged children, attributions of intent are not very good predictors of behavioural adjustment (Keane et al., 1990; Pettit et al., 1988), perhaps because children this age are developmentally not yet capable of discriminating between intentions and outcomes (i.e. if a negative outcome occurs it must be because the child causing the outcome did so intentionally) or, as suggested earlier, because balancing multiple bits of information is too cognitively complex. On the other hand, it appears that the ability to generate numerous and relevant solutions to social problems is a better predictor of social skills and competence among younger children (Mize & Ladd, 1988; Pettit et al., 1988; Rubin & Krasnor, 1986). This may reflect the relative variance in different aspects of processing that is accounted for by maturation versus experience during the preschool years. That is, early in development, when there are marked differences in rates of maturation among children of the same age, any stable individual differences in perception and attribution may be overshadowed by maturational variation. In contrast, differences among young children in strategy knowledge may be relatively less a function of maturation and more dependent on variations in experience and knowledge base.

With respect to stability, although some degree of cross-time coherence in processing patterns is implied in most contemporary models, there have been few efforts aimed at documenting patterns of stability/instability over time. In fact, only one published study of long-term stability in early-stage social information-processing could be located. Harrist et al. (1997) report cross-year correlations of 0.23 for encoding relevance and 0.25 for hostile attributions. This suggests that perceptual and attributional processes may be, at best, only modestly stable in the grade-school years.

Consideration of the developmental–salience issue requires the articulation of models that specify the general timetable for the emergence of perceptual and attributional processes germane to the development of aggression and conduct problems. Referring back to Fig. 11.1, it is plausible that generalized knowledge structures emerge first, as a consequence of early parent–child

relationships in interaction with children's biological capabilities. These structures direct attention to events in very general sorts of ways. It is only through
experience in social settings containing peers and others that children's expectations and knowledge structures become focused on situations that are personally meaningful and important, including social situations that are aversive
or ambiguous in nature or that have an 'attention-grabbing' character. From
these generalized knowledge structures, then, comes an experientially based set
of perceptual and attributional processes that serve as more proximal guides to
behaviour in circumscribed social situations. Only longitudinal research wed-
ding diverse theoretical orientations (e.g. attachment, scripts, social information-processing) will be able to provide answers to the key developmental
questions.

Reciprocal processes: experience, behaviour and cognition

The causal and temporal nature of the relation between processing and
behavioural outcome is in need of further study. Consistent with a causal
model of processing factors in aggression, there is some evidence from longitudinal research that processing problems antecede deviant behaviour (Dodge
et al., 1995), and some evidence from experimental research that manipulating
children's intent perceptions influences their relationships with peers (Rabiner
& Coie, 1989). In spite of these causally oriented findings, it remains quite
possible that processing patterns change in response to the kinds of experiences
that a child has with peers. Consider, for example, the case of the socially
rejected child. There is a strong correlation between aggression and peer
rejection, and longitudinal research suggests that an aggressive style tends
to lead to peer rejection (Coie & Dodge, 1998). Children who are rejected by
their peers also are known to have biases and deficits in social information-
processing (Crick & Dodge, 1994). However, not all rejected children are
aggressive and not all rejected children have problems in information processing. But the experience of rejection places children at risk for the development
of aggressive behavioural problems over time (Pettit, 1997), and this association
(i.e. between number of years of rejection and later aggression) appears to be
mediated by social information-processing biases and deficits (Dodge, in press).
This suggests a reciprocal cycle whereby processing both can lead to peer
rejection and aggression, and derive from peer rejection, leading to heightened
levels of aggression.

A proposed transactional–developmental model

There now is an extensive amount of empirical evidence supporting the
premise that the development of aggression and conduct problems follows

from cumulative transactions among characteristics of the child, such as temperament, sociocultural contexts, including economic resources and type of neighbourhood, parenting qualities, such as disciplinary effectiveness and monitoring, and degree of exposure to and involvement with deviant peers (Coie & Dodge, 1998). Dodge and colleagues (Dodge, in press) recently have proposed a model that describes how the cumulative impact of these individual, social and contextual factors on children's development of aggression and conduct problems may be understood in terms of proximal social information-processing mechanisms. A central tenet of the model is that child characteristics, sociocultural context and early social experiences operate on the development of conduct problems by shaping a child's social knowledge and characteristic styles of processing information about the social world. Consistent with the mediational models discussed earlier, it is proposed that perceptual and attributional processes (a) directly influence the development of conduct problems, (b) are acquired through early family and social experiences and (c) mediate the effects of risk factors on conduct problem outcomes.

In summary, emerging evidence suggests that social information-processing patterns – including perceptual and attributional processes – may provide clues as to why cumulative experiences with parents and peers may have enduring effects on children's behavioural and psychological adjustment. Of course, the social information-processing perspective also provides clues as to how the trajectory of increasing aggressiveness may be altered. Future research should be directed at refining conceptual formulations and improving measurement precision, particularly by focusing on the identification of those aspects of processing that are salient at differing points in development, and the life experiences that contribute to the evolution and maintenance of maladaptive processing patterns.

Acknowledgements

Preparation of this chapter was supported in part by NICHD grant HD 30572. The authors are grateful to Darrell Meece and Michael Criss for their helpful comments on an earlier version of the manuscript.

REFERENCES

Achenbach, T.M. (1985). *Assessment and Taxonomy of Child and Adolescent Psychopathology*. Newbury Park, CA: Sage.

Aydin, O. & Markova, I. (1979). Attribution tendencies of popular and unpopular children. *British Journal of Social and Clinical Psychology, 18*, 291–8.

Baldwin, M.W. (1992). Relational schemas and the processing of social information. *Psychological Bulletin, 112*, 461–84.

Bandura A. (1973). *Aggression: A Social Learning Analysis*. Englewood Cliffs, NJ: Prentice-Hall.

Bargh, J., Lombardi, W. & Higgins, E. (1988). Automaticity of chronically accessible constructs in Person × Situation effects on person perception: It's just a matter of time. *Journal of Personality and Social Psychology, 55*, 599–605.

Baron, R. & Kenny, D. (1986). The moderator-mediator variable distinction in social psychological research: conceptual, strategic, and statistical considerations. *Journal of Personality and Social Psychology, 51*, 1173–82.

Bates, J.E., Pettit, G.S. & Dodge, K.A. (1995). Family and child factors in stability and change in children's aggressiveness in elementary school. In J. McCord (Ed.), *Coercion and Punishment in Long-Term Perspective* (pp. 124–38). New York: Cambridge University Press.

Belsky, J., Spritz, B. & Crnic, K. (1996). Infant attachment security and affective-cognitive information processing at age 3. *Psychological Science, 7*, 111–14.

Bretherton, I., Ridgeway, D. & Cassidy, J. (1990). The role of internal working models in the attachment relationship: theoretical, empirical, and developmental considerations. In M. Greenberg, D. Cicchetti & E.M. Cummings (Eds.), *Attachment in the Preschool Years: Theory, Research, and Intervention* (pp. 273–310). Chicago: University of Chicago Press.

Cassidy, J., Kirsh, S.J., Scolton, K.L. & Parke, R.D. (1996). Attachment and representations of peer relationships. *Developmental Psychology, 32*, 892–904.

Coie, J.D. & Dodge, K.A. (1998). Aggression and antisocial behavior. In N. Eisenberg (Vol. Ed.) & W. Damon (Series Ed.), *Handbook of Child Psychology, Vol. 3. Social, Emotional, and Personality Development* (pp. 779–862). New York: John Wiley & Sons.

Crick, N.R. (1995). Relational aggression: The role of intent attributions, feelings of distress, and provocation type. *Development and Psychopathology, 7*, 313–22.

Crick, N.R. & Dodge, K.A. (1994). A review and reformulation of social information-processing mechanisms in children's adjustment. *Psychological Bulletin, 115*, 74–101.

Crick, N. R. & Dodge, K.A. (1996). Social information-processing mechanisms in proactive and reactive aggression. *Child Development, 67*, 993–1002.

Crick N.R. & Grotpeter, J. (1995). Relational aggression, gender, and social psychological adjustment. *Child Development, 66*, 710–22.

Crick, N.R. & Ladd, G.W. (1993). Children's perceptions of their peer experiences: attributions, loneliness, social anxiety, and social avoidance. *Developmental Psychology, 29*, 244–54.

Crittendon, P.M. & Ainsworth, M.D.S. (1989). Child maltreatment and attachment theory. In D. Cicchetti & V. Carlson (Eds.), *Child Maltreatment: Theory and Research on the Causes and Consequences of Child Abuse and Neglect* (pp. 432–63). New York: Cambridge University Press.

Dodge, K.A. (1980). Social cognition and children's aggressive behavior. *Child Development, 51*, 162–70.

Dodge, K.A. (1993). Social-cognitive mechanisms in the development of conduct disorder and depression. In L.W. Porter & M.R. Rosenweig (Eds.), *Annual Review of Psychology* (Vol. 44, pp. 559–84). Palo Alto, CA: Annual Reviews.

Dodge, K.A. (in press). Conduct disorder. In A. Sameroff, M. Lewis & S. Miller (Eds.), *Handbook of Development Psychopathology*. New York: Plenum Press.

Dodge, K.A., Bates, J.E. & Pettit, G.S. (1990). Mechanisms in the cycle of violence. *Science, 250,* 1678–83.

Dodge, K.A. & Feldman, E. (1990). Issues in social cognition and sociometric status. In S.R. Asher & J.D. Coie (Eds.), *Peer Rejection in Childhood* (pp. 119–55). New York: Cambridge University Press.

Dodge, K.A. & Frame, C.L. (1982). Social cognitive deficits and biases in aggressive boys. *Child Development, 53,* 620–35.

Dodge, K.A., Lochman, J.E., Harnish, J.D., Bates, J.E. & Pettit, G.S. (1997). Reactive and proactive aggression in school children and psychiatrically impaired chronically assaultive youth. *Journal of Abnormal Psychology, 106,* 37–51.

Dodge, K.A. & Newman, J.P. (1981). Biased decision making processes in aggressive boys. *Journal of Abnormal Psychology, 90,* 375–9.

Dodge, K.A., Pettit, G.S., Bates, J.E. & Valente, E. (1995). Social information-processing patterns partially mediate the effect of early physical abuse on later conduct problems. *Journal of Abnormal Psychology, 104,* 632–43.

Dodge, K.A., Pettit, G.S., McClaskey, C.L. & Brown, M. (1986). Social competence in children. *Monographs of the Society for Research in Child Development, 51* (1, Serial No. 213).

Dodge, K.A. & Price, J.M. (1994). On the relation between social information-processing and socially competent behavior in early school-aged children. *Child Development, 65,* 1385–97.

Dodge, K.A. & Somberg, D. (1987). Hostile attributional biases among aggressive boys are exacerbated under conditions of threats to the self. *Child Development, 58,* 213–24.

Dodge, K.A. & Tomlin, A.M. (1987). Utilization of self-schemata as a mechanism of interpretational bias in aggressive children. *Social Cognition, 5,* 280–300.

Downey, G. & Walker, E. (1989). Social cognition and adjustment in children at risk for psychopathology. *Developmental Psychology, 25,* 835–45.

Eisenberg, N., Guthrie, I., Fabes, R.A., et al. (1997). The relations of regulation and emotionality to resiliency and competent social functioning in elementary school children. *Child Development, 68,* 295–311.

Goetz, T.W. & Dweck, C.S. (1980). Learned helplessness in social situations. *Journal of Personality and Social Psychology, 39,* 246–55.

Gottman, J.M. (1986). Commentary: merging social cognition and behavior. *Monographs of the Society for Research in Child Development, 51* (1, Serial No. 213).

Gouze, K.R. (1987). Attention and problem solving as correlates of aggression in preschool males. *Journal of Abnormal Child Psychology, 15,* 181–97.

Graham, S. & Hudley, C. (1994). Attributions of aggressive and nonaggressive African American male early adolescents: a study of construct accessibility. *Developmental Psychology, 30,* 365–37.

Guerra, N.G. & Slaby, R.G. (1989). Evaluative factors in social problem solving by aggressive boys. *Journal of Abnormal Child Psychology, 17,* 277–89.

Harrist, A.W., Zaia, A., Bates, J.E., Dodge, K.A. & Pettit, G.S. (1997). Subtypes of social withdrawal in early and middle childhood. Behavioral and social-cognitive profiles across four years. *Child Development, 68,* 332–48.

Hart, C.H., Ladd, G.W. & Burleson, B. (1990). Children's expectations of the outcomes of social strategies: Relations with sociometric status and maternal disciplinary style. *Child Development*, *61*, 127–37.

Heider, F. (1958). *The Psychology of Interpersonal Relations*. New York: John Wiley & Sons.

Higgins, E.T. & Bargh, J.A. (1987). Social cognition and social perception. *Annual Review of Psychology*, *38*, 369–425.

Hinshaw, S.P. (1987). On the distinction between attentional deficits/hyperactivity and conduct problems/aggression in child psychopathology. *Psychological Bulletin*, *101*, 443–63.

Huesmann, L.R. (1988). An information-processing model for the development of aggression. *Aggressive Behavior*, *14*, 13–24.

Keane, S.P., Brown, K.P. & Crenshaw, T.M. (1990). Children's intention-cue detection as a function of maternal social behavior: Pathways to social rejection. *Developmental Psychology*, *26*, 1004–9.

MacKinnon-Lewis, C., Vollig, B., Lamb, M., et al. (1994). A cross-contextual analysis of boys' social competence: From family to school. *Developmental Psychology*, *30*, 325–33.

Main, M., Kaplan, N. & Cassidy, J. (1985). Security in infancy, childhood, and adulthood: a move to the level of representation. In I. Bretherton & E. Waters (Eds.), *Growing Points of Attachment Theory and Research. Monographs of the Society for Research in Child Development*, *50* (112, Serial No. 209), 66–104.

Meadows, S. (1993). *The Child as Thinker. The Development and Acquisition of Cognition in Childhood*. London: Routledge.

Mize, J. & Ladd, G.W. (1988). Predicting preschoolers' peer behavior and status from their interpersonal strategies: a comparison of verbal and enactive responses to hypothetical social dilemmas. *Developmental Psychology*, *24*, 782–8.

Mize, J. & Pettit, G.S. (1997). Mothers' social coaching, mother-child relationship style, and children's peer competence: is the medium the message? *Child Development*, *68*, 291–311.

Mize, J., Pettit, G.S. & Meece, D.W. (in press). Explaining the link between parenting behavior and children's peer competence: a critical examination of the 'mediating process' hypothesis. In K.A. Kerns, J.M. Contreras & A. Neal-Barnett (Eds.), *Family and Peers: Linking Two Social Worlds*. Westport, CT: Praeger.

Nasby, W., Hayden, B. & DePaulo, B.M. (1979). Attributional bias among aggressive boys to interpret unambiguous social stimuli as displays of hostility. *Journal of Abnormal Psychology*, *89*, 459–68.

Pettit, G.S. (1997). The developmental course of violence and aggression: mechanisms of family and peer influence. *Psychiatric Clinics of North America*, *20*, 283–99.

Pettit, G.S., Dodge, K.A. & Brown, M. (1988). Early family experience, social problem solving patterns, and children's social competence. *Child Development*, *59*, 107–20.

Quiggle, N., Garber, J., Panak, W. & Dodge, K.A. (1992). Social information-processing in aggressive and depressed children. *Child Development*, *63*, 1305–20.

Rabiner, D.L. & Coie, J.D. (1989). The effect of expectancy inductions on rejected children's acceptance by unfamiliar peers. *Developmental Psychology*, *25*, 450–7.

Rabiner, D.L., Lenhart, L. & Lochman, J.E. (1990). Automatic versus reflective social problem solving in relation to children's sociometric status. *Developmental Psychology*, *26*, 1010–16.

Rubin, K.H. & Krasnor, L.R. (1986). Social-cognitive and social behavioral perspectives on problem solving. In M. Perlmutter (Ed.), *Minnesota Symposium on Child Psychology* (Vol. 18, pp. 1–68). Hillsdale, NJ: Lawrence Erlbaum Associates.

Shank, R.C. & Abelson, R. (1977). *Scripts, Plans, Goals, and Understanding.* Hillsdale, NJ: Lawrence Erlbaum.

Slaby, R.G. & Guerra, N.G. (1988). Cognitive mediators of aggression in adolescent offenders: 1. Assessment. *Developmental Psychology, 24,* 580–8.

Suess, G.J., Grossman, K.E. & Sroufe, L.A. (1992). Effects of infant attachment to mother and father on quality of adaptation in preschool: from dyadic to individual organization of self. *International Journal of Behavioral Development, 15,* 43–65.

Thompson, R.A. (1994). Emotion regulation: a theme in search of definition. In N.A. Fox (Ed.), *The Development of Emotion Regulation: Biological and Behavioral Considerations* (pp. 25–52). *Monographs of the Society for Research in Child Development, 59* (2–3, Serial No. 240).

Waas, G.A. (1988). Social attributional biases of peer-rejected and aggressive children. *Child Development, 59,* 969–75.

Waldman, D. (1996). Aggressive boys' hostile perceptual and response biases: The role of attention and impulsivity. *Child Development, 67,* 1015–33.

Weiner, B. & Graham, S. (1994). An attributional approach to emotional development. In C.E. Izard, J. Kagan & B. Zajonc (Eds.), *Emotions, Cognitions, and Behavior* (pp. 167–91). New York: Cambridge University Press.

12

Attachment and conduct disorder

Michelle DeKlyen and Matthew L. Speltz

Introduction

After encountering several young thieves early in his clinical career, the psychiatrist John Bowlby sought some common thread in their backgrounds that might explain their behaviour (Bowlby, 1944). Bowlby mused that a parent's irritable and frustrating behaviour might lead not only to anger but also to an insatiable need for affection, or for things which might substitute for affection (Bowlby, 1944, p. 114); in turn, the child's hostility and greed might make the parent even more irritable and critical, establishing an interactional pattern reminiscent of Patterson's (1982) coercive cycle. Indeed, descriptions of many of the mothers of these young thieves suggested irritable, aggressive and critical parenting. However, on more careful inspection, the families of the thieving children did not appear to differ from those of other disturbed but nondelinquent children in terms of negative parenting or in the incidence of familial mental illness. One clear environmental factor did stand out in the histories of a subset of these thieves, characterized by Bowlby as 'affectionless' and detached, and that was the prolonged early separation of child and mother. This observation – of the apparently devastating effect of maternal deprivation on the social and moral development of children – set Bowlby on the course which was to result in his life work on attachment, separation and loss.

Attachment theory represented an alternative to both behavioural and psychoanalytic perspectives on human development, with the promise of providing new solutions to difficult questions about the genesis of social and antisocial behaviour. It supplied motivation and mechanisms for continuity between early and later experience. As do many novel theories, it attracted both passionate supporters and entrenched resistance.

In this chapter we first offer an overview of attachment theory, its basic tenets and measurement tools. The rationale for proposing a link between attachment and conduct disorder is then presented, along with a description of possible mechanisms of influence. Serious conduct problems frequently have their origins in early childhood and show considerable continuity over time (Moffitt, 1993; Robins, 1991). The attachment construct of cognitive–affective working models of relationships may help to explain this continuity. We then review research confirming modest but significant associations between attachment measures and problem behaviour, as well as other studies which point out the limitations of these measures. For example, attachment has generally been predictive for boys but not for girls, and within high risk but not community samples. These findings are consistent with an etiological model involving multiple pathways and multiple risk factors, of which insecure attachment is only one, and neither necessary nor sufficient (Greenberg et al., 1993). While theory has suggested that some insecure attachment strategies should be more likely than others to lead to conduct disorder, the data on this question are inconclusive.

Attachment theory has enlivened both theoretical debate and empirical investigation; however, important conceptual and measurement problems remain. Although a full consideration of these is beyond the scope of this chapter, some key issues and limitations involved in applying an attachment perspective to the study of conduct disorder are discussed next. These include the complexity of a multiple pathway model of disorder, the difficulty of teasing out the most 'active' ingredients among a number of highly intercorrelated risk factors (e.g. attachment, parent warmth, harsh parenting, family conflict, life stress, social support and parent psychopathology), as well as specific measurement questions. We close with a discussion of the treatment implications of attachment theory and a review of attachment-based intervention programmes and outcome studies.

Attachment theory and the systematic study of parent–child relationship quality

Attachment theory provides a unique framework for considering the development of conduct disorder in that it offers a macroanalytic, developmental and organizational perspective, incorporating behavioural, cognitive and affective aspects of the developing child's experience. It attempts to explain how early and continuing relationships might shape the child's expectations of others and his coping strategies. And, importantly, it provides systematic, qualitative and quantitative tools for assessing caregiving relationships and for testing important hypotheses linking these relationships to child outcomes.

The original impetus for Bowlby's theory of attachment was the explanation of psychopathology. Indeed his first speculations regarding the possible impact of early adverse experiences focused on antisocial behaviour among adolescents (Bowlby, 1944). Adapting ideas from ethology, systems, psychodynamic and learning theories, Bowlby (1969/1982) argued that infants and caregivers were innately predisposed to respond to one another in ways that serve to maximize the child's likelihood of survival, by promoting parent–child proximity in times of stress. The function of the attachment behavioural system was to provide protection to the infant, and its subjective 'set goal' was 'felt security'. Sensitive and responsive parenting during infancy was thought to facilitate the child's development of an expectation ('working model') that he would be cared for and responded to when necessary. This internal model of relationships would then serve to shape the child's perceptions of and responses within this and other relationships.

Central to attachment theory, then, are concerns for safety, and salient outcomes include the child's feelings of security and self-worth and his capacity to engage in close relationships. Not all aspects of the parent–child relationship pertain to attachment, and not all child outcomes are theoretically associated with attachment history. Thus, teaching, discipline and playful parent–child interactions serve distinct functions, separable from the attachment behavioural system, and many aspects of child development (e.g. language acquisition) are expected to be relatively unaffected by the attachment relationship (Sroufe, 1988). In the wake of researchers' enthusiasm, the specificity of attachment theory's claims have sometimes been lost sight of. However, Bowlby (1969/82) did explicitly propose that disturbances in attachment relations are a main cause of psychopathologies characterized by distrust or chronic anxiety, writing that individuals whose needs for security are not met come to view the world as 'comfortless and unpredictable, and they respond either by shrinking from it or doing battle with it' (Bowlby, 1973, p. 208). Such an image aptly describes many conduct-disordered children, although it is not exclusive to conduct disorder.

Although Bowlby viewed his theory as relevant across the life-span, his work initially focused attention on early childhood. To test aspects of the theory, Ainsworth developed a procedure called the Strange Situation to assess infant responses to stressful situations, including brief separations from their mothers (Ainsworth et al., 1978). She noted three distinct patterns of child behaviour, particularly during reunions. Some infants clearly sought to reestablish interaction with their mothers after separation, showing little tendency to avoid or resist contact (secure attachment). Others avoided their mothers (insecure-avoidant) or alternated between resistance and contact-seeking behaviours (insecure-ambivalent).

Early studies suggested that, cross-culturally, approximately 65% of normal infants were securely attached, 21% were avoidant and 14% ambivalent (van IJzendoorn & Kroonenberg, 1988); thus, while security is normative, a sizeable number of individuals are expected to be insecure. Classifications could be reliably assigned by trained observers and were systematically related to patterns of mother–child interactions observed in the home several months earlier (De Wolff & van IJzendoorn, 1997). Mothers of avoidant babies were more likely to have been insensitive to infant signals and to express dislike of physical contact, whereas mothers of resistant babies appeared inconsistent in responding to their infants. Mothers of secure babies were characterized by 'sensitive responsiveness' to infant signals. However, associations between 'sensitive responsive' maternal behaviours and infant security were modest (accounting for roughly 10% of the variance), leaving what van IJzendoorn (1995) has termed a 'transmission gap' in the explanation of how individual attachment styles develop. Temperament and genetic influences may play a role (Vaughn et al., 1992), but their influence is likely to be indirect, as indicated by frequent differences in attachment security of the same infant with mothers and fathers (Fox et al., 1991; van IJzendoorn, 1995).

These three categories fit all but a small number of infants. The unclassifiable cases were subsequently studied by Main & Solomon (1986), who concluded that most could be described by a fourth pattern, which they called disorganized/disoriented. This group of babies showed a variety of unusual behaviours upon reunion, often combining elements of avoidance and resistance, sometimes appearing confused, depressed or apprehensive. A disproportionate number came from families at risk because of maltreatment, maternal depression and/or poverty (Carlson et al., 1989; Lyons-Ruth et al., 1987; Spieker & Booth, 1988). Main & Hesse (1990) have argued that disorganization is a response to a fearful or fear-inspiring parent; because the child's presumed source of safety is also an occasion for fear, no strategy consistently provides a feeling of security.

The behaviours and underlying representations which characterize attachment relations at any given life stage depend upon the individual's cognitive, linguistic, social and affective development (Cicchetti et al., 1990). To extend attachment theory beyond infancy, it is necessary to shift attention to the cognitive–affective working models of attachment relationships that are thought to organize perceptual input and to engage the appropriate behavioural systems (Bretherton, 1985). These predictions are at the moment largely speculative but testable. If a child's experience has been that his mother will provide support when it is needed, he will probably readily approach her when he is distressed, suggesting an expectation of safety and responsiveness within the relationship. In contrast, the insecure-avoidant child learns not to approach his caregiver in times of stress, to avoid rejection. Because he has found that his mother is likely to distance herself further if he expresses anger or distress, these emotions may ultimately be shut out of consciousness. By limiting awareness of his feelings, however, he restricts his capacity to objectively appraise his experience. The insecure-ambivalent child, on the other hand, becomes hyper-vigilant and expressive, because he has learned that only in this way can he maintain proximity with an inconsistently attentive caregiver.

Working models of relationships are expected to become progressively resistant to change, because they create information processing biases and lead to behaviours which reinforce the models (Bowlby, 1969/1982; Main et al., 1985). They are not, however, immutable, and experiences which repeatedly contradict a working model may alter it, as suggested by the finding that major family transitions are often associated with predictable changes in child attachment classifications (Thompson et al., 1982; Vaughn et al., 1979).

Bowlby envisioned a direct correlation between specific attachment difficulties and psychopathological outcomes. Empirical investigation of these links has been delayed for perhaps three reasons. First, attachment measures were initially developed on normative, low risk samples. Secondly, disorders are often heterogeneous, with multiple and complex causes. Finally, establishing associations between attachment and identified psychopathology requires either (1) longitudinal studies with very large sample sizes and/or high-risk groups, or (2) the development of post-infancy measures of attachment.

In the past 15 years, measures have been developed to assess attachment in preschoolers (Cassidy et al., 1989; Crittenden, 1992), 5- and 6-year-olds (Main & Cassidy, 1988), adolescents (Armsden & Greenberg, 1987), and adults (Main & Goldwyn, 1994). Although the behavioural markers on which classification is based necessarily differ, incorporating verbalizations as well as new physical capacities, both the Cassidy & Marvin (1989) and Main & Cassidy (1988) measures have categories similar to those of the infancy measure. The major difference is that the disorganized category was expanded to include controlling behaviour, in response to Main's finding that most of the disorganized infants in her original, normative sample were quite controlling (either punitively or in a solicitous, caregiving manner) in reunions with their parents 5 years later. Crittenden's (1992) Miami system produces three somewhat different classifications (secure, defended, and coercive), with a significantly larger proportion of children tending to be classified insecure than is true within the infancy system.

The Adult Attachment Classification System (Main & Goldwyn, 1994) is based on the semi-structured Adult Attachment Interview (AAI; George et al., 1985), which asks subjects to describe early relationships with caregivers, changes in those relationships, experiences of loss and trauma and their impact on adult personality. Analysis of a transcript of the interview, with an emphasis on present state of mind and coherency of discourse, results in classifications of free/autonomous, dismissing, preoccupied and unresolved, analogous to the secure, avoidant, resistant and disorganized infant categories, respectively (Main et al., 1985). Other, questionnaire-based measures of adolescent and adult attachment have been developed, but to date, only the AAI has been empirically linked with other measures of attachment. Specifically, mothers' AAI classifications have been found to predict their infants' classifications in the Strange Situation several months later (Fonagy et al., 1991; van IJzendoorn, 1995). Although further study of the continuity of classification from one measure to the next is needed (see below), these new measures offer intriguing new possibilities for studying how the capacity for social relations develops.

Rationale for predicting a link between attachment and conduct disorder

Ample empirical evidence and a consensus among proponents of various theories identify parent–child relations as important in the development of conduct problems (Campbell, 1995; Kazdin, 1987; Shaw & Bell, 1993; and see Kiesner & Dishion, chapter 10, this volume). Whether based on microanalytic measures (Patterson et al., 1992) or organizational measures such as attachment (Lyons-Ruth et al., 1997; Speltz et al., 1995), significant, if modest, associations between parenting and child outcomes are found.

Positive parenting processes have been less often studied than have such negative aspects of the family environment as harsh discipline, conflict and maltreatment. Recently, there has been growing recognition that positive facets of parenting (e.g. warmth, positive involvement and secure child–parent attachment) independently affect the likelihood of antisocial behaviour. Mothers of children with behaviour problems have been found to be less warm (Eron et al., 1971; Olweus, 1980) and less positively involved (Gardner, 1987; Pettit & Bates, 1989; Russell & Russell, 1996) than other mothers. In a sample of high-risk youngsters, Wasserman et al. (1996) found positive parental involvement to be independently associated with fewer externalizing problems, even after negative aspects of parenting and monitoring were accounted for, both concurrently and prospectively. Patterson and his colleagues (1992), on the other hand, have reported that neither measures of positive involvement nor those of positive reinforcement predicted antisocial outcomes.

How might attachment concepts further our understanding of conduct disorders? Several positive parenting constructs (e.g. sensitivity, acceptance, warmth and responsiveness) are directly associated with parent–child attachment, which may therefore serve as a useful global variable, summarizing the history of caregiving quality. As Waters et al. (1993) have noted, however, attachment also correlates with many other family variables (stress, marital and biological), underlining the need to attend to the discriminant validity of measures and to alternative explanations for outcomes.

Specific mechanisms

Attachment theory suggests several specific processes that may be associated with the etiology or maintenance of conduct problems (Greenberg, 1999). The first of these occurs at the level of observable behaviour. Many of the early disruptive behaviours considered to be precursors of conduct disorder (e.g. tantrums, aggression and noncompliance) may be viewed as attachment-oriented strategies for gaining the attention and proximity of caregivers who are otherwise unresponsive. Although perhaps adaptive in the short term, these efforts may contribute to the development of aversive family interactions, increasing the likelihood of later conduct disorder. In a similar vein, Main & Hesse (1990) suggest that, in the absence of a coherent and predictable pattern of caregiving, the disorganized infant may attempt to take control of the parent–child relationship when stressed. Whereas this behaviour may improve the predictability of the relationship (Wahler & Dumas, 1986) and maintain a connection (albeit conflictual) with the parent, it may also evolve into the coerciveness characteristic of early conduct problems.

A second mechanism involves the development of cognitive–affective working models of relationships. As described above, these working models are believed to affect perception, cognition and motivation (Bretherton, 1985). Just as secure attachment establishes expectations of responsiveness, warmth and trust, setting the stage for reciprocal interactions, insecure attachment may play a causal role in later disorder through the development of working models characterized by mistrust, anger, anxiety and fear. This thinking fits well with Dodge's (1991) recent work (discussed in chapter 11 of this volume by Pettit et al.), which suggests that insecure attachment may lead to hostile attributional biases, resulting in reactive aggression. Research by Cassidy et al. (1996) indicates that, in contrast, secure children are more likely to express positive causal attributions and expectations.

Attachment may also contribute to the motivational processes involved in social intercourse (Richters & Waters, 1991). Maccoby & Martin (1983) argue that warm interactions and maternal responsiveness set the stage for developing compliance and internalized controls. Limit-setting and discipline are less likely to be effective in the absence of warm, responsive parent–child relationships, presumably because the child then cares less about pleasing the parent, fails to see the benefits of a reciprocal relationship, and does not internalize the values of a rejecting, unrewarding parent. Again, conduct disorder may be the ultimate outcome.

Attachment might affect later disorder through its impact on emotion regulation. The child learns to regulate emotions in the context of early parent–child interactions, for example, by turning away when overstimulated and returning with a smile when ready for more interaction. An insensitive, intrusive parent may not allow the child to modulate stimulation and an unresponsive one does not help the child achieve a desirable level of arousal. In either case, the child may learn a restricted and rigid set of rules for relating to others, either minimizing or heightening emotional awareness and/or expression in an effort to reach equilibrium (Cassidy, 1994). If a parent does not help a stressed child to manage his emotions effectively, that child may be left to his own, immature behavioural repertoire, perhaps including tantrums, aggression and other aversive behaviours.

The poorly regulated emotional system of insecure parent–child dyads may also affect neural organization. Although these ideas are quite speculative, some theorists posit that patterns of emotion regulation established in early childhood may substantially alter the fear conditioning processes in the amygdala (LeDoux, 1995), or the development of connections between the limbic system and the prefrontal cortex (Schore, 1996), particularly given a history of intense unregulated stress (e.g. abuse).

Fonagy et al. (1997) propose a mediating factor that involves both emotion regulation and motivational processes. Secure parent–child attachment may enhance the child's awareness of mental states (his own and others) and his reflective capacity. This 'mentalizing' facilitates relationship-building, by improving one's ability to understand and predict interpersonal behaviour, and inhibits malevolent acts because the individual is aware of their effect on others. Children who are deficient in their awareness of mental states may be less able to recognize and put in perspective their own emotions and more likely to violate the rights of others, for whom they lack empathy.

Evidence associating attachment with conduct problems

Research exploring the links between attachment and disordered behaviour can be divided into two groups, prospective studies which relate infant attachment to later outcomes and investigations assessing attachment concurrent with disorder.

Infant attachment and conduct problems

Early studies of preschoolers for whom infant attachment classifications were known provided tantalizing evidence that insecure attachment was associated with less compliance, more anger, poorer peer relations and less effective use of the support of caregivers (Matas et al., 1978; Sroufe, 1983). However, subsequent research seeking associations between early attachment and later externalizing behaviour problems produced mixed results. In low-risk convenience samples, with relatively low rates of both insecurity and psychopathology, no significant main effects were found (Bates et al., 1985, 1991; Fagot & Kavanagh, 1990; Lewis et al., 1984). In contrast, investigators studying populations with high social risk have provided evidence that, in the presence of other risk factors, attachment insecurity increases the likelihood of antisocial behaviour.

The Minnesota Mother–Child Project has followed a group of infants of primarily young, low SES, single mothers from birth into adolescence. Follow-up assessments in the preschool (Erickson et al., 1985; Troy & Sroufe, 1987), elementary school (Renken et al., 1989; Sroufe et al., 1990), and preadolescent periods (Urban et al., 1991) have consistently demonstrated that high-risk children with insecure infancy attachment classifications are more likely to have poor peer relations and symptoms of aggression and depression. Predictions from attachment to externalizing outcomes are stronger for boys than for girls.

These findings are consistent with the view that secure attachment may operate as a protective factor in high-risk environments and that insecure attachment combined with family adversity may contribute to later behaviour problems. They do not provide evidence for the differential effects of various kinds of insecurity; in the 10–11-year-old follow-up, for example, insecure-avoidant and insecure-ambivalent children were for the most part indistinguishable in outcome. However, initial attachment assessment of these youngsters did not include the disorganized classification, which may have limited its ability to delineate different pathways.

A number of recent studies have highlighted the role of disorganized classification in behaviour problem outcomes. In a high risk sample in which many mothers were depressed, 71% of preschoolers rated as hostile had been disorganized at 18 months of age (Lyons-Ruth et al., 1989). Furthermore, nine of the 16 disorganized children whose mothers had psychosocial problems were rated as hostile in kindergarten, compared to one of the 19 children without either risk factor. The combination of low infant intelligence and disorganized attachment was also predictive of clinically significant teacher-rated externalizing difficulties at age 7, again supporting a multirisk model

(Lyons-Ruth et al., 1997). Surprisingly, attachment did not predict mothers' ratings of their children's behaviour. In another follow-up study of this group, security at age 7 was shown to correlate with concurrent teacher ratings of externalizing behaviour, even after accounting for psychosocial risk and language scores; however, with this attachment measure the association between clinically significant problems and any one insecure classification was less clear (Easterbrooks et al., 1993). Small sample sizes (N = 45–50) must temper conclusions drawn from these studies.

Shaw and colleagues (Shaw & Vondra, 1995; Shaw et al., 1996) have also followed a high risk sample. Infant insecurity predicted behaviour problems at age 3 and age 5: whereas 60% (6 out of 10) of the children classified disorganized at 12 months of age showed clinically elevated levels of aggression, 31% of avoidant, 28% of ambivalent and only 17% of secure infants did so. Stability of attachment classification from 12 to 18 months was poor, and, although patterns of relations were similar for both sets of data, only a few predictions reached significance (e.g. 18-month but not 12-month security was related to age 3 externalizing, and disorganization predicted age 5 but not age 3 externalizing scores). In this sample of 100 infants, attachment was a meaningful predictor for boys, but not girls, and exerted a significant but small effect (acccounting for 10% of the variance in boys' externalizing scores at age 3).

Concurrent links between attachment and psychopathology

Because the base rate of serious behaviour problems is low, it is difficult to collect an infant sample large enough to provide a significant number of disordered youngsters. Investigations of high-risk populations represent one means of increasing the rate of later disorder; identifying a sample once early signs of disorder have appeared is another avenue for studying the influence of attachment on the development of problematic behaviour.

Three studies have examined concurrent attachment security in clinic-referred samples of children meeting criteria for oppositional defiant disorder (Greenberg et al., 1991; Speltz et al., 1990, 1999). Approximately 80% of the 50 clinic children in the first two cohorts were rated insecure. These included avoidant, ambivalent, controlling and insecure-other classifications. The controlling group was particularly large among the clinic boys, but the avoidant and insecure-other categories were also over-represented.

In a third, larger (N = 160) cohort of carefully matched clinic-referred and comparison boys, children with oppositional defiant disorder again had higher rates of concurrent insecurity (Speltz et al., 1999). This cohort differed from the first two in that the criteria for inclusion in the clinic group was lower (Child

Behavior Checklist aggression scores of 65 versus 70), and a smaller percentage (55%) of the clinic boys were classified insecure. The clinic group again included more controlling, avoidant and insecure-other boys than did the comparison group; no one insecure group stood out. Child attachment to fathers showed a pattern similar to that of attachment to mothers (DeKlyen et al., 1998). Being insecurely attached to both parents appeared to greatly increase risk; of the 18 youngsters classified insecure with both parents, 17 were clinic-referred. The suggestion by Fonagy et al. (1997) that children with incompatible working models of their mother and father (e.g. one secure and one insecure) are at greatest risk for psychopathology was not supported by these data. Fathers have rarely been included in studies linking attachment to problem behaviour. However, in a nonclinic sample, Suess et al. (1992) also found that problems were best predicted by knowledge of child's attachment to both mother and father.

A few facts should be noted. First, a number of the clinic-referred boys in these studies were securely attached with their parents, and others were avoidant during reunion, rather than controlling: insecurity is an element of some but not all pathways leading to early conduct disorder, and the reunion behaviour of disruptive boys is not merely a reflection of the oppositional disorder. In addition, some nonproblem boys were classified insecure: insecurity is not synonymous with pathology. Campbell (1990) has also noted that some highly aggressive and hyperactive boys appeared to have warm and trusting mother–child relationships. The one clinic study including girls (Speltz et al., 1990) found an association between attachment and problems only for boys. Finally, the finding that mothers' working model of attachment was highly concordant with child attachment in the Greenberg et al. (1991) cohort (DeKlyen, 1996) increases the probability that insecure child attachment preceded the first signs of disruptive behaviour problems. Other studies have related maternal attachment classification and children's behaviour problems as well (Constantino, 1996; Crowell et al., 1991).

Nonclinical samples have demonstrated similar links between concurrent attachment measures and school-age antisocial behaviour. Cohn (1990) reported that insecure 6-year-old boys were perceived as more aggressive by peers and rated by teachers as having more behaviour problems; this was not true of girls in the sample. Similarly, Turner (1991) found that 4-year-old boys (but not girls) concurrently classified as insecure were more aggressive, disruptive and attention-seeking in preschool than were secure boys. In a middle class group of 6-year-olds, children classified as controlling were rated more aggressive (Solomon et al., 1995) than avoidant, ambivalent and secure youngsters.

Insecure-controlling French–Canadian children aged 5 to 7 were also more likely to have problematic behaviour (teacher-rated) than were children with other classifications (Moss et al., 1996). Finally, Fagot & Pears (1996), using the Crittenden (1992) system for assessing preschool attachment, found that children classified coercive at age 3 displayed more behaviour problems at age 7 than did children labelled secure or defended.

The only empirical evidence linking the Adult Attachment Interview to concurrent adolescent or adult conduct problems is provided by Fonagy et al. (1997), who describe unpublished data confirming that most of the criminals in their sample were characterized by insecure classifications on the AAI.

Issues and limitations

We have argued that attachment relations may increase risk or buffer the effects of other risk factors in several specific ways. However, Bowlby's claim for attachment as a major cause of disorder now seems overly ambitious. Associations between attachment and behaviour problems tend to be modest, and multiple child and environmental factors – including temperament, gender, IQ, parental psychopathology and peer relations – play a role in determining antisocial behaviour.

Few childhood disorders have a single cause, and it is improbable that attachment insecurity alone will lead to disorder, although it may increase its likelihood (Sroufe et al., 1990). As a corollary, few disorders are likely to be eliminated by treating a single factor; even if powerful biological causes are implicated, the parent–child relationship may be a crucial focus for treatment (Rutter, 1982). To complicate matters, nonlinear relations may exist between risk factors and outcomes; for example, the rate of disorder may multiply as risk factors are added. Risk factors may also have differential influence during different developmental periods, with attachment perhaps playing an important role in the development of oppositional behaviour in early childhood, whereas parent monitoring and peer relations may become more critical in predicting antisocial outcomes later. Greenberg (in press) explores these and other considerations regarding the role of risk factors in developmental psychopathology.

Multifinality and equifinality

Attachment insecurity may increase the risk of psychopathology, but as previously noted, it is neither necessary nor sufficient to its expression: some secure individuals will show disorder, and some insecure individuals will not.

Insecurity may be a nonspecific risk factor, associated with a number of different forms of psychopathology, both externalizing and internalizing (Greenberg, in press; Rutter, 1985). Attachment theory suggests that this should be so, as different categories of insecurity are thought to be characterized by different representations of self, other and relationships, and with different styles of emotion regulation (outlined above). It has therefore been argued that specific categories of attachment should be associated with specific disorders (e.g. Fagot & Kavanagh, 1990; Lyons-Ruth, 1996; Rubin et al., 1991; Sroufe, 1983). However, as noted earlier, the evidence is mixed; our work, as well as that of others, indicates that multiple outcomes are associated with each category (multifinality), just as all categories of attachment may be represented in a sample of conduct disorder youngsters (equifinality).

Why might some children categorized, for example, as avoidant remain apparently untouched by pathology, others develop internalizing symptoms, others exhibit externalizing behaviours, and still others present with a combination of both? Subtypes within the avoidant classification might shed light on this question; however, reliability at this level of coding is often problematic and the number of cases usually too small to permit statistical analyses. Alternatively, accompanying risk factors may be determinative. Temperamental predispositions (towards high impulsivity, low reward dependence, and low anxiety, for example; Tremblay et al., 1994) may predispose some avoidant children to an antisocial outcome, whereas even-tempered children may be unlikely to exhibit conduct problems. Similarly, avoidance coupled with incompetent or harsh discipline strategies might provide a fertile ground for externalizing problems, whereas in the context of lax or guilt-inducing discipline it may more likely lead to anxiety or depression. Other risk factors that become more influential in middle and late childhood (e.g. neighbourhood quality, delinquent peers, school failure) may also play crucial roles in determining behaviour problems.

Although we have noted that all categories of attachment may be represented in a conduct disorder sample, this equifinality of outcome may be more apparent than real. It is possible that, as different types of the disorder become better delineated (e.g. socialized versus undersocialized, covert versus overt, early versus late onset), patterns relating each to specific attachment styles may be found. This would, however, require attachment data on larger samples of disordered youngsters than have as yet been available.

Intercorrelated risk factors

One of the challenges of conducting research in the real world with complex phenomena such as conduct disorder is the intricate web of interconnections among the many variables of interest. Depending upon one's theoretical bent one might focus on socioeconomic status, parent psychopathology, marital conflict, behaviour management strategies, or attachment, and find, in isolation, significant main effects. As Waters et al. (1993) warn, given a set of intercorrelated risk factors, it is crucial that causality not be uncritically attributed to one favoured variable. Fortunately, researchers are increasingly attempting to test multiple variables simultaneously to tease out mediating, moderating and unique effects. Thus, Shaw & Vondra (1995) found that 3-year-old boys' externalizing scores were mostly accounted for by attachment and mothers' depression scores, and not by temperament ratings. In recent analyses (Greenberg et al., in press) we have demonstrated the insecure attachment, positive and negative parenting, and child risk factors (but not family adversity) all contributed uniquely to the prediction of concurrent clinic referral for early behaviour problems.

However, large samples are required to test multifactorial models, and observational measures such as attachment are relatively expensive, limiting the number of studies in which such discriminating analyses are possible. It is clear that complex interaction effects exist, such that attachment quality may moderate or be moderated by other risks (Lyons-Ruth et al., 1997).

Belsky et al. (1998) argue that reported effect sizes may be small because parental influences have been averaged across children whose vulnerability to parenting varies. We have focused so far on variable-oriented analyses, which average effects over an entire sample, thus losing information about individual pathways. Our expectation, however, is that attachment will be an important contributor to the development of disorder for some individuals but not for others. Person-oriented analyses will be required to describe the discrete pathways associated with disorder and to determine whether outcomes for individuals characterized, for example, by insecure attachment and poor discipline differ from those for others who are at risk because of child characteristics (e.g. low IQ or attention deficits) and family adversity (e.g. low SES, single parenting or marital conflict). We are beginning to attempt such analyses in our longitudinal study of clinic-referred preschool boys (Greenberg et al., in press).

Placing attachment in a developmental context

Many questions persist concerning the process by which attachment interrelates with other risk factors. Poor discipline practices and insecure attachment might exert relatively independent, additive effects. Alternatively, insecure attachment may interfere with otherwise effective parenting (e.g. an insecure youngster may be less responsive to discipline because of less developed emotion regulation skills or reduced prosocial motivation); in this case, attachment might moderate the influence of parenting practices. Similarly, within the context of a secure parent–child attachment, a temperamentally impulsive or language-impaired child might acquire sufficient skill and support in emotion regulation that antisocial behaviours would be unlikely to become problematic. To the best of our knowledge, no data have yet been reported that specifically speaks to these questions.

Do the associations between early attachment and later outcomes represent an effect of attachment or continuity of environment? At least three scenarios are possible: (1) infancy experience impacts the young organism in ways that continue to influence interactions with the world despite later experiences (critical stage theory); (2) concurrent attachment working models will best predict outcomes, as attachment working models change over time in response to environmental changes; (3) because secure infant attachment is correlated with many measures of environmental 'goodness', the correlation of outcome with attachment is actually due to the continuity of other features of the environment; the best prediction of outcome will come from more proximal environmental measures. In an attempt to disentangle some of these effects, Sroufe et al. (1990) conducted several analyses with measures collected over a number of years. Infant attachment added to the prediction of teacher-rated preschool, but not elementary, competence after intermediary measures of home environment and child competence were accounted for. However, in a subsample of children who were extensively observed in a camp setting when they were 10–11 years old, attachment did contribute unique variance to ratings of social competence and emotional adjustment.

Measurement

Although attachment theory provides a useful framework for conceptualizing the emergence of conduct disorder, well-validated measures which allow continuous tracking of attachment relations from infancy through early adulthood do not yet exist. Classification based on the Strange Situation (Ainsworth et al., 1978) has been regarded as the 'gold standard' against which other measures have been validated, yet attempts to explain developmental discontinuities between 12- and 18-month assessments utilizing this system (Thompson et al., 1982; Vaughn et al., 1979; see also Shaw & Bell, 1993) are not entirely satisfying. Few reports exist on continuities between the infancy and preschool systems (but see Howes & Hamilton (1992) and Cicchetti & Barnett (1991)), in spite of initially encouraging data linking infancy and 6-year-old measures (Main & Cassidy, 1988) in a relatively stable normative sample. Some have chosen to focus on attachment in infancy, assessing the impact of this early measure to later development (e.g. Sroufe and his colleagues), whereas others anticipate that, as attachment remains salient across development, developmentally sensitive assessment of attachment at different stages should be feasible and useful (Cicchetti et al., 1990), particularly given demonstrated shifts in attachment as a result of theoretically meaningful changes in the caregiving environment; still others contend that continuity is not an appropriate expectation (Crittenden, 1992).

During the school years, as internal representations become more important and behavioural manifestations more subtle, a gap in established instrumentation appears, making it difficult to track developmental transformations. For late adolescence and adulthood, the AAI provides a tool whose association with parenting behaviour and child attachment has received considerable validation (van IJzendoorn, 1995), but there is little longitudinal data linking it with earlier attachment measures and experiences. It is not certain that the various attachment measures all tap the same construct.

Because current measures do not span the entire period over which conduct isorder develops, a comprehensive investigation of the involvement of attachment processes in its etiology and maintenance is not possible. Indeed, attachment theory is itself underdeveloped in accounting for transformations across the life-span. Bowlby's final stage, that of the 'goal-corrected partnership', is thought to begin around age 4, in the preschool years (Marvin, 1977), leaving a great deal of subsequent change unexplained. How do attachment relations and functions develop with the increasing capacities of the child, new parenting tasks and the child's broadening social horizons (school, peers, intimate partners, etc.)? Or does attachment, as currently defined, lose its significance as the child becomes more independent and capable of relying on himself?

Clinical applications of attachment theory to the treatment of conduct disorder

Despite research showing a range of psychological therapies to be effective in diminishing conduct problems in the short to medium term (Kazdin, chapter 15, this volume), in clinical practice these problems are often unresponsive to treatment. Substantial numbers of children are not helped, and new approaches to intervention are needed (Patterson et al., 1993). Attachment constructs offer the possibility of innovative methods of prevention and treatment which may prove useful.

There have been numerous case reports and treatment studies of interventions that either seek to improve the attachment status of high-risk infants by increasing parental responsiveness (Erickson et al., 1992; Juffer et al., 1997; Lieberman et al., 1991; van den Boom, 1994, 1995) or are designed to change some clinical symptom or disorder in older children or adolescents using a treatment that is said to follow from attachment theory (Delaney, 1991; Holland et al., 1993; Marvin, 1992; Speltz, 1990). In some cases, the conceptual linkage between intervention and attachment has been tenuous, based on little more than an emphasis on the importance of supportive relationships in the treatment of psychopathology.

Interventions designed to alter early attachment and its maternal antecedents are relevant to the prevention of conduct disorder, as they have targeted infants having many of the risk factors associated with early onset externalizing problems (e.g. family adversity, irritable temperament). These interventions can be divided into two types: those focusing almost exclusively on the mother, providing emotional support in the context of a long-term therapeutic relationship (e.g. Lieberman et al., 1991) and those emphasizing direct 'coaching' of the mother as she interacts with her infant, usually in a relatively short-term intervention (e.g. Project STEEP, using videotape feedback to help mothers read infant signals; Erickson et al., 1992). In a meta-analysis including both types of interventions, van IJzendoorn et al. (1995) found attachment-oriented treatments generally to be more effective in changing specific parental behaviours (e.g. sensitivity or contingency during interaction with the infant or child) than in changing children's attachment classifications. It was further evident that short-term, skills-oriented interventions involving the young child were more effective than longer, more intensive therapeutic interventions focused on mothers.

In the most persuasive of these studies, van den Boom (1994) selected middle-class Dutch infants showing relatively high irritability at 6 months and randomly assigned their mothers to either a skill-based intervention or a no treatment group. The intervention was based on a four-stage model of maternal responsiveness (perceiving infant signals, interpreting infant signals, selecting an appropriate response, and implementing the response). Techniques such as imitation of infant behaviour and silence during infant gaze aversion were modelled and reinforced during a 3-month intervention. Follow-up assessment at 12 months revealed a significant effect of intervention on attachment classification (62% secure in the intervention group versus 22% secure in the control group). Results at 18 months were similar, and another assessment at age 3 found greater maternal responsiveness and child cooperative behaviour among intervention participants, an effect that was mediated by attachment status (van den Boom, 1995). Despite the relatively small number of subjects (31 secure and 19 insecure infants in the intervention group and 11 secure and 39 insecure infants in the control group at 12 months) and the need for replication, the potential of this intervention is obvious, particularly given the temperamental vulnerability of these infants.

Much less is known about attachment-related treatments for older children presenting with early or fully developed forms of conduct disorder. Speltz (1990) described an extension of a standard parent training intervention for preschoolers with externalizing behaviour problems that emphasized maternal responsiveness during child-directed play and parent–child negotiation of conflict, based on Bowlby's notion of the 'goal-corrected partnership'. However, no outcome data were reported. Delaney (1991) has detailed a therapeutic strategy for working with 'attachment-disordered' youth, essentially a diagnostic term for antisocial behaviour coupled with sociopathy (i.e. blatant disregard for others' feelings and welfare and 'counterfeit' emotionality). Delaney's approach begins with verbal confrontations designed to force the child's verbalization of the negative working model. This is followed by more typical cognitive–behavioural techniques that attempt to replace negative 'self-talk' about attachment relationships (e.g. 'I am worthless'; 'Others are unresponsive and unreliable') with more adaptive cognitive–affective messages. This approach is also lacking empirical validation.

DeKlyen (1996) has suggested that parent attachment status, determined by the AAI, may have implications for the assignment of families to different types of parent training interventions for children with early onset conduct problems. For example, parents with secure working models of attachment may benefit from a standard parent training programme focusing primarily on behaviour management skills, whereas a parent with a dismissing, preoccupied or unresolved attachment may require supplemental treatment strategies aimed at clarifying for the parent the distinctions between past and present attachment relationships. Such parents may have difficulty attending to and processing the specifics of their child's behaviour because their interpersonal perceptions are so clouded by unresolved aspects of previous events and relationships (Strand & Wahler, 1996). Speltz (1990) described one method for working with such parents, by engaging them in discussions of potential linkages between the parent–child relationship and the parents' other close relationships, as the parent watches and is questioned about selected videotaped interactions between themselves and their child.

To our knowledge, the use of the AAI for selecting and planning parent training interventions has not been systematically investigated. However, one study of clinic children with externalizing behaviour problems found that parent attachment status interacted with pretreatment problem severity to explain significant variance in child outcomes following a standard parent training programme (Routh et al., 1995); parent training had more positive impact on children whose parents had secure attachment status. The strongest associations with poor outcomes 2 to 4 years later were with unresolved maternal attachment, the analogue of disorganized infant status. However, very small numbers (total N = 37) render this a tentative finding.

One programme for adolescents with conduct disorder, called the Response Programme (Holland et al., 1993), traces its conceptual roots to attachment theory. This 30-day residential programme is followed by intensive, long-term outreach services in the community that attempt to directly alter the youth's social ecology. For example, a close relationship between the adolescent and an adult role model in a work setting might be fostered. An uncontrolled follow-up study (Moretti et al., 1994) indicated significant reductions in adult- and youth-reported symptoms. However, the programmes' goals and procedures – although certainly compatible with attachment theory – seem not to differ substantially from other community outreach programmes emphasizing supportive social relationships for troubled youth (Henggler et al., 1986).

Overall, the clinical application of attachment theory to conduct problems is at a very early stage of development. There are several promising directions that deserve further investigation. Skills-oriented coaching programmes for parents of high-risk infants may prove to be an effective method for the prevention of conduct problems, if their effects can be shown to maintain through the age period when clinically significant problems are typically first observed (ages 4 to 6). Van den Boom's (1995) report that infant outcomes in her programme were mediated by child attachment status suggests a causal link between attachment security and the development of prosocial behaviour; more studies of this nature are needed. Other areas deserving investigation are the use of the AAI to assign parents to varying types of parent training and of structured interviews and videotape feedback to improve the social information processing of unresolved, dismissing and preoccupied parents.

Conclusion

This chapter has presented an overview of attachment theory and its potential value in explaining the development of conduct disorder. Particular attention was given to possible mechanisms, empirical support and the limitations of this explanatory model. Finally, some clinical implications for the treatment of conduct-disordered youth were discussed. While strong claims for attachment as a main effect have not received support, in a multifactorial, multipathway model it has proven to have some predictive utility. Furthermore, the theory has enriched our thinking about the processes which might lead to disorder and ways of effectively intervening.

REFERENCES

Ainsworth, M.D.S., Blehar, M.C., Waters, E. & Wall, S. (1978). *Patterns of Attachment*. Hillsdale, NJ: Lawrence Erlbaum.

Armsden, G.C. & Greenberg, M.T. (1987). The Inventory of Parent and Peer Attachment: Individual differences and their relationship to psychological well-being in adolescence. *Journal of Youth and Adolescence, 16*, 427–54.

Bates, J.E., Bayles, K., Bennett, D.S., Ridge, B. & Brown, M.M. (1991). Origins of externalizing behavior problems at eight years of age. In D.J. Pepler & K.H. Rubin (Eds.), *The Development and Treatment of Childhood Aggression* (pp. 93–120). Hillsdale, NJ: Lawrence Erlbaum.

Bates, J.E., Maslin, C.A. & Frankel, K.A. (1985). Attachment security, mother-child interaction, and temperament as predictors of behavior-problem ratings at age three years. In I. Bretherton & E. Waters (Eds.), *Growing Points of Attachment Theory and Research. Monographs of the Society for Research in Child Development, 50*, 167–93.

Belsky, J., Hsieh, K.-H. & Crnic, K. (1998). Mothering, fathering, and infant negativity as antecedents of boys' externalizing problems and inhibition at age 3 years: Differential suscepti- bility to rearing experience? *Development and Psychopathology, 10*, 301–20.

Belsky, J. & Nezworski, T. (1988). *Clinical Implications of Attachment*. Hillsdale, NJ: Lawrence Erlbaum.

Bowlby, J. (1944). Forty-four juvenile thieves: Their characters and home-life. *International Journal of Psycho-Analysis, 1*, 19–52, 107–27.

Bowlby, J. (1969/1982). *Attachment and Loss: Vol. 1. Attachment* (2nd Edn). New York: Basic Books.

Bowlby, J. (1973). *Attachment and Loss: Vol. 2. Separation*. New York: Basic Books.

Bretherton, I. (1985). Attachment theory: Retrospect and prospect. In I. Bretherton & E. Waters (Eds.), *Growing Points of Attachment Theory and Research. Monographs of the Society for Research in Child Development, 50*, 3–35.

Campbell, S.B. (1990). *Behavior Problems in Preschool Children: Clinical and Developmental Issues*. New York: Guilford Press.

Campbell, S.B. (1995). Behavior problems in preschool children: A review of recent research. *Journal of Child Psychology and Psychiatry, 36*, 113–49.

Carlson, V., Cicchetti, D., Barnett, D., & Braunwald, K. (1989). Disorganized/disoriented attachment relationships in maltreated infants. *Developmental Psychology, 25*, 525–31.

Cassidy, J. (1994). Emotion regulation: Influences of attachment relationships. In N.A. Fox (Ed.), *The development of emotion regulation: biological and behavioral considerations. Monographs of the Society for Research in Child Development, 59* (2–3, Serial No. 240), 228–49.

Cassidy, J., Kirsch, S.J., Scolton, K. & Parke, R.D. (1996). Attachment and representation of peer relationships. *Developmental Psychology, 32*, 892–904.

Cassidy, J., Marvin, R.S. & the MacArthur Working Group on Attachment (1989). *Preschool Attachment Assessment System*. Coding Manual. MacArthur Working Group.

Cicchetti, D. & Barnett, D. (1991). Attachment organization in maltreated preschoolers. *Development and Psychopathology, 3*, 397–411.

Cicchetti, D., Cummings, M., Greenberg, M. & Marvin, R.S. (1990). An organizational perspective on attachment beyond infancy: implications for theory, measurement, and research. In M.T. Greenberg, D. Cicchetti & E.M. Cummings (Eds.), *Attachment in the Preschool Years: Theory, Research, and Intervention* (pp. 3–49). Chicago: University of Chicago Press.

Cohn, D.A. (1990). Child-mother attachment of six-year-olds and social competence at school. *Child Development, 61*, 152–62.

Constantino, J.N. (1996). Intergenerational aspects of the development of aggression: A preliminary report. *Developmental and Behavioral Pediatrics, 17*, 176–82.

Crittenden, P.M. (1992). Quality of attachment in the preschool years. *Development and Psychopathology, 4*, 209–41.

Crowell, J.A. & Feldman, S.S. (1988). Mothers' internal working models of relationships and children's behavioral and developmental status: A study of mother-child interaction. *Child Development, 59*, 1273–85.

Crowell, J.A., O'Connor, E., Wollmers, G., Sprafkin, J. & Rao, U. (1991). Mothers' conceptualizations of parent–child relationships: Relation to mother–child interaction and child behavior problems. *Development and Psychopathology, 3*, 431–44.

DeKlyen, M. (1996). Disruptive behavior disorders and intergenerational attachment patterns: A comparison of normal and clinic-referred preschoolers and their mothers. *Journal of Consulting and Clinical Psychology, 64*, 357–65.

DeKlyen, M., Speltz, M.L. & Greenberg, M.T. (1998). Fathering and early onset conduct problems: Positive and negative parenting, father–son attachment, and the marital context. *Clinical Child and Family Psychology Review, 1*, 3–21.

Delaney, R.J. (1991). *Fostering Changes: Treating Attachment-disordered Foster Children*. Oklahoma City: Wood 'N' Barnes.

De Wolff, M.S. & van IJzendoorn, M.H. (1997). Sensitivity and attachment: A meta-analysis on parental antecedents of infant attachment. *Child Development, 68*, 571–91.

Dodge, K.A. (1991). The structure and function of reactive and proactive aggression. In D.J. Pepler & K.H. Rubin (Eds.), *The Development and Treatment of Childhood Aggression* (pp. 201–18). Hillsdale, NJ: Lawrence Erlbaum.

Easterbrooks, M.A., Davidson, C.E. & Chazan, R. (1993). Psychosocial risk, attachment, and behavior problems among school-aged children. *Development and Psychopathology, 5*, 389–402.

Erickson, M.F., Korfmacher, J. & Egeland, B. (1992). Attachments past and present: Implications for therapeutic intervention with mother-infant dyads. *Development and Psychopathology, 4*, 495–507.

Erickson, M.F., Sroufe, L.A. & Egeland, B. (1985). The relationship between quality of attachment and behavior problems in preschool in a high-risk sample. In I. Bretherton & E. Waters

(Eds.), *Growing Points of Attachment Theory and Research. Monographs of the Society for Research in Child Development, 50*, 147–66.

Eron, L.D., Walder, L.O. & Lefkowitz, M.M. (1971). *Learning of Aggression in Children*. Boston, MA: Little, Brown, & Co.

Fagot, B.I. & Kavanagh, K. (1990). The prediction of antisocial behavior from avoidant attachment classifications. *Child Development, 61*, 864–73.

Fagot, B.I. & Pears, K.C. (1996). Changes in attachment during the third year: Consequences and predictions. *Development and Psychopathology, 8*, 721–33.

Fonagy, P., Steele, H. & Steele, M. (1991). Maternal representations of attachment during pregnancy predict the organization of infant–mother attachment at one year of age. *Child Development, 62*, 891–905.

Fonagy, P., Target, M., Steele, M., et al. (1997). Morality, disruptive behavior, borderline personality disorder, crime, and their relationship to security of attachment. In L. Atkinson & K.J. Zucker (Eds.), *Attachment and Psychopathology*. New York: Guilford Press.

Fox, N.A., Kimmerly, N.L. & Schafer, W.D. (1991). Attachment to mother/attachment to father: A meta-analysis. *Child Development, 62*, 210–25.

Gardner, F.E.M. (1987). Positive interaction between mothers and conduct-problem children: Is there training for harmony as well as fighting? *Journal of Abnormal Child Psychology, 15*, 283–93.

George, C., Kaplan, N. & Main, M. (1985). *Adult Attachment Interview*. Unpublished manuscript, Department of Psychology, University of California at Berkeley.

Greenberg, M.T. (1999). Attachment and psychopathology in childhood. In J. Cassidy & P.R. Shaver (Eds.), *Handbook of Attachment: Theory, Research and Clinical Applications* (pp. 469–96). New York: Guilford Press.

Greenberg, M.T., Speltz, M.L. & DeKlyen, M. (1993). The role of attachment in the early development of disruptive behavior problems. *Development and Psychopathology, 5*, 191–213.

Greenberg, M.T., Speltz, M.L., DeKlyen, M. & Endriga, M.C. (1991). Attachment security in preschoolers with and without externalizing behavior problems: A replication. *Development and Psychopathology, 3*, 413–30.

Greenberg, M.T., Speltz, M.L., DeKlyen, M. & Jones, K. (in press). Correlates of clinic referral for early conduct problems: Variable vs. person-oriented analyses. The differential role of risk for predicting clinic referral for early conduct problems. *Development and Psychopathology*.

Henggler, S.W., Rodick, J., Borduin, C., et al. (1986). Multisystemic treatment of juvenile offenders: Effects on adolescent behavior and family interaction. *Developmental Psychology, 22*, 132–41.

Holland, R., Moretti, M.M., Verlaan, V. & Peterson, S. (1993). Attachment and conduct disorder: The Response Program. *Canadian Journal of Psychiatry, 38*, 420–31.

Howes, C. & Hamilton, C.E. (1992). Children's relationships with child care teachers: Stability and concordance with parental attachments. *Child Development, 63*, 867–78.

Juffer, F., van IJzendoorn, M.H. & Bakermans-Kranenburg, M.J. (1997). Intervention in transmission of insecure attachment: A case study. *Psychological Reports, 80*, 531–43.

Kazdin, A.E. (1987). *Conduct Disorders in Childhood and Adolescence. Developmental Clinical Psychology and Psychiatry Series, Vol. 9*. Newbury Park, CA: Sage.

LeDoux, J.E. (1995). Emotion: Clues from the brain. *Annual Review of Psychology, 46*, 209–35.

Lewis, M., Feiring, C., McGuffog, C. & Jaskir, J. (1984). Predicting psychopathology in 6-year-olds from early social relations. *Child Development, 55*, 123–36.

Lieberman, A.F., Weston, D.R. & Pawl, J.H. (1991). Preventive intervention and outcome with anxiously attached dyads. *Child Development, 62*, 199–209.

Lyons-Ruth, K. (1996). Attachment relationships among children with aggressive behavior problems: The role of disorganized early attachment patterns. *Journal of Consulting and Clinical Psychology, 64*, 64–73.

Lyons-Ruth, K., Connell, D., Zoll, D. & Stahl, J. (1987). Infants at social risk: Relations among infant maltreatment, maternal behavior, and infant attachment behavior. *Developmental Psychology, 23*, 223–32.

Lyons-Ruth, K., Easterbrooks, M.A. & Davidson Cibelli, C.E. (1997). Infant attachment strategies, infant mental lag, and maternal depressive symptoms: Predictors of internalizing and externalizing problems at age 7. *Developmental Psychology, 33*, 681–92.

Lyons-Ruth, K., Zoll, D., Connell, D. & Grunebaum, H.V. (1989). Family deviance and family disruption in childhood: Associations with maternal behavior and infant maltreatment during the first years of life. *Development and Psychopathology, 1*, 219–36.

Maccoby, E.E. & Martin, J.A. (1983). Socialization in the context of the family: Parent-child interaction. In E.M. Hetherington (Ed.), *Handbook of Child Psychology: Vol. 4. Socialization, Personality, and Social Development* (pp. 469–546). New York: John Wiley & Sons.

Main, M. & Cassidy, J. (1988). Categories of response to reunion with the parent at age 6: Predictable from infant attachment classifications and stable over a 1-month period. *Developmental Psychology, 24*, 415–42.

Main, M. & Goldwyn, R. (1994). *Adult Attachment Interview Classification System*. University of California at Berkeley.

Main, M. & Hesse, E. (1990). Parents' unresolved traumatic experiences are related to infant disorganized attachment status: Is frightened and/or frightening parental behavior the linking mechanism? In M.T. Greenberg, D. Cicchetti & E.M. Cummings (Eds.), *Attachment in the Preschool Years* (pp. 161–82). Chicago: University of Chicago.

Main, M., Kaplan, N. & Cassidy, J. (1985). Security in infancy, childhood, and adulthood: A move to the level of representation. In I. Bretherton & E. Waters (Eds.), *Growing Points of Attachment Theory and Research. Monographs of the Society for Research in Child Development, 50*, 66–104.

Main, M. & Solomon, J. (1986). Discovery of an insecure-disorganized/disoriented attachment pattern. In T.B. Brazelton & M. Yogman (Eds.), *Affective Development in Infancy* (pp. 95–124). Norwood, NH: Ablex.

Marvin, R.S. (1977). An ethological–cognitive model for the attenuation of mother-child attachment behavior. In T.M. Alloway, L. Krames & P. Piner (Eds.), *Children's Planning Strategies, No. 18: New Directions in Child Development*. San Francisco: Josey-Bass.

Marvin, R.S. (1992). Attachment and family systems-based intervention in developmental psychopathology. *Development and Psychopathology, 4*, 697–711.

Matas, L., Arend, R. & Sroufe, L.A. (1978). Continuity of adaptation in the second year: The relationship between quality of attachment and later competence. *Child Development, 49*, 547–56.

Moffitt, T.E. (1993). 'Life-course persistent' and 'adolescence-limited' antisocial behavior: A developmental taxonomy. *Psychological Review, 100*, 674–701.

Moretti, M.M., Holland, R. & Peterson, S. (1994). Long term outcome of an attachment-based program for conduct disorder. *Canadian Journal of Psychiatry, 39*, 360–9.

Moss, E., Parent, S., Gosselin, C., Rousseau, D. & St-Laurent, D. (1996). Attachment and teacher-reported behavior problems during the preschool and early school-age period. *Development and Psychopathology, 8*, 511–26.

Olweus, D. (1980). Familial and temperamental determinants of aggressive behavior in adolescent boys: A causal analysis. *Developmental Psychology, 16*, 644–60.

Patterson, G.R. (1982). *Coercive Family Process*. Eugene, OR: Castalia.

Patterson, G.R., Dishion, T.J. & Chamberlain, P. (1993). Outcomes and methodological issues relating to treatment of antisocial children. In T.R. Giles (Ed.), *Effective Psychotherapy: A Handbook of Comparative Research* (pp. 43–88). New York: Plenum Press.

Patterson, G.R., Reid, J.B. & Dishion, T.J. (1992). *Antisocial Boys*. Eugene, OR: Castalia.

Pettit, G.S. & Bates, J.E. (1989). Family interaction patterns and children's behavior problems from infancy to four years. *Developmental Psychology, 25*, 413–20.

Renken, B., Egeland, B., Marvinney, D., Mangelsdorf, S. & Sroufe, L.A. (1989). Early childhood antecedents of aggression and passive-withdrawal in early elementary school. *Journal of Personality, 57*, 257–81.

Richters, J.E. & Waters, E. (1991). Attachment and socialization: The positive side of social influence. In M. Lewis & S. Feinman (Eds.), *Social Influences and Socialization in Infancy* (pp. 185–213). New York: Plenum Press.

Robins, L.N. (1991). Conduct disorder. *Journal of Child Psychology and Psychiatry, 32*, 193–212.

Routh, C.P., Hill, J.W., Steele, H., Elliott, C.E. & Dewey, M.E. (1995). Maternal attachment status, psychosocial stressors and problem behaviour: Follow-up after parent training courses for conduct disorder. *Journal of Child Psychology and Psychiatry, 36*, 1179–98.

Rubin, K.H., Hymel, S., Mills, R.S.L. & Rose-Krasnor, L. (1991). Conceptualizing different developmental pathways to and from social isolation in childhood. In D. Cicchetti & S.L. Toth (Eds.), *Internalizing and Externalizing Expressions of Dysfunction: Rochester Symposium on Developmental Psychopathology*. Vol. 2 (pp. 91–122). Hillsdale, NJ: Lawrence Erlbaum.

Russell, A. & Russell, G. (1996). Positive parenting and boys' and girls' misbehavior during a home observation. *International Journal of Behavioral Development, 19*, 291–307.

Rutter, M. (1982). Prevention of children's psychosocial disorder: Myth and substance. *Pediatrics, 70*, 883–94.

Rutter, M. (1985). Resilience in the face of adversity: Protective factors and resistance to psychiatric disorder. *British Journal of Psychiatry, 147*, 598–611.

Schore, A.N. (1996). The experience-dependent maturation of a regulatory system in the orbital prefrontal cortex and the origin of developmental psychopathology, *Development and Psychopathology, 8*, 59–87.

Shaw, D.S. & Bell, R.Q. (1993). Developmental theories of parental contributors to antisocial behavior. *Journal of Abnormal Child Psychology, 21*, 493–518.

Shaw, D.S., Owens, E.B., Vondra, J.I., Keenan, K. & Winslow, E.B. (1996). Early risk factors and pathways in the development of early disruptive behavior problems. *Development and Psycho-pathology, 8*, 679–700.

Shaw, D.S. & Vondra, J.I. (1995). Infant attachment security and maternal predictors of early behavior problems: A longitudinal study of low-income families. *Journal of Abnormal Child Psychology, 23*, 335–57.

Solomon, J., George, C. & De Jong, A. (1995). Children classified as controlling at age 6: Evidence of disorganized representational strategies and aggression at home and at school. *Development and Psychopathology, 7*, 447–63.

Speltz, M.L. (1990). The treatment of preschool conduct problems: An integration of behavioral and attachment concepts. In M.T. Greenberg, D. Cicchetti & M. Cummings (Eds.), *Attachment in the Preschool Years: Theory, Research and Intervention* (pp. 399–426). Chicago: University of Chicago Press.

Speltz, M.L., DeKlyen, M., & Greenberg, M.T. (1999). Attachment in boys with early onset conduct problems. *Development and Psychopathology, 11*, 269–89.

Speltz, M.L., DeKlyen, M., Greenberg, M.T. & Dryden, M. (1995). Clinic referral for Opposi-tional Defiant Disorder: Relative significance of attachment and behavioral variables. *Journal of Abnormal Child Psychology, 23*, 487–507.

Speltz, M.L., Greenberg, M.T. & DeKlyen, M. (1990). Attachment in preschoolers with disrup-tive behavior: A comparison of clinic-referred and nonproblem children. *Development and Psychopathology, 2*, 31–46.

Spieker, S.J. & Booth, C.L. (1988). Maternal antecedents of attachment quality. In J. Belsky & T. Nezworski (Eds.), *Clinical Implications of Attachment Theory* (pp. 95–135). Hillsdale, NJ: Law-rence Erlbaum.

Sroufe, L.A. (1983). Infant-caregiver attachment and patterns of adaptation in preschool: The roots of maladaptation and competence. In M. Perlmutter (Ed.), *Minnesota Symposia in Child Psychology*, (Vol. 16, pp. 41–81). Hillsdale, NJ: Lawrence Erlbaum.

Sroufe, L.A. (1988). The role of infant-caregiver attachment in development. In J. Belsky & T. Nezworski (Eds.), *Clinical Implications of Attachment* (pp. 18–39). Hillsdale, NJ: Lawrence Erlbaum.

Sroufe, L.A., Egeland, B. & Kreutzer, T. (1990). The fate of early experience following develop-mental change: Longitudinal approaches to individual adaptation in childhood. *Child Develop-ment, 61*, 1363–73.

Strand, P.S. & Wahler, R.G. (1996). Predicting maladaptive parenting: Role of maternal object relations. *Journal of Clinical Child Psychology, 25*, 43–51.

Suess, G.J., Grossmann, K.E. & Sroufe, L.A. (1992). Effects of infant attachment to mother and father on quality of adaptation in preschool: From dyadic to individual organisation of self. *International Journal of Behavioural Development, 15*, 43–65.

Thompson, R.A., Lamb, M.E. & Estes, D. (1982). Stability of infant–mother attachment and its relationship to changing life circumstances in an unselected middle-class sample. *Child Develop-ment, 53*, 144–8.

Tremblay, R.E., Pihl, R.O., Vitaro, F. & Dobkin, P.L. (1994). Predicting early onset of male antisocial behavior from preschool behavior. *Archives of General Psychiatry, 51*, 732–9.

Troy, M. & Sroufe, L.A. (1987). Victimization among preschoolers: The role of attachment relationship history. *Journal of the American Academy of Child and Adolescent Psychiatry, 26,* 166–72.

Turner, P. (1991). Relations between attachment, gender, and behavior with peers in the preschool. *Child Development, 62,* 1475–88.

Urban, J., Carlson, E., Egeland, B. & Sroufe, L.A. (1991). Patterns of individual adaptation across childhood. *Development and Psychopathology, 3,* 445–60.

van den Boom, D.C. (1994). The influence of temperament and mothering on attachment and exploration: An experimental manipulation of sensitive responsiveness among lower-class mothers with irritable infants. *Child Development, 65,* 1457–77.

van den Boom, D.C. (1995). Do first-year intervention effects endure? Follow-up during toddlerhood of a sample of Dutch irritable infants. *Child Development, 66,* 1798–816.

van IJzendoorn, M.H. (1995). Associations between adult attachment representations and parent–child attachment, parental responsiveness, and clinical status: A meta-analysis on the predictive validity of the Adult Attachment Interview. *Psychological Bulletin, 117,* 387–403.

van IJzendoorn, M.H., Juffer, F. & Duyvesteyn, M.G.C. (1995). Breaking the intergenerational cycle of insecure attachment: A review of the effects of attachment-based interventions on maternal sensitivity and infant security. *Journal of Child Psychology and Psychiatry, 36,* 225–48.

van IJzendoorn, M.H. & Kroonenberg, P.M. (1988). Cross-cultural patterns of attachment. A meta-analysis of the Strange Situation. *Child Development, 59,* 147–56.

Vaughn, B., Egeland, B., Sroufe, L.A. & Waters, E. (1979). Individual differences in infant-mother attachment at twelve and eighteen months: Stability and change in families under stress. *Child Development, 50,* 971–5.

Vaughn, B., Stevenson-Hinde, J., Waters, E., et al. (1992). Attachment security and temperament in infancy and early childhood: Some conceptual clarifications. *Developmental Psychology, 28,* 463–73.

Wahler, R.G. & Dumas, J.E. (1986). 'A chip off the old block': Some interpersonal characteristics in coercive children across generations. In P. Strain, M.J. Guralnick & H.M. Walker (Eds.), *Children's Social Behavior: Development, Assessment, and Modification* (pp. 49–91). New York: Academic Press.

Wartner, U.G., Grossmann, K., Fremmer-Bombik, E. & Suess, G. (1994). Attachment patterns at age six in south Germany: Predictability from infancy and implications for preschool behavior. *Child Development, 65,* 1014–27.

Wasserman, G.A., Miller, L.S., Pinner, E. & Jaramillo, B. (1996). Parenting predictors of early conduct problems in urban, high-risk boys. *Journal of the American Academy of Child and Adolescent Psychiatry, 35,* 1227–36.

Waters, E., Posada, G., Crowell, J. & Keng-Ling, L. (1993). Is attachment theory ready to contribute to our understanding of disruptive behavior problems? *Development and Psychopathology, 5,* 215–24.

13

Friends, friendships and conduct disorders

Frank Vitaro, Richard E. Tremblay and William M. Bukowski

Scope and overview

A developmental perspective

Friends have been recognized as a potent source of influence on children's social, cognitive and emotional development (Hartup & Sancilio, 1986). Friendship is already important as a context of development during the preschool years, although it is second to the family context (Howes, 1988; Ladd et al., 1996). By pre- and early adolescence, friends (mostly same-gender) become a strong source of influence (Berndt, 1979; Steinberg, 1986; Sullivan, 1953). Together with the influence of the larger peer group the influence of friendships remains operative throughout adolescence. The increasing influence of peers and friends from childhood to adolescence corresponds with a decrease in parental influence (Furman & Robins, 1985). During this time, the conception, determinants and function of friendship also evolve (Aboud & Mendelson, 1996). Throughout this chapter, we adopt a developmental perspective concordant with the previous description to understand whether and how friends or peers might influence children's/adolescents' conduct disorder.

Many studies have considered peer influence in group contexts such as gangs (ex: Elliott et al., 1985; Thornberry et al., 1993). Others have focused on dyadic contexts such as friendship (Dishion et al., 1995a; Tremblay et al., 1995; Vitaro et al., 1997). Within the latter, some have considered all possible friendship dyads, others have included only very best friends, and yet others have used only mutual friends. Whereas close friends may exert stronger influences on children than exerted by other peers (e.g. acquaintances) (Newcomb & Bagwell, 1995; Savin-Williams & Berndt, 1990), the influence of other peers may also be significant. Hence their influences may add to or even equal the more intense influence from close friends. Few authors considered both perspectives in the same study.

Features of friendships may also vary across developmental periods. In

346

comparison to their relationships with nonfriends, school-age children evidence higher levels of positive engagement (i.e. having social contact, talking, cooperating, and expressing positive affect such as smiling, looking, laughing and touching) with their friends (mutual or unilateral) than preschool children (see Newcomb & Bagwell, 1995). In turn, early adolescents tend to express more positive engagement and more relationship properties (i.e. more similarity, more equality, less dominance, more mutual liking and more loyalty) than school-age children. On the other hand, mutual friends experience more positive engagement than acquaintances at all three age levels examined by Newcomb & Bagwell (preschool, primary school and early adolescence). Friends also succeed in resolving conflicts and avoiding new conflicts more than acquaintances. Finally, during primary school and early adolescence, mutual friends express more relationship properties than acquaintances. All in all, these results suggest that the intensity and quality of friendship increase with age. These findings apply essentially to normally developing children. As it will be shown later, it is not clear whether aggressive children with behaviour problems (i.e. conduct disorder, aggressiveness, disruptiveness, delinquency, antisociality) experience a similar progression of friendship quality with their probably deviant friends. On the contrary, conflicts may be generated more often and may not be resolved in a satisfactory way. Moreover, positive engagement and relationship properties may prove poorer than with non-deviant friends. Children with behaviour problems, on the other hand, might be highly influentiable by their deviant friends. In such conditions, the possible negative features of conduct-disordered children's friendships may represent a training ground for undesirable behaviours and impact negatively on their behavioural trajectory. Paradoxically, if children with behaviour problems experience positive engagement with their deviant friends and if their relationship properties are similar to conventional children's friendships, then the influence of deviant friends might actually be increased (Agnew, 1991; Wills & Vaughan, 1989). Hence, although in general friendships might promote children's emotional, social and cognitive development, it is important to take into account the qualitative features of these friendships as well as the characteristics of the friends when considering the possible influence of deviant friends on children's psychosocial development (Hartup, 1996). In addition, deviant friends may exert a stronger influence on children who are already prone to such influences because of personal (i.e. antisocial or aggressive behavioural profile), social (i.e. rejection from conventional peers), familial (i.e. rejection or low monitoring from parents) or contextual (i.e. transition into high school) factors. These possible moderators of the links between friends' characteristics and friendship features, on one hand, and children's subsequent maladjustment, on the other, will be detailed later in the chapter. Congruent with Moffitt's (1993) theoretical position, it will be argued that friends might help explain late onset conduct disorder but not its early onset counterpart.

A basic premise of much of the theory and research we discuss here is the view that friendships constitute an important developmental context. Friendships are environments that are organized around shared activities and result from the affective bond and the behavioural habits and goals of the two friends. Friends influence each other via several means, especially their co-construction of the behavioural standards that come to underlie their interactions. By choosing to be a friend of a particular peer, a child chooses a particular environment in which to develop. In this way, the individual child and the child's friendship experiences are conceptually distinct but in some ways difficult to disentangle. This theme, namely the relationship between children and their friendship experiences, forms the centrepiece for much of the discussion in this chapter.

Friends may be important because of their presence or their absence. Having a deviant friend may influence children's behaviour problems through socializing processes while, as a result of peer rejection, conventional peers may deprive rejected children of positive socializing experiences. Consequently, peer rejection may foster resentment towards conventional peers and foster association with deviant peers, leading, ultimately to initiation or escalation in behaviour problems. Parker & Asher (1987) reviewed studies that investigated how peer rejection may lead to delinquency or other types of adjustment problems. The present chapter will not focus on rejection from conventional peers but rather on the role of deviant friends in explaining the development of adjustment problems. Peer popularity will be included only to better understand affiliation with deviant peers.

Finally, most studies focused only on boys' maladjustment as it might be related to their friends' deviancy. Those that included girls often failed to distinguish friends' influences on boys' and girls' developmental patterns separately. Because of the scarcity of data on girls, differences between boys and girls will be highlighted when they have been found. It is indeed possible that girls might be influenced by deviant friends more than boys because they value social relationships more than boys (Hartup, 1993) and because their friendships are characterized by more intimacy and closeness than boys (Bukowski et al., 1994). In turn, these qualitative features of friendship might moderate (i.e. amplify) friends' influence, as already suggested.

Some methodological issues

The first selection of studies to be reported in this chapter included those that used a definition and a measure of conduct disorder concordant to the DSM. However, because of the scarcity of these studies and because of the conceptual similarity between conduct disorder and delinquency, studies exploring the role of friends on delinquency or related externalizing behaviours (e.g. anti-sociality, violence or aggressiveness), whether assessed in a categorical or a continuous way, were also included. This decision was justified on the basis that instruments designed to assess delinquency, antisociality, or conduct disorder often share several items, many of which refer to aggressive behaviour, theft, vandalism and truancy (Elliott et al., 1989; Patterson, 1992). Consequently, the labels of conduct disorder, delinquency, antisociality or aggressiveness were used interchangeably depending on the original terms used by the authors of the studies considered. Other conditions such as ADHD often co-occur with aggressiveness, antisociality, conduct disorder or delinquency (see Hinshaw, 1987). However, few studies have considered the presence of these additional personal dispositions as possible moderators of the link between friends' deviancy and subjects' deviancy. For example, disruptive children who have an attention deficit–hyperactivity problem may be prone to more influence from deviant friends because they are more socially active or because they are more rejected by conventional peers than disruptive children who are not hyperactive-inattentive. These aspects will be underlined in the few studies that included them.

Studies that used a longitudinal approach to investigate the role of deviant friends on delinquency and related conduct disorder were preferred to cross-sectional studies. Cross-sectional studies cannot disentangle the direction of the links between variables and thus cannot explain the role deviant friends might play on the development of delinquency and conduct disorder. To examine the effect of a presumed causal variable (i.e. friends) on a presumed effect (i.e. conduct disorder/delinquency), some temporal separation between them is needed. Longitudinal data make this separation possible. However, the relationship between the variables remain correlational. The direction of the causal relationships between these variables, if any, can be clarified by experimental manipulations of the presumed cause (i.e. friends) but the manipulation of 'friends' is not easily achieved and is probably unethical. Accordingly, experimental studies of this sort are unlikely.

Most authors rely on participants to assess their friends' characteristics and their own conduct disorder or delinquency levels. This use of a single inform-ant runs the risk of monomethod bias (Cook & Campbell, 1979) and it may obscure the similarity between participants' and friends' deviancy (see Bauman & Ennett, 1996). For example, Elliott & Voss (1974) observed an overestimation and an underestimation of friends' delinquency, respectively, among delinquent and nondelinquent respondents. Few authors have used different sources to assess friends' and participants' characteristics. Parents, teachers and peers have been sometimes used to assess participants' and friends' deviancy but this procedure does not entirely eliminate a possible confounding effect due to the possible stereotyped rating of friends based on the rating of target subjects themselves. As Thornberry & Krohn (1996) noted, friends themselves have been rarely interviewed directly about their deviant behaviours. In cases when such a procedure was adopted, friends were typically limited to the school context. In other cases individual friends were not identified and assessed individually. Instead, authors have relied on the global rating of the clique of peers with whom participants associated. In conclusion, very few studies have relied on target participants' and their friends' own reports of deviant behaviours with no limitations on friends' origin.

In regard to the measurement of friends' behaviour, some authors collected data on friends' delinquency/conduct disorder whereas others relied on analogue measures of participants' or friends' deviance such as aggressiveness or relational problems. Few authors have controlled for SES variables despite the established link between SES and access to deviant friends and delinquent behaviours/conduct disorder. There is a need also to control for initial behavioural dispositions when assessing the contribution of deviant friends in the development of delinquent behaviours. Early disruptive behaviours predict delinquency and conduct disorder and may also explain the links between teenagers' conduct problems and the selection of friends with similar conduct problems. However, given that even early antisocial behaviour may be influenced by peers (Farver, 1996), early behavioural dispositions may themselves, at least partially, result from peers' influence (in addition to parental, siblings and temperamental factors).

Consequently, we need studies that start with very young children and look at the dynamic and reciprocal manner in which children's evolving behavioural characteristics predict their selection of friends and in which friends' changing characteristics explain children's evolution on conduct problems, thus controlling for children's and friends' previous characteristics at each new step. No study to our knowledge has yet adopted such a developmental–interactional perspective.

Influence (role) of deviant friends on conduct disorder

Four theoretical models regarding the role of deviant friends on the development of delinquency have been proposed: Peer influence, Individual characteristics, Social interactional, and a Mixed model. Each will be outlined in this section.

Peer influence model

The Peer influence model has been variously referred to as the Social facilitation, Cultural deviance, Differential association, or Socialization model depending on whether one refers to the psychological, sociological or criminological literature. It views deviant friends as a causal necessity for the development of delinquency (Cohen, 1977; Elliott et al., 1985; Johnson et al., 1987; Sutherland, 1947). This model suggests that ineffective parenting leads to association with deviant peers which, in turn, mediates the link between ineffective parenting (or childhood behaviour problems related to ineffective parenting) and later delinquency. Concordant with social learning principles, initiation in delinquency is acquired through exposure to deviant peers, and continuation or escalation of delinquency is explained by the modelling or the social reinforcement from peers for deviant values, attitudes and behaviours (Akers et al., 1979; Sutherland, 1947). In support of the Peer influence model, some authors have shown that most adolescents become involved with delinquent peers before exhibiting delinquency behaviours (Elliott et al., 1989; Simons et al., 1994). For example, Elliott et al. (1985) found that the association with delinquent peers was the only variable, other than prior delinquency, to have a strong influence on subsequent delinquency. This finding holds for males and females, as well as for minor or serious delinquency. Similarly, Coie et al. (1995) used survival analysis to demonstrate that the first arrest for those early adolescents in deviant peer groups begins at or after the time at which deviant peer associations are assessed. Another illustration comes from a study by Keenan et al. (1995) who found that exposure to deviant peers resulted in subsequent engagement in delinquent behaviour for previously nondelinquent male adolescents. Finally, Thornberry et al. (1993) found that gang members reported more delinquent behaviours than nongang members only during the time they belonged to a gang, not before joining the gang nor after dropping out of it.

Individual characteristics model

In contrast, the Individual characteristics model (also referred to as the Social control or Selection model) views deviant friends as an epiphenomenon which plays no (causal) role on the development of delinquency. Instead, the Individual characteristics perspective suggests that antisocial or aggressive behaviours (which may result from ineffective parenting) lead independently to both delinquency and association with deviant peers (Gottfredson & Hirschi, 1990). From this perspective association with deviant peers is a byproduct of behaviour problems and does not help explain delinquency. In fact, selection of deviant friends follows initiation of deviant behaviours through a process of mutual attraction between children who tolerate or value deviant behaviours and attitudes (Cairns et al., 1988). At least two studies indicate that deviant peer association does not predict later delinquency after accounting for prior deviance. Coie et al. (1995) found that for both sexes, aggressiveness and previous delinquency during early adolescence predicted later delinquency (police arrests), with no influence of associations with deviant peers. Conversely aggressiveness during mid-childhood predicted association with deviant peers. Similarly, Tremblay et al. (1995) found that friends' characteristics did not mediate the association between antisocial behaviours during childhood and delinquency during mid-adolescence for boys with mutual friends in the classroom. Affiliation with deviant peers and delinquency appeared to be related only because of their common link to early antisocial behaviour. Once early antisocial behaviour was controlled for in statistical analyses, the relationship disappeared. It is worth noting that both studies that did not report a contribution of deviant peers or deviant friends in the prediction of delinquency above and beyond personal dispositions used low SES inner city samples. As suggested by Coie et al. (1995) many participants in their low SES inner-city subjects were involved in cliques that contain at least a few members that get into trouble. Many participants were themselves involved in aggressive behaviours. Consequently, the proportion of cliques or friends that would be considered deviant can be high in these low SES samples relative to middle-class peer contexts. The high prevalence of aggression and association with deviant friends might explain the noninfluence of these variables on subsequent delinquency or conduct disorder.

Despite their seemingly clear-cut and opposing positions, the Peer influence and the Individual characteristics models make concessions to each other, opening the door to more nuanced perspectives such as the Social interactional and the Mixed model perspectives discussed below. For example, Gottfredson & Hirschi (1990) granted that associations with deviant peers might facilitate the development of delinquency in individuals who already have antisocial tendencies. Conversely, Elliott (1994) admitted that, contrary to what would be expected according to the Social facilitation model, delinquency preceded the association with deviant friends for some youths.

Recently, Elliott & Menard (1996) identified a developmental sequence which integrates elements of the Peer influence model and the Individual characteristics model. First, delinquent friends influence initiation of minor delinquency. Second, having been involved in minor delinquency influences a further association with more severely delinquent friends. Finally, involvement with very delinquent friends results in an escalation to even greater delinquent behaviours. Consequently, it is possible that deviant friends are mostly important during early adolescence with respect to initiation of minor delinquency and during middle adolescence regarding initiation or escalation toward serious delinquency.

Social interactional model

The Social interactional perspective (also referred to as the Facilitation or the Social enhancement model) views the affiliation with deviant peers or friends as a moderator variable (Dishion, 1990a, b; Patterson et al., 1989). Deviant friends are not necessary for high-risk children to become delinquent. That is, anti-social or aggressive children become associated with deviant peers and seek out peer contexts that accept deviant behaviours (Cairns et al., 1988). In turn, antisocial youths who affiliate with deviant peers become even more deviant. Affiliation with deviant peers, then, amplifies the link between early antisocial behaviour (due to poor family management practices and exacerbated by peer rejection and school failure) and later delinquency. High-risk children can become delinquent without such affiliations. Although these affiliations are not causal, they make the path toward delinquency easier to travel. The Social interactional model implies a statistical interaction between personal attributes (i.e. aggression) and peers' deviancy in predicting later conduct problems or delinquency. In addition, the breakdown of the interaction should reveal that peers' deviancy contributes to risk only or mostly for deviant (i.e. aggressive) children. Dishion et al. (1995b) termed the process whereby antisocial children merge together and mutually socialize towards increasing levels of delinquency, trait confluence. This view is similar to the one expressed by Elliott & Menard (1996). One notable exception, however, exists between the two perspectives. This exception refers to the starting point in the process of reciprocal and dynamic socialization between individuals and their friends. For Elliott & Menard (1996) the starting point is peer influence (i.e. capitalizing on a socialization process from deviant peers). In contrast, for Dishion and colleagues the starting point seems to be the children's personal (and familial) dispositions (i.e. capitalizing on a selection of similar peers' process).

Hence, according to the Social interactional model, the initial and most influential predictor of later delinquency remains the children's aggressiveness.

In support of this model, Simons et al. (1994) found that for young adolescent males with oppositional/defiant disorders, this behavioural pattern predicted their involvement with deviant friends, which in turn predicted criminal justice system involvement. In addition, these authors found an interaction between children's oppositional/defiant behavioural pattern and their association with deviant friends: criminal justice system involvement was highest for those youths who were oppositional/defiant and had deviant friends. Proponents of the Social interactional model argue that deviant friends reinforce and model deviant attitudes and behaviours. Moreover, antisocial youths coerce each other into deviant behaviour (Dishion et al., 1994a, d).

Farver (1996) showed that, already by age 4, preschoolers associate within cliques based on behavioural similarity with respect to such dimensions as aggressiveness and social competence. Moreover, those who were involved in mutual friendships manifested more aggressive behaviours. Unfortunately, this author could not assess the impact of this association with aggressive friends on subsequent aggressiveness because of her cross-sectional design.

Nonetheless, one conclusion from Farver's (1996) study is clear: it is already too late by early or mid-adolescence to disentangle the interplay between selection processes (through peer preference) and socialization processes (through peer influence) in our attempt to explain deviant trajectories, because these processes have been probably ongoing since early childhood. At most, we can access parts of the moving system of interplay through the relatively narrow window that longitudinal studies over periods of 2 or 3 years provide (cross-sectional studies would only provide snapshots and would be useless in this respect). In other words, trying to disentangle these processes to find the initial spark of an antisocial trajectory necessarily involves longitudinal studies of peer interactions from infancy. Unfortunately, most researchers looked at this process once it was already well established by early- or mid-adolescence. Very few studies have tried to look at this process much earlier in order to try to uncover its initial sparks. The rare exceptions might not have gone back far enough in the developmental history of individuals or did not use a longitudinal approach. As it stands now, aggressive children establish reciprocal patterns of mutually supportive interactions that serve to support and promote aggressive–antisocial behaviours and this dynamic system of reciprocal influence may be operative as early as the first social interactions in infancy and early toddlerhood.

Mixed model

Vitaro et al. (1997) have recently proposed a complementary alternative interpretation of the preceding models. The Mixed model posits that children who are highly aggressive throughout childhood, some of whom correspond to Moffitt's (1993) early-onset/life-course-persistent delinquents, will become early delinquents by virtue of their personal dispositions (which may result from exposure to deviant parents or siblings, harsh discipline, or some other family or temperamental factors, but without the mediating role of deviant peers, consistent with the Individual characteristics model). For these children, deviant peers can still amplify their initial delinquent tendencies. For the moderately/unstable aggressive children, who probably correspond to Moffitt's (1993) late onset/adolescence-limited delinquents, exposure to deviant peers would be a necessary condition for becoming delinquent (consistent with the Peer influence model). Their personal dispositions (or other family characteristics) would not be sufficient for them to become delinquent. They need support from deviant peers. Hence, the children for whom deviant peers play an important role during early adolescence (for initiating delinquency) and throughout adolescence (for escalating in delinquent behaviours) might well be the adolescence-limited or late conduct-disordered youth. In other words there should be a curvilinear relationship between children's aggressive tendencies and friends' aggression in the prediction of children's aggressive behaviour. Those children who have a strong predisposition or a very low predisposition toward aggression will behave aggressively or nonaggressively, respectively, regardless of whether their friends are aggressive. Children who are at the midrange in aggressive predisposition, however, will show higher or lower levels of aggression as a function of whether their friends are aggressive.

The process of late onset conduct disorder through the influence of deviant peers might be particularly salient for girls. This speculative statement is based on data indicating that (a) by adolescence the prevalence of behaviour problems in girls is as high as in boys although it was much lower during childhood (Zoccolillo, 1993) and (b) there is a tendency for early maturing girls to affiliate with older deviant males (Caspi et al., 1993; Magnusson et al., 1985; Stattin & Magnusson, 1990). These associations result in an increase in conduct problems during adolescence.

In some respects, the Mixed model concurs with the Peer influence model when it focuses on the initiation of delinquency in moderately/unstable aggressive children who are candidates for late delinquency. In other respects, it is consistent with the Individual characteristics model when considering initiation of delinquency for highly/stable aggressive children who might be early-starters. Finally, escalation in delinquency for the highly/stable aggressive children during adolescence would be more congruent with the Social interactional model.

The Mixed model fits data reported by Simons et al. (1994) indicating that affiliation with deviant peers was the contributing factor to delinquency for late-starters whereas it had only a moderating role for early-starters. In the latter case, behaviour problems were the strongest predictor for later delinquency. Studies that reported data congruent with the Peer influence model might have included mostly late-starter candidates. Conversely, studies supportive of the Individual characteristics or Social interactional models (both consider the primacy of children's personal dispositions in explaining initiation of delinquency), might have included mostly high risk samples with many early starters. Consequently, all theoretical perspectives and their underlying process mechanisms (i.e. peer influence, peer preference or peer enhancement) might be equally operative but would not apply to the same individuals.

The Mixed model helps explain recent findings reported by Fergusson & Horwood (1996). These authors found that peer influences partially mediated the link between early conduct problems and delinquency. At the same time, they found a moderate direct link between early conduct problems and delinquency. Each effect may have been contributed by different groups of subjects; for some subjects, peer influences may have been important (i.e. moderately conduct-disordered subjects at risk of becoming the adolescence-limited delinquents), for others, this may not have been the case (i.e. highly conduct-disordered subjects at risk for life-course persistent delinquency). However, these authors did not test for such a possibility. All in all, it may well be that the differences between the Social interactional model and the Mixed model are more apparent than real and result from the method used by the proponents of each perspective. The Social interactional model uses mostly a variable-oriented approach that ends up showing that deviant peers can 'globally' moderate the 'global' link between individual dispositions and later conduct disorders. 'Globally' and 'global', here, refer to the fact that these effects apply equally (or linearly) throughout the sample of subjects. Conversely, the Mixed model uses mostly a person-oriented approach (Bergman & Magnusson, 1987). This approach is more suited for analysing the processes of interest at the level of individuals, some processes being operative for some individuals and others for other individuals, without the necessity of an 'averaging' process throughout all individuals.

The possibility that only some types of children are susceptible to deviant friends' influences might also explain why some researchers have found weak or nonsignificant effects of friends' characteristics when predicting changes in adolescents' deviant norms or behaviours over time, particularly when friends' characteristics were not assessed through adolescents' self-reports (Berndt & Keefe, 1995; Graham et al., 1991).

Some research findings are, however, apparently difficult to reconcile with the Mixed model. For example, Keenan et al. (1995) found that exposure to deviant peers for previously delinquency-free children who were in grades 4 and 7 resulted in subsequent onset of disruptive and delinquent behaviours. However, all the children who became disruptive and delinquent after exposure to deviant friends may all have been candidates for adolescence-limited delinquency since none of them manifested disruptive behaviours at the beginning of the study. Consequently, these findings partly support and partly disprove the Peer influence and the Individual characteristics models, respectively. A similar suggestion can be made in reference to the findings from Elliott & Menard (1996) who only considered subjects reporting no delinquent behaviours at the beginning of their study. Elliott (1994) reported that the most probable path toward the initiation of delinquency for nondelinquent 11- and 12-year-olds begins with deviant peer association. This path was even more dramatic when serious delinquency was considered. Again, these results, although very supportive of the Peer influence model, might only apply to the children who did not yet develop delinquent behaviours or externalizing problems by early adolescence; in other words for late-starters.

Who associates with deviant friends and why

Behavioural similarity is a strong predictor of mutual attraction and aggressive children are attracted to each other (Boivin & Vitaro, 1995; Cairns et al., 1988). As early as grade 1, and even in preschool, aggressive–antisocial children affiliate with each other and form well identified cliques to which children themselves are able to refer (Dishion et al., 1994c; Farver, 1996). Attraction through similarity may also operate at the psychosexual level rather than at the purely behavioural level. For example, early maturing girls are attracted to older, deviant, male peers. In addition, friends who are already similar prior to friendship formation tend to become even more similar over the course of their relationship (Epstein, 1983; Kandel, 1978).

Despite similarities between friends, behavioural homophily is far from complete. Correlation coefficients between youths' and friends' aggressive-disruptive behaviour are moderate at best (Dishion et al., 1994a; Fergusson & Horwood, 1996). Vitaro et al. (1997) found that about one out of five highly disruptive boys had clearly nondisruptive mutual friends, although the majority had disruptive mutual friends. Moreover, an almost equal proportion of conforming boys associated with highly disruptive mutual friends. Understanding why some children associate with deviant friends may be helpful for prevention efforts, in light of the possible negative influence of deviant friends on children's behaviours. Indeed, it may prove easier to manipulate factors that predict affiliation with deviant friends than to counterbalance such influences once affiliations have been established or to try to modify such affiliations. Surprisingly, few studies have addressed the question of why most aggressive and some nonaggressive children associate with deviant friends, beyond the behavioural similarity explanation.

Peer rejection

After controlling for children's antisocial behaviour and school problems, rejection from conventional peers was found to predict children's association with deviant friends (Dishion et al., 1991). Physical maturation can also contribute to this process, for both sexes (Dishion et al., 1999; Stattin & Magnusson, 1990). However, as shown by Cairns et al. (1988), most aggressive children and adolescents are not rejected by all their peers. Instead, many aggressive children form cliques that include other aggressive (and possibly rejected) peers. Furthermore, they form reciprocated friendships within these cliques. Consequently, aggressive-antisocial children might be rejected by conventional peers but still actively involved in cliques and in friendships with other aggressive-antisocial peers. Rejection from conventional peers and association with antisocial peers can thus be viewed as complementary and partially independent experiences contributing to deviant behaviour. They might also have interactive effects. For example, rejection by conventional peers might potentiate the influence of deviant friends while acceptance by conventional peers may protect from the influence of deviant peers. Finally, in contexts where aggression is normative or valued, it may be positively rather than negatively related to popularity (Boivin et al., 1995; Coie et al., 1995). In such circumstances, it may well be popularity rather than rejection that might be positively related to deviant peer association as reported by Coie et al. (1995).

Parental processes

Lack of bonding to parents or poor family management practices, such as low monitoring or supervision, may constitute another factor contributing to affiliation with deviant peers. Dishion et al. (1991) showed that poor monitoring made a significant contribution in predicting association with deviant peers two years after controlling for pre-adolescent's antisocial behaviour and low peer acceptance. However, Snyder et al. (1986) had shown previously that the relative influence of parental monitoring and discipline and children's personal dispositions (i.e. lack of social skills and antisocial attitudes) in predicting association with deviant peers varies with age. Elliott et al. (1985) used poor bonding to parents to explain the association with deviant peers. Moreover, in accordance with the Peer influence model, they showed that such an association mediated the link between poor bonding and later delinquency. In contrast, the Individual characteristics model (Gottfredson & Hirschi, 1990; Hirschi, 1969) predicts that low bonding to parents would foster low self-control and, therefore, contribute directly to the development of deviant behaviours.

An integrated developmental model to explain association with deviant peers has been described by Patterson et al. (1992). This model represents the first part of the Interactional model described earlier with reference to the role of deviant friends in the initiation of delinquency. According to this model, poor parenting interacts with a difficult temperament and results in behaviour problems which the child transfers to other social environments, such as the school or peer relations. In turn, behaviour problems become inter-related with school difficulties and peer rejection. Finally, the rejected children avoid environments (i.e. school, home) and people (i.e. conventional peers, adults) that serve as punishment agents and seek social settings and social agents (i.e. deviant friends) that are supportive of their characteristics and interests. As shown recently by Brendgen et al. (1998), low self-esteem may be involved as a mediating psychological factor in the process linking negative parent–child relationships, behavioural dispositions, and low acceptance from peers to affiliation with deviant friends.

No authors, to our knowledge, have investigated the influence of parental characteristics (i.e. antisocial personality, depression) on their children's association with deviant friends. If influential, these characteristics might operate through lowered supervision. They might also operate through a modelling process as, for example, antisocial parents might be involved with other antisocial adults (Doyle & Markiewicz, 1996). In addition, a good relationship with an antisocial parent might contribute positively, rather than negatively, to an association with deviant peers, as suggested by data reported by Andrews et al. (1997).

Finally, bonding to parents or parents' management practices may also moderate the influence of deviant peers on children's conduct problems. For example, Mason et al. (1994) reported that a positive mother–adolescent relationship attenuated the influence of friends' deviancy on participants, whereas father's absence magnified the impact of friends' deviancy. The amount of time spent with the family also seems to counteract the influence of delinquent friends. This moderating effect of time spent with parents can be explained through reduced access to delinquent peers or increased exposure to parent law-abiding behaviours (Warr, 1993b). Warr (1993b) also contributed data showing that affective attachment to parents (i.e. communication and emotional closeness) does not reduce the potentially negative effect of deviant friends towards delinquency for those teenagers who are already exposed to deviant friends. However, parental attachment might inhibit the establishment of deviant friendships, which, indirectly, might still contribute to preventing delinquency. Conversely, the link between low parental attachment and teenagers' delinquent behaviours seemed mediated by their affiliation with deviant friends. Most of the studies showing a moderating or mediating effect of parental influence, however, did not control for participants' initial level of conduct problems. Hence, positive attachment to parents or time spent with the family may reflect the children's positive personal dispositions. Moreover the existing studies asked participants to rate their peers' behaviour problems, referring to the peer group in general instead of specific friends or best friend. The participants also rated their relationship with their parents. Contrary to previous findings, Hoge et al. (1994) and Keenan et al. (1995) reported the absence of an interaction between family relationship variables and association with deviant peers in predicting severe delinquency. These contradictory results suggest that the issue is far from resolved.

Dual role of friends

A plethora of studies have investigated the impact of deviant friends on subsequent delinquency. In contrast, very few studies explored the protective effect of conventional peers with at-risk children. In one such study, Brown et al. (1986) found that nondeviant friends influence children not to engage in antisocial behaviours. However, Vitaro et al. (1997) found no protective effect of conventional friends on disruptive boys' trajectories towards delinquency during early adolescence.

Even fewer studies looked at the impact of absence of friends on the development of children's delinquency. Given that aggressive-antisocial children report almost as many friends and are involved in peer clusters in almost the same proportion as nonaggressive-nonantisocial children (Boivin & Vitaro, 1995; Cairns et al., 1988), a stringent criterion such as mutuality (Bukowski & Hoza, 1989) must be used in order to generate a sufficient number of (aggressive-antisocial) children with no real (i.e., mutual) friends. According to the Peer influence and Social interactional models, absence of friends should protect against initiation or escalation of delinquency, especially since most overt and some covert delinquent acts occur in the company of peers (Miller, 1982; Reiss, 1986). In contrast, it should make no difference according to the Individual characteristics perspective. Vitaro et al. (1997) showed that highly disruptive boys with no friends were not more nor less delinquent than their counterparts with deviant mutual friends, although they were more at risk for delinquency because of their poor academic functioning and highly disruptive behaviours.

Rejection by conventional peers can also contribute to the initiation or escalation of delinquency because it may lead to an association of the rejected child with deviant children, part of whom may be outside the school system. In support of this hypothesis, De Rosier et al. (1994) showed that chronic peer rejection is associated with heightened levels of aggression in school. Further-more, Kupersmidt et al. (1995) found that rejected children who reported relatively higher levels of conflict with their best friend were more likely to be delinquent than rejected children who reported low or moderate conflict, although they tended to be less aggressive. The authors interpreted these findings by suggesting that rejected children who reported high levels of conflict with their best friend actually had a real best friend and participated in a delinquent peer group. In contrast, rejected children with low levels of conflict may have had a less close relationship with their best friend and lacked the skills to be socially involved. Hence, low levels of conflict may reflect severe deficits in social skills. Such deficits, in turn, seem to protect against delinquency since they would hinder friendships with other aggressive/deviant children as well as with normal peers. In addition, low levels of conflict might reflect better problem-solving capabilities. In this study, the authors also reported that having a friend did not protect against delinquency whereas friends' aggressive-ness contributed beyond peer rejection and other social variables in the prediction of delinquency.

Finally, only one study (Brendgen et al., 2000) has verified if deviant friends buffer children against internalizing problems although they might put them at risk for delinquent behaviours. In general, a close relationship with a best friend inhibits the decrease in self-esteem associated with peer rejection or loneliness (Bukowski & Hoza, 1989; Vernberg, 1990). It also decreases depressive feelings in depressed children who manage to establish a mutual friendship over their school years (Allen et al., 1995). However, having a mutual friend did not prevent internalizing problems or a decrease in self-esteem in rejected children (Hoza et al., 1995; Vandell & Hembree, 1994). Brendgen et al. (1998, 2000) found similar results for children with deviant friends: having mutual (deviant) friends did not buffer them against an increase in depressive feelings over a

1-year period (i.e. between ages 12 and 13) in comparison to children with no friends.

Features of friendships

Previous findings tend to suggest that the quality of friendship and social interactions between aggressive-antisocial or rejected children and their deviant peers may lack some important features to foster well-being in individuals. These aspects have been largely neglected, most authors focusing on the qualities of friends or quantity of deviant friends, ignoring the qualities of friendships such as intimacy, conflict, stability, etc. as potential sources of influence on adjustment (Sullivan, 1953). This perspective has been rarely applied to the explanation of the influence of friends on delinquency and conduct disorder. However, recent studies have shown that the influence of deviant friends is stronger if the children are satisfied with the relationship (Agnew, 1991; Kupersmidt et al., 1995). In general, however, the friendships of delinquent youth possess fewer positive features (i.e. support, validation and feelings of security) and more negative features (i.e. coercion, conflicts) in comparison to friendships of nondelinquent youth (see Marcus, 1996 for a review).

Given the relative lack of positive features in friendships with deviant youth, it is not surprising that these friendships do not buffer children against internalizing problems. Moreover, due to the presence of the negative features, such as dominance, coercion and unresolved conflict, it is reasonable to suppose that friendship itself (and the interactional process it involves) contributes to aggressive-deviant behaviour above and beyond friends' characteristics.

In support of the previous speculations, Berndt & Keefe (1995) reported data with normal children showing that negative friendship features increased self-reported disruption at school and were concurrently related to low self-esteem. In addition, Buhrmester & Yin (1997) recently reported that increases in aggression, delinquency, substance use, loneliness, and depression between grade 6 and grade 8 were predicted by poor quality friendship (i.e. a composite score of low positive features such as disclosure, support, approval, satisfaction and companionship, and high negative features such as conflict, criticism, pressure, exclusion and power), after controlling for grade 6 adjustment measures. Comparatively, only subjects' school behavioural problems and delinquency were predicted by the corresponding characteristics of their sixth grade friends, suggesting that friendship features might be more influential on subsequent adjustment than friends' characteristics. These authors, however, did not assess the relative, additive and interactive influence that friendship features and friends' behavioural characteristics might have had on adolescents' adjustment.

Theorists with a sociological–criminological perspective such as Sutherland (1947) and Warr (1993a) have emphasized other features of friendship as possibly contributing to the influence of deviant friends (in accordance to the Peer influence model). Number of deviant friends, time spent in company of deviant friends, age of first exposure to deviant friends, importance of friends to the subjects, and subjects' commitment or loyalty to their friends are all possible features that might enhance friends' influence. Warr (1993a) presented data showing that both first age of exposure to deviant friends and duration of exposure (in number of years) contributed toward predicting age 17 self-reported delinquency. Notably, however, amongst adolescents with similar duration of exposure to deviant friends, those who acquired delinquent friends most recently reported highest levels of delinquent behaviours. First age of exposure to deviant friends and duration of exposure were not, however, independent since association with deviant friends, once started, tends to remain stable although specific friends might vary. Warr (1993a) also presented data showing that the age distribution of delinquency during adolescence parallels age-related changes in the importance and allegiance to peers as well as the amount of time spent in their company. Both aspects reach their zenith during the middle-to-late teens, falling thereafter.

Features of friendship can also act as moderators of deviant friends' influence on externalizing problems. Although positive features such as attachment, companionship or closeness are positively related to adolescents' social adjustment (Furman, 1996) and have been found to be negatively related to delinquency (Buhrmester, 1990), they may still bear a negative potential by amplifying the influence of friends' deviancy on subjects' delinquency as shown by Agnew (1991) and Wills & Vaughan (1989). Some authors, however (Kupersmidt et al., 1995), found no interactions between friendship features such as support or conflict and best friends' aggressiveness in predicting delinquency. Given that the quality of aggressive children's friendships may be lower than nonaggressive children's friendships, more research is needed to clarify how the positive and the negative aspects of aggressive children's friendships with their possible deviant friends can moderate the impact of the influence of deviant friends, if any.

Putative mechanisms of influence

The models we have discussed so far are predicated on the idea that friends exert a negative impact on children's behaviours through coercion, reinforcement of deviant behaviours, support and expression of attitudes supportive of the use of aggression, modelling of negative behaviours and training of conflict behaviours with no problem-solving strategies.

Berndt and colleagues (Berndt, 1989; Berndt & Keefe, 1995) have shown that early adolescents who have negative interactions with friends (i.e. conflicts, etc.) report more disruptive behaviours at the end of the school year even after controlling for initial levels of disruptiveness. Berndt (1996) interprets this finding by suggesting that children who practice a negative-conflictual style of interaction with friends actually learn to tease, argue and insist on their own way in conflicts. They may transfer these new disruptive behaviours to the interactions with their teachers and classmates. This process may be even more operative between children who are aggressive-disruptive and who lack social problem solving strategies (Dodge, 1993). Coercion theory, proposed by Patterson (1982) to explain how negative social exchanges between parents and children may train the latter to become disruptive, may very well be used to explain negative interchanges between friends. In support to the coercion process between delinquent children, Windle (1994) found that delinquent children's friendships are characterized by a dominant-submissive relationship in comparison to friendships of nondelinquent children, which are more egalitarian. Dishion et al. (1994a) also found that antisocial boys tended to be more bossy with their friends and more frequently involved in coercive exchanges than conventional boys. In line with this, Kupersmidt et al. (1995) showed that conflict with a best friend predicts delinquency beyond what is already predicted by measures of peer rejection and best friend's aggressiveness. Consequently, as suggested previously, it is possible that the negative features of aggressive children's friendships with their deviant friends directly influence these children's problematic behavioural profile through coercion training.

Deviant friends may also train children's antisocial behaviours through reinforcement of deviant behaviours, as illustrated by data from Dishion and collaborators and reviewed in more detail in their chapter of this volume. By directly observing videotaped discussions in group sessions devoted to teaching problem-solving strategies to problem youths, these authors found that groups where peers supported and reinforced (through laughter or positive nonverbal feedback) rule breaking talk actually resulted in increases in subsequent delinquent behaviour and substance use, even after controlling for prior levels of these behaviours (Dishion & Andrews, 1995; Dishion et al., 1995a, 1996). In another study, Dishion et al. (1994b; cited in Dishion et al., 1995b) noted that antisocial boys elicited less positive reactions from their friends following normative talk than normal boys with their friends. However, antisocial and conventional boys and their friends tended to laugh equally after rule-breaking verbal suggestions. This was interpreted as evidence for differential reinforcement for rule-breaking behaviours in antisocial dyads.

Warr & Stafford (1991) noted that peers' behaviours (what they do) was more influential on teenagers' delinquency than their attitudes (what they thought). However, deviant friends may still influence children's problem-solving strategies by formulating or demonstrating attributional biases, negative emotional reactions, valorization of aggression, or verbalization of aggressive solutions (Crick & Dodge, 1994). Recently, Brendgen et al. (1999) reported data indicating that children with aggressive friends tended to adopt more aggressive solutions in response to ambiguous provocation situations, even after controlling for their initial social-cognitive conflict solution strategies.

On the other hand, most antisocial teenagers desist from delinquency during early adulthood. This turning point in development follows turning away from delinquent peers (Mulvey & Aber, 1988), possibly because they get involved in a romantic relationship (Nagin & Farrington, 1992). However, this path may apply only to late-starters–adolescence limited delinquents. For early-starters or life-persistent delinquents, establishment of a romantic relationship may not result in reduced delinquency because (a) it is not followed by a de-association from deviant peers, (b) the romantic partner might also be antisocial as a process of assortative mating would predict, (c) early onset delinquents might not need the help of peers to initiate their delinquent behaviours, as suggested by the Mixed model or the Individual characteristics model, so that de-association from deviant peers will have few if any consequences.

Friends and prevention/intervention of conduct disorders

Prevention/intervention studies are a good strategy to manipulate risk or protective factors (e.g. by reducing association with deviant friends or increasing association with conventional friends) in order to test their causal links with delinquency (Loeber & Farrington, 1995). Indeed, a study aimed at improving friends' characteristics or friendship quality and using an experimental design offers a real possibility to test causal links. Improving friends' characteristics for at-risk children should lead to a reduction in delinquency according to the Peer

influence model but no changes whatsoever according to the Individual characteristics model. Intermediate or mixed results would be expected according to
the Interaction or the Mixed model: for example, delinquency should be
reduced in the prevention/intervention group but for a subgroup of children
only (i.e. the late-starters or the moderately disruptive only). On the other
hand, a reduction of delinquency in the prevention/intervention group would
be expected only if friends' characteristics have been improved in the short
term according to the Social facilitation model, whereas no such changes are
predicted by the Social control perspective.

Despite its theoretical and clinical usefulness, few studies have tried to
manipulate directly friends' characteristics as a means of preventing/reducing
delinquency. A notable exception comes from Feldman & Caplinger (1983)
who used nondeviant peers to successfully influence delinquent boys' trajectories. These authors, however, crossed their group composition variable (i.e.
exposed to nondeviant peers or not exposed to nondeviant peers) with two
other variables (i.e. two types of treatment and two levels of experience for
trainers). Consequently, it was not possible to assess the mere influence of the
exposure-to-nondeviant-peers variable since no interactions between variables
were examined by the authors.

Vitaro et al. (1999) demonstrated that the impact of a prevention programme
for disruptive boys achieved its aims of preventing later conduct disorder
through its impact on reduced disruptiveness and its impact on friends' selection (i.e. boys from the prevention programme selected less deviant friends
than boys in the control group). In turn, friends' characteristics partially
mediated the link between early reduction in disruptive behaviours and later
reduction in conduct disorder.

Many researchers have paired children either with a friend or with a
nonfriend and then compared their behaviour or their partners' behaviour
under controlled conditions (Hartup et al., 1993; Nelson & Aboud, 1985).
Azmitia & Montgomery (1993) found that problem solving improved more
following task cooperation with a friend than with a nonfriend. Furthermore,
these authors showed that performance on a problem solving task was positively related to conflict resolution during the cooperative session. However, if
child and friend lack problem solving strategies but experience conflict repeatedly, as seems to be the case between delinquent friends (Marcus, 1996), they
might actually train inappropriate behaviours, as suggested previously. In
addition, children and their friends might reinforce each other's deviant behaviours, as shown by Dishion et al. (1996). Consequently, it might be difficult to

involve deviant children's friends in an intervention designed to reduce delinquency without first modifying target children's and friends' problem solving strategies, attitudes towards deviant behaviours and interactional style in their friendships. The iatrogenic effects reported by Dishion & Andrews (1995), who grouped together antisocial youths for social skills training, some of whom might have become friends, support the previous speculations. Similarly, Dishion et al. (1999) found that part of the negative effects of the Somerville prevention study were attributable to the grouping of disruptive boys in summer camps. On the other hand, it might be advisable to modify the propensity of aggressive children to form cliques as early as possible (i.e. during the preschool years) (Farver, 1996). This can be achieved by including prosocial peers in 'forced' playgroups. However, this strategy would run the risk that aggressive children negatively influence conventional peers. One way to avoid such a possible adverse influence might be to devise playgroups or cooperative work groups in the classroom that would include a high ratio of conventional peers relative to deviant children. In such groups, however, deviant children might run the risk of being rejected. Consequently, it appears difficult or unethical to (a) expose deviant children to other deviant children while trying to improve all the participants' skills because of the potential for iatrogenic effects; (b) expose deviant children to conventional children (and hope that some become friends) because of the potential risk of negative influence on conventional children or social rejection of antisocial children.

This situation might help explain the dearth of clinical–experimental studies trying to influence the selection of friends, modify friends' characteristics, or improve friendship quality directly. It remains nonetheless possible to try to influence these processes by improving target children's and their friends' problem solving strategies and behaviour and by improving parents' monitoring skills with regard to their children's selection of friends. Another possible and interesting strategy has been proposed by Coie & Jacobs (1993). These authors suggest influencing deviant peer leaders by providing them with opportunities to associate with attractive youth idols and to do so publicly in circumstances where they endorse nonviolent and nonrisk-taking behaviour. If successful, these peer leaders' new attitudes and behaviours would influence the other members of deviant peer groups provided they gain access to personal valorization for such behaviours. The first major challenge of influencing successfully the peer leaders' behaviours and attitudes is, however, still awaiting empirical support.

Friends' influence on girls' maladjustment

The influence of deviant friends on girls' conduct disorder is yet mostly unknown, as most studies included only males. A notable exception in that respect is a study by Magnusson et al. (1985) who found that early maturing girls reported more delinquency than girls who were on-time or late maturers. They also had older male friends (who were mostly deviant). Finally, within the group of early maturing girls, those with older male friends were involved in even more delinquency than those with same-age friends or with no friends. Despite the previous findings, little is known about friends' influence on female delinquent behaviours in comparison to male delinquency. As already suggested earlier in the chapter, given that conduct-disordered girls are almost as prevalent during adolescence as conduct-disordered boys but much less during childhood (Robins, 1986; Zoccolillo, 1993), it is plausible to speculate that conduct-disordered girls belong to the late onset/adolescence-limited delinquent category proportionately more than conduct-disordered boys. Consequently, peer influence for girls might be even more important than for boys especially since girls typically enter mixed-age and mixed-sex peer groups earlier than boys (Stattin et al., 1989). These speculations are in line with the Peer influence and the Mixed models. However, in conformity with the Individual characteristics model, early maturing girls that are the most prone to peer influence (especially from older males outside the school system) tend to have more adjustment problems and more frequent norm violations than nonearly maturers (Caspi et al., 1993; Caspi & Moffitt, 1991; Simmons & Blyth, 1987; Stattin & Magnusson, 1990).

Another possible basis for the suggestion that girls are more susceptible to peer influence than boys comes from data showing that girls' friendships during adolescence are characterized by greater intimacy and loyalty than boys' (Berndt, 1982; Savin-Williams & Berndt, 1990). Consequently, it is possible that girls may be more prone to peer influence during early adolescence (including deviant older boys' influence) than boys (Kandel, 1986; Margulies et al., 1977). Some authors, however, reported data not supporting this view (Urberg et al., 1991). Clearly, more research is needed to clarify this issue.

Future directions and conclusions

Previous sections underscored some of the issues future research should address: the need for multivariate-longitudinal studies that take into account several sources of socialization simultaneously, additively and interactively: peers, but also parents, teachers and siblings. Siblings' influence might be particularly relevant, especially during infancy and toddlerhood because the processes involved are reminiscent of the processes involved in peer relationship (e.g. conflict and support) (Loeber & Tangs, 1986; Patterson, 1986; Stormshak et al., 1996). Contrary to predictions of the Individual characteristics model (Gottfredson & Hirschi, 1990; Hirschi, 1969), most studies that investigated the relative contribution of peer and family (i.e. monitoring, supervision, disciplinary practices) influences on delinquency found that peers were the primary source of influence (Agnew, 1991; Akers et al., 1979; Elliott et al., 1985). However, these studies are biased in favour of peers since they used early adolescent or adolescent samples who are particularly sensitive to peers. In support of this notion, a meta-analysis by Lipsey & Derzon (1998) showed that antisocial peers was the second best predictor of serious delinquency during adolescence and early adulthood, provided it was assessed by age 12 or later. Conversely, when assessed before age 12, antisocial peers ranked last amongst a series of about 20 predictors. However, their conclusion about the non-contribution of friends' deviancy before age 12 was based on a very small number of studies.

Researchers should also focus on the common, complementary, and unique contributions from best friends and from other social contexts such as close friends, cliques or the more general peer group. The impact of each of these contexts on subjects' delinquency may vary greatly depending on their convergence with respect to norm-breaking behaviours and attitudes. They should also adopt a stringent definition of friendship as proposed by some researchers (Bukowski & Hoza, 1989). Finally, they should consider the level of intimacy and other features of the relationship between friends in addition to the friendship involvement or the number of close friends (Urberg et al., 1997).

We also need experimental manipulations to test causal links and process variables involved in friends' influence (i.e. friends' characteristics, friendship quality and interactional style). We suggest 'experimental manipulations' during the preschool years by arranging playgroups that would bring aggressive children away from their aggressive friends and close to nonaggressive friends (who are less at risk of rejecting them and also possibly more influential than other classmates). It would be important that the ratio of nonaggressive to aggressive children be clearly in favour of the former. The preschool period seems an interesting period because friendships are volatile and modifiable without negative reactions from the children, teachers' collaboration and parents' permission might be easier to obtain, the educative context is more focused on socialization than academic learning objectives and, finally, ethical problems appear more surmountable than with older children. Yet, as indicated previously, selection and socialization processes are already operative during the preschool years. Furthermore, the presence of (presumed nondeviant) friends and positive features of friendships during the preschool years have been related to young children's early school social and academic adjustment (Ladd, 1990; Ladd et al., 1996). Transition periods from preschool to primary school and, although with more difficulty, between primary and secondary school can also be other possibilities for such manipulations. In these contexts it would be useful to capitalize on all moderating variables that could maximize nonaggressive friends' influence (i.e. social status, quality of the friendship etc.), as it is important to continue to explore the (protective) factors that could diminish the impact of deviant friends on children's deviancy. Prevention efforts might be aimed at influencing these moderating variables of all sorts (i.e. personal, familial, social, etc.) rather than trying to avoid or diminish exposure to deviant friends directly (which may prove difficult as argued previously).

Finally, we need to distinguish the influence of deviant friends on subtypes of conduct disorder. Keenan et al. (1995) found similar results with overt and covert types of delinquent behaviours. However, Coie et al. (1996) found that the impact of deviant peer associations (after controlling for previous aggressive behaviours) was greater on serious offending than on minor delinquency. Serious delinquency included felony theft, felony assault, robbery and arson.

Concluding comments

(a) Having friends may be very positive on children's socio-emotional, socio-cognitive and social development as shown by many authors (see Bukowski et al., 1996). However, dependent on their personal characteristics and the quality of the friendship or the feedback they contribute, friends may be detrimental on the development of externalizing and, possibly, internalizing behaviour problems.

(b) There are possible cultural and ethnic differences in the way friends' characteristics, friendship qualities and delinquent trajectories are related. These need to be taken into account in future studies.

(c) Many investigators have explored the influence of deviant friends on problem behaviours that are related, yet distinct, from conduct disorder. These other problem behaviours include, for example, drug use (Curran et al., 1997; Kandel, 1978) and dropping out of school (Cairns et al., 1989; Elliott & Voss, 1974). These authors raised theoretical and methodological issues similar to the ones raised in the present chapter. The integration of these studies would broaden the perspective of friends' influence on psychosocial maladjustment beyond our current view.

(d) Four different theoretical models have been offered to help explain peers' influence on deviant behavioural trajectories. The Individual characteristics model views peers as incidental in the trajectory leading from early disruptive behaviours to later conduct disorders. The Peer influence model, on the contrary, views peers as playing a mediating role: without their presence, conduct disorders would not develop. The Social interactional model suggests that peers play a moderating role: they amplify the risk for conduct disorders in children with behaviour problems. Finally, the Mixed model proposes that all three previous models can be operative depending on the children's personal dispositions or family characteristics: deviant peers might be necessary for some children, incidental for others, or facilitative for still others.

The contradictions between studies trying to support one specific model might originate, at least partly, from methodological issues. For example, the models which promote children's personal dispositions as the explanatory triggering factor of the causal chain of events leading to later conduct disorder tend to use high-risk samples (based on children's personal characteristics or social–familial condition). Many children in such samples are candidates for early onset delinquency and a proportion of them are life-course persistent antisocial children. Conversely, studies showing the primacy of deviant peers in support of the Peer influence model tend to use samples of children with no prior history of delinquent antisocial behaviour during childhood. Many children in these samples are candidates for late onset delinquency and very few can be categorized as life-course-persistent delinquents. A proportion of them would rather be categorized as adolescence-limited delinquents. Finally, studies supportive of the Mixed model tend to include all children from community samples, some of whom are prone to peer influence and others not. The studies in this category that use a variable-oriented approach tend to support some partial mediation of deviant peers and conclude direct effects of personal dispositions towards later delinquency and conduct disorders. Similarly, those who adopt a person-oriented approach tend to report peer influence for some children, and a direct link between early personal dispositions and later delinquency-conduct disorders for others.

REFERENCES

Aboud, F.E. & Mendelson, M. J. (1996). Determinants of friendship selection and quality: Developmental perspectives. In W.M. Bukowski, A.F. Newcomb & W.W. Hartup (Eds.), *The Company They Keep: Friendship in Childhood and Adolescence* (pp. 87–112). Cambridge: Cambridge University Press.

Agnew, R. (1991). The interactive effects of peer variables on delinquency. *Criminology, 29*, 47–72.

Akers, R.K., Krohn, M.D., Lanza-Kaduce, L. & Radosevich, M. (1979). Social learning and deviant behavior. A specific test of a general theory. *American Sociological Review, 44,* 636–55.

Allen, E.A., Hoye, W., Blakely, B. & Rholes, W.S. (1995). Friendship and peer group acceptance: Relationships with depressive symptoms in middle childhood (abstract). *Proceedings of the Society for Research in Child Development, USA,* 270.

Andrews, J.A., Hops, H. & Duncan, S.C. (1997). Adolescent modeling of parent substance use: The moderating effect of the relationship with the parent. *Journal of Family Psychology, 11,* 259–70.

Azmitia, M. & Montgomery, R. (1993). Friendship, transactive dialogues, and the development of scientific reasoning. *Social Development, 2,* 202–21.

Bauman, K.E. & Ennett, S.T. (1996). Peer influence on adolescent drug use. *American Psychologist, 49,* 820–2.

Bergman, L.R. & Magnusson, D. (1987). A person approach to the study of the development of adjustment problems: An empirical example and some research consideration. In D. Magnusson & A. Öhman (Eds.), *Psychopathology: An Interactional Perspective* (pp. 383–401). New York: Academic Press.

Berndt, T.J. (1979). Developmental changes in conformity to peers and parents. *Developmental Psychology, 15,* 608–16.

Berndt, T.J. (1982). The features and effects of friendship in early adolescence. *Child Development, 53,* 1447–60.

Berndt, T.J. (1989). Obtaining support from friends in childhood and adolescence. In D. Belle (Ed.), *Children's Social Networks and Social Supports* (pp. 308–31). New York: John Wiley & Sons.

Berndt, T.J. (1996). Exploring the effects of friendship quality on social development. In W.M. Bukowski, A.F. Newcomb & W.W. Hartup (Eds.), *The Company They Keep: Friendships in Childhood and Adolescence* (pp. 346–65). Cambridge: Cambridge University Press.

Berndt, T.J. & Keefe, K. (1995). Friends' influence on adolescents' adjustment to school. *Child Development, 66,* 1312–29.

Boivin, M., Dodge, K.A. & Coie, J.D. (1995). Individual-group behavioral similarity and peer status in experimental play groups: The social misfit revisited. *Journal of Personality and Social Psychology, 69,* 269–79.

Boivin, M. & Vitaro, F. (1995). The impact of peer relationships on aggression in childhood: Inhibition through coercion or promotion through peer support. In J. McCord (Ed.), *Coercion and Punishment in Long-term Perspectives* (pp. 183–97). Cambridge: Cambridge University Press.

Brendgen, M., Bowen, F., Rondeau, N. & Vitaro, F. (1999). Effects of friends' characteristics on children's social cognitions. *Social Development, 8,* 41–51.

Brendgen, M., Vitaro, F. & Bukowski, W.M. (1998). Affiliation with delinquent friends: Contributions of parents, self-esteem, delinquent behavior, and peer rejection. *Journal of Early Adolescence, 18,* 244–65.

Brendgen, M., Vitaro, F. & Bukowski, W. M. (2000). Deviant friends and early adolescents' emotional and behavioural adjustment. *Journal of Research on Adolescence, 10,* 173–89.

Brown, B.B., Lohr, M.J. & McClenahan, E.L. (1986). Early adolescents' perceptions of peer pressure. *Journal of Early Adolescence, 6,* 139–54.

Buhrmester, D. (1990). Intimacy of friendship, interpersonal competence, and adjustment during preadolescence and adolescence. *Child Development*, 61, 1101–11.

Buhrmester, D. & Yin, J. (1997, April). A longitudinal study of friends' influence on adolescents' adjustment (program). Proceedings of the Society for Research in Child Development, USA, 100.

Bukowski, W.M. & Hoza, B. (1989). Popularity and friendship: Issues in theory, measurement, and outcome. In T. Berndt & G. Ladd (Eds.), *Peer Relationships in Child Development* (pp. 15–45). New York: John Wiley & Sons.

Bukowski, W.M., Hoza, B. & Boivin, M. (1994). Measuring friendship quality during pre- and early adolescence: The development and psychometric properties of the friendship qualities scale. *Journal of Social and Personal Relationships*, 11, 471–84.

Bukowski, W.M., Newcomb, A.F. & Hartup, W.W. (1996). *The Company They Keep: Friendship in Childhood and Adolescence*. Cambridge: Cambridge University Press.

Cairns, R.B., Cairns, B.D. & Neckerman, H.J. (1989). Early school dropout: Configurations and determinants. *Child Development*, 60, 1437–52.

Cairns, R.B., Cairns, B.D., Neckerman, H.J., Gest, S.D. & Gariépy, J.-L. (1988). Social networks and aggressive behavior: Peer support or peer rejection? *Developmental Psychology*, 24, 815–23.

Caspi, A., Lynam, D., Moffitt, T.E. & Silva, P.A. (1993). Unraveling girls' delinquency: Biological, dispositional, and contextual contributions to adolescent misbehavior. *Developmental Psychology*, 29, 19–30.

Caspi, A. & Moffitt, T.E. (1991). Individual differences are accentuated during periods of social change: The sample case of girls at puberty. *Journal of Personality and Social Psychology*, 61, 157–68.

Cohen, J. (1977). *Statistical Power Analysis for the Behavioral Sciences*. New York: Academic Press.

Coie, J.D. & Jacobs, M.R. (1993). The role of social context in the prevention of conduct disorder. *Development and Psychopathology*, 5, 263–75.

Coie, J.D., Miller-Johnson, S., Terry, R., Maumary-Gremaud, A. & Lochman, J.E. (1996). The influence of deviant peers on types of adolescent delinquency (abstract). *Proceedings of the American Society for Criminology, USA*, 48, 209.

Coie, J.D., Terry, R., Miller-Johnson, S. & Lochman, J. (1995). Longitudinal effects of deviant peer groups on criminal offending in late adolescence (abstract). *Proceedings of the American Society of Criminology, USA*, 47, 217.

Coie, J.D., Terry, R., Zabriski, A. & Lochman, J. (1995). Early adolescent social influences on delinquent behavior. In J. McCord (Ed.), *Coercion and Punishment in Long-term Perspectives* (pp. 229–44). Cambridge: Cambridge University Press.

Cook, T.D. & Campbell, D.T. (1979). *Quasi-experimentation: Design and Analysis Issues for Field Settings*. Chicago: Rand McNally.

Crick, N.R. & Dodge, K.A. (1994). A review and reformulation of social information-processing mechanisms in children's social adjustment. *Psychological Bulletin*, 115, 74–101.

Curran, P.J., Stice, E. & Chassin, L. (1997). The relation between adolescent alcohol use and peer alcohol use: A longitudinal random coefficients model. *Journal of Consulting and Clinical Psychology*, 65, 130–40.

De Rosier, M.E., Kupersmidt, J.B. & Patterson, C.J. (1994). Children's academic and behavioral adjustment as a function of the chronicity and proximity of peer rejection. *Child Development, 65*, 1799–813.

Dishion, T.J. (1990*a*). The family ecology for boys' peer relations in middle childhood. *Child Development, 61*, 874–92.

Dishion, T.J. (1990*b*). Peer context of troublesome behavior in children and adolescents. In P. Leone (Ed.), *Understanding Troubled and Troublesome Youth* (pp. 128–53). Beverly Hills, CA: Sage.

Dishion, T.J. & Andrews, D.W. (1995). Preventing escalation in problem behaviors with high-risk young adolescents: Immediate and 1-year outcomes. *Journal of Consulting and Clinical Psychology, 63*, 538–48.

Dishion, T.J., Andrews, D.W. & Crosby, L. (1994*a*). Antisocial boys and their friends in early adolescence: Relationship characteristics, quality, and interactional processes. *Child Development, 66*, 139–51.

Dishion, T.J., Andrews, D.W., Patterson, G.R. & Poe, J. (1994*b*). *Adolescent antisocial boys and their friends: Accounting for behavioral confluence*. Unpublished manuscript, Oregon Social Learning Center, Eugene.

Dishion, T.J., Capaldi, D., Spracklen, K.M. & Li, F. (1995*a*). Peer ecology of male adolescent drug use. Special Issue: Developmental processes in peer relations and psychopathology. *Development and Psychopathology, 7*, 803–24.

Dishion, T.J., Duncan, T.E., Eddy, J.M., Fagot, B.I. & Fetrow, R. (1994*c*). The world of parents and peers: Coercive exchanges and children's social adaptation. *Social Development, 3*, 255–68.

Dishion, T.J., French, D.C. & Patterson, G.R. (1995*b*). The development and ecology of antisocial behavior. In D. Cicchetti & D.J. Cohen (Eds.), *Developmental Psychopathology*, (Vol. 2, pp. 421–71). New York: John Wiley & Sons.

Dishion, T.J., McCord, J. & Poulin, F. (1999). When interventions harm: Peer groups and problem behavior. *American Psychologist, 54*, 755–64.

Dishion, T.J., Patterson, G.R. & Griesler, P.C. (1994*d*). Peer adaptations in the development of antisocial behavior: A confluence model. In L.R. Huesmann (Ed.), *Aggressive Behavior: Current Perspectives* (pp. 61–95). New York: Plenum Press.

Dishion, T.J., Patterson, G.R., Stoolmiller, M. & Skinner, M.L. (1991). Family, school, and behavioral antecedents to early adolescent involvement with antisocial peers. *Developmental Psychology, 27*, 172–80.

Dishion, T.J., Spracklen, K.M., Andrews, D.W. & Patterson, G.R. (1996). Deviancy training in male adolescents' friendships. *Behavior Therapy, 27*, 373–90.

Dodge, K.A. (1993). Social-cognitive mechanism in the development of conduct disorder and depression. *Annual Review of Psychology, 44*, 559–84.

Doyle, A.B. & Markiewicz, D. (1996). Parents' interpersonal relationships and children's friendships. In W.M. Bukowski, A.F. Newcomb & W.W. Hartup (Eds.), *The Company They Keep: Friendship in Childhood and Adolescence* (pp. 115–36). Cambridge: Cambridge University Press.

Elliott, D.S. (1994). Longitudinal research in criminology: Promise and practice. In E.G.M. Weitekamp & H.-J. Kerner (Eds.), *Cross-national Longitudinal Research on Human Development and Criminal Behavior* (pp. 189–201). Dordrecht, The Netherlands: Kluwer Academic.

Elliott, D.S., Huizinga, D. & Ageton, S.S. (1985). *Explaining Delinquency and Drug Use*. Beverly Hills, CA: Sage.

Elliott, D.S., Huizinga, D. & Menard, S. (1989). *Multiple Problem Youth: Delinquency, Substance Abuse and Mental Health Problems*. New York: Springer-Verlag.

Elliott, D.S. & Menard, S. (1996). Delinquent friends and delinquent behavior: Temporal and developmental patterns. In J.D. Hawkins (Ed.), *Delinquency and Crime: Current Theories* (pp. 28–67). Cambridge: Cambridge University Press.

Elliott, D.S. & Voss, H.L. (1974). *Delinquency and Dropout*. Lexington, MA: Lexington Books.

Epstein, J.L. (1983). The influence of friends in achievement and affective outcomes. In J.L. Epstein & N. Karweit (Eds.), *Friends in School: Patterns of Selection and Influence in Secondary Schools* (pp. 177–200). New York: Academic Press.

Farver, J.A.M. (1996). Aggressive behavior in preschoolers' social networks: Do birds of a feather flock together? *Early Childhood Research Quarterly, 11*, 333–50.

Feldman, R.A. & Caplinger, T.E. (1983). The St-Louis experiment: Treatment of antisocial youths in prosocial peer groups. In J.R. Kluegel (Ed.), *Evaluating Juvenile Justice* (pp. 121–48). Beverly Hills, CA: Sage.

Fergusson, D.M. & Horwood, L.J. (1996). The role of adolescent peer affiliations in the continuity between childhood behavioral adjustment and juvenile affendings. *Journal of Abnormal Child Psychology, 24*, 205–21.

Furman, W. (1996). The measurement of friendship perception: Conceptual and methodological issues. In W.M. Bukowski, A.F. Newcomb & W.W. Hartup (Eds.), *The Company They Keep: Friendship in Childhood and Adolescence* (pp. 41–65). New York: Cambridge University Press.

Furman, W. & Robins, P. (1985). What's the point? Issues in the selection of treatment objectives. In B.H. Schneider, K.H. Rubin, & J.E. Ledingham (Eds.), *Children's Peer Relations: Issues in Assessment and Intervention* (pp. 41–56). New York: Springer-Verlag.

Gottfredson, M.R. & Hirschi, T. (1990). *A General Theory of Crime*. Stanford, CA: Stanford University Press.

Graham, J.W., Marks, G. & Hansen, W.B. (1991). Social influence processes affecting adolescent substance use. *Journal of Applied Psychology, 76*, 291–8.

Hartup, W.W. (1993). Adolescents and their friends. In B. Larson (Ed.), *Close Friendships in Adolescence* (pp. 3–22). San Francisco: Josey Bass.

Hartup, W.W. (1996). The company they keep: Friendships and their development significance. *Child Development, 67*, 1–13.

Hartup, W.W., French, D.C., Laursen, B., Johnston, M.K. & Ogawa, J.R. (1993). Conflict and friendship relations in middle childhood: Behavior in a closed-field situation. *Child Development, 64*, 445–54.

Hartup, W.W. & Sancilio, M.F. (1986). Children's friendships. In E. Schopler & G.B. Mesibov (Eds.), *Social Behavior in Autism*. New York: Plenum Press.

Hinshaw, S.P. (1987). On the distinction between attentional deficits/hyperactivity and conduct problems/aggression in child psychopathology. *Psychological Bulletin, 101*, 443–63.

Hirschi, T. (1969). *Causes of Delinquency*. Berkeley, CA: University of California Press.

Hoge, R.D., Andrews, D.A. & Leschied, A.W. (1994). Tests of three hypotheses regarding the predictors of delinquency. *Journal of Abnormal Child Psychology, 22*, 547–59.

Howes, C. (1988). Peer interaction of young children. *Monographs of the Society for Research in Child Development, 53*(217).

Hoza, B., Molina, B., Bukowski, W.M. & Sippola, L.K. (1995). Aggression, withdrawal and measures of popularity and friendships as predictors of internalizing and externalizing problems during early adolescence. *Development and Psychopathology, 7*, 787–802.

Johnson, R.E., Marcos, A.C. & Bahr, S. (1987). The role of peers in the complex etiology of drug use. *Criminology*, 323–40.

Kandel, D.B. (1978). Homophily, selection, and socialization in adolescent friendships. *American Journal of Sociology, 84*, 427–36.

Kandel, D.B. (1986). Processes of peer influences in adolescence. In R.K. Silbereisen, K. Eyferth & G. Rudinger (Eds.), *Development as Action in Context: Problem Behavior and Normal Youth Development* (pp. 203–27). Berlin: Springer-Verlag.

Keenan, K., Loeber, R., Zhang, Q., Stouthamer-Loeber, M. & Van Kammen, W.B. (1995). The influence of deviant peers on the development of boys' disruptive and delinquent behavior: A temporal analysis. *Development and Psychopathology, 1*, 715–26.

Kupersmidt, J.B., Burchinal, M. & Patterson, C.J. (1995). Developmental patterns of childhood peer relations as predictors of externalizing behavior problems. *Development and Psychopathology, 7*, 825–43.

Ladd, G.W. (1990). Having friends, keeping friends, making friends, and being liked by peers in the classroom: Predictors of children's early school adjustment? *Child Development, 61*, 312–31.

Ladd, G.W., Kochenderfer, B.J. & Coleman, C.C. (1996). Friendship quality as a predictor of young children's early school adjustment. *Child Development, 67*, 1103–18.

Lipsey, M. W. & Devzon, J. H. (1998). Predictors of violent or serious delinquency in adolescence and early adulthood: A synthesis of longitudinal research. In R. Loeber & D. P. Farrington (Eds), *Serious and Violent Juvenile Offenders: Risk Factors and Successful Interventions* (pp. 86–105). Thousand Oaks, CA: Sage.

Loeber, R. & Farrington, D.P. (1995). Longitudinal approaches in epidemiological research of conduct problems. In F.C. Verhulst & H.M. Koot (Eds.), *The Epidemiology of Child and Adolescent Psychopathology* (pp. 309–36). New York: Oxford University Press.

Loeber, R. & Tangs, T. (1986). The analysis of coercive chains between children, mothers, and siblings. *Journal of Family Violence, 1*, 51–70.

Magnusson, D., Stattin, H. & Allen, V.L. (1985). Biological maturation and social adjustment processes from mid-adolescence to adulthood. *Journal of Youth and Adolescence, 14*, 276–83.

Marcus, R.F. (1996). The friendships of delinquents. *Adolescence, 21*, 145–58.

Margulies, R.Z., Kessler, R.C. & Kandel, D.B. (1977). A longitudinal study of onset of drinking among high-school students. *Journal of Studies on Alcohol, 38*, 897–912.

Mason, C.A., Cauce, A.M., Gonzales, N. & Hiraga, Y. (1994). Adolescent problem behavior: The effect of peers and the moderating role of father absence and the mother-child relationship. *American Journal of Community Psychology, 22*, 723–43.

Miller, W.B. (1982). Gangs, groups, and serious youth crime. In R. Giallombardo (Ed.), *Juvenile Delinquency: A Book of Readings* (pp. 311–28). 4th edn. New York: John Wiley & Sons.

Moffitt, T.E. (1993). Adolescence-limited and life-course persistent antisocial behavior: A developmental taxonomy. *Psychological Review, 100*, 674–701.

Mulvey, E.P. & Aber, M.S. (1988). Growing out of delinquency: Development and desistance. In R. Jenkins & W. Brown (Eds.), *The Abandonment of Delinquent Behavior: Promoting the Turn Around*. New York: Praeger.

Nagin, D. & Farrington, D.P. (1992). The onset and persistence of offending. *Criminology, 30*, 501–23.

Nelson, J. & Aboud, F.E. (1985). The resolution of social conflict between friends. *Child Development, 56*, 1009–17.

Newcomb, A.F. & Bagwell, C.L. (1995). Children's friendship relations: A meta-analytic review. *Psychological Bulletin, 117*, 306–47.

Parker, J.G. & Asher, S.R. (1987). Peer relations and later personal adjustment: Are low-accepted children at risk? *Psychological Bulletin, 102*, 357–89.

Patterson, G.R. (1982). *Coercive Family Process*. Eugene, OR: Castalia Press.

Patterson, G.R. (1986). The contribution of siblings to training for fighting: A microsocial analysis. In D. Olweus, J. Block & M. Radke-Yarrow (Eds.), *Development of Antisocial and Prosocial Behavior: Research, Theory, and Issues* (pp. 235–61). New York: Academic Press.

Patterson, G.R. (1992). Developmental changes in antisocial behavior. In R.D. Peters, R.J. McMahon & V.L. Quinsey (Eds.), *Aggression and Violence throughout the Life Span* (pp. 52–82). Newbury Park, CA: Sage.

Patterson, G.R., DeBaryshe, B.D. & Ramsey, E. (1989). A developmental perspective on antisocial behavior. *American Psychologist, 44*, 329–35.

Patterson, G.R., Reid, J.B. & Dishion, T.J. (1992). *Antisocial Boys*. Eugene, OR: Castalia.

Reiss, A.J., Jr. (1986). Co-offender influences on criminal careers. In A. Blumstein, J. Cohen, J.A. Roth & C.A. Visher (Eds.), *Criminal Careers and Career Criminals*, (Vol. II, pp. 121–60). Washington, DC: National Academy Press.

Robins, L.N. (1986). The consequences of Conduct Disorder in girls. In D. Olweus, J. Block & M. Radke-Yarrow (Eds.), *Development of Antisocial and Prosocial Behavior*. Orlando, FL: Academic Press.

Savin-Williams, R.C. & Berndt, T.J. (1990). Friendships and peer relations. In S.S. Feldman & G. Elliott (Eds.), *At the Threshold: The Developing Adolescent* (pp. 277–307). Cambridge, MA: Harvard University Press.

Simmons, R.G. & Blyth, D.A. (1987). *Moving into Adolescence: The Impact of Pubertal Change and School Context*. New York: Aldine.

Simons, R.L., Wu, C., Conger, R.D. & Lorenz, F.O. (1994). Two routes to delinquency: Differences between early and late starters in the impact of parenting and deviant peers. *Criminology, 32*, 247–75.

Snyder, J., Dishion, T.J. & Patterson, G.R. (1986). Determinants and consequences of associating with deviant peers during preadolescence and adolescence. *Journal of Early Adolescence, 6*, 29–48.

Stattin, H., Gustafson, S.B. & Magnusson, D. (1989). *Peer Influences on Adolescent Drinking: A Social Transition Perspective*. Report from the Department of Psychology, University of Stockholm, number 693.

Stattin, H. & Magnusson, D. (1990). *Pubertal Maturation in Female Development*. Hillsdale, NJ: Lawrence Erlbaum.

Steinberg, L. (1986). Latchkey children and susceptibility to peer pressure: An ecological analysis. *Developmental Psychology, 22,* 433–9.

Stormshak, E.A., Bellanti, C.J. & Bierman, K.L. (1996). The quality of sibling relationships and the development of social competence and behavioral control in aggressive children. *Developmental Psychology, 32,* 79–89.

Sullivan, H.S. (1953). *The Interpersonal Theory of Psychiatry.* New York: Norton.

Sutherland, E. (1947). *Principles of Criminology.* 3rd edn. Philadelphia: Lippincott.

Thornberry, T.P. & Krohn, M.D. (1996). Peers, drug use, and delinquency. In D. Stoff, J. Breiling & J.D. Maser (Eds.), *Handbook of Antisocial Behavior.* New York: John Wiley & Sons.

Thornberry, T.P., Krohn, M.D., Lizotte, A.J. & Chard-Wierschem, D. (1993). The role of juvenile gangs in facilitating delinquent behavior. *Journal of Research in Crime and Delinquency, 30,* 55–87.

Tremblay, R.E., Mâsse, L., Vitaro, F. & Dobkin, P.L. (1995). The impact of friends' deviant behavior on early onset of delinquency: Longitudinal data from 6 to 13 years of age. *Development and Psychopathology, 7,* 649–67.

Urberg, K.A., Cheng, C. & Shyu, S. (1991). Grade changes in peer influence on adolescent cigarette smoking: A comparison of two measures. *Addictive Behaviors, 16,* 21–8.

Urberg, K.A., Degirmencioglu, S.M. & Pilgrim, C. (1997). Close friend and group influence on adolescent cigarette smoking and alcohol use. *Developmental Psychology, 33,* 834–44.

Vandell, D. & Hembree, S. (1994). Peer social status and friendship: Predictors of children's social and academic adjustment. *Merrill-Palmer Quarterly, 40,* 461–77.

Vernberg, E.M. (1990). Psychological adjustment and experiences with peers during early adolescence: Reciprocal, incidental, or unidirectional relationships? *Journal of Abnormal Child Psychology, 18,* 187–98.

Vitaro, F., Brendgen, M., Pagani, L., Tremblay, R.E. & McDuff, P. (1999). Disruptive behavior, peer association, and conduct disorder: Testing the developmental links through early intervention. *Development and Psychopathology, 11,* 287–304.

Vitaro, F., Tremblay, R.E., Kerr, M., Pagani, L. & Bukowski, W.M. (1997). Disruptiveness, friends' characteristics, and delinquency in early adolescence: A test of two competing models of development. *Child Development, 68,* 676–89.

Warr, M. (1993a). Age, peers, and delinquency. *Criminology, 31,* 17–40.

Warr, M. (1993b). Parents, peers, and delinquency. *Social Forces, 7,* 247–64.

Warr, M. & Stafford, M. (1991). The influence of delinquent peers: What they think or what they do? *Criminology, 29,* 851–66.

Wills, T.A. & Vaughan, R. (1989). Social support and substance use in early adolescence. *Journal of Behavioral Medicine, 12,* 321–39.

Windle, M. (1994). A study of friendship characteristics and problem behavior among middle adolescents. *Child Development, 65,* 1764–77.

Zoccolillo, M. (1993). Gender and the development of Conduct Disorder. *Development and Psychopathology, 5,* 65–78.

14

Continuities and discontinuities of development, with particular emphasis on emotional and cognitive components of disruptive behaviour

Rolf Loeber and John Coie

This chapter concerns continuities and discontinuities in disruptive behaviour disorder, including oppositional defiant disorder (ODD) and conduct disorder (CD). It takes as its starting point a series of reviews on the stability of disruptive behaviour (Caspi & Moffitt, 1995; Coie & Dodge, 1998; J.D. Hawkins et al., 1998; Lahey et al., 1992, 1997; Lipsey & Derzon, 1998; Loeber, 1982, 1991; Loeber & Dishion, 1983; Loeber & Stouthamer-Loeber, 1987; Maughan & Rutter, 1998) showing quite high continuities between childhood, adolescent and adult manifestations of disruptive behaviours, including delinquency and antisocial personality disorder. This chapter expands the prior reviews by addressing the following questions:

(1) What are some of the main findings on the prediction of disruptive behaviour, and what are the caveats to be kept in mind when interpreting figures on the continuity of disruptive behaviour?

(2) Why is it important to understand heterotypic continuity of disruptive behaviour?

(3) What are psychiatric models of continuity and escalation in disruptive behaviour?

(4) Are there multiple pathways to serious symptoms of disruptive behaviour?

(5) What are the emotional and cognitive factors that are thought to influence the stability of disruptive behaviour?

It should be understood that there are many different factors that influence the continuity of disruptive behaviour. In this volume, neurochemistry and brain factors are reviewed by Herbert & Martinez (chapter 4), genetic factors by Simonoff (chapter 8), environmental influences by Maughan (chapter 7) and neuropsychological aspects are reviewed by Lynam & Henry (chapter 9). The final part of the present chapter will complement these accounts by concentrating on the ways in which emotional and cognitive factors may contribute to continuities in disruptive behaviour.

Predictors, degree of continuities and caveats

Many studies on the development of children's disruptive behaviour have emphasized the relatively high stability (i.e. continuity) of disruptive behaviour including aggression (Caspi et al., 1987; Haapasalo & Tremblay, 1994; Farrington, 1991, 1994; Loeber, 1982, 1991; Loeber et al., 1989; Olweus, 1979; Pulkkinen, 1992; Tremblay et al., 1991). Often, authors cite Olweus's (1979) review showing that the correlation between early and later aggression on average is 0.63 (0.79 when corrected for attenuation), which approximates the stability of intelligence over time.

There is empirical evidence that the prediction of disruptive behaviour can be enhanced by knowledge of certain behavioural precursors (Loeber, 1982): (a) an early onset of disruptive behaviour in males, compared to a later onset; (b) disruptive behaviour occurring in multiple settings, rather than in a single setting; (c) a high variety of disruptive behaviour compared to single disruptive behaviours; and (d) a high frequency of the disruptive behaviour compared to a low frequency.

Research shows that predictors of disruptive behaviour and delinquency can be found in the individual (e.g. impulsivity, or oppositional behaviour, discussed later), the family (e.g. parents' child rearing practices, parental psychopathology), the peer group (e.g. associations with delinquent peers, gang membership), the school (poor school motivation, poor educational performance), and the neighbourhood (neighbourhood crime, poverty etc.). None of the separate predictors is able to forecast later disruptive behaviour well. Instead, accumulation of risk factors substantially enhances predictability (Loeber & Farrington, 1998).

The most thorough review of predictors of serious and violent offending has been undertaken by Lipsey & Derzon (1998). Their meta-analysis has shown that early predictors of serious and violent offending tend to differ from later predictors. The strongest, potentially modifiable predictors of serious and violent offending evident between ages 6–11 are nonserious delinquent acts, aggression, substance use, low family socio-economic status and antisocial parents. In contrast, among the strongest at ages of 12 and 14 are lack of strong social ties, antisocial peers, nonserious delinquent acts, poor school attitude and performance, and psychological conditions such as impulsivity. Juveniles to whom the strongest predictor variables apply are 5–20 times more likely to engage in subsequent serious and violent offending than those without such predictor variables. Many of the same risk factors that predict adolescent delinquency and violence also predict substance abuse, dropping out of school, early sexual involvement and teen pregnancy.

Additionally, studies show that the risk of engaging in serious and violent juvenile offending (SVJ) is greatly enhanced when youth join a gang or become drug dealers. Gang members, while representing a minority of the juvenile population, are responsible for the majority of serious delinquent acts. Rates of SVJ offending increase after joining a gang and decrease after leaving a gang (Thornberry, 1998). Similarly, rates of SVJ offending increase after youth start to deal in drugs and decrease after they stop dealing in drugs (Van Kammen et al., 1994).

Different interpretations of continuity

The continuity of disruptive behaviour can be interpreted in several ways, ranging from inherent differences among individuals in their criminal propensity, to continuities in risk (and protective) factors. Individuals are thought to differ in their criminal propensity (Nagin & Land, 1993), also called criminal potential (Nagin & Farrington, 1992), and this propensity is thought to be stable over time (Nagin & Paternoster, 1991). In a second version of this theme, continuity is thought to reflect state dependency (Nagin & Paternoster, 1991) in which prior delinquent acts may increase the probability of future offending through, for example, a reduction in inhibitions against engaging in delinquent acts.

These notions can be contrasted with conceptualizations that continuity is not absolute and that levels of delinquency may change as a result of the interaction between individual characteristics, environment, and risk experience, which is sometimes referred to as cumulative continuity (Caspi & Moffitt, 1995; Rutter et al., 1998). In this interpretation of continuity, causes are seen as residing both in the individual and in his/her environment, and the degree of continuity is thought to depend on the interaction between an individual's predisposing characteristics and his or her exposure to risk factors (Kolvin et al., 1990; Nijboer & Weerman, 1998). The stepping stone interpretation of continuity (Farrington, 1986) is a variant on this theme, and proposes that manifestations of disruptive behaviour may change over time, but that juveniles' escalation from minor to more serious forms of disruptive behaviour reflects the presence of external factors. In contrast, de-escalation in offending is associated with absence of risk factors and the presence of protective factors

(Sampson & Laub, 1993). In summary, recent studies are advancing the notion that individuals differ in their continuity of disruptive behaviour, and that some of these individual differences derive from individuals' exposure to risk and protective factors.

Some caveats

The evidence for the stability and predictability of disruptive behaviour is quite impressive, and provides support for the idea that early disruptive children are a worthy target for preventive interventions. However, disruptive behaviour is a complex phenomenon and several caveats apply to our conclusions about the continuity of the behaviour. The first concerns issues of measurement. Two rather different examples illustrate some of the complexities involved. First, most of the evidence for the continuity of aggression or antisocial behaviour comes from studies in which ratings of aggression by parents, teachers or peers provide the dependent measure. However, such ratings are not necessarily correlated with direct observations of the same behaviours. In one of the few published studies linking direct observations to teacher and peer ratings of aggression, Coie & Dodge (1998) reported on the school-based observations of 302 first and third grade children. Each child was observed for a total of 60 minutes in 5-minute blocks distributed across several days. Although teacher ratings and peer nominations of aggressive behaviour were significantly correlated ($r = 0.43$ for first graders, $r = 0.59$ for third graders), neither teacher nor peer scores were significantly correlated with observed frequencies of aggression for individual children. The most likely explanation for these findings is that even as time-consuming a sampling framework as was used with this large sample was not adequate to capture a representative sampling of individual children's aggressive acts. The point is that aggressive acts occur relatively infrequently, and may require a time-sampling framework that is much more demanding of observational resources than was employed in these studies.

The same applies to conduct problems, which are often episodic and can vary in their presence from year to year (Baicker-McKee, 1990; Lahey et al., 1995; Loeber, 1991; Verhulst & van der Ende, 1992). Lahey et al. (1995) showed that the continuity in a diagnosis of conduct disorder increased as the window of time in which the diagnosis took place also increased. In a sample of clinic-referred boys referred over a period of four years, half (51%) of the boys who met criteria for conduct disorder in any given year also met criteria for conduct disorder the following year. Similar results of 50% continuity have been reported elsewhere (Graham & Rutter, 1973; Robins, 1966). However, when the interval between assessments was longer, the stability over time was much higher: 88% of the boys initially diagnosed with conduct disorder were diagnosed again with conduct disorder over the next three years. The results indicate that cumulative continuity, compared to point-by-point continuity, tends to be higher. Second, apparent desistence or cessation of disruptive behaviour actually may only mean temporary interruption of the behaviour. Therefore, a fuller understanding about the continuity of disruptive behaviour is only possible when a longer time frame is taken into account. Thus, conclusions about the stability of disruptive behaviour are much dependent on methods of measurements and analysis used, and on the time frame considered.

The second caveat concerns informants and measurement error. Maughan & Rutter (1998) reviewed studies from different informants on disruptive child behaviour, and concluded that different methods of combining information from informants can produce different stability estimates. Further, such estimates are affected by measurement error: the lower the error, the higher the stability estimate.

Another important point concerns the ways in which definitions of disruptive behaviour change across the broad span of development from early childhood to adulthood. The fact that oppositional behaviour by boys peaks in the early to middle childhood period simply reflects the fact that children begin to challenge parental authority in the toddler period. Similarly, minor forms of aggression, including physical fighting, tend to peak in the early school years and decrease with age, particularly during adolescence (Greene et al., 1973; Loeber, 1985; Richards, 1981; Straus et al., 1980). On the other hand, perhaps owing primarily to increased physical size and strength and access to weapons, serious forms of aggression tend to increase in prevalence from childhood to early adulthood, even though the absolute frequency of aggressive activity decreases from middle childhood to late adolescence (Loeber, 1985; Loeber & Stouthamer-Loeber, 1998).

What these differing developmental patterns in the prevalence of differing types of disruptive behaviour imply for any interpretation of stability coefficients is that such coefficients represent heterotypic continuity (i.e. continuity between functionally different behaviours, such as aggression and theft) rather than continuity of the same form of behaviour across time. In general, youth who engage in one form of disruptive behaviour earlier in life are typically involved in other negative forms of antisocial behaviour in later life (Robins, 1966). In fact, parent, teacher and self-ratings of disruptive behaviours have shown that cross-sectionally most disruptive behaviours are intercorrelated (Jessor & Jessor, 1977; Loeber et al., 1998b). However, factor analyses usually show that several factors can be distinguished, such as oppositional behaviour, overt behaviour and covert behaviour (Fergusson et al., 1994). As a rule overt disruptive behaviour, such as aggression and violence, involves direct confrontation with victims and infliction or threat of physical harm, whereas covert, nonviolent forms of delinquency such as theft or fraud do not involve direct confrontation, but are concealing or sneaky in nature.

Meta-analyses of the factor analytic studies have demonstrated that the interrelations can be quantified according to one or more dimensions of disruptive acts. Loeber & Schmaling (1985) and Frick et al. (1993) found evidence for a dimension defined by two poles, an overt disruptive pole and a covert disruptive pole, with several forms of disobedience being positioned in the middle of this dimension. In addition, Frick et al. (1993) found evidence for a second dimension that they have entitled destructive-nondestructive behaviour.

Escalation from earlier disruptive behaviour to conduct disorder

A key question with respect to the stability of disruptive behaviour is which of the less serious disruptive behaviours constitute stepping stones to a diagnosis of conduct disorder. Psychiatry, because of its reliance on diagnoses, tends to conceptualize juveniles' escalation in disruptive acts in terms of molar diagnostic units, with little reference to the developmental aspects of individual symptoms. In contrast, developmental psychologists and criminologists have focused more on the developmental aspects of specific behaviours or symptoms. We need to examine the utility of each approach. We will review oppositional defiant disorder (ODD), attention deficit hyperactivity disorder (ADHD), and aggression as precursors to conduct disorder (CD). In addition, we will consider early symptoms of antisocial personality disorder (APD).

Oppositional defiant disorder and attention deficit hyperactivity disorder

Figure 14.1 shows the most common hypothesized developmental order of disruptive disorders. ODD often is seen as a precursor to CD, which in turn is seen as a precursor to APD (with the understanding that as currently formulated in DSM–IV, a diagnosis of CD precludes a diagnosis of ODD; in contrast, a diagnosis of APD assumes the presence of CD; American Psychiatric Association, 1994). In addition several prospective studies have demonstrated a developmental relation between ADHD and CD (Gittelman et al., 1985); however, since ODD is often comorbid with ADHD, a key question is whether ODD and ADHD are both equally predictive of the onset of CD, or whether

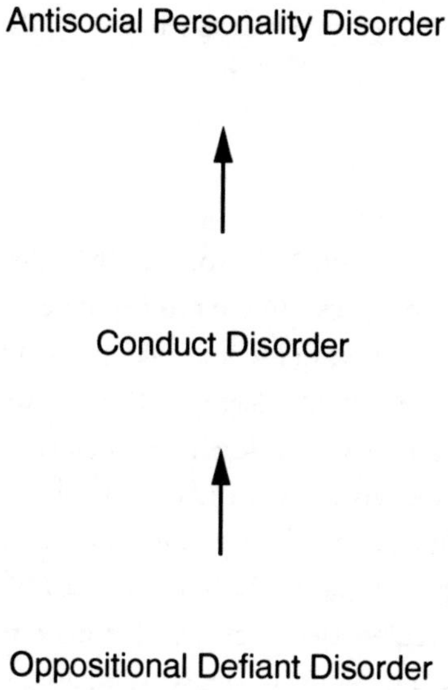

Antisocial Personality Disorder

↑

Conduct Disorder

↑

Oppositional Defiant Disorder

Fig. 14.1. Assumed development order of disruptive behaviour disorders and antisocial personality disorder (based on DSM–IV, American Psychiatric Association, 1994).

one or the other is the more important predictor. Loeber et al. (1995) investigated this in a follow-up over 6 years of the same sample already reported on by Lahey et al. (1995). They found that boys who developed CD had a higher number of ODD symptoms than boys who did not develop CD. Logistic regression showed that ODD, among other factors, predicted the onset of CD. In contrast, ADHD only predicted an early onset of CD (for further evidence, see Lahey et al., in press). We postulate that the impulsive/hyperactive rather than the inattentive component of ADHD is implicated in this predictive relationship. Whether these results also apply to the development of CD in girls remains to be seen.

Aggression

In the study of juveniles' escalation to CD, it is possible that there are certain individual symptoms that are particularly associated with the onset of the full disorder. Loeber et al. (1995) systematically examined all 13 symptoms of CD, and found that physical aggression was the only individual symptom which in univariate analyses predicted the onset of CD (however, physical fighting was not a predictor in logistic regression). We attach significance to this finding, because physical fighting often emerges early in life (Loeber et al., 1989; Tremblay et al., 1991), is somewhat stable over time (Olweus, 1979), and predicts disruptive behaviour and APD later (Loeber et al., in press; Robins, 1966).

Early antisocial personality symptoms

Conduct disorder is seen as a precursor to antisocial personality disorder (American Psychiatric Association, 1994). The question we raise is the extent to which symptoms of APD already are present early in life and may predict those CD cases who are likely to qualify for APD later in life. Some of the research we will review concerns the concept of psychopathy (Cleckley, 1976; Hare, 1991), which is related to the diagnosis of APD, but also has some unique elements.

Frick et al. (1994), in a study of clinic-referred, preadolescent children, examined the presence of symptoms of psychopathy. Factor analyses of their new child instrument of psychopathy revealed two factors: Callous Unemotional and Impulsivity-Conduct Problems. The two factors were related to the diagnoses of ODD and CD, and to dimensional ratings of delinquency and aggression. Lynam (1997) examined many of the features of psychopathy in boys from the middle sample (N = 508) of the Pittsburgh Youth Study at ages 12–13. This is a longitudinal study of a randomly selected sample of boys in Pittsburgh public schools. After a screening procedure, boys were followed up at half-yearly intervals on six occasions. Results revealed that boys with psychopathic characteristics, compared to those without these features, were more likely to be serious and stable offenders, to be impulsive, and to score high on teacher ratings of externalizing and internalizing problems. The crucial question as to whether these boys are 'fledgling psychopaths' who will be future cases of APD, remains to be addressed. However, it is quite plausible that there is continuity between early symptoms of APD or psychopathy early in life and later manifestations of the syndromes. There is great utility in determining this, because of the importance of identifying those cases of CD that are more likely to progress to APD. Additionally, data on such life-course linkages can provide empirical justification for a better specification of CD in future revisions of the diagnostic systems. It should be noted, however, that developmental associations among ODD, CD and APD are by necessity rather molar and crude. We will now examine a more overarching conceptualization.

Multiple pathways to serious symptoms of conduct disorder

The conceptualization of ODD or ADHD as a precursor to the onset of CD basically represents a single pathway model to deviance, and therefore poorly reflects individual differences in disruptive development. Specifically, we need to be able to explain why it is that some youth become engaged in both serious overt and covert disruptive behaviours, while others become involved in serious covert or overt behaviours only (Loeber & Stouthamer-Loeber, 1998). Thus, conduct disorder is a concept that is overly broad, and does not well reflect individual differences in disruptive behaviour. For that reason, we prefer to break down long-term prediction into smaller and less broad steps and examine pathway(s) to more serious outcomes. A developmental pathway is defined as the behavioural development of a group of individuals that is different from the behavioural development of other group(s) of individuals (Loeber et al., 1997).

In order to better address individual differences in the development of disruptive behaviour, we raise the question of whether juveniles' escalation to serious outcomes can best be represented by a single pathway or multiple pathways (Dishion et al., 1995; Loeber et al., 1993; Patterson, 1982; Patterson et al., 1998). A first step for the specification of pathways is to demonstrate developmental sequences in the order of onset of disruptive behaviours.

Development sequences

One of the important questions in the study of disruptive behaviour is whether development of symptoms takes place in a random or in a predictable fashion. An example of an orderly development is when the onset of symptom A is usually preceded by the onset of symptom B, and where the reverse order is much less common. The evidence for developmental sequences in symptoms of disruptive behaviour is dealt with extensively in other publications and is only summarized briefly here (see Elliott, 1994; Huizinga, 1995; Kelley et al., 1997; Loeber et al., 1992, 1993, 1997, 1998*a*; Tolan, 1998; Tolan & Gorman-Smith, 1998).

Overall, the research literature on sequences of disruptive behaviour indicates that: (a) the onset of less serious symptoms tends to occur prior to the onset of more serious disruptive symptoms; (b) some behaviours such as frequent arguing and annoying others have very similar ages of onset and, therefore, can be grouped into the same behavioural category; and (c) developmental patterns can be broken down most distinctly into three domains of overt, covert and authority conflict problems. Among overt conduct problems, the earliest appearing behaviours are minor aggression, followed by physical fighting and then more serious forms of violence such as weapon use and rape. For the covert behaviours, the developmental sequence consists of minor

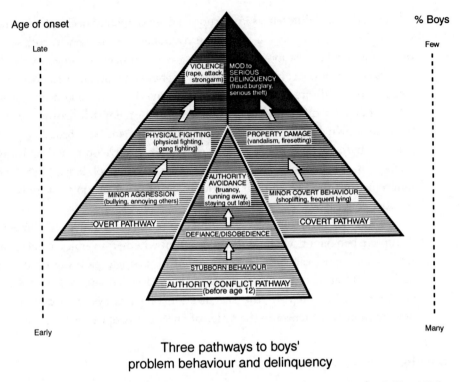

Fig. 14.2. Three developmental pathways to serious disruptive behaviours (Loeber & Hay, 1994).

covert behaviours, followed by property damage (firesetting or vandalism), which in turn is followed by moderate to serious forms of delinquency. Conflict with authority figures is a category that includes serious disobedience but also avoidant behaviours, such as truancy and running away from home, by which juveniles attempt to withdraw from the supervision and control of adults (Loeber & Stouthamer-Loeber, 1998). For authority conflict, behaviours tend to have the earliest onset, followed by defiance, which in turn is followed by authority avoidance (truancy, running away, staying out late at night). Findings suggest that the latter sequences best applied to youth prior to age 12.

Multiple pathways

Developmental sequences refer to group data, and do not necessarily imply that individuals' development takes place in an orderly fashion. The concept of developmental pathways best captures individuals' trajectories in diverse disruptive symptoms over time (Fig. 14.2). Recent findings show that the greatest majority of boys fit the postulated sequences (meaning that boys would show steps in accordance with the postulated order of the pathway, while not fitting the reverse ordering, e.g. step 1 after step 2). Some boys, a minority, skipped steps but maintained the overall sequence (e.g. from step 1 to step 3, omitting step 2). Another way of evaluating pathways is to show that most of those in a pathway entered the pathway at the first step, fewer at the second step, and fewest at the last step. Again, the evidence is that persistently disruptive boys demonstrated this pattern more than temporarily disruptive boys who experimented with disruptive behaviour (Loeber et al., 1997).

Thus far, we have considered evidence that boys begin the three pathways in the same order, but do not necessarily complete all the steps in a pathway. This fact is contrary to the much accepted notion among clinicians and researchers that once boys become deviant in one way, they become deviant in many other ways. It should be understood, however, that individuals can be on several pathways at the same time. Individuals whose disruptive behaviour is limited to a single pathway are quite uncommon in clinic referred samples; instead, clinic-referred youth often show the more versatile behaviours characteristic of their having advanced on several pathways simultaneously. These would be the youth who show the pattern of diverse offending. On the other hand, population samples, with a lower proportion of seriously affected individuals, are bound to show more individuals in individual pathways.

Several replications have buttressed the validity of the three pathways in different male populations, including African-Americans and Hispanics (Loeber et al., 1997, 1998a; Tolan, 1998; Tolan & Gorman-Smith, 1998). Recently, the findings have also been linked to another body of literature that emphasizes the distinction between early onset, life-course persistent delinquents (showing 'tenacious stability across time and in diverse circumstances') and adolescent-limited delinquents (characterized by an onset and desistance of delinquency during adolescence) (Moffitt, 1993, p. 685). Analyses by Tolan et al. (unpublished data) have shown those males who progress to higher and more serious steps in the overt and covert pathways tend to have an earlier age of onset of disruptive behaviour compared to those who do not progress to serious steps in the two pathways.

Risk factors and continuity and escalation in disruptive behaviour

Caspi & Moffitt (1995) have outlined a sequence of major factors that could account for the continuity of individuals' disruptive behaviours across the life course. The dynamic underlying their explanation of continuity or escalation in the development of antisocial behaviour is that early risk factors set the stage for greater vulnerability to succeeding factors. For example, genetic factors and prenatal brain injury may lead to greater impulsivity, automatic reactivity or deficient verbal skills and executive functioning in the first few years of life. Each of these brain-related vulnerabilities can be linked to child behaviour problems that would stress the management capabilities of most parents. A second set of risk factors can be categorized in terms of the child and family environment. Family poverty, neighbourhood crime, low social support and limited community resources serve to stress parenting effectiveness. Parents themselves may be poorly prepared to raise their children, owing to their own psychopathology, prior history of antisocial behaviour or immaturity. This second set of risk factors is often correlated with the first set, increasing the overall risk dimension multiplicatively. In this latter circumstance, person–environment interactions can create the kind of problematic child rearing environment that Patterson and his colleagues (Patterson et al., 1992) refer to as a coercive family system. Out of this early parent–child socialization experience emerge a number of cognitive and emotional patterns of risk that can become stable individual risk factors. These stable individual characteristics can evoke 'reciprocal, sustaining responses from others in ongoing social interaction, thereby reinstating the [disruptive] behaviour pattern across the individual's life course whenever the relevant interactive situations are replicated' (Caspi et al., 1989, p. 375). Furthermore, individuals have different propensities to select those environments that help to perpetuate their behaviour. In the remainder of this chapter we will attempt to provide an explication of some of the cognitive and emotional processes that promote increased disruptive behaviour among individuals.

General emotional and cognitive factors associated with disruptive behaviour

Prior work on the significance of emotional and cognitive functioning for the development of antisocial behaviour has focused on general aspects of cognitions and emotions (see also Angold & Costello, chapter 6, this volume). Two general emotional factors that have been related to antisocial behaviour are insufficient arousal and emotional reactivity. The need to increase one's arousal level has been connected to sensation seeking and risk-taking behaviour (Newman & Wallace, 1992). Juveniles are thought to persist more in their disruptive behaviour when they score high on indices of sensation seeking. Sensation seeking has been linked to physiological under-arousal, as evidenced by low heart-rate and low galvanic skin response (Raine, 1993).

A second general emotional factor emerges from studies of child abuse (Cummings et al., 1991; Luntz & Widom, 1994). Early exposure to physical abuse, coupled with high conflict among parents may lead children to have difficulty with the regulation of emotions, particularly anger. Dodge and his colleagues (Dodge et al., 1995) have traced early physical abuse to some of the specific cognitive and emotion regulation problems that predict aggression in middle childhood. It is, therefore, plausible to hypothesize that crimes of rage may be related to this second general emotional factor.

Some research on cognitive factors in disruptive behaviour is predicated on the fact that, on average, delinquents have lower intelligence than nondelinquents. This relationship tends to hold even when controlling for socioeconomic factors and race (Lynam et al., 1993) or factors determining the detection of delinquency (Moffitt & Silva, 1988). Some researchers have focused on the poor cognitive control over behaviour that characterizes many delinquents. There is a consensus among research findings that poor self-control and impulsivity are replicated in many delinquent acts (Gottfredson & Hirschi, 1990; Moffitt, 1993).

It should be noted, however, that low intelligence, poor impulsive or self-control, and sensation seeking are very broad concepts that do not reveal which specific emotional or cognitive processes are associated with particular types of disruptive behaviour. A major problem with these concepts, and those deriving from moral development (Smetana, 1990; Turiel, 1998), is that they are nonspecific, and do not address well why some juveniles engage in covert acts only, others in overt acts, and a third group in both covert and overt acts, and in that specific manner contribute to the continuity of the disruptive behaviour. Furthermore, the portrayal of disruptive and delinquent juveniles as intellectually and emotionally impaired and showing deficits in self-control, although applicable to a proportion of delinquents, is overly simplistic. One category of antisocial individual delinquents (psychopaths) has above average intelligence (Cleckley, 1976). They and experienced delinquents often show considerable self-control to achieve antisocial acts. Experienced criminals (including persistent conduct-disordered youth) have been described as having 'a great deal of technical and interpersonal skill and knowledge relevant to specific crime opportunities' (Carroll & Weaver, 1986, p. 22). It is our hope that a focus on specific cognitive patterns and emotions will provide greater insight into particular types of antisocial behaviour and serve to explain continuities and discontinuities within the larger framework of disruptive problems. Before reviewing specific emotional and cognitive processes, we will first present a matrix of different types of disruptive behaviours, which is relevant for a better differentiation of emotional and cognitive aspects of disruptive behaviour.

A matrix of emotional and cognitive aspects of disruptive behaviours

We selected a matrix of two dimensions of disruptive behaviour, i.e. overt-covert and reactive-proactive disruptive behaviour (Table 14.1), to illustrate shared and distinct emotional and cognitive processes contributing to each of the behaviours. Although some of the aspects of the matrix have been re-searched, we hope that the remaining aspects will elicit future research. We will briefly discuss the two dimensions and then review emotional and cogni-tive processes thought to be pertinent to the disruptive behaviours.

Findings supporting the behavioural distinction between overt and covert disruptive behaviour have already been alluded to (Frick et al., 1993; Loeber & Schmaling, 1985). In addition, researchers have distinguished between reac-tive and proactive aggression (Dodge & Coie, 1987). Reactive aggression involves a response to antecedent conditions of provocation and is primarily interpersonal and hostile in nature, usually accompanied by the expression of anger. Proactive aggression is directed at self-serving outcomes that involve interpersonal dominance or instrumental gain. Dodge & Coie (1987) demon-strated that although most boys identified by peers as highly aggressive ex-hibit both forms of aggression, some boys are predominantly proactive in their aggression, whereas other boys are predominantly reactive (see also Vitaro et al., 1998). Within the proactive aggression category we make a distinction between instrumental aggression and aggression that is predatory or aimed at bullying or intimidation (this is akin to Hartup's (1974) distinction between hostile and instrumental aggression, and Lorenz's (1966) distinction between affective and instrumental aggression). In instrumental aggression, the conflict centres around the perpetrator's forceful removal of money or goods from the victim (as in grabbing things, strongarming, robbery). By contrast, noninstrumental aggression refers to aggression in which the perpe-trator inflicts pain or humiliation on others, without forceful extraction of money or goods. Childhood and adolescent bullying fit the latter category as do most forms of sexual assault. Both cognitions and emotions need to be examined within this matrix of disruptive behaviours (Orbio de Castro & Bosch, 1998-99).

Although the proactive versus reactive distinction has been applied only to aggressive acts until now, we think that it might usefully be applied to covert conduct problems as well, such as lying and deception. Juveniles can reactively lie in order to escape detection and the consequent anticipated punishment for their misdeeds. In contrast, proactive deception involves premeditated lying to obtain money, goods or favours, as in the case of fraud. In addition, juveniles may use proactive deception in order to enact planned misbehaviour at a later point in time, to meet their desire for increased autonomy, or to engage in adult-type behaviours (such as alcohol use or early sexual activity). Most theft (i.e. the illegal acquisition of goods through, for example, shoplifting or burglary) appears of a covert, presumably proactive nature (Frick et al., 1993; Loeber & Schmaling, 1985). However, some acts of theft, especially among children, may be reactive and retaliatory in nature.

In the covert category of disruptive behaviour, we include relational aggression, which in recent years has received increased research attention (Crick & Grotpeter, 1995). Relational aggression can be reactive when the person attempts to get even with someone by gossiping about them or scheming to exclude them from existing social relationships. Relational aggression can also be proactive in that it can be used to gain social advantage over a perceived rival (as in the case of jealousy), to inflict social injury on another person, or to provide amusement to the self or others. Some relational aggression overlaps with the lying category, but here the lying is not motivated to protect oneself from punishment or scrutiny or to cheat someone out of money or possessions.

Table 14.1 shows that property damage (vandalism or fire setting) can be displayed either in an overt or covert manner, depending on the perpetrator's intention to claim responsibility for the damage. However, research shows that most property damage takes place in a covert fashion (Frick et al., 1993; Loeber & Schmaling, 1985). Also, property damage can be reactive or proactive. As to the former, young children may destroy property of playmates in retaliation for a real or imagined grievance. An example of proactive property damage is when juvenile gang members will deface property or 'turf' of rival groups in order to intimidate rivals and demarcate gang territory.

Specific emotions and cognitions associated with overt–covert and reactive–proactive dimensions of disruptive behaviour

It is our thesis that emotions and cognitions co-occurring with disruptive behaviour differ according to whether the acts concern overt or covert anti-social behaviours, and whether they involve reactive or proactive strategies. For reasons of space, we will not review moral cognitions that are said to be relevant for the learning of aggression (see for example Guerra et al., 1994).

Table 14.1 contains our hypotheses about underlying cognitive and emotional mechanisms that are thought to operate during the commission of these different antisocial acts. Although we have attempted to distinguish between the cognitive and emotional components of these activities, it is not our

Table 14.1. Overview of behavioural, emotional and cognitive aspects of the most common overt and covert disruptive behaviours

General disruptive behaviour	Specific behaviours	Emotions	Examples of cognitions
Overt behaviour			
Reactive	*Aggression* (verbal aggression, threats, physical aggression)	Anger, revenge, anxiety over continued victimization	Attribution of hostile intent to other person
	Property damage (vandalism, firesetting)	Anger, revenge	Attribution of hostile intent. Belief that property damage is justified and one will be able to get away with it
Proactive	*Noninstrumental aggression* (bullying, intimidation, predatory physical fighting, violence, sexual assault)	Need for dominance, high arousal	Belief that aggression is acceptable and successful mode of achieving goals and belief that one's own material needs are more important than those of the victim
	Instrumental aggression (grabbing things, intimidation, strongarming, robbery)	Need for dominance, need for arousal, appetitive emotion	Belief that one's own material needs are more important than those of victims
	Property damage (vandalism, firesetting)	High arousal	
Covert behaviour			
Reactive	*Retaliatory theft*	Anger, revenge	Attribution of hostile intent to other, belief that act is justified and one will be able to get away with it
	Property damage (vandalism, firesetting)	Anger, revenge	
	Relational aggression (spreading rumours, ostracism, anonymous letter writing, obscene telephone calls, revealing another person's secrets)	Jealousy, anxiety about detection/punishment; dissimulation, facial control	

Table 14.1. (*cont.*)

General disruptive behaviour	Specific behaviours	Emotions	Examples of cognitions
Proactive	*Deception* (lying, conning, fraud, actions to increase autonomy from adults)	Dissimulation of intentions, simulation of emotions to mislead others, postural and facial control, avoidance behaviour	
	Unprovoked theft *Property damage* (vandalism; firesetting; falsely claim insurance money)	Appetitive emotion	Belief that others can do without the things/money they have. Belief that one's covert behaviour will be successful in deception
	Relational aggression (spreading rumours, ostracism, anonymous letter writing, obscene telephone calls, revealing another person's secrets)	Anger, revenge, dissimulation, postural and facial control	

contention that cognitive and emotional factors are separable. In fact, we regard them usually as interrelated dimensions of the same reaction or process.

Overt disruptive behaviour

The interrelation between emotion and cognition can clearly be seen in the analysis of overt reactive disruptive behaviour. Reactive aggression, by definition, occurs in response to provocation, whether real or imagined, and the motivation to behave aggressively in retaliation may be immediate or may build up over time as recent events are interpreted in light of prior interactions. Children who are prone to reactive aggression are more likely than other children to make hostile attributions about the other person's intentions toward the self when this person is associated with a negative event for the self (Dodge & Coie, 1987; Dodge et al., 1986; Pettit et al., chapter 11, this volume). Such an interpretation of the other's intention leads to anger and the desire to retaliate. These latter emotional reactions to perceived hostile intent are common to virtually all children (Dodge, 1980), since the hostile intent of the other justifies one's own aggression; but not all children reach these conclusions under the same circumstances. Reactive aggression, more so than proactive aggression, leads to peer rejection (Price & Dodge, 1989) and peer rejection increases a child's hostile attribution tendencies and reactive aggression. This cycle partially explains the persistence of reactive aggression developmentally.

Individuals who are caught up in the throes of what they feel is justifiable anger may be less calculating about the immediate consequences of their aggressive acts. Therefore, they may be less calculating about whether the target of their aggression will retaliate or not, and may not think about the consequences of their behaviour as much as those youth who are involved in proactive aggression (Crick & Dodge, 1996). However, it is our supposition that some element of self-control differentiates those who use physical aggression to retaliate from those who reactively engage in property damage. The latter individuals tend to calculate the degree to which the other person will experience harm or loss by these acts, but either out of fear of immediate (or more effective) retaliation by the other or out of fear of apprehension, they choose to get even by acts of vandalism, fire setting and other forms of property damage. Because these individuals display their angry retaliation toward other people by means of property damage, we hypothesize that they engage in some evaluation of the consequences of their acts in the same way that proactively aggressive youth do. Thus, we propose that they believe their acts are justified and that they are likely to be successful.

The attribution of hostile intent mechanism and its correlated emotion of anger is less characteristic of children whose aggression is predominantly proactive. Proactively aggressive youth are more apt to hold positive beliefs about aggression (Guerra et al., 1995) and to have more positive expectations of its effectiveness (Perry et al., 1986). These beliefs and expectations may be based on actual experiences in life. In childhood, proactive aggression is associated with bullying and acts of aggression related to achieving social dominance. Bullying, as distinguished from simply establishing oneself in the social dominance hierarchy, may involve a serious lack of empathy for victims and a gratification from inflicting and observing pain that suggests an early lack of social bonding.

Although we think that similar cognitions and emotions may be implicated in proactive and reactive forms of aggression and property damage shown in

Table 14.1, we think there may be other cognitive or emotional elements involved in instrumental aggression; however, there is no evidence to support these conclusions as yet. Instrumental aggression may be motivated by appetitive factors and justified to the self by beliefs that one's own material needs are more important than those of the victim or that it is common practice to gratify one's own needs in this way.

Covert disruptive behaviour

Several of the same cognitions and emotions implicated in overt disruptive behaviour may also apply to covert disruptive behaviours. To some extent, all acts of aggression involve the calculation of costs and benefits (Kornadt, 1984). The motivation prompted by revenge, appetitive factors, or the need for excitement is usually balanced against calculations of resistance or retaliation by the victim or apprehension and punishment by authorities. Overt acts reflect a minimalization of the latter concerns, whereas covert acts are designed to avoid retaliation or punishment. To some extent, this decision may involve an appraisal of situational circumstances by all would-be aggressors, but individual factors may also be significant. Individuals who are more disposed to anxiety about consequences would be more likely to turn to covert acts. In the case of physical aggression, lack of physical strength and ability, as well as heightened concern over physical well-being, may be important determinants of covert antisocial acts.

Most covert acts of theft are motivated by appetitive concerns and involve the acquisition of material goals or money. To justify these acts to the self, an individual must evaluate his or her own needs as greater than those of the victim or have been socialized to the acceptability of taking what one can successfully get away with. The calculation of success and avoidance of apprehension are at issue here also, although there are forms of unprovoked theft (kleptomania) that seem to minimize these factors. An important emotional factor for youth who steal is the excitement and elevated arousal that reinforces covert acts such as burglary and shoplifting. Retaliatory theft which is less common, on the other hand, is motivated by similar emotions and cognitions as reactive aggression, namely, a young thief's anger over the belief that the victim intentionally harmed him or her and deserves retribution. Because of concerns over punishment, particularly if the victim is more powerful than oneself, this retaliation may take the form of theft or property damage. Either of these acts deprive the victim of the use of the property. In the case of theft, there is the additional gratification of acquiring the victim's property. In the case of property damage, the physical act of destroying something belonging to the victim may produce a source of gratification to the offending individual.

Proactive acts of deception may share important emotional and cognitive components with proactive theft, to the extent that they both involve the illegal acquisition of money or goods. Acts of fraud also may involve additional emotional and cognitive elements. Lying and deception entail control over one's emotions in order to be successful. In some cases, this involves the postural and facial dissimulation of emotion, as well as good control over anxiety. It is our contention that to achieve this control requires a certain belief in the justifiability of this behaviour, either by denying the harm one is doing to the other person or by placing one's own needs over those of others. It is also probable that these activities satisfy the need for emotional arousal, since individuals with generally heightened automatic arousal would have difficulty managing the deception.

We have added one category, relational aggression, to the covert list because it has increased research attention, especially among females (Crick & Grotpeter, 1995). Some of relational aggression overlaps with the lying category, but here the lying is not motivated to protect oneself from punishment or scrutiny, in the reactive case, or to cheat someone out of money or possessions, in the proactive case. Instead, relational aggression can serve a reactive goal by getting even with someone by gossiping about them or scheming to exclude them from existing social relationships. Crick (1995) has demonstrated that relational aggression is connected with the same hostile attribution bias as is reactive physical aggression, suggesting that relational aggression is predominantly reactive in nature. Relational aggression may also be proactive in that it can be used to gain social advantage over a perceived rival or, as in the case of bullying or predation, simply to inflict social injury on another person or to provide amusement to the self or others.

Implications for research and interventions

We have argued that emotional and cognitive processes play important roles in the persistence of disruptive behaviour, and that, conversely, these factors are crucial in comprehending the discontinuity of that behaviour over time. We also have argued that emotional and cognitive processes affect disruptive behaviour differently depending on whether the behaviour involves overt or covert acts, or whether the motivation is reactive or proactive in nature.

Admittedly, the research evidence is strongest for cognitions related to overt behaviour (especially aggression), and virtually nonexistent for covert behaviour. There are several other aspects that warrant researchers' attention. Firstly, developmental aspects of cognitions pertaining to disruptive behaviour can profitably be studied from the 'Theory of mind' perspective, that is the ability of children to attribute mental states to themselves and to others to explain and predict behaviour (Astington et al., 1988). Although some attempt has been made to apply this conceptualization to aggressive behaviours in childhood (Happé & Frith, 1996), no attempt appears to have been made to link this to covert acts.

Secondly, there are important sex differences in emotions and cognitions concerning overt and covert disruptive behaviours. There is a consensus that girls' aggression is less common than boys' aggression (Maccoby & Jacklin, 1974), but these differences disappear once provocation is taken into account (Bettencourt & Miller, 1996), and may be smaller once social and indirect forms of aggression are known. However, on the level of serious violence, adolescent males exceed females in all studies (Loeber & Farrington, 1998). The emotional and cognitive processes that can explain why girls are less violent still remain to be investigated. One hypothesis is that girls have more fears for the negative consequences of physical confrontations, or that confrontation elicits negative emotions, and that when girls engage in more proactive forms of covert activities aimed at harming others, they avoid negative emotions commonly associated with direct confrontation.

Thirdly, developmental aspects of emotions and cognitions need to be investigated. For example, there is a degree of emotional sophistication required for deception (Saarni, 1989; Underwood et al., 1992) and juveniles' capacity for sophisticated deception increases with age. Increasing skill at deception and avoidance of adult sanctions may be one of the ways that deviant peers train each other for greater participation and success in antisocial activity (Dishion et al., 1994). Likewise, their understanding of possession rules improves from childhood through adolescence (Loeber & Hay, 1994).

Fourthly, the contextual and cultural aspects of cognitions associated with disruptive behaviour need more attention. Although the justification for theft has not been studied in cognitive processing terms, as it has for proactive aggression, there is anecdotal evidence that some children may grow up in a context of poverty that places less negative connotations on the theft since it provides for basic survival needs. It may prove true that a greater belief in the justifiability of theft will differentiate individuals who are more consistently involved in stealing than those who are not. A second motivational consideration to be considered from a contextual point of view is the excitement and elevated arousal that reinforces covert acts. It may be the case that high crime neighbourhoods alter the meaning of these activities and that they become part of the rite of passage among youth. As such, the emotional consequences of these activities may be altered.

Fifthly, improved knowledge of emotions and cognitions pertaining to specific disruptive behaviour should be related to the relative persistence or desistance of behaviour. For example, reactive and proactive disruptive behaviour have different implications for the consistency of disruptive behaviour. For proactive disruptive behaviour that serves to create personal advantage or acquisition of goods or money, consistency would be highest where need is great and the perception of success relative to failure or cost is high. Alternatively, where proactive antisocial activity creates heightened arousal one would expect strong interindividual differences so long as measurement of the behaviour extends across a sufficiently lengthy interval to include multiple opportunities for the behaviour to be displayed.

Finally, we see knowledge of emotional and cognitive components of disruptive behaviour as a first step toward improving interventions to reduce disruptive behaviour. The more we learn about emotional and cognitive processes associated with the persistence of disruptive behaviour, the better such aspects can be incorporated in interventions. Although correlational and survey evidence is useful, the ultimate utility of improved knowledge of cognitive and emotional aspects of disruptive behaviour is improved interventions.

Acknowledgements

We are grateful to Erica Spokart for preparing the references. The study was supported by grants from the National Institute of Drug Abuse (DA411018), the National Institute of Mental Health (MH50778), and the Office of Juvenile Justice and Delinquency Prevention (96-MU-FX-0012). Points of view or opinions in this document are those of the authors and do not necessarily represent the official position of OJJDP, the Department of Justice, NIMH or NIDA.

REFERENCES

American Psychiatric Association (1994). *Diagnostic and Statistical Manual of Mental Disorders* (4th Edn). Washington, DC: American Psychiatric Association.

Astington, J.W., Harris, P.L. & Olson, D.R. (Eds.) (1988). *Developing Theories of Mind*. New York: Cambridge University Press.

Baicker-McKee, C. (1990). *Saints, sinners, and prodigal sons: An investigation of continuities and discontinuities in antisocial development*. PhD dissertation. Virginia: University of Virginia.

Bettencourt B.A. & Miller, N. (1996). Gender differences in aggression as a function of provocation: A meta-analysis. *Psychological Bulletin, 119*, 422–47.

Carroll, J. & Weaver, F. (1986). Shoplifters' perception of crime opportunities: A process-tracing study. In D.B. Cornish & R.V. Clarke (Eds.), *The Reasoning Criminal: Rational Choice Perspectives on Offending*, pp. 20–38. New York: Springer-Verlag.

Caspi, A., Elder, G.H. & Bem, D.J. (1987). Moving against the world: Life-course patterns of explosive children. *Developmental Psychology, 23*, 308–13.

Caspi, A., Behm, D.J. & Elder, G.H. (1989). Continuities and consequences of interactional styles across the life course. *Journal of Personality, 57*, 375–406.

Caspi, A. & Moffitt, T.E. (1995). The continuity of maladaptive behavior: From description to understanding in the study of antisocial behavior. In D. Cicchetti & D.J. Cohen (Eds.), *Developmental Psychopathology*, Vol. 2 (pp. 472–511). New York: John Wiley & Sons.

Cleckley, H. (1976). *The Mask of Sanity* (5th edn). St. Louis, MO: Mosby.

Coie, J.D. & Dodge, K.A. (1988). Multiple sources of data on social behavior and social status in the school: Across-age comparison. *Child Development, 59*, 815–29.

Coie J.D. & Dodge, K.A. (1998). Aggression and antisocial behavior. In N. Eisenberg (Ed.), *Handbook of Child Psychology, Fifth Edition, Volume 3: Social, Emotional and Personality Development* (pp. 779–862). New York: John Wiley & Sons.

Crick, N.R. (1995). Relational aggression: The role of intent attributions, feelings of distress, and provocation type. *Developmental Psychopathology, 7*, 313–22.

Crick, N.R. & Dodge, K.A. (1996). Social information-processing mechanisms in reactive and proactive aggression. *Child Development, 67*, 993–1002.

Crick, N.R. & Grotpeter, J.K. (1995). Relational aggression, gender, and social-psychological adjustment. *Child Development, 66*, 710–22.

Cummings, E.M., Hennessy, K.D., Rabideau, G.J. & Cicchetti, D. (1991). Responses of physically abused boys to inter-adult anger involving their mothers. *Development and Psychopathology, 6*, 31–41.

Dishion, T.J., French, D.C. & Patterson, G.R. (1995). The development and ecology of antisocial behavior. In D. Cicchetti & D.J. Cohen (Eds.), *Developmental Psychopathology* (Vol. 2, pp. 421–71). New York: John Wiley & Sons.

Dishion, T.J., Patterson, G.R. & Griesler, P.C. (1994). Peer adaptations in the development of antisocial behavior. In L.R. Huesmann (Ed.), *Aggressive Behavior: Current Perspectives* (pp. 61–95). New York: Plenum Press.

Dodge, K.A. (1980). Social cognition and children's aggressive behavior. *Child Development, 81,* 162–70.

Dodge, K.A. & Coie, J.D. (1987). Social information-processing factors in reactive and proactive aggression in children's peer groups. *Journal of Personality and Social Psychology, 53,* 1146–58.

Dodge, K.A., Pettit, G.S., Bates, J.E. & Valente, E. (1995). Social information processing patterns partially mediate the effect of early physical abuse on later conduct problems. *Journal of Abnormal Psychology, 104,* 632–43.

Dodge, K.A., Pettit, G.S., McClaskey, C.L. & Brown, M.M. (1986). Social competence in children. *Monographs of the Society for Research in Child Development, 51* (2, Serial No. 213).

Elliott, D.S. (1994). Longitudinal research in criminology: promise and practice. In E.G.M. Weitekamp & H.J. Kerner (Eds.), *Cross-national Longitudinal Research on Human Development and Criminal Behavior* (pp. 189–201). Dordrecht, The Netherlands: Kluwer.

Farrington, D.P. (1986). Stepping stones to adult criminal careers. In D. Olwens, J. Block & M.R. Yarrow (Eds.), *Development of Antisocial and Prosocial Behavior* (pp. 359–83). New York: Academic Press.

Farrington, D.P. (1991). Childhood aggression and adult violence: Early precursors and later life outcomes. In D.J. Pepler & K.H. Rubins (Eds.), *The Development and Treatment of Childhood Aggression.* Hillsdale, NJ: Lawrence Erlbaum.

Farrington, D.P. (1994). Childhood, adolescent, and adult features of violent males. In L.R. Huesmann (Ed.), *Aggressive Behavior: Current Perspectives* (pp. 215–40). New York: Plenum Press.

Fergusson, D.M., Horwood, L.J. & Lynskey, M.T. (1994). Structure of DSM–III–R criteria for disruptive childhood behaviors: confirmatory factor models. *Journal of the American Academy of Child and Adolescent Psychiatry, 33,* 1145–57.

Frick, P.J., Lahey, B.B., Loeber, R., et al. (1993). Oppositional defiant disorder & conduct disorder: I. Meta-analytic review of factor analyses. *Clinical Psychology Review, 13,* 319–40.

Frick, P.J., O'Brien, B.S., Wootton, J.M. & McBurnett, K. (1994). Psychopathy and conduct problems in children. *Journal of Abnormal Psychology, 103,* 700–7.

Gittelman, R., Mannuzza, S., Shenker, R. & Bonagura, N. (1985). Hyperactive boys almost grown up. *Archives of General Psychiatry, 42,* 937–47.

Gottfredson, M.R. & Hirschi, T. (1990). *A General Theory of Crime.* Stanford, CA: Stanford University Press.

Graham, P. & Rutter, M.L. (1973). Psychiatric disorders in the young adolescent: A follow-up study. *Proceedings of the Royal Society of Medicine, 66,* 1226–9.

Greene, E.L., Langner, T.S., Herson, J.H., et al. (1973). Some methods of evaluating behavioral variations in children 6 to 18. *Journal of the American Academy of Child Psychiatry, 12,* 531–53.

Guerra, N.G., Huesmann, L.R. & Hanish, L. (1995). The role of normative beliefs in children's social behavior. In N. Eisenberg (Ed.), *Review of Personality and Social Psychology, Development, and Social Psychology: The Interface* (pp. 140–58). Thousand Oaks, CA: Sage.

Guerra, N.G., Nucci, L. & Huesmann, L.R. (1994). Moral cognition and childhood aggression. In R. L. Huesmann (Ed.), *Aggressive Behavior. Current Perspectives* (pp. 13–33). New York: Plenum Press.

Haapasalo, J. & Tremblay R.E. (1994). Physically aggressive boys from ages 6 to 12: family background, parenting behavior, and prediction of delinquency. *Journal of Consulting and Clinical Psychology, 62,* 1044–52.

Happé, F. & Frith, U. (1996). Theory of mind and social impairment in children with conduct disorder. *British Journal of Developmental Psychology, 14,* 385–98.

Hare, R.D. (1991). *The Hare Psychopathy Checklist – Revised.* Toronto, Canada: Multi-Health Systems.

Hartup, W.W. (1974). Aggression in childhood: Developmental perspectives. *American Psychologist, 29,* 336–41.

Hawkins, D.F., Laub, J.H. & Lauritsen, J.L. (1998). Race, ethnicity, and serious juvenile offending. In R. Loeber & D. Farrington (Eds.), *Serious and Violent Juvenile Offenders: Risk Factors and Successful Interventions* (pp. 13–29). Thousands Oaks, CA: Sage.

Hawkins, J.D., Herrenkohl, T., Farrington, D. P., et al. (1998). A review of predictors of youth violence. In R. Loeber & D.P. Farrington (Eds.), *Serious and Violent Juvenile Offenders: Risk Factors and Successful Interventions* (pp. 106–46). Thousand Oaks, CA: Sage.

Huizinga, D.H. (1995). Developmental sequences in delinquency. In L. Crockett & A. Crouter (Eds.), *Pathways Through Adolescence* (pp. 15–34). Mahwah, NJ: Lawrence Erlbaum.

Jessor, R. & Jessor, S.L. (1977). *Problem Behavior and Psychosocial Development.* New York: Academic Press.

Kelley, B.T., Loeber, R., Keenan, K. & DeLamatre, M. (1997). *Developmental Pathways in Boys' Disruptive and Delinquent Behavior.* Washington, DC: Office of Juvenile Justice and Delinquency Prevention, U.S. Department of Justice.

Kolvin, I., Miller, F.J.W., Scott, D.M., Gatzanis, S.R.M. & Fleeting, M. (1990). *Continuities of deprivation? The Newcastle 1000 family study.* Aldershot: Avebury.

Kornadt, H.J. (1984). Motivation theory of aggression and its relation to social psychological approaches. In A. Mummendy (Ed.), *Social Psychology of Aggression: From Individual Behavior to Social Interaction* (pp. 21–31). New York: Springer.

Lahey, B.B., Loeber, R., Hart, E.L., et al. (1995). Four-year longitudinal study of conduct disorder in boys: Patterns and predictors of persistence. *Journal of Abnormal Psychology, 104,* 83–93.

Lahey, B.B., Loeber, R., Quay, H.C., Frick, P.J. & Grimm, J. (1992). Oppositional defiant and conduct disorder: Issues to be resolved for DSM–IV. *Journal of the American Academy of Child and Adolescent Psychiatry, 31,* 539–46.

Lahey, B.B., Loeber, R., Quay, H.C., Frick, P.J. & Grimm, J. (1997). Oppositional defiant disorder and conduct disorder. In T.A. Widiger, A.J. Frances, H.A. Pincus, et al. (Eds.), *DSM–IV Sourcebook* (Vol. 3, pp. 189–209). Washington DC: American Psychiatric Association.

Lahey, B.B., McBurnett, K. & Loeber, R. (in press). Are attention-deficit/hyperactivity disorder and oppositional defiant disorder developmental precursors to conduct disorder? In M. Lewis & A. Sameroff (Eds.), *Handbook of Developmental Psychopathology* (Vol. 2). New York: Plenum Press.

Lipsey, M.W. & Derzon, J.H. (1998). Predictors of violent or serious delinquency in adolescence and early adulthood: A synthesis of longitudinal research. In R. Loeber & D. Farrington (Eds.), *Serious and Violent Juvenile Offenders: Risk Factors and Successful Interventions* (pp. 86–105). Thousand Oaks, CA: Sage.

Loeber, R. (1982). The stability of antisocial and delinquent child behavior. *Child Development, 53,* 1431–46.

Loeber, R. (1985). Patterns and development of antisocial child behavior. In G.J. Whitehurst (Ed.), *Annals of Child Development* (Vol. 2, pp. 77–116). Greenwich, CT: JAI Press.

Loeber, R. (1991). Antisocial behavior: More enduring than changeable? *Journal of the American Academy of Child and Adolescent Psychiatry, 31,* 393–7.

Loeber, R., DeLamatre, M., Keenan, K. & Zhang, Q. (1998a). A prospective replication of developmental pathways in disruptive and delinquent behavior. In R. Cairns, L. Bergman & J. Kagan (Eds.), *Methods and Models for Studying the Individual* (pp. 185–215). Thousands Oaks, CA: Sage.

Loeber, R. & Dishion, T.J. (1983). Early predictors of male delinquency: A review. *Psychological Bulletin, 94,* 68–99.

Loeber, R. & Farrington, D.P. (Eds.) (1998). *Serious and Violent Juvenile Offenders: Risk Factors and Successful Interventions.* Thousand Oaks, CA: Sage.

Loeber, R., Farrington, D.P., Stouthamer-Loeber, M. & Van Kammen, W.B. (1998b). *Antisocial Behavior and Mental Health Problems: Explanatory Factors in Childhood and Adolescence.* Mahwah, NJ: Lawrence Erlbaum.

Loeber, R., Green, S.M., Keenan, K. & Lahey, B.B. (1995). Which boys will fare worse? Early predictors of the onset of conduct disorder in a six year longitudinal study. *Journal of the American Academy of Child and Adolescent Psychiatry, 34,* 499–509.

Loeber, R., Green, S.M. & Lahey, B.B. (in press). Risk factors of adult antisocial personality in adulthood. In J. Coid & D.P. Farrington (Eds.), *Primary Prevention of Adult Antisocial Personality.* Cambridge: Cambridge University Press.

Loeber, R., Green, S.M., Lahey, B.B., Christ, M.A.G. & Frick, P.J. (1992). Developmental sequences in the age of onset of disruptive child behaviors. *Journal of Child and Family Studies, 1,* 21–41.

Loeber, R. & Hay, D.F. (1994). Developmental approaches to aggression and conduct problems. In M. Rutter and D.F. Hay (Eds.), *Development Through Life: A Handbook for Clinicians* (pp. 488–516). Oxford: Blackwell Scientific Publications.

Loeber, R., Keenan, K. & Zhang, Q. (1997). Boys' experimentation and persistence in developmental pathways toward serious delinquency. *Journal of Child & Family Studies, 6,* 321–57.

Loeber, R. & Schmaling, K. (1985). Empirical evidence for overt and covert patterns of antisocial conduct problems. *Journal of Abnormal Child Psychology, 13,* 337–52.

Loeber, R. & Stouthamer-Loeber, M. (1987). Prediction. In H.C. Quay (Ed.), *Handbook of Juvenile Delinquency* (pp. 325–82). New York: John Wiley & Sons.

Loeber, R. & Stouthamer-Loeber, M. (1998). Development of juvenile aggression and violence. Some common misconceptions and controversies. *American Psychologist, 53,* 242–59.

Loeber, R., Tremblay, R.E., Gagnon, C. & Charlebois, P. (1989). Continuity and desistance in disruptive boys' early fighting in school. *Development & Psychopathology, 1,* 39–50.

Loeber, R., Wung, P., Keenan, K., et al. (1993). Developmental pathways in disruptive child behavior. *Development & Psychopathology, 5,* 101–32.

Lorenz, K. (1966). *On Aggression.* New York: Harcourt.

Luntz, B.K. & Widom, C.J. (1994). Antisocial personality disorders in abused and neglected children grown up. *American Journal of Psychiatry, 151,* 670–4.

Lynam, D.R. (1997). Pursuing the psychopath: Capturing the fledgling psychopath in a nomological net. *Journal of Abnormal Psychology, 106,* 425–38.

Lynam, D., Moffitt, T. & Stouthamer-Loeber, M. (1993). Explaining the relation between IQ and delinquency: Class, race, test motivation, school failure, or self control? *Journal of Abnormal Psychology, 102,* 187–96.

Maccoby, E.E. & Jacklin, C.M. (1974). *The Psychology of Sex Differences.* Stanford: Stanford University Press.

Maughan, B. & Rutter, M. (1998). Continuities and discontinuities in antisocial behavior from childhood to adult life. In T.H. Ollendick & R.J. Prinz (Eds.), *Advances in Clinical Child Psychology* (Vol. 20, pp. 1–47). New York: Plenum Press.

Moffitt, T.E. (1993). Adolescence-limited and life-course-persistent antisocial behavior: a developmental taxonomy. *Psychology Review, 100,* 674–701.

Moffitt, T.E. & Silva, P.A. (1988). IQ and delinquency: A direct test of the differential detection hypothesis. *Journal of Abnormal Psychology, 97,* 330–3.

Nagin, D.S. & Farrington, D.P. (1992). The stability of criminal potential from childhood to adulthood. *Criminology, 30,* 235–60.

Nagin, D.S. & Land K.S. (1993). Age, criminal careers, and population heterogeneity: specification and estimation of a nonparametric, mixed poisson model. *Criminology, 31,* 327–62.

Nagin, D.S. & Paternoster, R. (1991). On the relationship of past to future participation in delinquency. *Criminology, 29,* 163–89.

Newman, J.P. & Wallace, J.F. (1992). Three pathways to impulsive behavior: Implications for violence and aggression. In *Proceedings: Fourth Symposium on Violence and Aggression.* Saskatchewan: University of Saskatchewan and Regional Psychiatric Centre.

Nijboer, J.A. & Weerman, F.M. (1998). Delinquente carrières van jongens. Variërende gedragspatronen in de adolescentieperiode. *Justitiële Verkenningen* (The Hague, Netherlands), *24,* 26–43.

Olweus, D. (1979). Stability of aggressive reaction patterns in males. *American Psychological Bulletin, 86,* 852–7.

Orbio de Castro, B. & Bosch, J. D. (1998–99). Sociale-informatieverwerking door jongens met gedragsproblemen. *Jaarboek Ontwikkelingspsychologie, orthopedagogiek en kinderpsychiatrie, 3,* 212–41.

Patterson, G.R. (1982). *A Social Learning Approach: Coercive Family Process* (Vol. 3). Eugene, OR: Castalia Publishing Company.

Patterson, G.R., Forgatch, M.S., Yoerger, K.L. & Stoolmiller, M. (1998). Variables that initiate and maintain an early-onset trajectory for juvenile offending. *Development and Psychopathology, 10,* 531–47.

Patterson, G.R., Reid, J.B. & Dishion, T.J. (1992). *Antisocial Boys.* Eugene, OR: Castalia.

Perry, D.G., Perry, L.C. & Rasmussen, P. (1986). Cognitive social learning mediators of aggression. *Child Development, 57,* 700–11.

Price, J.M. & Dodge, K.A. (1989). Reactive and proactive aggression in childhood: Relations to peer status and social context dimensions. *Journal of Abnormal Child Psychology, 17,* 455–71.

Pulkkinen, L. (1992). Life-styles in personality development. *European Journal of Personality, 6,* 139–55.

Raine, A. (1993). *The Psychopathology of Crime.* San Diego, CA: Academic Press.

Richards, P. (1981). Quantitative and qualitative sex differences in middle-class delinquency. *Criminology, 18,* 5–28.

Robins, L.N. (1966). *Deviant Children Grow Up: A Sociological and Psychiatric Study of Sociopathic Personality.* Baltimore: Williams & Wilkins.

Rutter, M., Giller, H. & Hagel, A. (1998). *Antisocial Behavior by Young People.* Cambridge: Cambridge University Press.

Saarni, C. (1989). Children's understanding of strategic control of emotional expression in social transactions. In C. Saarni & P.L. Harris (Eds.), *Children's Understanding of Emotion* (pp. 181–208). Cambridge: Cambridge University Press.

Sampson, R.J. & Laub, J.H. (1993). *Crime in the Making. Pathways and Turning Points through Life.* Cambridge, MA: Harvard University Press.

Smetana, J.G. (1990), Morality and conduct disorder. In M. Lewis & S.M. Miller (Eds), *Handbook of Developmental Psychopathology* (pp. 157–79). New York: Plenum Press.

Straus, M.A., Gelles, R.J. & Steinmetz, S.K. (1980). *Behind Closed Doors: Violence in the American Family.* Garden City, NY: Anchor.

Thornberry, T. (1998). Membership in youth gangs and involvement in serious and violent offenders. In R. Loeber & D. Farrington (Eds.), *Serious and Violent Juvenile Offenders: Risk Factors and Successful Interventions* (pp. 147–66). Thousand Oaks, CA: Sage.

Tolan, P.H. (1998). Voorspellers van gewelddadig gedrag bij jongeren. In W. Koops & W. Slot (Eds.), *Van lastig tot misdadig* (pp. 52–64). Houten/Diegem, The Netherlands: Bohn Stafleu Van Loghum.

Tolan, P.H. & Gorman-Smith, D. (1998). Development of serious and violent offending careers. In R. Loeber & D. Farrington (Eds.), *Serious and Violent Juvenile Offenders: Risk Factors and Successful Intervention* (pp. 68–87). Thousands Oaks, CA: Sage.

Tremblay, R.E., Loeber, R., Gagnon, C., et al. (1991). Disruptive boys with stable and unstable high fighting behavior patterns during junior elementary school. *Journal of Abnormal Child Psychology, 19,* 285–300.

Turiel, E. (1998). The development of morality. In N. Eisenberg (Ed.), *Handbook of Child Psychology: Social, Emotional, and Personality Development,* 5th edition (pp. 863–932). New York: John Wiley & Sons.

Underwood, M.K., Coie, J.D. & Herbsman, C.R. (1992). Display rules for anger and aggression in school-age children. *Child Development, 63,* 366–80.

Van Kammen, W.B., Maguin, E. & Loeber, R. (1994). Initiation of drug selling and its relationship with illicit drug use and serious delinquency in adolescent boys. In E.G.M. Weitekamp & H.J. Kerner (Eds.), *Cross-National Longitudinal Research on Human Development and Criminal Behavior* (pp. 229–41). Dordrecht, The Netherlands: Kluwer.

Verhulst, F.C. & van der Ende, J. (1992). Six-year stability of parent-reported problem behavior in an epidemiological sample. *Journal of Abnormal Child Psychology, 20,* 595–610.

Vitaro, F., Gendreau, P.L., Tremblay, R.E. & Oligny, P. (1998). Reactive and proactive aggression differentially predict later conduct problems. *Journal of Child Psychology and Psychiatry, 39*, 377–85.

15

Treatment of conduct disorders

Alan E. Kazdin

Among the many points detailed in previous chapters, we have learned that conduct disorder is one of the most frequent bases of clinical referral in child and adolescent treatment services, has relatively poor long-term prognosis, and is transmitted across generations. Because children with conduct disorder often traverse multiple social services (e.g. special education, mental health, juvenile justice), the disorder is one of the most costly mental disorders in the United States (Robins, 1981). (Children will be used to refer to both children and adolescents. When pertinent to the discussion, a distinction will be made and referred to accordingly.) Clearly, there is an urgent need to develop effective intervention programmes. At the same time, developing effective treatments for conduct disorder is daunting. The very nature of the disorder and the many facets with which it is associated portend many obstacles in merely delivering treatment let alone achieving therapeutic change. Nevertheless, within the past two decades, significant advances have been made in treatment. The present chapter reviews and evaluates advances in the treatment of conduct disorder. Promising treatments are presented and evaluated. Each of the treatments was selected because it has been carefully evaluated in controlled clinical trials. In addition to evaluating specific techniques, limitations of current treatment research and models of delivering service to conduct disordered youth are also discussed.

Key characteristics to consider in relation to treatment

From a treatment perspective, conduct disorder represents an array of child, parent, family and contextual conditions. These other conditions, apart from the central symptoms of the disorder, may significantly influence delivery and effectiveness of treatment. Consider briefly salient domains that are relevant to treatment.

Heterogeneity of the disorder

Conduct disorder encompasses heterogeneous and multifaceted problems. In the *Diagnostic and Statistical Manual of Mental Disorders* (DSM–IV; American

Psychiatric Association, 1994), the diagnosis is reached if the child shows at least three of the 15 symptoms within the past 12 months, with at least one symptom evident within the past 6 months. The symptoms of Conduct Disorder include bullying others, initiating fights, using a weapon, being physically cruel to others or to animals, stealing while confronting a victim, destroying property, breaking into others' property, stealing items of nontrivial value, staying out late, running away, lying, deliberate firesetting and truancy. Clearly, children who meet the diagnostic criteria can vary greatly in the specific symptom combinations they present, leaving aside variations in severity and duration of individual symptoms and overall impairment. Even if children present similar symptom patterns, we know that they may be quite different in the paths that led them to that point (Moffitt et al., 1996). That is, there are quite different clinical presentations of conduct disorder and when there are similar presentations, there can be quite different developmental histories.

The diagnostic criteria are not invoked in discussing treatments in the present chapter for two reasons. First and foremost, the vast majority of studies have not used any formal diagnostic system in recruiting or selecting participants. Diverse criteria are used (e.g. clinical referral to inpatient or outpatient services for antisocial behaviour, extreme scores on parent checklists, adjudication). Second and perhaps more significant, there is no clear evidence that the diagnostic criteria represent a cut-off or level at which clinical dysfunction begins. Indeed, evidence suggests that the need for treatment, impairment and long-term deleterious outcomes characterize children who fall below the threshold for meeting a diagnosis for the disorder (Offord et al., 1992). Consequently, for purposes of this chapter, conduct disorder (lower case) will be used to encompass children who engage in antisocial and aggressive behaviour and evince significant impairment. The proper noun, Conduct Disorder, will be reserved for instances in which criteria for a diagnosis (e.g. DSM–IV) are met.

Associated features

If one were to consider 'only' the symptoms of conduct disorder and the persistence of impairment, the challenge of identifying effective treatments would be great enough. However, the presenting characteristics of children and their families usually raise a number of other considerations that are central to treatment. Consider characteristics of children, parents, families and contexts that are associated with conduct disorder as a backdrop for later comments on treatment.

Children who meet criteria for Conduct Disorder are likely to meet criteria for other disorders as well, as discussed in a prior chapter. Several other associated features are likely to be relevant to treatment. Children with conduct disorder are also likely to show academic deficiencies, as reflected in achievement level, grades, being left behind in school, early termination from school, and deficiencies in specific skill areas such as reading (Kazdin, 1995b). Children with the disorder are likely to show poor interpersonal relations, as reflected in diminished social skills in relation to peers and adults and higher levels of peer rejection. Conduct-disordered children also are likely to show a variety of deficits and distortions in their cognitive and attributional processes and cognitive problem-solving skills. In general, there are many domains likely to be implicated in regard to child functioning. For treatment to be effective, more will need to be addressed within the child's repertoire than the core symptoms of the disorder.

Several parent and family characteristics are associated with conduct disorder (see Kazdin, 1995b; Robins, 1991; Stoff et al., 1997). Criminal behaviour and alcoholism are two of the stronger and more consistently demonstrated parental characteristics. Parent disciplinary practices and attitudes, especially harsh, lax, erratic and inconsistent discipline practices, often characterize the parents. Dysfunctional relations are also evident, as reflected in less acceptance of their children, less warmth, affection, and emotional support, and less attachment, compared to parents of nonreferred youth. Less supportive and more defensive communications among family members, less participation in activities as a family and clearer dominance of one family member are also evident. In addition, unhappy marital relations, interpersonal conflict and aggression characterize the parental relations of antisocial children. Poor parental supervision and monitoring of the child and knowledge of the child's whereabouts also are associated with conduct disorder. The parent factors can greatly influence whether the parents bring their child to, remain in, and profit from treatment.

Finally, conduct disorder is associated with a variety of untoward living conditions such as large family size, overcrowding, poor housing and disadvantaged school settings (Kazdin, 1995b). Many of the untoward conditions in which families live place stress on the parents or diminish their threshold for coping with everyday stressors. The net effect can be evident in parent–child interaction in which parents inadvertently engage in patterns that sustain or accelerate antisocial and aggressive interactions (Dumas & Wahler, 1983; Patterson et al., 1991).

Quite often the child's dysfunction is embedded is a larger context that cannot be neglected in conceptual views about the development, maintenance and course of conduct disorder nor in the actual delivery of treatment. For example, at our outpatient clinical service (Yale Child Conduct Clinic), it is likely that a family referred for treatment will experience a subset of these characteristics: financial hardship (unemployment, significant debt, bankruptcy), untoward living conditions (dangerous neighbourhood, small living quarters), transportation obstacles (no car or car in frequent repair, state provided taxi service), psychiatric impairment of one of the parents, stress related to significant others (former spouses, boyfriends or girlfriends), and adversarial contact with an outside agency (schools, youth services, courts).

Child, parent, family and contextual characteristics are highlighted merely to place the disorder in a broader perspective. At the same time, the discussion does not convey the flavour of the cases that come to treatment. Consider two brief vignettes that better convey the contexts and situations in which conduct disorder is embedded. The vignettes are drawn from cases referred to an outpatient clinic devoted to the treatment of children (ages 3–13) seen for conduct disorder.

Two brief case vignettes
Vignette 1: family values
In this case, the mother was referred to our clinic by her son's school because of his high rate of fighting and repeated school suspensions. The mother telephoned our clinic and scheduled an appointment for an intake evaluation. She did not show up nor did she call to cancel or reschedule the appointment. There was no answer at her residence and no further contact was made with her at this time. About 4 months later, she called again, scheduled another appointment, and a few days later she and her 10-year-old son came to the clinic and completed the intake evaluation. As part of the conversation during the day of assessment, the clinician asked about the prior call about 4 months earlier, and noted how good it was that she came to the clinic on this second occasion. The mother apologized for not showing up for the prior appointment. She stated that she was unable to come in because she 'broke a family rule'. Of course, the clinician asked what that rule was. The mother reported that she and her husband, and for that matter a number of their relatives, often shoot each other (with guns). However, there is one family rule, 'You *never* shoot someone in public'. The mother said, she broke this rule, some neighbours saw her shoot her husband, and she spent 3 months in prison. Now that she is out of prison, she said she is ready for her son to begin treatment.

Vignette 2: multiple sources of dysfunction and stress

In another one of our cases, the mother was a single parent with two young boys (ages 2 and 4). She came to treatment because her older son was engaging in relatively severe and uncontrollable aggressive behaviour, including hitting, kicking and biting of his younger sibling. The mother was currently diagnosed as clinically depressed and was on medication for depression. She had a prior suicide attempt and at the time of intake was at risk for suicide, based on her reporting of suicidal ideation. Her boyfriend is the father of the two children. He lives nearby and calls her a couple of times a week. In these calls, he demands that she come over so he can see the children. During these visits, the father engages the mother in what she refers to as 'forced sex' (rape) while the two children watch. In principle, the mother could have refused the visits. However, the boyfriend said that if she did not comply, he would stop paying the money due to her for child support, take the children away in a custody battle, kill himself, and come over to the house and kill her and two children. His threats of violence were to be taken seriously; he had a prior arrest record for assault and brandishes a gun. The father fuelled the mother's fears regarding loss of the children. He said that he would take the children in a custody battle in the courts. The mother, who was in psychotherapy for depression and suicidal ideation, said that she could end it all by just driving the children and herself over a cliff. Our involvement in the case was for the treatment of the older child and his aggressive behaviour.

General comments

These vignettes are not extreme examples in the day-to-day business of clinical care of conduct disorder children and their families, as would be readily acknowledged by others involved in clinical practice. The vignettes underscore a central point, namely, quite often the child's dysfunction is embedded in a larger context that cannot be neglected in conceptual views about the development, maintenance and course of conduct disorder nor in the actual delivery of treatment.

Conduct disorder is often conceived as a dysfunction of children and adolescents. The accumulated evidence regarding the symptom constellation, risk factors and course over childhood, adolescence and adulthood attests to the heuristic value of focusing on the individual. At the same time, there is a child-parent-family-context *gestalt* that includes multiple and reciprocal influences that affect each participant (child and parent) and the systems in which they operate (family, school). For treatment to be effective, it is likely that multiple domains will have to be addressed.

Current treatments of choice

Overview

Many different treatments have been applied to conduct-disordered children, including psychotherapy, pharmacotherapy, psychosurgery, home, school and community-based programmes, residential and hospital treatment, and social services (Brandt & Zlotnick, 1988; Brestan & Eyberg, 1998; Dumas, 1989; United States Congress, 1991). Of the over 550 documented psychotherapies available for children and adolescents (Kazdin, 2000), the vast majority have not been studied. Among those that have, none has been shown to controvert conduct disorder and its long-term course.

There is increased interest in identifying treatments that have support on their behalf (Nathan & Gorman, 1998; Roth & Fonagy, 1996). The terms 'validated', 'empirically supported', and 'evidence based' have been used to delineate these interventions for adults (see Chambless et al., 1996; Task Force on Promotion and Dissemination of Psychological Procedures, 1995) and children and adolescents (Bennett-Johnson, 1996; Kazdin & Weisz, 1998; Lonigan et al., 1998). Although criteria have varied, the thrust of these efforts has been to identify treatments that have been shown to produce change in randomized controlled outcome studies with clinically referred samples. Replicating treatment effects in multiple studies and showing that treatment effects are enduring (over some follow-up period) are also included in discussions of criteria for empirically based treatments (Chambless & Hollon, 1998). The criteria that are invoked to decide whether a treatment is empirically supported raise many questions (e.g. ought some outcome measures count more than others, are posttreatment comparisons sufficient or should follow-up be considered; how many replications are needed to establish a technique). And, even if treatments meet currently invoked criteria, our knowledge base of how treatment works and for whom is paltry (Kazdin, 1997). Nevertheless, the context is important to consider as well. The vast majority of treatments in use have never been evaluated empirically (Kazdin, 1988, 2000). The four treatments highlighted below have been effective in treating conduct disorder and are among the most well established treatments in light of criteria mentioned above.

Parent management training

Background and underlying rationale

Parent management training (PMT) refers to procedures in which parents are trained to alter their child's behaviour in the home. The parents meet with a therapist or trainer who teaches them to use specific procedures to alter interactions with their child, to promote prosocial behaviour, and to decrease deviant behaviour. Training is based on the general view that conduct problem behaviour is inadvertently developed and sustained in the home by maladaptive parent–child interactions. There are multiple facets of parent–child interaction that promote aggressive and antisocial behaviour. These patterns include directly reinforcing deviant behaviour, frequently and ineffectively using commands and harsh punishment, and failing to attend to appropriate behaviour (Patterson, 1982; Patterson et al., 1992).

It would be misleading to imply that the parent generates and is solely responsible for the child–parent sequences of interactions. Influences are bidirectional, so that the child influences the parent as well (Bell & Harper, 1977; Lytton, 1990). Indeed, in some cases, the children engage in deviant behaviour to help prompt the interaction sequences. For example, when parents behave inconsistently and unpredictably (e.g. not attending to the child in the usual ways), the child may engage in some deviant behaviour (e.g. whining, throwing some object) which increases the likelihood that the parent will respond in more predictable ways (Wahler & Dumas, 1986). Essentially, inconsistent and unpredictable parent behaviour is an aversive condition for the child; terminating this condition negatively reinforces the child's deviant behaviour. However, the result is also to increase parent punishment of the child.

Among the many interaction patterns, those involving coercion have received the greatest attention (Patterson et al., 1992). Coercion refers to deviant behaviour on the part of one person (e.g. the child) which is rewarded by another person (e.g. the parent). Aggressive children are inadvertently rewarded for their aggressive interactions and their escalation of coercive behaviours, as part of the discipline practices that sustain aggressive behaviour. Several studies, involving clinic and nonclinic samples, cross-sectional and longitudinal designs, and randomized controlled clinical trials, have shown that inept parenting practices predict deviant child behaviour and that changing these practices has significant impact on child functioning (Dishion & Andrews, 1995; Dishion et al., 1992; Forgatch, 1991). Overall, parenting practices can play a significant role in the development and amelioration of aggressive and antisocial behaviour.

The general purpose of PMT is to alter the pattern of interchanges between parent and child so that prosocial, rather than coercive, behaviour is directly reinforced and supported within the family. This requires developing several different parenting behaviours, such as establishing the rules for the child to follow, providing positive reinforcement for appropriate behaviour, delivering mild forms of punishment to suppress behaviour, negotiating compromises, and other procedures. These parenting behaviours are systematically and progressively developed within the sessions in which the therapist shapes (develops through successive approximations) parenting skills. The programmes that parents eventually implement in the home also serve as the basis for the focus of the sessions in which the procedures are modified and refined.

The methods to alter parent and child behaviour are based on principles and procedures of operant conditioning. Operant conditioning, elaborated by B. F. Skinner (1938) in animal laboratory research, describes and explains how behaviour can be acquired and influenced by a variety of stimuli and consequences. Beginning in the late 1950s and early 1960s, extensions of this work led to applications across a broad range of settings (psychiatric hospitals, rehabilitation facilities, nursing homes, special education and regular classrooms, the military, business and industry) (Kazdin, 1978, 1994a). Experimental demonstrations have repeatedly shown that persons (e.g. parents, teachers, peers, hospital and institutional staff) directly in contact with others (e.g. patients, students, residents and inmates) can be trained to administer consequences for behaviour and to achieve therapeutic changes. Early applications with children focused on mental retardation, autism and special problems in institutional or special education settings. Many extensions in the home focused on everyday concerns of parents rather than clinical dysfunction or impairment (e.g. tantrums, thumbsucking, toileting, completing homework, complying with requests). Applications in the home, begun initially in the late 1960s and early 1970s (Hanf, 1969), stimulated a vigorous line of research that continues today.

Characteristics of treatment

Although many variations of PMT exist, several common characteristics can be identified. Treatment is conducted primarily with the parent(s) who implement several procedures at home. The parents meet with a therapist who teaches them to use specific procedures to alter interactions with their child, to promote prosocial behaviour, and to decrease deviant behaviour. Parents are trained to identify, define and observe problem behaviours in new ways. Careful specification of the problem is essential for the delivery of reinforcing or punishing consequences and for evaluating if the programme is achieving the desired goals. The treatment sessions provide concrete opportunities for parents to see how the techniques are implemented, to practice and refine use of the techniques (e.g. through extensive role-playing), and to review the behaviour-change programmes implemented at home. Parent-managed reinforcement programmes for child deportment and performance at school, completion of homework, and activities on the playground are routinely included, with the assistance of teachers, as available.

In most PMT programmes, one parent (usually the mother) comes to treatment due to scheduling issues (e.g. employment of the other parent) but also due to the high rate of single-parent families among conduct-problem children. Requiring two parents to attend treatment is not essential for therapeutic change and has not led to enhanced outcomes (Horton, 1984). However, this has not been thoroughly studied. Also, participation of both parents, rather than just one, is confounded with many other variables (e.g. marital conflict, stress, family income) that do contribute to clinical outcomes, as discussed later. As treatment is implemented, concrete efforts usually are made to integrate the parent who does not attend sessions in the programme carried out at home.

Duration of treatment has varied depending on the severity of child dysfunction. Programmes for young, mildly oppositional children usually last from 6–8 weeks. With clinically referred conduct-disordered children, the programmes usually last from 12–25 weeks. It is difficult to provide a firm statement of the required duration of treatment because of two competing trends, namely, efforts to develop more abbreviated and more cost-effective variations of treatment, on the one hand (Thompson et al., 1996) and to combine PMT with other treatment modalities (multimodal treatments), on the other hand (Webster-Stratton, 1996).

Overview of the evidence

Parent management training is one of the most well researched therapy techniques and has been evaluated in scores of randomized controlled outcome trials with children and adolescents varying in age (e.g. 2–17 years old) and severity of oppositional and conduct problems (Graziano & Diament, 1992; Kazdin, 1997b; Miller & Prinz, 1990; Patterson et al., 1993; Serketich & Dumas, 1996). Indeed, a recent review of treatments for conduct disorder identified PMT as the only intervention that is well established, i.e. has been shown to be effective in independently replicated controlled clinical trials (Brestan & Eyberg, 1998). Although many researchers contributed to the extensive literature on behalf of PMT, several research programmes (e.g. Eyberg, University of Florida; Forehand, University of Georgia; Patterson, Oregon Social Learning Research Center; Webster-Stratton, University of Washington) have made special inroads in developing the treatment, assessing factors that contribute to change, evaluating follow-up and replicating treatment effects across multiple samples (Eyberg & Boggs, 1989; Forgatch, 1991; McMahon & Wells, 1989; Webster-Stratton, 1996). The outcome studies support several conclusions:

Σ   PMT has led to marked improvements in child behaviour in parent and teacher reports of deviant behaviour, direct observation of behaviour at home and at school, and institutional records (e.g. school truancy, police contacts, arrest rates, institutionalization).

Σ   The magnitude of change has placed conduct problem behaviours to within nonclinic levels of functioning at home and at school, based on normative data from nonreferred peers (e.g. same age, sex).

Σ   Treatment gains have been maintained in several studies 1–3 years after treatment, although one programme reported maintenance of gains 10–14 years later (Long et al., 1994).

Σ   Improvements in child behaviours not focused on directly, on behaviours of siblings in the home and in maternal psychopathology, particularly depression, have also been documented. Occasionally, marital satisfaction and family cohesion improve following treatment, but data on these outcomes are sparse.

Considerable attention has been devoted to identifying parent and family characteristics that contribute to outcome. Family socioeconomic disadvantage, marital discord, high parental stress and low social support, single-parent families, harsh punishment practices, parent history of antisocial behaviour predict: (1) who remains in treatment; (2) the magnitude of change among those who complete treatment; and (3) the extent to which changes are maintained at follow-up (Dadds & McHugh, 1992; Dumas & Wahler, 1983; Kazdin, 1995a; Webster-Stratton & Hammond, 1990). Those families at greatest risk often respond to treatment, but the magnitude of effects is attenuated as a function of the extent to which these factors are present. Among child characteristics, more severe and chronic antisocial behaviour and comorbidity predict reduced responsiveness to treatment (Kazdin, 1995a; Ruma et al., 1996).

Characteristics of treatment also contribute to outcome. Providing parents with in-depth knowledge of social learning principles, rather than just teaching them the techniques, improves outcomes. Also, including mild punishment (e.g. brief time out from reinforcement) along with reinforcement programmes in the home enhances treatment effects (Kazdin, 1985). These components are now standard in most PMT programmes. Processes within treatment have also been studied to identify who responds to treatment. Measures of parent resistance (e.g. parents saying, 'I can't', 'I won't') correlate with parent discipline practices at home; changes in resistance during therapy predict changes in parent behaviour. Moreover, specific therapist ploys during the sessions (e.g. reframing, confronting) can overcome or contribute to resistance (Patterson & Chamberlain, 1994). This work begins to identify ways to enhance the administration of PMT.

In much of the outcome research, PMT has been administered to families individually in clinic settings. Group administration has been facilitated greatly by the development of videotaped materials that present themes, principles and procedures to the parents of conduct problem children (see Webster-Stratton, 1996). Randomized controlled trials have shown that video-based treatment, particularly in group format and when supplemented with therapist-led discussions, leads to clinically significant changes at posttreatment and that these changes are maintained at follow-up 1 and 3 years later.

PMT has been extended to community settings to bring treatment to those persons least likely to come to or remain in treatment. PMT is effective and highly cost-effective when provided in small parent groups in neighbourhoods where the families reside (Cunningham et al., 1995; Thompson et al., 1996). Occasionally, community-based has been more effective than clinic-based treatment. Of course, it is not clear that one form of treatment can replace another for all children. Yet, community applications may permit dissemination of treatment to families that otherwise might not attend the usual mental health services.

Overall evaluation
Perhaps the most important point to underscore is that no other technique for conduct disorder probably has been studied as often or as well in controlled trials as has PMT (Brestan & Eyberg, 1998). The outcome evidence makes PMT one of the most promising treatments. Related lines of work bolster the evidence. First, the study of family interaction processes that contribute to antisocial behaviour in the home and evidence that changing these processes alters child behaviour provide a strong empirical base for treatment. Second, the procedures and practices that are used in PMT (e.g. various forms of reinforcement and punishment practices) have been widely and effectively applied outside the context of conduct disorder. For example, the procedures have been applied with parents of children with autism, language delays, developmental disabilities, medical disorders for which compliance with special treatment regimens is required, and with parents who physically abuse or neglect their children (Kazdin, 1994b). Third, a great deal is known about the procedures and parameters of delivery that influence the effectiveness of reinforcement and punishment practices. Consequently, very concrete recom-

mendations can be provided to change behaviour and to alter programmes when behaviour change has not occurred.

Several resources are available to facilitate use of PMT clinically and in research. Treatment manuals are available for clinicians and convey the structure, content and flow of treatment sessions (Forehand & McMahon, 1981; Forgatch & Patterson, 1989; Patterson & Forgatch, 1987; Sanders & Dadds, 1993). Books and pamphlets are also available for parents (Forehand & Long, 1996; Patterson, 1976) that convey basic concepts and show how to apply various techniques. Already mentioned were videotapes that can also be used by professionals to guide group PMT. In short, several training materials are available for professionals as well as their clients.

Several limitations of PMT can be identified as well. First, PMT makes several demands on the parents, such as mastering educational materials that convey major principles underlying the programme, systematically observing deviant child behaviour and implementing specific procedures at home, attending weekly sessions and responding to frequent telephone contacts made by the therapist. For some families, the demands may be too great to participate in treatment. Interestingly, within the approach several procedures (e.g. shaping parent behaviour through reinforcement) provide guidelines for developing parent compliance and the desired response repertoire in relation to their children.

Second, perhaps the greatest limitation or obstacle in using PMT is that there are few training opportunities for professionals to learn the approach. Training programmes in child psychiatry, clinical psychology and social work are unlikely to provide exposure to the technique, much less opportunities for formal training. PMT requires mastery of social learning principles and multiple procedures that derive from them (Cooper et al., 1987; Kazdin, 1994a). For example, the administration of reinforcement by the parent in the home (to alter child behaviour) and by the therapist in the session (to change parent behaviour) requires more than passing familiarity with the principle and the parametric variations that dictate its effectiveness (e.g. need to administer reinforcement contingently, immediately, frequently, to use varied and high quality reinforcers; prompting, shaping). The requisite skills in administering these within the treatment sessions can be readily trained but they are not trivial.

Finally, the applicability of PMT to adolescents, as compared with children, is less clear. PMT has reduced offence rates among delinquent adolescents (Bank et al., 1991) and school behavioural problems and substance use among adolescents at risk for serious conduct problems (Dishion & Andrews, 1995). In the Bank et al. (1991) study, the impact of treatment, relative to intensive family therapy, group therapy and drug counselling, was modest over posttreatment and 3-year follow-up. Analyses from other studies suggest that adolescents respond less well to PMT, when compared with preadolescents (Dishion & Patterson, 1992), but this effect may be accounted for by severity of symptoms at pretreatment (Ruma et al., 1996). Adolescents referred for treatment tend to be more severely and chronically impaired than preadolescents; once severity is controlled, age does not influence outcome. In light of limited applications with adolescents, the strength of conclusions about the efficacy of PMT applies mainly to preadolescent children.

Cognitive problem-solving skills training

Background and underlying rationale

Cognitive processes refer to a broad class of constructs that pertain to how the individual perceives, codes and experiences the world. Individuals who engage in conduct disorder behaviours, particularly aggression, have been found to show distortions and deficiencies in various cognitive processes. These deficiencies are not merely reflections of intellectual functioning. Several cognitive processes have been studied. Examples include generating alternative solutions to interpersonal problems (e.g. different ways of handling social situations), identifying the means to obtain particular ends (e.g. making friends) or consequences of one's actions (e.g. what could happen after a particular behaviour); making attributions to others of the motivation of their actions; perceiving how others feel; and expectations of the effects of one's own actions (see Pettit et al., chapter 11, this volume; Shirk, 1988; Spivack & Shure, 1982). Deficits and distortion among these processes relate to teacher ratings of disruptive behaviour, peer evaluations and direct assessment of overt behaviour (Lochman & Dodge, 1994; Rubin et al., 1991).

An example of cognitive processes implicated in conduct disorder can be seen in the work on attributions and aggressive behaviour. Aggression is not merely triggered by environmental events, but rather through the way in which these events are perceived and processed. The processing refers to the child's appraisals of the situation, anticipated reactions of others and self-statements in response to particular events. Attribution of intent to others represents a salient cognitive disposition critically important to understanding aggressive behaviour. Aggressive children and adolescents tend to attribute hostile intent to others, especially in social situations where the cues of actual intent are ambiguous (see Crick & Dodge, 1994). Understandably, when situations are initially perceived as hostile, children are more likely to react aggressively. Although many studies have shown that conduct-disordered children experience various cognitive distortions and deficiencies, the specific contribution of these processes to conduct disorder, as opposed to risk factors with which they may be associated (e.g. untoward living conditions, low IQ) has not been established. Nevertheless, research on cognitive processes among aggressive children has served as a heuristic base for conceptualizing treatment and for developing specific treatment strategies.

Characteristics of treatment

Problem-solving skills training (PSST) consists of developing interpersonal cognitive problem-solving skills. Although many variations of PSST have been applied to conduct problem children, several characteristics usually are shared. First, the emphasis is on how children approach situations, i.e. the thought processes in which the child engages to guide responses to interpersonal situations. The children are taught to engage in a step-by-step approach to solve interpersonal problems. They make statements to themselves that direct attention to certain aspects of the problem or tasks that lead to effective solutions. Second, behaviours that are selected (solutions) to the interpersonal situations are important as well. Prosocial behaviours are fostered through modelling and direct reinforcement as part of the problem-solving process. Third, treatment utilizes structured tasks involving games, academic activities and stories. Over the course of treatment, the cognitive problem-solving skills are increasingly applied to real-life situations. Fourth, therapists usually play an active role in treatment. They model the cognitive processes by making verbal self-statements, apply the sequence of statements to particular problems, provide cues to prompt use of the skills, and deliver feedback and praise to develop correct use of the skills. Finally, treatment usually combines several different procedures including modelling and practice, role-playing, and reinforcement and mild punishment (loss of points or tokens). These are deployed in systematic ways to develop increasingly complex response repertoires of the child.

Overview of the evidence

Several outcome studies have been completed with impulsive, aggressive and conduct-disordered children and adolescents (see Baer & Nietzel, 1991; Durlak et al., 1991 for reviews). Cognitively based treatments have significantly reduced aggressive and antisocial behaviour at home, at school and in the community. At follow-up, these gains have been evident up to 1 year later. Many early studies in the field (e.g. 1970–80s) focused on impulsive children and nonpatient samples. Since that time, several studies have shown treatment effects with inpatient and outpatient cases (Kazdin, 1993; Kendall, 1991; Pepler & Rubin, 1991).

There is only sparse evidence that addresses the child, parent, family, contextual or treatment factors that influence treatment outcome. Evidence suggests that older children (> 10–11 years of age) profit more from treatment than younger children, perhaps due to their cognitive development (Durlak et al., 1991). However, the basis for differential responsiveness to treatment as a function of age has not been well tested. Conduct-disordered children who show comorbid diagnoses, academic delays and dysfunction and lower reading achievement, and who come from families with high levels of impairment (parent psychopathology, stress and family dysfunction) respond less well to treatment than children with less dysfunction in these domains (Kazdin, 1995a). However, these child, parent and family characteristics may influence the effectiveness of several different treatments for conduct-disordered children rather than PSST in particular. Much further work is needed to evaluate factors that contribute to responsiveness to treatment.

Overall evaluation

There are features of PSST that make it an extremely promising approach. Several controlled outcome studies with clinic samples have shown that cognitively based treatment leads to therapeutic change. Basic research in developmental psychology continues to elaborate the relation of maladaptive cognitive processes among children and adolescents and conduct problems that serve as underpinnings of treatment (Crick & Dodge, 1994; Shirk, 1988). An advantage of the approach is that versions of treatment are available in manual form (Feindler & Ecton, 1986; Finch et al., 1993; Shure, 1992). Consequently, the treatment can be evaluated in research and explored further in clinical practice.

Critical questions remain to be addressed in research. Primary among these is the role of cognitive processes in clinical dysfunction. Evidence is not entirely clear showing that a specific pattern of cognitive processes characterizes children with conduct problems, rather than adjustment or externalizing problems more generally. Also, although evidence has shown that cognitive processes change with treatment, evidence has not established that change in these processes mediates or is responsible for improvements in treatment outcome. Thus, the basis for therapeutic change has yet to be established. Although central questions about treatment and its effects remain to be resolved, PSST is highly promising in light of its effects in several controlled outcome studies with conduct-disordered children.

Functional family therapy

Background and underlying rationale

Functional family therapy (FFT) reflects an integrative approach to treatment that has relied on systems, behavioural and cognitive views of dysfunction (Alexander et al., 1994; Alexander & Parsons, 1982). Clinical problems are conceptualized from the standpoint of the functions they serve in the family as a system, as well as for individual family members. The assumption is made that problem behaviour evident in the child is the only way some interpersonal functions (e.g. intimacy, distancing, support) can be met among family members. Maladaptive processes within the family are considered to preclude a more direct means of fulfilling these functions. The goal of treatment is to alter interaction and communication patterns in such a way as to foster more adaptive functioning. Treatment is also based on learning theory and focuses on specific stimuli and responses that can be used to produce change. Social-learning concepts and procedures, such as identifying specific behaviours for change and reinforcing new adaptive ways of responding, and empirically evaluating and monitoring change are included in this perspective. Cognitive processes refer to the attributions, attitudes, assumptions, expectations and emotions of the family. Family members may begin treatment with attributions that focus on blaming others or themselves. New perspectives may be needed to help serve as the basis for developing new ways of behaving.

The underlying rationale emphasizes a family systems approach. Treatment strategies draw on findings that underlie PMT in relation to maladaptive and coercive parent–child interactions, discussed previously. FFT views interaction patterns from a broader systems view that focuses also on communication patterns and their meaning. As an illustration of salient constructs, research underlying FFT has found that families of delinquents show higher rates of defensiveness in their communications, both in parent–child and parent–parent interactions, blaming and negative attributions, and also lower rates of mutual support compared to families of nondelinquents (see Alexander & Parsons, 1982). Improving these communication and support functions is a goal of treatment.

Characteristics of treatment

FFT requires that the family see the clinical problem from the relational functions it serves within the family. The therapist points out interdependencies and contingencies between family members in their day-to-day functioning and with specific reference to the problem that has served as the basis for seeking treatment. Once the family sees alternative ways of viewing the problem, the incentive for interacting more constructively is increased.

Treatment is designed to increase reciprocity and positive reinforcement among family members, to establish clear communication, to help specify behaviours that family members desire from each other, to negotiate constructively and to help identify solutions to interpersonal problems. In therapy, family members identify behaviours they would like others to perform. Responses are incorporated into a reinforcement system in the home to promote adaptive behaviour in exchange for privileges. However, the primary focus is within the treatment sessions where family communication patterns are altered directly. During the sessions, the therapist provides social reinforcement (verbal and nonverbal praise) for communications that suggest solutions to problems, clarify problems or offer feedback.

Overview of the evidence

Relatively few outcome studies have evaluated FFT (see Alexander et al., 1994). The available studies have focused on difficult to treat populations (e.g. adjudicated delinquent adolescents, multiple offender delinquents) and have produced relatively clear effects. In controlled study comparisons, FFT has led to greater change than other treatment techniques (e.g. client-centred family groups, psychodynamically oriented family therapy) and various control conditions (e.g. group discussion and expression of feeling, no-treatment control groups). The benefits of treatment have been reflected in improved family communication and interactions and lower rates of referral to and contact of youth with the courts. Moreover gains have been evident in separate studies up to 2.5 years after treatment.

Research has examined processes in therapy to identify in-session behaviours of the therapist and how these influence responsiveness among family members (Alexander et al., 1976; Newberry et al., 1991). For example, providing support and structure and reframing (recasting the attributions and bases of a problem) can influence family member responsiveness and blaming of others. The relations among such variables are complex insofar as the impact of various types of statements (e.g. supportive) can vary as a function of gender of the therapist and family member. Evidence of change in processes proposed to be critical to FFT (e.g. improved communication in treatment, more spontaneous discussion) supports the conceptual view of treatment.

Overall evaluation

Several noteworthy points can be made about FFT. First, the outcome studies indicate that FFT can alter conduct problems among delinquent youth. Several studies have produced consistent effects. Second, the evaluation of processes that contribute to family member responsiveness within the sessions as well as outcome represents a line of work rarely seen among treatment techniques for children and adolescents. Some of this process work has extended to laboratory (analogue) studies to examine more precisely how specific types of therapist statements (e.g. reframing) can reduce blaming among group members (Morris et al., 1991). Third, a treatment manual has been provided (Alexander & Parsons, 1982) to facilitate further evaluation and extension of treatment.

Further work extending FFT to children and to clinic populations would be of interest in addition to the current work with delinquent adolescents. Also, further work on child, parent and family characteristics that moderate outcome would be a next logical step in the existing research programme. Finally, primarily the investigators who pioneered treatment have conducted the few studies available. Replication by others would be important as a way of further establishing the technique.

Multisystemic therapy

Background and underlying rationale

Multisystemic therapy (MST) is a family-systems based approach to treatment (Henggeler & Borduin, 1990; Henggeler et al., 1998). Family approaches maintain that clinical problems of the child emerge within the context of the family and focus on treatment at that level. MST expands on that view by considering the family as one, albeit a very important, system. The child is embedded in a number of systems including the family (immediate and extended family members), peers, schools and neighbourhood. For example, within the context of the family, some tacit alliance between one parent and child may contribute to disagreement and conflict over discipline in relation to the child. Treatment may be required to address the alliance and sources of conflict in an effort to alter child behaviour. Also, child functioning at school may involve limited and poor peer relations; treatment may address these areas as well. Finally, the systems approach entails a focus on the individual's own behaviour insofar as it affects others. Individual treatment of the child or parents may be included in treatment.

Because multiple influences are entailed by the focus of the treatment, many different treatment techniques are used. Thus, MST can be viewed as a package of interventions that are deployed with children and their families. Treatment procedures are used on an 'as needed' basis directed toward addressing individual, family and system issues that may contribute to problem behaviour. The conceptual view focusing on multiple systems and their impact on the individual serves as a basis for selecting multiple and quite different treatment procedures.

Characteristics of treatment

Central to MST is a family-based treatment approach. Several therapy techniques (e.g. joining, reframing, enactment, paradox and assigning specific tasks)
are used to identify problems, increase communication, build cohesion and
alter how family members interact. The goals of treatment are to help the
parents develop behaviours of the adolescent, to overcome marital difficulties
that impede the parents' ability to function as parents, to eliminate negative
interactions between parent and adolescent, and to develop or build cohesion
and emotional warmth among family members.

MST draws on many other techniques as needed to address problems at the
level of individual, family and extrafamily. As prominent examples, PSST, PMT
and marital therapy are used in treatment to alter the response repertoire of the
adolescent, parent–child interactions at home and marital communication,
respectively. In some cases, treatment consists of helping the parents address a
significant domain through practical advice and guidance (e.g. involving the
adolescent in prosocial peer activities at school, restricting specific activities
with a deviant peer group). Although MST includes distinct techniques of other
approaches, it is not a mere amalgamation of them. The focus of treatment is
on interrelated systems and how they affect each other. Domains may be
addressed in treatment (e.g. parent unemployment) because they raise issues
for one or more systems (e.g. parent stress, increased alcohol consumption) and
affect how the child is functioning (e.g. marital conflict, child discipline practices).

Overview of the evidence

Several outcome studies have evaluated MST, primarily with delinquent adolescents with arrest and incarceration histories that include violent crime (e.g.
manslaughter, aggravated assault with intent to kill). MST has led to greater
reductions in delinquency and emotional and behavioural problems and improvements in family functioning in comparison to other procedures, including
'usual services' provided to adolescents (e.g. probation, court-ordered activities
that are monitored such as school attendance), individual counselling and
community-based eclectic treatment (e.g. Borduin et al., 1995; Henggeler et al.,
1986, 1992, 1998). Follow-up studies up to 2, 4 and 5 years later with separate
samples have shown that MST adolescents have lower arrest rates than those
who receive other services (Henggeler, 1994).

Treatment influences critical processes proposed to contribute to deviant
behaviour (Mann et al., 1990). Specifically, parents and teenagers show a
reduction in coalitions (e.g. less verbal activity, conflict and hostility) and

increases in support, and parents show increases in verbal communication and decreases in conflict. Moreover, decreases in adolescent symptoms are positively correlated with increases in supportiveness and decreases in conflict between the mother and father. This work provides an important link between theoretical underpinnings of treatment and outcome effects.

The evidence on behalf of MST has several strengths. The focus on children who are severely impaired (delinquent adolescents with a history of arrest) provides a strong test of treatment. Treatment effects have been replicated across adolescents with different types of problems (e.g. sexual offences, drug use) and with parents who engage in physical abuse or neglect (Borduin et al., 1990; Brunk et al., 1987). Follow-up data have been provided that are much more extensive (up to 5 years later) than what is available for most treatments. Also, the outcome measures have included socially important indices of effectiveness (e.g. arrest records, reinstitutionalization). Another strength is the conceptualization of conduct problems at multiple levels, namely, as dysfunction in relation to the individual, family and extrafamilial systems and the transactions among these. In fact, youths with conduct problems experience dysfunction at multiple levels including individual repertoires, family interactions and extrafamilial systems (e.g. peers, schools, employment among later adolescents). MST begins with the view that many different domains are likely to be relevant; they need to be evaluated and then addressed as needed in treatment.

Several questions or challenges of the approach are noteworthy. First, precisely what techniques are or are not included in the approach need to be made explicit. Second, the decision-making process regarding what treatments to use in a given case is not clear. The guidelines available for the therapist are somewhat general (e.g. focus on developing positive sequences of behaviours between systems such as parent and adolescent) (Henggeler, 1994). Providing interventions as needed is very difficult without a consistent way to assess what is needed, given inherent limits of decision making and perception, even among trained professionals. Third, the administration of MST is demanding in light of the need to provide several different interventions in a high quality fashion. Individual treatments (e.g. PSST, PMT) alone are difficult to provide; multiple combinations invite problems related to providing treatments of high quality, strength, and integrity.

Overall evaluation

MST has provided multiple replications across problems, therapists and settings (Henggeler et al., 1995, 1998). This shows that the treatment and methods of decision making can be extended and that treatment effects are reliable. The same team of researchers has conducted the replications. Replications by others not involved with the original development of the programme is the next logical step. The treatment has already impressive evidence in its behalf and is undergoing further treatment trials. The central issue is understanding what treatment components to provide to whom, how the decisions are made, and to identify whether these rules can be reliable implemented across settings and investigators. These questions ought not detract from the promising evidence that has been provided and the consistency of the outcomes.

Comments on the current evidence

The four interventions highlighted here are among the most well established for the treatment of conduct disorder. Each treatment has controlled trials in its behalf, has replications of treatment effects, and has assessed outcome over the course of follow-up, at least up to a year, but often longer. Moreover, the techniques have been evaluated with children whose aggressive and antisocial behaviour have led to impairment and referral to social services (e.g. clinics, hospitals, courts). In the context of child and adolescent psychotherapy research in general, these characteristics are notable exceptions (Durlak et al., 1995; Kazdin et al., 1990a).

It is possible to make distinctions among the techniques and to provide further comments about their application. Among the techniques covered, PMT is the most well established treatment. This is due in part to the scope of the outcome studies, but also because of the research underlying treatment application (e.g. the role of parent-discipline practices in child antisocial behaviour). Also, the treatment techniques are based on principles and procedures derived from operant conditioning and a great deal is known about their effects in experimental and applied contexts. Among the techniques, FFT is currently the least well studied. PSST and MST continue to receive attention in the literature.

Identifying four promising treatments will raise the obvious questions, namely, among these which is the most effective and when and for whom ought the options be applied. These questions cannot be answered in an informed way at present for three reasons: (1) comparative studies directly contrasting any two or more of the promising treatments have yet to be reported, (2) the samples and recruitment procedures have varied widely among the four treatments and (3) little work is available on moderating variables that would identify which among the treatments works for whom. A few tentative guidelines can be provided. With preadolescent children, PMT is likely to be preferred in light of some evidence that it is especially effective for this age group; MST and FFT have been applied with older, delinquent adolescents and might be treatments of choice with this group. Rather than arguing on the basis of very weak evidence for which among the four treatments might be applied in any given situation, the more stark discrimination is probably the one worth underscoring. It is unclear when another treatment ought to be applied that is not included in this set of promising treatments. Individual and general family counselling, relationship therapy and psychodynamically oriented treatments are still applied in clinical work, although at best none has been identified as even approaching empirically supported treatments (Brestan & Eyberg, 1998).

The discussion has focused on single-modality treatments, with the exception of MST. Conduct-problem children and their families often present multiple problems, as noted at the outset of the chapter. No single treatment modality, however beneficial, is likely to be sufficient. Consequently, efforts have been made to vary treatment or to combine treatment with other procedures. One variation of PMT has been to provide supplementary sessions that address parent and family stressors and conflict often associated with conduct problems. PMT, supplemented with such sessions, compared to PMT alone, has reduced dropping out of treatment, improved clinical outcomes of the children, and increased positive communication and collaboration between the parents (Dadds et al., 1987; Griest et al., 1982; Prinz & Miller, 1994; Webster-Stratton, 1994). PMT has also been combined with PSST; evidence suggests that this combination is more effective than PMT alone, although limited research is available on this point (Kazdin et al., 1992; Webster-Stratton, 1996).

Combined treatments are usually considered as an obvious strategy for the treatment of conduct problems. Yet, there are reasons to proceed cautiously with treatment combinations. First, combined treatments are not always positive or neutral in their effects. In one study, PMT supplemented with adolescent group treatment led to worse outcomes at follow-up than PMT alone (Dishion & Andrews, 1995), a finding possibly due to the untoward peer influences (e.g. engaging in substance use) such groups may foster. Second, combined treatments often consist of diluted versions of the constituent treatments that form the combination. That is, two treatments are squeezed into a space (e.g. number of sessions, weeks or months of treatment) that are otherwise used for one treatment. Unless the duration of treatment is extended to accommodate the full regimens of individual treatments, there are a priori reasons to be concerned about what a combined version can accomplish.

Finally, we know that many youth can profit from single-modality treatments such as PMT or PSST, even though the combination may be superior for many youth. Clearly the task is to identify who can profit from single modality treatments and who requires a combined treatment approach (Kazdin, 1996a). Combined treatments are more costly and there is no need to apply them in cases where they are not likely to provide a significant increment in outcome benefits.

Limitations of the evidence

Assessment of outcome domains

Even though the treatments reviewed above have made remarkable gains, they also bear limitations worth highlighting. A significant issue for each of the treatments and indeed for child therapy research more generally pertains to the focus of outcome assessment. In the majority of child therapy studies, child symptoms are the exclusive focus of outcome assessment (Kazdin et al., 1990a). Obviously, reductions in core symptoms of conduct disorder are critical. Because most children referred clinically are likely to have comorbid disorders, reductions across a broad range of symptoms is important to demonstrate. Even so, other domains such as prosocial behaviour and academic functioning are likely to be important as well. Indeed, they may relate to current and long-term adjustment (Asher & Coie, 1990).

Perhaps the greatest single deficit in the evaluation of treatment is absence of attention to impairment, i.e. the extent to which the individual's functioning in everyday life is impeded. For a child or adolescent, meeting role demands at home and at school, interacting prosocially and adaptively with others, and being restricted in the settings, situations and experiences in which one can function can vary considerably among children with a given disorder or problem. Impairment is related to, but distinguishable from, symptoms or meeting criteria for a disorder (Sanford et al., 1992) and contributes significantly to the likelihood that a child is referred for mental health services (Bird et al., 1990). A significant issue from the standpoint of treatment is the extent to which functioning is impaired initially and improved by treatment. Assessing impairment and moving individuals toward reduced impairment may be a considerable accomplishment of treatment. By singling out impairment, I do not intend to imply that one criterion (impairment) ought to replace another (symptoms). Just the opposite, a broad range of outcome criteria is relevant in developing and identifying effective treatments.

Beyond child functioning, parent and family functioning may also be relevant. Parents and family members of conduct-disordered children often experience dysfunction (e.g. psychiatric impairment and marital conflict). Also, the problem behaviours of the child often are part of complex, dynamic and reciprocal influences that affect all relations in the home. Consequently, parent and family functioning and the quality of life for family members are relevant outcomes and may be appropriate goals for treatment.

In general, there are many outcomes that are of interest in evaluating treatment. From existing research we already know that the conclusions reached about a given treatment can vary depending on the outcome criterion. Within a given study, one set of measures (e.g. child functioning) may show no differences between two treatments but another measure (e.g. family functioning) may show that one treatment is clearly better than the other (Kazdin et al., 1989, 1992; Szapocznik et al., 1989). Thus, in examining different outcomes of interest, we must be prepared for different conclusions that these outcomes may yield.

Magnitude and durability of therapeutic change

Promising treatments have achieved change, but do changes make a difference in the lives of the treated children? Clinical significance refers to the practical value or importance of the effect of an intervention, that is, whether it makes any 'real' difference to the patients or to others with whom they interact (Kazdin, 1998). Clinical significance is important because it is quite possible for treatment effects to be statistically significant, but not to have impact on most or any of the cases in a way that improves their functioning or adjustment in daily life.

There are several ways to evaluate clinical significance, including: (a) the extent to which or whether initially deviant children return to normative levels of functioning on standardized measure; (b) the amount of change individuals make from pre- to posttreatment, in standard deviation units, on the outcome measures; (c) whether children no longer meet criteria for a diagnosis at the end of treatment; (d) whether others in contact with the client judge the difference to be important or obvious; and (e) changes on measures of clear social interest (e.g. arrest, truancy, rehospitalization) (Kazdin, 1998). The most common method is to consider the extent to which children function at normative levels at the end of treatment (i.e. compared to same age and sex peers who are functioning well). This is particularly useful as a criterion in relation to children and adolescents because base rates of emotional and behavioural problems can vary greatly as a function of age. Promising treatments occasionally have shown that treatment returns individuals to normative levels in relation to behavioural problems and prosocial functioning at home and at school. However, the majority of studies have not invoked clinical significance as an outcome criterion (Kazdin et al., 1990a).

Although the goal of treatment is to effect clinically significant change, other less dramatic goals are not trivial. For many conduct-disordered children, symptoms may escalate, comorbid diagnoses (e.g. substance abuse, depression) may emerge and family dysfunction may increase. Also, such children are at risk for teen marriage, dropping out of school, and running away. If treatment were to achieve stability in symptoms and family life and to prevent or delimit future dysfunction, that would be a significant achievement. The reason evaluation is so critical to the therapeutic enterprise is to identify whether treatment makes a difference because 'making a difference' can have many meanings that are important in the treatment of conduct disorder.

In addition to magnitude of change, significant questions remain about the durability of change. Promising treatments have included follow-up assessment, usually up to a year after treatment. Yet, conduct disorder has a poor long-term prognosis, so it is especially important to identify whether treatment has enduring effects. Much longer follow-up evaluations are needed than those currently available. Follow-up data are important in part because the conclusions about the effects of different treatments may vary greatly, depending on when the assessments are conducted (Kolvin et al., 1981; Meyers et al., 1996; Newman et al., 1997). Thus, even if two techniques are equally effective immediately after treatment, the course of change during follow-up may differ considerably. It may be unrealistic to demand long-term follow-up from all treatment trials. In its stead, data can be collected on two or a few occasions after treatment (e.g. each spanning several months) to identify the function or course of change once treatment has terminated. The trajectory provided by these data points does not necessarily convey the long-term impact, but provides excellent information about the likely course. Apart from conclusions about treatment, follow-up may provide important information that permits differentiation among children. Over time, children who maintain the benefits of treatment may differ in important ways from those who do not. Understanding who responds and who responds more or less well to a particular treatment can be very helpful in understanding, treating and preventing conduct disorder.

Attrition and subject selection bias

Follow-up data are invariably difficult to obtain, but perhaps especially so because aggression and antisocial behaviour are associated with higher rates of dropping out (Capaldi & Patterson, 1987; Kaminer et al., 1992). Dropping out of treatment has broader effects than those associated with follow-up. In child and adolescent therapy research, among families that begin treatment, 40–60% terminate prematurely (Kazdin, 1996b; Wierzbicki & Pekarik, 1993).

Many parent and family factors predict premature termination from treatment, including socioeconomic disadvantage, characteristics of the family constellation (younger mothers, single-parent families), high parent stress, adverse child-rearing practices (e.g. harsh punishment, poor monitoring and supervision of the child), and parent history of antisocial behaviour (Kazdin et al., 1993, 1994). Child characteristics that predict early termination from treatment include comorbidity (multiple diagnoses and symptoms across a range of disorders), severity of delinquent and antisocial behaviour, and poor academic functioning. The accumulation of these factors places families at increased risk for dropping out of treatment within the first few weeks of treatment. Interestingly, many of the child, parent and family factors that predict premature termination from treatment are the same factors that portend a poor response to treatment and poor long-term prognosis (Dadds & McHugh, 1992; Dumas & Wahler, 1983; Kazdin, 1995a; Webster-Stratton, 1985; Webster-Stratton & Hammond, 1990).

The cases who terminate early are those who evince the greatest impairment in parent, family and child characteristics. In clinical work, the usual impression is that individuals who drop out of treatment are much worse off than those who have remained in treatment. Our own work suggests that this is true, but due primarily to the fact that those who drop out are more severely impaired to begin with (Kazdin et al., 1994). The matter is complex insofar as our most recent work suggests that a small proportion of families who drop out have significantly improved, and a small proportion of families who have completed treatment have not significantly improved (Kazdin & Wassell, 1998). Although there may be many reasons why families drop out of treatment, our work has suggested that families often experience many barriers to participation in treatment, including stressors and obstacles associated with coming to treatment, perceptions that treatment is demanding or not especially relevant to the child's problems, and a poor relationship of the parent with the therapist (Kazdin et al., 1997a, b).

Attrition raises significant issues for interpretation of the outcome research. Attrition or loss of participants can affect virtually all facets of experimental validity by altering random composition of the groups and group equivalence (internal validity), limiting the generality of findings to a special group (e.g. those subjects who are persistent or especially compliant) (external validity), raising the prospect that the intervention, combined with special subject characteristics, accounts for conclusions (external and construct validity), and reducing sample size and power or by systematically changing the variability within the sample (statistical conclusion validity) (see Kazdin, 1998). In the usual study, data analyses are used to show that dropouts are not different from the nondropouts or that dropouts from one group are no different from dropouts from another group. However, this is not particularly helpful in interpreting the results in light of the small sample sizes for such comparisons. For the outcome studies reviewed previously, the impact of attrition is difficult to evaluate. Obviously, there are very few treatment outcome data on dropouts (Kazdin et al., 1994). If it is the case that more severe cases drop out, then conclusions about the benefits of treatment may need to be tempered.

Developmental issues and perspectives

A conspicuous limitation of current evidence is the absence of research that integrates developmental perspectives and issues with treatment. That is, among the promising treatments and lines of research, there is little attention to the relative utility of different treatments for youth at different points in development or how a given treatment might be modified in light of develop- mental considerations. Conceptual integration of developmental themes re- lated to such areas as social and cognitive development, attachment, sibling relations, for example, with treatment would be very important.

The closest the literature comes to developmental issues has been the evaluation of age as a variable in relation to treatment outcome. As noted previously, parent training has been found to be more effective for younger children than for adolescents (Dishion & Patterson, 1992) and problem-solving skills training has been found to be more effective for older children than for younger children (Durlak et al., 1991). These effects are not well-established and multiple factors likely to be confounded with age would need to be partialled out. For example, the prevalence rates of conduct disorder for boys and girls and the types of conduct problems vary by age.

As a general guideline, broad constructs such as age may be a useful beginning point for research. Yet, it is important to disaggregate broad con- structs, to identify individual components and their contribution to the out- come, and to understand processes involved that account for the relations. If age is included as a variable, it is preferable to identify and to assess specific processes or components that are predicted to underlie age-related effects, to hypothesize and to specify why the differences or effects would occur, and then to show the relation of these processes to the outcomes or dependent measures. Treatment research has yet to look at processes associated with and responsible for therapeutic change, leaving aside those that might be specifically processes that are associated with different phases, levels or types of development.

There is keen interest in the developmentally relevant distinction of early (childhood) and late (adolescent) onset conduct disorder, as mentioned further later. This distinction may prove to be very important. An issue of significance in the treatment literature is the fact that most conduct-disordered children who come for treatment are child-onset cases (e.g. between the ages of 6–11). Subtyping this group may prove to be quite important. In our own work, severity of dysfunction (e.g. number of conduct problem symptoms), how early the onset is, and number of symptoms from other disorders (e.g. another to consider comorbidity) relate to treatment responsiveness, but these distinctions have not been widely studied nor are conceptually very enlightening nor developmentally informed. Much more work is needed related to child development and decision making about which treatments to apply and when over the course of development.

General comments

In light of the above comments, clearly even the most promising treatments have several limitations. Yet, it is critical to place these in perspective. As noted previously, the most commonly used treatments in clinical practice have rarely been tested in controlled outcome studies showing that they achieve therapeutic change in referred (or nonreferred) samples of children with conduct disorder (Kazdin et al., 1990a, b). Many forms of behaviour therapy have a rather extensive literature showing that various techniques (e.g. reinforcement programmes, social skills training) can alter aggressive and other antisocial behaviours (Kazdin, 1985; McMahon & Wells, 1989). Yet, the focus has tended to be on isolated behaviours, rather than a constellation of symptoms. Also, durable changes among clinical samples rarely have been shown.

Pharmacotherapy represents a line of work of some interest. For one reason, stimulant medication (e.g. methylphenidate), frequently used with children diagnosed with Attention-Deficit/Hyperactivity Disorder, has some impact on aggressive and other antisocial behaviours (see Hinshaw, 1994). This is interesting in part because such children often have a comorbid diagnosis of Conduct Disorder. Still no strong evidence exists that stimulant medication can alter the constellation of symptoms (e.g. fighting, stealing) associated with conduct disorder. A review of various medications for aggression in children and adolescents has raised possible leads, but the bulk of research consists of uncontrolled studies (see Campbell & Cueva, 1995; Stewart et al., 1990).

Controlled studies (e.g. random assignment, placebo-controls) have shown anti-aggressive effects with some medications (e.g. lithium; Campbell et al., 1995) but not others (e.g. carbamazepine; Cueva et al., 1996). Reliable psychopharmacological treatments for aggression, leaving aside the constellation of conduct disorder (e.g. firesetting, stealing and so on), remain to be developed.

Clearly it is premature to consider only a few candidates as viable options for the treatment of conduct disorder and none of the treatments mentioned here ought to be ruled out as potential treatments. The current status of the literature provides an excellent base for evaluating treatment. It is clear that any new interventions or combinations of existing interventions that are proposed, ought to be compared against one of the treatments highlighted earlier. We know that PMT, PSST, FFT and MST can achieve marked changes, that they have often surpassed the impact of various forms of standard or routine clinical care, and no treatment. New treatments have these promising interventions as a viable comparison condition.

Developing more effective treatments

Predictors of treatment response

We have known for many years that the critical question of psychotherapy is not what technique is effective, but rather what technique works for whom, under what conditions and as administered by whom (Kiesler, 1971; Paul, 1967). The adult psychotherapy literature has focused on a range of questions to identify factors (e.g. patient, therapist, treatment process) that contribute to outcome. The child and adolescent therapy research has been devoted almost exclusively to questions about treatment technique, with scant attention to the role of child, parent, family and therapist factors that may moderate outcome (Kazdin et al., 1990a).

In the case of conduct disorder, a few studies have looked at who responds to treatment, mostly in the context of parent management training and problem-solving skills training. Although much more work is needed, current evidence suggests that many of the risk factors for onset of conduct disorder and poor long-term prognosis play a role in responsiveness to treatment (Dumas & Wahler, 1983; Kazdin, 1995a; Webster-Stratton, 1985). Early onset and more severe child antisocial behaviour, comorbid diagnoses, child academic impairment, socioeconomic disadvantage, single-parent families, parental stress (perceived) and life events, and parent history of antisocial behaviour in their childhood portend limited responsiveness to treatment. Our own work has shown that even those children with multiple risk factors still improve with treatment, but the changes are not as great as those achieved for cases with fewer risk factors. Currently, we do not know whether these factors affect responsiveness to any treatment or to particular forms of treatment.

In current subtyping of conduct-disordered youths, early (childhood) and later (adolescent) onset conduct disorder are distinguished (Hinshaw et al., 1993; Moffitt, 1993). Early-onset conduct-disordered children are characterized by aggressive behaviour, neuropsychological dysfunction (in 'executive' functions), a much higher ratio of boys to girls, and a poor long-term prognosis. Later-onset adolescents (onset at about age 15) are characterized more by delinquent activity (theft, vandalism), a more even distribution of boys and girls and a more favourable prognosis. The subtype and associated characteristics are by no means firmly established (Moffitt, 1993; Patterson et al., 1989). Moreover, the subtyping is of little help in distinguishing among the vast array of child-onset cases. Yet, at present, different ways of subtyping may be worth pursuing as a way of predicting response to treatment.

Addressing comorbidity

Comorbidity has been conceived of rather narrowly, namely, the presence of two or more disorders. In relation to treatment research and practice, there may be value in extending the notion more broadly. It is likely that children have many symptoms from many different disorders, even though they might not meet the criteria for each of the disorders. Indeed, in our research we have found the total number of symptoms across the range of disorders to be a more sensitive predictor of treatment outcome than the presence of comorbid disorders or the number of diagnoses. Although the number of disorders may be important, symptoms across the full range of disorders is noteworthy as well.

It may be useful to expand the notion of comorbidity well beyond psychiatric symptoms and diagnoses in light of the domains of impairment affected by the disorder. These domains can include other disorders (e.g. depression, substance abuse), learning difficulties (specific reading disorders, language delays, learning disability), dysfunctional peer relations (e.g. rejection, absence of prosocial friends), and perhaps deficits in prosocial activities (e.g. participation in school, athletic and extracurricular events). Problems or dysfunctions in each of these domains, apart from conduct disorder symptoms themselves, can influence the effects of treatment and long-term prognosis.

At present, research has not provided guidelines for how to address comorbid conditions. Indeed, much of the treatment research has eschewed diagnosis, so the number or proportions of youth who meet criteria for any disorder is usually unclear (Kazdin et al., 1990a). We can say very little at this point about whether comorbid conditions invariably influence outcome, whether the influence and direction of that influence vary by the specific comorbid condition, and how to alter treatment in light of these conditions. This area of work represents a major deficiency in the knowledge base among even the most promising treatments for conduct disorder.

New models of delivering treatment

The model of treatment delivery in current research is to provide a relatively brief and time-limited intervention. In child therapy research, the usual regimen of treatment is 8–10 sessions (Kazdin et al., 1990a). For several clinical dysfunctions or for a number of children with a particular dysfunction such as conduct disorder, the course of maladjustment may be long-term. In such cases, the notion of providing a brief, time-limited treatment may very much limit outcome effects. Even if a great combination of various psychotherapies were constructed, administration in the time-limited fashion might have the usual, checkered yield. More extended and enduring treatment in some form may be needed to achieve clinically important effects with the greatest number of children. Two ways of delivering extended treatment illustrate the point.

The first variation might be referred to as a continued-care model. The model of treatment delivery that may be needed can be likened to the model used in the treatment of diabetes mellitus. With diabetes, ongoing treatment (insulin) is needed to ensure that the benefits of treatment are sustained. The benefits of treatment would end with discontinuation of treatment. Analogously, in the context of conduct disorder, a variation of ongoing treatment may be needed. Perhaps after the child is referred, treatment is provided to address the current crises and to have impact on functioning at home, at school and in the community. After improvement is achieved, treatment is modified rather than ended. At that point, the child could enter into maintenance therapy, i.e. continued treatment perhaps in varying schedules ('doses'). Treatment would continue but perhaps on a more intermittent basis. Continued treatment in this fashion has been effective in treating recurrent depression in adults (Frank et al., 1992) and has evidence as an effective model for treating depression in children (Kroll et al., 1996). Obviously, the use of ongoing treatment is not advocated in cases where there is evidence that brief and time-limited treatment is effective. Beginning with a model of brief and time-limited treatment may be quite reasonable, but alternative models ought to be tested as well.

A variation of continued treatment might be referred to as a dental-care model. An alternative to continued treatment is to provide treatment followed by systematic case monitoring. After initial treatment and demonstrated improvement in functioning in everyday life, treatment is suspended. At this point, the child's functioning begins to be monitored regularly (e.g. every 3 months) and systematically (with standardized measures). The assessment need not involve an extensive battery, but may reflect screening items to assess functioning of the child at home and at school. Treatment could be provided as needed based on the assessment data or emergent issues raised by the family, teachers, or others. This is similar to the model for dental care in the United States in which 'check-ups' are recommended every 6 months; an intervention is provided if, and as, needed based on these periodic checks.

Obviously, the use of ongoing treatment is not advocated in cases where there is evidence that short-term treatment is effective. A difficulty with most of the research on treatment of conduct disorder, including treatments reviewed previously, is that they are relatively brief and time limited. Without considering alternative models of delivery, current treatments may be quite limited in the effects they can produce. Although more effective treatments are sorely needed, the way of delivering currently available treatments ought to be reconsidered.

Conclusions

The treatment challenges that conduct disorder poses are well known. The children referred for treatment often experience dysfunction and impairment in multiple domains, including comorbid disorders, learning and academic difficulties, dysfunctional peer relations and deficits in prosocial activities. Family morbidity is no less significant for developing and evaluating treatment for conduct disorder. There is likely to be a high rate of dysfunction among family members and deleterious influences (e.g. risk factors) in the contexts in which children live (e.g. low socioeconomic status, high levels of stress, poor or violent neighbourhoods). It is not necessarily the case that all influences need to be addressed in treatment. At the same time, child, parent and contextual influences cannot be neglected either in the formulation of treatment or the evaluation of potential moderators of treatment outcome.

Treatment of conduct disorder has progressed significantly. There are promising treatments with evidence on their behalf, based on randomized controlled trials with clinical samples; treatment effects have been replicated and follow-up data up to a few years support the effects of treatment. Among available treatments for conduct disorder, clearly parent management training, problem-solving skills training, functional family therapy and multisystemic therapy are the treatments of choice. It is of course one thing to note that some techniques have much more and better evidence on their behalf and that treatments have led to significant changes, but quite another to note that we have effective treatments for conduct disorder. There are still basic questions that remain, even among the most promising treatments. We do not know the long-term effects of treatment, the individuals for whom some treatments are likely to be effective and how the techniques achieve their change. Unfortunately, treatment research tends to ignore these questions (see Kazdin, 1997a, 2000).

Significant issues remain to be addressed to accelerate advances in treatment. Evaluating multiple outcome domains, the clinical impact of treatment effects, and long-term maintenance were three areas identified as priorities. Until research better evaluates these issues, we cannot yet say that one intervention can ameliorate conduct disorder and overcome the poor long-term prognosis. On the other hand, much can be said. Treatments are currently available with strong evidence on their behalf. This evidence provides an important set of comparison conditions as investigators propose new techniques and variations and combinations of existing techniques for the treatment of conduct disorder. Any new technique that can be shown to surpass the effects of those obtained with PMT, PSST, FFT or MST in randomized controlled trials, with clinic samples, and follow-up data would be a major advance. The current data also provide important information for clinical application particularly in a climate where there is a keen interest in validated or empirically based treatments (Nathan & Gorman, 1998; Roth & Fonagy, 1996; Task Force on Promotion and Dissemination of Psychological Procedures, 1995). It is important that current results serve as a guide to clinical practice. Much of what is practiced in clinical settings is based on psychodynamically oriented treatment, general relationship counselling and family therapy (other than FFT and MST, highlighted previously). These and other procedures, alone and in various combinations in which they are often used, have rarely been evaluated empirically. The absence of evidence is not tantamount to ineffectiveness. At the same time, promising treatments reviewed in this chapter have advanced considerably and ought to serve as the initial treatment of choice.

Acknowledgements

Completion of this paper was facilitated by support from the Leon Lowenstein Foundation, the William T. Grant Foundation and the National Institute of Mental Health. Support for this work is gratefully acknowledged.

REFERENCES

Alexander, J.F., Barton, C., Schiavo, R.S. & Parsons, B.V. (1976). Systems-behavioral intervention with families of delinquents: Therapist characteristics, family behavior, and outcome. *Journal of Consulting and Clinical Psychology, 44*, 656–64.

Alexander, J.F., Holtzworth-Munroe, A. & Jameson, P.B. (1994). The process and outcome of marital and family therapy research: review and evaluation. In A.E. Bergin & S.L. Garfield (Eds.), *Handbook of Psychotherapy and Behavior Change* (4th edn, pp. 595–630). New York: John Wiley & Sons.

Alexander, J.F. & Parsons, B.V. (1982). *Functional Family Therapy.* Monterey, CA: Brooks/Cole.

American Psychiatric Association (1994). *Diagnostic and Statistical Manual of Mental Disorders* (4th edn) (DSM–IV). Washington, DC: APA.

Asher, S.R. & Coie, J.D. (Eds.) (1990). *Peer Rejection in Childhood.* New York: Cambridge University Press.

Baer, R.A. & Nietzel, M.T. (1991). Cognitive and behavioral treatment of impulsivity in children: A meta-analytic review of the outcome literature. *Journal of Clinical Child Psychology, 20*, 400–12.

Bank, L., Marlowe, J.H., Reid, J.B., Patterson, G.R. & Weinrott, M.R. (1991). A comparative evaluation of parent-training interventions for families of chronic delinquents. *Journal of Abnormal Child Psychology, 19*, 15–33.

Bell, R.Q. & Harper, L. (1977). *Child Effects on Adults.* New York: John Wiley & Sons.

Bennett-Johnson, S. (1996). *Task Force on Effective Psychosocial Interventions: A Lifespan Perspective – A Report to the Division 12 Board.* Washington, DC: American Psychological Association.

Bird, H.R., Yager, T.J., Staghezza, B., et al. (1990). Impairment in the epidemiological measurement of psychopathology in the community. *Journal of the American Academy of Child and Adolescent Psychiatry, 29*, 796–803.

Borduin, C.M., Henggeler, S.W., Blaske, D.M. & Stein, R. (1990). Multisystemic treatment of adolescent sexual offenders. *International Journal of Offender Therapy and Comparative Criminology, 34*, 105–13.

Borduin, C.M., Mann, B.J., Cone, L.T., et al. (1995). Multisystemic treatment of serious juvenile offenders: Long-term prevention of criminality and violence. *Journal of Consulting and Clinical Psychology, 63*, 569–78.

Brandt, D.E. & Zlotnick, S.J. (1988). *The Psychology and Treatment of the Youthful Offender.* Springfield, IL: Charles C. Thomas.

Brestan, E.V. & Eyberg, S.M. (1998). Effective psychosocial treatment of conduct-disordered children and adolescents: 29 years, 82 studies, and 5275 kids. *Journal of Clinical Child Psychology, 27*, 180–9.

Brunk, M., Henggeler, S.W. & Whelan, J.P. (1987). A comparison of multisystemic therapy and parent training in the brief treatment of child abuse and neglect. *Journal of Consulting and Clinical Psychology, 55*, 311–18.

Campbell, M., Adams, P.B., Small, A.M., et al. (1995). Lithium in hospitalized aggressive children with conduct disorder: A double-blind and placebo-controlled study. *Journal of the American Academy of Child and Adolescent Psychiatry, 34,* 445–53.

Campbell, M. & Cueva, J.E. (1995). Psychopharmacology in child and adolescent psychiatry: A review of the past seven years. Part II. *Journal of the American Academy of Child and Adolescent Psychiatry, 34,* 1262–72.

Capaldi, D. & Patterson, G.R. (1987). An approach to the problem of recruitment and retention rates for longitudinal research. *Behavioral Assessment, 9,* 169–87.

Chambless, D.L. & Hollon, S. (1998). Defining empirically supported therapies. *Journal of Consulting and Clinical Psychology, 66,* 7–18.

Chambless, D.L., Sanderson, W.I.C., Shoham, V., et al. (1996). An update on empirically validated treatments. *Clinical Psychologist, 49,* 5–18.

Cooper, J.O., Heron, T.E. & Heward, W.L. (1987). *Applied Behavior Analysis.* Columbus, OH: Merrill.

Crick, N.R. & Dodge, K.A. (1994). A review and reformulation of social information processing mechanisms in children's social adjustment. *Psychological Bulletin, 115,* 74–101.

Cueva, J.E., Overall, J.E., Small, A.M., et al. (1996). Carbamazepine in aggressive children with conduct disorder: A double-blind and placebo controlled study. *Journal of the American Academy of Child and Adolescent Psychiatry, 35,* 480–90.

Cunningham, C.E., Bremner, R. & Boyle, M. (1995). Large group community-based parenting programs for families of preschoolers at risk for disruptive behaviour disorders: Utilization, cost effectiveness, and outcome. *Journal of Child Psychology and Psychiatry, 36,* 1141-59.

Dadds, M.R. & McHugh, T.A. (1992). Social support and treatment outcome in behavioral family therapy for child conduct problems. *Journal of Consulting and Clinical Psychology, 60,* 252–9.

Dadds, M.R., Schwartz, S. & Sanders, M.R. (1987). Marital discord and treatment outcome in behavioral treatment of child conduct disorders. *Journal of Consulting and Clinical Psychology, 55,* 396–403.

Dishion, T.J. & Andrews, D.W. (1995). Preventing escalation in problem behaviors with high-risk young adolescents: Immediate and 1-year outcomes. *Journal of Consulting and Clinical Psychology, 63,* 538–48.

Dishion, T.J. & Patterson, G.R. (1992). Age effects in parent training outcomes. *Behavior Therapy, 23,* 719–29.

Dishion, T.J., Patterson, G.R. & Kavanagh, K.A. (1992). An experimental test of the coercion model: Linking theory, measurement, and intervention. In J. McCord & R.E. Tremblay (Eds.), *Preventing Antisocial Behavior* (pp. 253–82). New York: Guilford Press.

Dumas, J.E. (1989). Treating antisocial behavior in children: Child and family approaches. *Clinical Psychology Review, 9,* 197–222.

Dumas, J.E. & Wahler, R.G. (1983). Predictors of treatment outcome in parent training: Mother insularity and socioeconomic disadvantage. *Behavioral Assessment, 5,* 301–13.

Durlak, J.A., Fuhrman, T. & Lampman, C. (1991). Effectiveness of cognitive-behavioral therapy for maladapting children: A meta-analysis. *Psychological Bulletin, 110,* 204–14.

Durlak, J.A., Wells, A.M., Cotten, J.K. & Johnson, S. (1995). Analysis of selected methodological issues in child psychotherapy research. *Journal of Clinical Child Psychology, 24,* 141–8.

Eyberg, S.M. & Boggs, S.R. (1989). Parent training for oppositional-defiant preschoolers. In C.E. Schaefer & J.M. Briesmeister (Eds.), *Handbook of Parent Training: Parents as Co-therapists for Children's Behavior Problems* (pp. 105–32). New York: John Wiley & Sons.

Feindler, E.L. & Ecton, R.B. (1986). *Adolescent Anger Control: Cognitive–Behavioral Techniques.* Elmsford, NY: Pergamon.

Finch, A.J., Jr., Nelson, W.M. & Ott, E.S. (1993). *Cognitive–Behavioral Procedures with Children and Adolescents: A Practical Guide.* Needham Heights, MA: Allyn & Bacon.

Forehand, R. & Long, N. (1996). *Parenting the Strong-willed Child.* Chicago: Contemporary Books.

Forehand, R. & McMahon, R.J. (1981). *Helping the Noncompliant Child: A Clinician's Guide to Parent Training.* New York: Guilford Press.

Forgatch, M.S. (1991). The clinical science vortex: A developing theory of antisocial behavior. In D.J. Pepler & K.H. Rubin (Eds.), *The Development and Treatment of Childhood Aggression* (pp. 291–315). Hillsdale, NJ: Lawrence Erlbaum.

Forgatch, M. & Patterson, G. (1989). *Parents and Adolescents Living Together – Part 2: Family Problem Solving.* Eugene, OR: Castalia Publishing Company.

Frank, E., Johnson, S. & Kupfer, D.J. (1992). Psychological treatments in prevention of relapse. In S.A. Montgomery & F. Rouillon (Eds.), *Long-term Treatment of Depression* (pp. 197–228). Chichester: John Wiley & Sons.

Graziano, A.M. & Diament, D.M. (1992). Parent behavioral training: An examination of the paradigm. *Behavior Modification, 16,* 3–38.

Griest, D.L., Forehand, R., Rogers, T., et al. (1982). Effects of parent enhancement therapy on the treatment outcome and generalization of a parent training program. *Behaviour Research and Therapy, 20,* 429–36.

Hanf, C. (1969). *A two-stage program for modifying maternal controlling during mother-child interaction.* Paper presented at the meeting of the Western Psychological Association, Vancouver, British Columbia.

Henggeler, S.W. (1994). *Treatment Manual for Family Preservation using Multisystemic Therapy.* Charleston, SC: Medical University of South Carolina, South Carolina Health and Human Services Finance Commission.

Henggeler, S.W. & Borduin, C.M. (1990). *Family Therapy and Beyond: A Multisystemic Approach to Teaching the Behavior Problems of Children and Adolescents.* Pacific Grove, CA: Brooks/Cole.

Henggeler, S.W., Melton, G.B. & Smith, L.A. (1992). Family preservation using multisystemic therapy: An effective alternative to incarcerating serious juvenile offenders. *Journal of Consulting and Clinical Psychology, 60,* 953–61.

Henggeler, S.W., Rodick, J.D., Borduin, C.M., et al. (1986). Multisystemic treatment of juvenile offenders: Effects on adolescent behavior and family interaction. *Developmental Psychology, 22,* 132–41.

Henggeler, S.W., Schoenwald, S.K. & Pickrel, S.A.G. (1995). Multisystemic therapy: Bridging the gap between university- and community-based treatment. *Journal of Consulting and Clinical Psychology, 63,* 709–17.

Henggeler, S.W., Schoenwald, S.K., Borduin, C.M., Rowland, M.D. & Cunningham, P.B. (1998).

Multisystems Treatment of Antisocial Behaviour in Children and Adolescents. New York: Guilford Press.

Hinshaw, S.P. (1994). *Attention Deficits and Hyperactivity in Children*. Thousand Oaks, CA: Sage.

Hinshaw, S.P., Lahey, B.B. & Hart, E.L. (1993). Issues of taxonomy and comorbidity in the development of conduct disorder. *Development and Psychopathology, 5*, 31–49.

Horton, L. (1984). The father's role in behavioral parent training: A review. *Journal of Clinical Child Psychology, 13*, 274–9.

Kaminer, Y., Tarter, R.E., Bukstein, O.G. & Kabene, M. (1992). Comparison between treatment completers and noncompleters among dually diagnosed substance-abusing adolescents. *Journal of the American Academy of Child and Adolescent Psychiatry, 31*, 1046–9.

Kazdin, A.E. (1978). *History of Behavior Modification: Experimental Foundations of Contemporary Research*. Baltimore: University Park Press.

Kazdin, A.E. (1985). *Treatment of Antisocial Behavior in Children and Adolescents*. Homewood, IL: Dorsey Press.

Kazdin, A.E. (1988). *Child Psychotherapy: Developing and Identifying Effective Treatments*. Needham Heights, MA: Allyn & Bacon.

Kazdin, A.E. (1993). Treatment of conduct disorder: Progress and directions in psychotherapy research. *Development and Psychopathology, 5*, 277–310.

Kazdin, A.E. (1994a). *Behavior Modification in Applied Settings* (5th edn). Pacific Grove, CA: Brooks/Cole.

Kazdin, A.E. (1994b). Psychotherapy for children and adolescents. In A.E. Bergin & S.L. Garfield (Eds.), *Handbook of Psychotherapy and Behavior Change* (4th edn, pp. 543–94). New York: John Wiley & Sons.

Kazdin, A.E. (1995a). Child, parent, and family dysfunction as predictors of outcome in cognitive–behavioral treatment of antisocial children. *Behaviour Research and Therapy, 33*, 271–81.

Kazdin, A.E. (1995b). *Conduct Disorder in Childhood and Adolescence* (2nd edn). Thousand Oaks, CA: Sage.

Kazdin, A.E. (1996a). Combined and multimodal treatments in child and adolescent psychotherapy: Issues, challenges, and research directions. *Clinical Psychology: Science and Practice, 3*, 69–100.

Kazdin, A.E. (1996b). Dropping out of child psychotherapy: Issues for research and implications for practice. *Clinical Child Psychology and Psychiatry, 1*, 133–56.

Kazdin, A.E. (1997a). A model for developing effective treatments: Progression and interplay of theory, research, and practice. *Journal of Clinical Child Psychology, 26*, 114–29.

Kazdin, A.E. (1997b). Parent management training: Evidence, outcomes, and issues. *Journal of the American Academy of Child and Adolescent Psychiatry, 36*, 1349–56.

Kazdin, A.E. (1998). *Research Design in Clinical Psychology* (3rd edn). Needham Heights, MA: Allyn & Bacon.

Kazdin, A.E. (2000). *Psychotherapy of Children and Adolescents: Directions for Research and Practice*. New York: Oxford University Press.

Kazdin, A.E., Bass, D., Ayers, W.A. & Rodgers, A. (1990a). Empirical and clinical focus of child and adolescent psychotherapy research. *Journal of Consulting and Clinical Psychology, 58*, 729–40.

Kazdin, A.E., Bass, D., Siegel, T. & Thomas, C. (1989). Cognitive–behavioral treatment and relationship therapy in the treatment of children referred for antisocial behavior. *Journal of Consulting and Clinical Psychology, 57*, 522–35.

Kazdin, A.E., Holland, L. & Crowley, M. (1997a). Family experience of barriers to treatment and premature termination from child therapy. *Journal of Consulting and Clinical Psychology, 65*, 453–63.

Kazdin, A.E., Holland, L., Crowley, M. & Breton, S. (1997b). Barriers to Participation in Treatment Scale: Evaluation and validation in the context of child outpatient treatment. *Journal of Child Psychology and Psychiatry, 38*, 1051–62.

Kazdin, A.E., Mazurick, J.L. & Bass, D. (1993). Risk for attrition in treatment of antisocial children and families. *Journal of Clinical Child Psychology, 22*, 2–16.

Kazdin, A.E., Mazurick, J.L. & Siegel, T.C. (1994). Treatment outcome among children with externalizing disorder who terminate prematurely versus those who complete psychotherapy. *Journal of the American Academy of Child and Adolescent Psychiatry, 33*, 549–57.

Kazdin, A.E., Siegel, T.C. & Bass, D. (1990b). Drawing upon clinical practice to inform research on child and adolescent psychotherapy: A survey of practitioners. *Professional Psychology: Research and Practice, 21*, 189–98.

Kazdin, A.E., Siegel, T. & Bass, D. (1992). Cognitive problem-solving skills training and parent management training in the treatment of antisocial behavior in children. *Journal of Consulting and Clinical Psychology, 60*, 733–47.

Kazdin, A.E. & Wassell, G. (1998). Treatment completion and therapeutic change among children referred for outpatient therapy. *Professional Psychology: Research and Practice, 29*, 332–40.

Kazdin, A.E. & Weisz, J.R. (1998). Identifying and developing empirically supported child and adolescent treatments. *Journal of Consulting and Clinical Psychology, 66*, 19–36.

Kendall, P.C. (Ed.). (1991). *Child and Adolescent Therapy: Cognitive–Behavioral Procedures*. New York: Guilford Press.

Kiesler, D.J. (1971). Experimental designs in psychotherapy research. In A.E. Bergin & S.L. Garfield (Eds.), *Handbook of Psychotherapy and Behavior Change: An Empirical Analysis* (pp. 36–74). New York: John Wiley & Sons.

Kolvin, I., Garside, R.F., Nicol, A.E., et al. (1981). *Help Starts Here: The Maladjusted Child in the Ordinary School*. London: Tavistock.

Kroll, L., Harrington, R., Jayson, D., Frazer, J. & Gowers, S. (1996). Pilot study of continuation cognitive–behavior therapy for major depression in adolescents. *Journal of the American Academy of Child and Adolescent Psychiatry, 35*, 1156–61.

Lochman, J.E. & Dodge, K.A. (1994). Social-cognitive processes of severely violent, moderately aggressive, and nonaggressive boys. *Journal of Consulting and Clinical Psychology, 62*, 366–74.

Long, P., Forehand, R., Wierson, M. & Morgan, A. (1994). Does parent training with young noncompliant children have long-term effects? *Behaviour Research and Therapy, 32*, 101–7.

Lonigan, C.J., Elbert, J.C. & Johnson, S.B. (1998). Empirically supported psychosocial interventions for children: An overview. *Journal of Clinical Child Psychology, 27*, 138–45.

Lytton, H. (1990). Child and parent effects in boys' conduct disorder: A reinterpretation. *Developmental Psychology, 26*, 683–97.

Mann, B.J., Borduin, C.M., Henggeler, S.W. & Blaske, D.M. (1990). An investigation of systemic conceptualizations of parent–child coalitions and symptom change. *Journal of Consulting and Clinical Psychology, 58*, 336–44.

McMahon, R.J. & Wells, K.C. (1989). Conduct disorders. In E.J. Mash & R.A. Barkley (Eds.), *Treatment of Childhood Disorders* (pp. 73–132). New York: Guilford Press.

Meyers, A.W., Graves, T.J., Whelan, J.P. & Barclay, D. (1996). An evaluation of television-delivered behavioral weight loss program. Are the ratings acceptable? *Journal of Consulting and Clinical Psychology, 64*, 172–8.

Miller, G.E. & Prinz, R.J. (1990). Enhancement of social learning family interventions for child conduct disorder. *Psychological Bulletin, 108*, 291–307.

Moffitt, T.E. (1993). The neuropsychology of conduct problems. *Development and Psychopathology, 5*, 135–51.

Moffitt, T.E., Caspi, A., Dickson, N., Silva, P. & Stanton, W. (1996). Childhood-onset versus adolescent onset antisocial conduct problems in males; Natural history from ages 3–18. *Development and Psychopathology, 8*, 399–424.

Morris, S.M., Alexander, J.F. & Turner, C.W. (1991). Do reattributions reduce blame? *Journal of Family Psychology, 5*, 192–203.

Nathan, P.W. &. Gorman, J.M. (Eds.) (1998). *A Guide to Treatments that Work*. New York: Oxford University Press.

Newberry, A.M., Alexander, J.F. & Turner, C.W. (1991). Gender as a process variable in family therapy. *Journal of Family Psychology, 5*, 158–75.

Newman, M.G., Kenardy, J., Herman, S. & Taylor, C.B. (1997). Comparison of palmtop-computer-assisted brief cognitive–behavioral treatment to cognitive–behavioral treatment for panic disorder. *Journal of Consulting and Clinical Psychology, 65*, 178–83.

Offord, D., Boyle, M.H., Racine, Y.A., et al. (1992). Outcome, prognosis, and risk in a longitudinal follow-up study. *Journal of the American Academy of Child and Adolescent Psychiatry, 31*, 916–23.

Patterson, G.R. (1976). *Living with Children: New Methods for Parents and Teachers* (revised). Champaign, IL: Research Press.

Patterson, G.R. (1982). *Coercive Family Process*. Eugene, OR: Castalia.

Patterson, G.R., Capaldi, D. & Bank, L. (1991). An early starter model for predicting delinquency. In D.J. Pepler & K.H. Rubin (Eds.), *The Development and Treatment of Childhood Aggression* (pp. 139–68). Hillsdale, NJ: Lawrence Erlbaum.

Patterson, G.R. & Chamberlain, P. (1994). A functional analysis of resistance during parent training therapy. *Clinical Psychology: Science and Practice, 1*, 53–70.

Patterson, G.R., DeBaryshe, B.D. & Ramsey, E. (1989). A developmental perspective on antisocial behavior. *American Psychologist, 44*, 329–35.

Patterson, G.R., Dishion, T.J. & Chamberlain, P. (1993). Outcomes and methodological issues relating to treatment of antisocial children. In T.R. Giles (Ed.), *Handbook of Effective Psychotherapy* (pp. 43–87). New York: Plenum Press.

Patterson, G.R. & Forgatch, M. (1987). *Parents and Adolescents Living Together – Part 1: The Basics*. Eugene, OR: Castalia Publishing Company.

Patterson, G.R., Reid, J.B. & Dishion, T.J. (1992). *Antisocial Boys*. Eugene, OR: Castalia.

Paul, G.L. (1967). Outcome research in psychotherapy. *Journal of Consulting Psychology, 31,* 109–18.

Pepler, D.J. & Rubin, K.H. (Eds.) (1991). *The Development and Treatment of Childhood Aggression.* Hillsdale, NJ: Lawrence Erlbaum.

Prinz, R.J. & Miller, G.E. (1994). Family-based treatment for childhood antisocial behavior: Experimental influences on dropout and engagement. *Journal of Consulting and Clinical Psychology, 62,* 645–50.

Robins, L.N. (1981). Epidemiological approaches to natural history research: Antisocial disorders in children. *Journal of the American Academy of Child Psychiatry, 20,* 566–680.

Robins, L.N. (1991). Conduct disorder. *Journal of Child Psychology and Psychiatry, 32,* 193–212.

Roth, A. & Fonagy, P. (1996). *What Works for Whom: A Critical Review of Psychotherapy Research.* New York: Guilford Press.

Rubin, K.H., Bream, L.A. & Rose-Krasnor, L. (1991). Social problem solving and aggression in childhood. In D.J. Pepler & K.H. Rubin (Eds.), *The Development and Treatment of Childhood Aggression* (pp. 219–48). Hillsdale, NJ: Lawrence Erlbaum.

Ruma, P.R., Burke, R.V. & Thompson, R.W. (1996). Group parent training: Is it effective for children of all ages? *Behavior Therapy, 27,* 159–69.

Sanders, M.R. & Dadds, M.R. (1993). *Behavioral Family Intervention.* Needham Heights, MA: Allyn & Bacon.

Sanford, M.N., Offord, D.R., Boyle, M.H., Peace, A. & Racine, Y.A. (1992). Ontario Child Health Study: Social and school impairments in children aged 6–16 years. *Journal of the American Academy of Child and Adolescent Psychiatry, 31,* 60–7.

Serketich, W.J. & Dumas, J.E. (1996). The effectiveness of behavioral parent training to modify antisocial behavior in children: A meta-analysis. *Behavior Therapy, 27,* 171–86.

Shirk, S.R. (Ed.). (1988). *Cognitive Development and Child Psychotherapy.* New York: Plenum Press.

Shure, M.B. (1992). *I Can Problem Solve (ICPS): An Interpersonal Cognitive Problem Solving Program.* Champaign, IL: Research Press.

Skinner, B.F. (1938). *The Behavior of Organisms: An Experimental Analysis.* New York: Appleton-Century.

Spivack, G. & Shure, M.B. (1982). The cognition of social adjustment: Interpersonal cognitive problem solving thinking. In B.B. Lahey & A.E. Kazdin (Eds.), *Advances in Clinical Child Psychology* (Vol. 5, pp. 323–72). New York: Plenum Press.

Stewart, J.T., Myers, W.C., Burket, R.C. & Lyles, W.B. (1990). A review of the psychopharmacology of aggression in children and adolescents. *Journal of the American Academy of Child and Adolescent Psychiatry, 29,* 269–77.

Stoff, D.M., Breiling, J. & Maser, J.D. (Eds.) (1997). *Handbook of Antisocial Behavior.* New York: John Wiley & Sons.

Szapocznik, J., Rio, A., Murray, E., et al. (1989). Structural family versus psychodynamic child therapy for problematic Hispanic boys. *Journal of Consulting and Clinical Psychology, 57,* 571–8.

Task Force on Promotion and Dissemination of Psychological Procedures (1995). Training in and dissemination of empirically validated psychological treatments: Report and recommendations. *Clinical Psychologist, 48,* 3–23.

Thompson, R.W., Ruma, P.R., Schuchmann, L.F. & Burke, R.V. (1996). A cost-effectiveness evaluation of parent training. *Journal of Child and Family Studies*, *5*, 415–29.

United States Congress, Office of Technology Assessment. (1991). *Adolescent Health*. (OTA-H-468). Washington, DC: US Government Printing Office.

Wahler, R.G. & Dumas, J.E. (1986). Maintenance factors in coercive mother–child interactions: The compliance and predictability hypotheses. *Journal of Applied Behavior Analysis*, *19*, 13–22.

Webster-Stratton, C. (1985). Predictors of treatment outcome in parent training for conduct disordered children. *Behavior Therapy*, *16*, 223–43.

Webster-Stratton, C. (1994). Advancing videotape parent training: A comparison study. *Journal of Consulting and Clinical Psychology*, *62*, 583–93.

Webster-Stratton, C. (1996). Early intervention with videotape modeling: Programs for families of children with oppositional defiant disorder or conduct disorder. In E.D. Hibbs & P. Jensen (Eds.), *Psychosocial Treatment Research of Child and Adolescent Disorders: Empirically Based Strategies for Clinical Practice* (pp. 435–74). Washington, DC: American Psychological Association.

Webster-Stratton, C. & Hammond, M. (1990). Predictors of treatment outcome in parent training for families with conduct problem children. *Behavior Therapy*, *21*, 319–37.

Wierzbicki, M. & Pekarik, G. (1993). A meta-analysis of psychotherapy dropout. *Professional Psychology: Research and Practice*, *24*, 190–5.

16

The prevention of conduct disorder: a review of successful and unsuccessful experiments

David LeMarquand, Richard E. Tremblay and Frank Vitaro

'There is probably no area of behaviour or psychiatric disorder riper for an experimental design than conduct problems'. Lee Robins (Robins, 1992, p. 11) based this opinion on the following arguments: (1) the population at risk is known, (2) we have the appropriate instruments to measure the presence of the problem, (3) there is a large window of opportunity (from age 10 to 16) to evaluate their occurrence and (4) a number of hypothetical causal agents have been identified which are good candidates for prevention: disorganized neighbourhoods, family adversity, poor parenting, cognitive and emotional deficits. Many other calls have been made for preventive trials over several decades, because corrective interventions have not been shown to be generally successful, and because preventive experiments appear the best means of testing hypothetical causes of conduct disorder (Bovet, 1951; Cabot, 1940; Earls, 1986; Farrington et al., 1986; Lipton et al., 1975; McCord, 1978; Tonry et al., 1991).

The aims of this chapter were to identify well designed preventive trials, assess their effectiveness and give examples of successful and unsuccessful interventions in the prevention of conduct problems in children. We expected that a significant research effort had been put forward to implement preventive interventions, since the hypothetical causal agents and the developmental course of conduct disorder have been identified and re-identified over more than a century (Andry, 1960; Carpenter, 1851; Glueck & Glueck, 1934; Hart, 1910; Jenkins & Glickman, 1947; Pitkanen, 1969; Quetelet, 1833; Robins, 1966; Rutter et al., 1981; Shaw & McKay, 1942). Surprisingly, we found relatively few preventive intervention experiments specifically targeting conduct disorder, and still fewer with adequate design characteristics such as random assignment and sufficiently long-term follow-ups to investigate distal outcomes. We actually did not find one adequately designed prevention experiment of conduct disorder which used the DSM or ICD criteria of conduct disorder to assess the effectiveness of the intervention with at least a 1 year follow-up. Despite the dearth of well-designed preventive intervention trials in this area, the first was initiated over 50 years ago, and there has been a distinct resurgence of interest in this area in recent years.

We were able to identify only 20 published experiments which met our minimal methodological requirements. First, the preventive experiments had to be implemented with nonreferred children, to distinguish prevention from treatment experiments. The term 'prevention' is generally reserved for those interventions occurring before the initial onset of a disorder, i.e. before an individual fulfils the criteria for a disorder (Mrazek & Haggerty, 1994). Second, studies were chosen if participants were ages 12 and under at the start of the intervention, to emphasize that the interventions were implemented before the actual onset of the disorder. Third, studies were included if follow-up periods were a minimum of 1 year, to test whether prevention experiments would demonstrate their intended distal effects. We wanted to choose a longer follow-up period as a minimum (3 or 5 years), however this would have reduced the number of available studies to only 13. Finally, only studies employing random assignment, or quasi-experimental designs (pre–post measures in intervention and adequate control groups) were included.

The 20 studies we selected are summarized in Table 16.1. They are arranged first according to intervention type, be they universal, selective or indicated (Gordon, 1983, 1987). A universal preventive intervention is applied to an entire population; a selective preventive intervention is applied to individuals at above average risk for a disorder primarily due to environmental factors; and an indicated preventive intervention is one applied to asymptomatic individuals who manifest a risk factor related to their personal disposition which places them at high risk for the development of a disorder. Indicated preventive interventions can be applied to asymptomatic individuals with markers as well as to symptomatic individuals early in the course of a disorder whose symptoms are not severe enough to warrant a diagnosis (Mrazek & Haggerty, 1994). In Table 16.1, preventive interventions are classified as selective if the participants manifest an environmental risk factor (i.e. a moderating variable, such as poverty) placing them at higher risk for the development of disruptive behaviour. Preventive interventions are classified as indicated if the participants are manifesting personal risk factors (e.g. disruptive behaviour, low IQ). Within intervention type, the studies are arranged according to descending age at which the intervention was implemented. The results represent those at most recent follow-up, unless otherwise specified. Interestingly, only nine of the 20 studies were designed to prevent conduct problems specifically.

Included in Table 16.1 are effect sizes (ESs), calculated for three different types of outcome measures: (a) externalizing behaviour, generally teacher- or parent-rated questionnaire measures of disruptive behaviour; (b) delinquency, representing self-report or officially recorded criminality; and (c) aversive behaviour, representing observer-rated disruptive behaviour. The overall ES for a study represents the average of all ESs calculated for all disruptive behaviour outcome measures. ESs represent the mean of the control group subtracted from the mean of the intervention group, and divided by the pooled within-group standard deviation, and are unweighted (Hedges & Olkin, 1985). They are calculated so that positive scores reflected improvement in the intervention group relative to the controls. ESs of 0.2 are generally considered small, 0.5 medium, and 0.8 large (Cohen, 1977).

Effect sizes were not calculated for one of the studies due to a lack of required data in the report. Slightly more studies in Table 16.1 found positive effects of preventive interventions on disruptive behaviour outcomes. Note however the wide variability in effect sizes, ranging from large effect sizes favouring the intervention group (0.87 for Lochman et al., 1993) to effect sizes indicating the control group did better relative to the intervention group (e.g. −0.31 for Szapocznik et al., 1989). As well, there is wide variability in the types of measures of disruptive behaviour employed. The majority of studies focused on participants who remained in treatment, however in two studies, an intention-to-treat approach was used: analyses included all participants available at follow-up, regardless of attrition from the intervention. Half of the studies included attrition analyses comparing participants assessed at follow-up versus those who dropped out either during the treatment or follow-up period.

Variability can also be observed in the target populations and the content of the intervention programmes. According to Gordon's (1987) classification two studies were considered universal interventions because they were applied to entire populations of children entering school. Eight studies were classified selective interventions since the targets were individuals at high risk due to environmental factors, while the last ten studies were labelled indicated interventions since the targeted children were considered at risk because of personal dispositions.

The two universal interventions targeted children who were age 6 years at the start of the intervention, however one intervention lasted 2 years while the other lasted 6 years. The eight selective interventions targeted preschool children: two targeted pregnant women, one lasting 3 years and the other 5.5 years; five targeted infants and lasted from 8 months to 5 years; while one targeted 4–5-year-olds and lasted 4 months. The ten indicated interventions targeted children aged 3 to 12 years old: three targeted 3–4-year-olds and lasted from 3 months to 2 years; two targeted 7-year-olds, one lasted 10 weeks, the

Table 16.1. Descriptive summary of the preventive intervention studies reviewed

Authors	Sample size at pretest (I = intervention; C = control)	Age at intervention (years)	Design	Type of intervention	Description of intervention	Context of intervention	Length of intervention	Follow-up: length; sample size	Results for disruptive behaviour (I vs. C, at most recent follow-up ES=effect size)	Other results (for intervention group, compared to controls, at latest assessment)
1. Kellam et al. (1994); Dolan et al. (1993)	693 girls and boys; 153 Good Behaviour Game (GBG), 163 Mastery Learning (ML), 377 C	6.6	Random assignment of school classrooms	Universal	GBG: teachers trained to reward teams of children for refraining from maladaptive behaviour. ML: increasing children's academic performance	School	2 years	4 years; 590 children	Externalizing behaviour (ES = 0.08) Decreased teacher-rated aggressive behaviour in males in GBG group with high baseline aggression relative to combined ML and control groups	Decreased depression, shyness; increased school achievement
2. Hawkins et al. (1999); Seattle Development Project	643 (316 girls); 156 full I, 267 late I, 220 C	6	1st graders in 1 school assigned to full I, in 2nd school to C, and in 6 other schools random assignment to full I or C; 5th graders in 18 schools added to late I or C groups	Universal	Teacher training in proactive classroom management, interactive teaching, cooperative learning; parent training in child behaviour management skills; child training in cognitive and social skills by teachers	School, family	6 years	6 years; 598 (299 girls); 149 full I, 243 late I, 206 C	Delinquency (ES = 0.18) Full I students show significantly less self-reported violent delinquency, officially-recorded school misbehaviour Full I students tend toward reduced self-report nonviolent delinquency, police arrests, and official court records	Full I students demonstrate better academic functioning, reduced substance use, and reduced sexual misbehaviour
3. Webster-Stratton (1998)	426 (202 girls); 296 I, 130 C	Mean = 4.7 years	Random assignment of Head Start centres	Selective; Head Start children, many with multiple risk factors for conduct problems	Parent training; fostering parental competence and increasing parents' involvement in children's Head Start preschool experiences teacher training; supporting parents' classroom involvement, strengthening teacher's behavioural management skills	School	4 months	1 year; 296; 189 I, 107 C	Overall ES = −0.06 Externalizing behaviour (ES = 0.01) No differences on mother- or teacher-reported externalizing problems Aversive behaviour (ES = −0.25) Observer-rated home deviant and noncompliant behaviours tended to be lower in both intervention and control groups, with slightly greater reduction in intervention group	Mothers more positive, nurturing, reinforcing and competent, more consistent discipline and appropriate limit-setting; fewer criticisms, less harsh discipline, less physically and verbally negative discipline Children more positive affect, prosocial behaviours; less noncompliance, negative affect

Study	N	Age at start	Assignment	Selection	Intervention	Setting	Duration	Age/N at outcome	Externalizing behaviour	Other outcomes
4. Johnson & Walker (1987); Houston Parent-Child Development Center	Approx. 235 families in five yearly cohorts	1	Random assignment	Selective; low family income, low education, low SES families	Education, parent training, nursery school	Home, day care	2 years	5 to 8 years, 139; 51 (25 girls) I, 88 (47 girls) C	Externalizing behaviour (ES = 0.45) Decreased teacher-rated acting out (obstinacy, disruptiveness, fighting)	Higher teacher-rated considerateness
5. Clarke & Campbell (1998); The Abecedarian Project	111 (59 girls); 57 I, 54 C	Mean = 4.4 m	Random assignment	Selective; children at risk for suboptimal cognitive development due to poverty, social stress	Preschool emphasizing cognitive and motor development, social and self-help skills, and language skills	Daycare	5 years	13 years; 105, 54 I, 51 C	Delinquency (ES = 0.03) No differences in officially-recorded adult criminal charges and arrests (including proportion charged, mean number of charges, mean number of arrests)	At age 15, higher IQ, higher academic achievement, lower proportion of students retained in a grade at least once, higher graduation rate
6. McCarton et al. (1997); Infant Health & Development Program	985 (499 girls), 377 I, 608 C	Birth	Random assignment	Selective; low birth weight infants	Parent training on child development, day care	Home, day care	3 years	5 years; 874 (441 girls); 336 I, 538 C	Externalizing behaviour (ES = -0.05) No change in mother-reported externalizing behaviour	Heavier low birth weight intervention group had higher IQs, better math achievement and vocabulary vs. controls
7. Seitz et al. (1985); Yale Child Welfare Research Project	36 (14 girls); 18 I (7 girls), 18 C (7 girls)	Birth	Matched C group recruited after I complete (no random assignment)	Selective; mothers at poverty level	Education, medical support, parent training, day care	Home, day care	2.5 years	10 years	Externalizing behaviour (ES = 0.80) Better school adjustment (including fewer teacher-rated serious acting out problems, negative attributes); less truancy	Decreased service usage Increased family socioeconomic status Improved parenting style
8. Stone et al. (1988); Mailman Center Program	131 boys and girls; 58 I, 73 C	Birth	Random assignment of teenage mothers	Selective; infants of low SES teenage mothers	Caregiving, developmental milestones information; instruction in infant stimulation exercises	Home, nursery	8 months	5 to 8 years, 61 (28 girls); 31 I, 30 C	Externalizing behaviour (ES = -0.09) No differences on mother-reported number or intensity of child problem behaviors	No group differences on maternal self-esteem, child academic functioning, or child social/emotional functioning

Table 16.1. (cont.)

Authors	Sample size at pretest (I = intervention; C = control)	Age at intervention (years)	Design	Type of intervention	Description of intervention	Context of intervention	Length of intervention	Follow-up: length; sample size	Results for disruptive behaviour (I vs. C, at most recent follow-up ES=effect size)	Other results (for intervention group, compared to controls, at latest assessment)
9. Olds et al. (1997, 1998); Elmira Home Visitation Study	400 pregnant mothers; 184 tx1 + tx2; 100 tx3; 116 tx4	Prenatal	Random assignment	Selective; low SES, single young (<19 years) mothers	tx1 + tx2: sensory and developmental screening, transportation; tx3: tx1 + tx2 plus nurse visits during pregnancy; tx4: tx3 plus nurse visits to age 2, focusing on promoting healthy behaviour in mothers, the care parents provide to their children, maternal personal life-course development	Home	30 months	13 years	Delinquency (ES = na) In total sample, greater incidence of times stopped by police in tx4 vs tx1 + tx2; fewer self-reported arrests, convictions and parole violations in tx4 vs tx1 + tx2 and tx3 vs tx1 + tx2. In low-SES, unmarried subsample, fewer self-reported times ran away in tx4 vs tx1 + tx2 and tx3 vs tx1 + tx2, fewer mother-reported arrests in tx4 vs tx1 + tx2 Externalizing behaviour (ES = na) No differences in self-, parent-, or teacher-reported externalizing behaviour	Children of tx4 women in the low-SES unmarried subsample had fewer sexual partners, less alcohol and cigarette consumption, and less impairment due to alcohol and drugs Women in tx4 had improved health-related behaviour, reduced rates of child abuse/neglect, welfare dependence, fewer subsequent pregnancies, fewer alcohol/drug problems, and less criminal involvement
10. Lally et al. (1988); Syracuse University Family Development Research Program	216 boys and girls; 108 I, 108 C	Pre-natal (2nd trimester)	Matched control group established after intervention group (no random assignment)	Selective; offspring of poor single-parent teens (mean age = 18)	Parent training, education (language acquisition skills, creativity), nutrition, health and safety, fostering mother–child relationship	Day care, home	5.5 years	At post tx, 156; 82 I, 74 C; 10 year follow-up, 119; 65 I; 54 C	Delinquency (ES = 0.49) Fewer on probation, less severity of recorded offences (including aggressive behaviour and physical assault)	Lower costs of antisocial behaviour (court, probation, placement, detention costs) Higher IQ (at age 3 only), better social behaviour, greater school achievement, more positive self-evaluation

Study	Sample	Age	Design	Target	Intervention	Setting	Follow-up intervals	Results	Additional results
11. McCord (1978, 1992); Cambridge-Somerville Youth Study	650 boys; 325 I, 325 C	Mean = 10.5	Random assignment of matched boys	Indicated; boys headed for trouble	Counselling; home visits; tutoring; referrals to health care; extracurricular activities; parent training	Family, community	5.5 years / 31 years. 506 boys; 253 I, 253 C	Delinquency (ES = −0.08) Higher rates of court-recorded criminal activity	Higher self-report rates of alcoholism, physical ailments Higher proportion of more serious psychiatric diagnoses
12. Lochman (1992)	145 boys: 31 anger-coping (AC) intervention, 52 untreated aggressives (UA), 62 nonaggressives (NON)	9–12	Random assignment of some cohorts	Indicated; teachers nominated the most aggressive boys	Cognitive-behavioural, anger control	School	4–5 months / 2.5–3.5 years	Overall ES = −0.01 Delinquency (ES = 0.06) No differences in self-report delinquency (including crimes against persons, general theft) between AC and UA boys Aversive behaviour (ES = −0.22) No differences in observer-rated disruptive-aggressive off-task behaviour	Increased problem solving ability, self-esteem in AC boys Lower substance use in AC boys
13. Kolvin et al. (1986); Newcastle-upon-Tyne Study	592 boys and girls. Junior cohort: 67 at-risk controls (ARC), 69 parent counselling (JPC), 74 play group therapy (PG), 60 nurture work (NW). Senior cohort: 92 maladjusted controls (MC), 83 parent counselling (PC), 73 senior group therapy (SG), 74 behaviour modification (BM)	Junior 7–8; 11–12	Random assignment	Indicated; peer-rated as isolated or rejected; poor readers, having behaviour problems, high absenteeism, or neuroticism	JPC, PC: casework with families, consultations with teachers; PG: play and reflection of feelings; NW: compensatory and enrichment activities, support from mental health professionals, behavioural shaping; SG: traditional group therapy; BM: defining goals, social reinforcement techniques, behavioural prescriptions	School, home	4–16 months / 20–32 months	Externalizing behaviour (ES = 0.26) Junior: PG decreased aggregate and teacher-rated antisocial behaviour vs other three groups; PG and NW decreased parent-rated antisocial behaviour vs other two groups Senior: BM decreased parent-rated antisocial behaviour vs MC; SG decreased teacher-rated antisocial behaviour vs. MC; SG and BM tended to decrease aggregate antisocial behaviour vs. PC and MC	Junior: PG decreased aggregate neurotic behaviour vs ARC at final follow-up Senior: SG and BM show decreased aggregate neurotic behaviour vs PC and MC at final follow-up

Table 16.1. (cont.)

Authors	Sample size at pretest (I = intervention; C = control)	Age at intervention (years)	Design	Type of intervention	Description of intervention	Context of intervention	Length of intervention	Follow-up: length; sample size	Results for disruptive behaviour (I vs. C, at most recent follow-up ES=effect size)	Other results (for intervention group, compared to controls, at latest assessment)
14. Szapocznik et al. (1989)	69 Hispanic boys; 26 structural family therapy (SFT), 26 individual psychodynamic child therapy (IPCT), 17 C	Mean = 9 y, 2 m	Random assignment	Indicated; 32% ODD, 30% anxiety disorders, 16% CD, 12% adjust. disorders, 10% other	SFT: modification of maladaptive interactional patterns; IPCT: expression of feelings, limit setting, insight and transference interpretation; C: recreational activities	Clinic	17–19 weeks (hours)	1 year, 58; 23 SFT, 21 IPCT, 14 C	Externalizing behaviour (ES = −0.31) Maintenance of decreased mother-reported externalizing behaviour in all three groups observed at post-tx, but no group differential: no change in mother-rated conduct disorder or socialized aggression	Decreases in emotional problems in both tx conditions at post-tx, maintained at follow-up
15. Lochman et al. (1993)	52 boys and girls; 9 aggressive-rejected intervention (ARI), 17 rejected-only intervention (RI), 9 aggressive-rejected control (ARC), 17 rejected-only control (RC)	9 (4th grade)	Random assignment	Indicated; aggressive and/or rejected children	Positive social skill training, cognitive-behavioural strategies to promote nonimpulsive problem solving	Elementary school	6 months	1 year, 44; 7 ARI, 17 RI, 6 ARC, 14 RC	Externalizing behaviour (ES = 0.87) Lower teacher-rated aggression in ARI vs ARC; no difference between RI and RC Trend for lower peer-rated aggression in ARI vs ARC and RI vs RC	ARI higher teacher-rated prosocial behaviour vs ARC Trend for higher peer-rated social acceptance for ARI vs ARC
16. Bierman et al. (1987)	32 boys in instructions (I), prohibitions (P), instructions and prohibitions (IP), or control (C) groups (2 × 2 design)	Mean = 7 y, 7 m	Random assignment	Indicated; peer-nominated as negative and displayed negative peer interactions	Instructions to promote positive social behaviour, and/or prohibitions to reduce negative behaviour	School	10 weeks	1 year; 8 I, 7 P, 8 IP, 6 C	Externalizing behaviour (ES = 0.17) No changes in teacher and peer aggression ratings	No changes in play ratings, positive or negative peer nominations, or partner ratings

Study	Sample	Age	Design	Target population	Intervention	Setting	Duration	Follow-up	Results	
17. Tremblay et al. (1995); Montréal Longitudinal-Experimental Study	166 boys; 43 I, 123 combined attention/observation and no treatment C	7	Random assignment	Indicated; low SES boys who scored high on disruptiveness	Parent training in effective child rearing; social skills training for children	Home, school	2 years	6 years	Overall ES = 0.06 Externalizing behaviour (ES = −0.04) Trend toward less teacher-rated disruptive behaviour at ages 10 to 13 Delinquency (ES = 0.11) Less self-reported delinquent behaviours 1 to 6 years after end of intervention No difference in court registered delinquent offences	Larger proportion (vs pooled control group) in age-appropriate regular classrooms from ages 10 to 12 No differences in boys' perceptions of punishment or supervision by parents
18. Strayhorn & Weidman (1991)	105 (59 girls); 55 I, 50 C	3 y, 9 m	Random assignment	Indicated; adverse SES children with disruptive behaviour	Parent training, involving improving communication, positive reinforcement, effective punishment	Clinic	Approx. 3 months	1 year, 45 I, 39 C	Externalizing behaviour (ES = 0.45) Trend for less teacher-rated hostile-aggressive behaviour	Less teacher-rated hyperactivity; trend for less teacher-rated anxious behaviour, parent-rated externalizing and anxious behaviour
19. Schweinhart et al. (1993); High/Scope Perry Preschool Study	123 (51 girls); 58 (25 girls) I, 65 (26 girls) C	3–4	Pairing on IQ followed by random assignment	Indicated; lower IQ children of low SES families	Enhancing cognitive development through daily preschool and teacher home visits	School, home	1–2 years	22 years	Delinquency (ES = 0.35) Fewer mean officially-recorded lifetime arrests No differences on self-report misconduct variables	Higher IQ, greater school achievement, more high school graduands, higher yearly income, higher % home owners, fewer received social services
20. Schweinhart & Weikart (1997); High/Scope Preschool Curriculum Study	68 (37 girls); 23 Direct Instruction (DI), 22 High/Scope (HS), 23 Nursery School (NS)	3–4	Random assignment	Indicated; lower IQ children of low SES families	DI (programmed-learning) approach: teacher-initiated activities HS (open-framework) approach: teacher and child planned & initiated activities NS (child-centred) approach: child-initiated activities	School, home	1–2 years	18 years, 52; 19 DI, 14 HS, 19 NS	Delinquency (ES = 0.22) DI had higher self-report mean frequency of work suspensions (ES = 0.22 for self-report delinquency variables, HS vs other two groups) DI had higher officially-recorded lifetime arrests, adult arrests, felony arrests (specifically property felonies) and property misdemeanour arrests (ES = 0.21 for officially-recorded lifetime arrests, juvenile and adult, HS vs other two groups)	DI had more years special education for emotional disturbance, had done less volunteer work, and had older cars vs other two groups; DI had more sources of irritation, less co-habitation with spouses, lower highest year of schooling planned, fewer member with checking accounts vs HS group, more members remaining in Ypsilanti vs NS

other 2 years; five targeted 9–12-year-olds and lasted from 4 months to 5.5 years.

Variability can also be observed in the length of the follow-ups (1 year to 31 years), the type of outcome measured, and, most importantly, the content of the interventions. Six studies provided quality day care, seven studies provided social skills or social-cognitive skill training, five studies tried to enhance academic skills, two offered psychodynamic psychotherapy, 13 provided parenting skills training, one provided family therapy, one provided peer training, four provided teacher training, and one provided social case work. None targeted the school or the community environment.

Being confronted by such diversity in type of participants, content and duration of programmes, duration of follow-up assessments, and observed effects, for only 20 studies, we came to the conclusion that, based on the best set of studies we could find, there was no way we could definitively point to the best strategies for preventing conduct disorder. Each study appears to be unique. Scientists in this field have yet to provide clear replications of successful interventions. It should also be recalled that not one of the 20 studies used DSM or ICD criteria to assess the impact of the intervention.

In the following pages we describe in some detail experiments which were successful in reducing conduct problems, and some that were not. This should highlight experiments which should be replicated and those which should not. When available we chose one for each broad age group. We also selected interventions with long-term follow-ups. Following this, we discuss some hypothesized mechanisms mediating the salutary effects of interventions on conduct problems, briefly outline some large-scale ongoing preventive interventions and discuss design and implementation issues.

Preventive experiments that reduced conduct problems

During the elementary school years

Hawkins and colleagues (Hawkins et al., 1999) have recently reported a 6-year follow-up of the Seattle Social Development Project which found significant effects of an intervention designed to prevent negative outcomes in adolescence. This universal prevention experiment included a 6-year full intervention group (grades one through six), a 2-year late intervention group (grades five and six), and a no-treatment control group. The design was quasi-experimental. Initially, in six schools, entering first grade students were randomly assigned to intervention or control classrooms. A seventh school was assigned as a full intervention and an eighth was assigned as a full control. Four years later, in grade five, the sample was expanded to augment the control group and include a second experimental group (the late intervention group). The intervention was multi-modal, including teacher training on proactive classroom management, interactive teaching and cooperative learning; teacher training in interpersonal cognitive problem solving (teaching children to think through interpersonal problems, explore alternative responses); child training in resisting undesirable social influences and generating positive alternatives; and parent training in child behaviour management skills. Outcome was measured primarily through self-report and official school and community records.

Results at 6-year follow-up are encouraging (Hawkins et al., 1999). The full intervention group demonstrated fewer violent delinquent acts, and tended towards less nonviolent delinquency, self-report arrests and officially recorded juvenile delinquency, compared to controls. Additionally, there were improvements in other spheres for the full intervention group. Relative to the control group, the full intervention group demonstrated better academic functioning and school behaviour, reduced substance use and reduced sexual misbehaviour. The late intervention group fell between the full intervention and control groups on a number of outcome measures, suggesting 'dose-response' effects.

During the preschool years

The best evidence of long-term preventive intervention success are the two studies from the High/Scope Foundation, the Perry Preschool Study (Schweinhart et al., 1993) and the Preschool Curriculum Comparison Study (Schweinhart & Weikart, 1997). In the Perry Preschool Study, 123 children were randomly assigned to either a preschool or no-preschool group. The preschool model was the High/Scope curriculum (described below). In the Preschool Curriculum Comparison Study, 68 children were randomly assigned to one of three groups, representing distinct preschool models: Direct Instruction, High/Scope or Nursery School interventions. The Direct Instruction preschool programme represented a programmed-learning approach in which the teacher initiated activity and the child responded. The emphasis was on academic achievement. The Nursery School programme represented a child-centred approach in which the child initiated activity and the teacher responded. The focus was on social, rather than intellectual, development. The High/Scope model represented an open-framework approach in which both the teacher and child initiated activities. The emphasis was on planning, doing and reviewing one's actions within a stimulating environment, with teachers playing a supportive role, encouraging intellectual, social and physical development. In both studies, the preschool interventions lasted one to two years (depending on the cohort), and consisted of preschool for two and one-half hours on weekday mornings and a one and one-half hour home visit to each mother and child on weekday afternoons. In the Perry Preschool Study, home visits were weekly, in the Preschool Curriculum Study, home visits were every other week. The Perry Preschool Study participants have been followed for 22 years, to age 27; the Preschool Curriculum Study participants have been followed for 18 years, to age 23.

Results from both studies suggest positive effects of preschool on criminality later in life. In the Perry Preschool Study, the preschool programme significantly reduced officially recorded lifetime arrests and teacher-rated misconduct, with less of an effect on self-rated misconduct. In the Preschool Curriculum Comparison Study, both the High/Scope preschool model and the Nursery School curriculum showed reduced levels of self-report and officially recorded delinquency compared to the Direct Instruction group. Each of the studies had significant positive effects on other aspects of functioning as well (see Table 16.1).

Overall, these two studies are methodologically sound. They have been criticized for their low sample sizes and reliance on self-report and officially recorded delinquency. Despite these issues, however, the two studies have demonstrated a significant impact on delinquency and crime from 18 to 24 years after the end of the intervention. The results suggest that early childhood intervention, primarily cognitive-behavioural in nature, can reduce antisocial behaviour in the long-term. It would be very interesting and extremely important to know the mechanisms through which these interventions impacted on their distal outcomes. This issue is addressed later in this chapter.

During infancy

The Houston Parent–Child Development Center (PCDC) project (Johnson & Walker, 1987) was a selective intervention experiment implemented with low income Mexican–American families. Designed to promote social and intellectual competence, the goals of the Houston PCDC also included the prevention of behaviour problems. Families were randomly assigned to the programme or control conditions. Programme and control group sizes at the start of the study are not reported in the 5- to 8-year follow-up (Johnson & Walker, 1987). Attrition rates are reported at 50% for both the programme and control groups, and it is stated that there was no evidence of differential attrition, although no supporting analyses are presented.

The intervention began when the children were one year old and lasted two years. In the first year, it involved home visits focusing on child development, parenting skills and the development of a home learning environment. In the second year, children and their mothers came to the centre to learn child management, cognitive development and communication skills. Periodically, mothers learned home management skills while their children were in nursery school. The 5- to 8-year follow-up (summarized in Table 16.1) demonstrated decreases in teacher-rated acting out problems in the programme group relative to controls.

Recently, Johnson (personal communication) has reported on a 6- to 13-year follow-up of the Houston PCDC project. Two hundred and forty-four children out of a possible 389 were followed up (89 of 153 programme children, 155 of 236 control children). Preliminary analyses suggest that the programme children demonstrated reduced mother-rated externalizing behaviour, but there were no differences on teacher-rated aggression/hostility between the programme and control groups. There was also no difference in mother-reported delinquency (although note that the only delinquent act reported by the mothers was school truancy). Thus there appears to be evidence that the programme had a positive effect on disruptive behaviour (as assessed by the mothers), although the absence of a difference in aggression/hostility from more unbiased observers (i.e. teachers) is unfortunate.

During pregnancy

The Elmira Home Visitation Study (Olds et al., 1997, 1998) provided sensory and developmental screening, free transportation for prenatal and well-child care through to the child's second birthday, as well as home visits from a nurse during pregnancy until the child was 2 years old (termed 'Treatment 4'). This combination of services was compared to two control groups offering either the sensory and developmental screening and transportation only (termed 'Treatments 1 and 2'), or the screening and transportation plus nurse visits during pregnancy only ('Treatment 3'). The nurses emphasized improving women's health-related behaviours, parent child care and parent's personal development.

Assignment of the 400 participating families to groups was random. The intervention was selective in nature, as women who were less than 19 years old, unmarried or of low socioeconomic status were chosen. Participants were registered in the study prior to the 25th week of gestation. Participants have been followed up for 13 years past the end of the intervention.

The majority of the significant differences between Treatments 1 and 2 and Treatment 4 were found in a subsample of women who were both unmarried and from low-socioeconomic households at registration during pregnancy.

This subsample represented the authors' operationalization of a group with higher stress levels and fewer personal resources to manage the stress. Within this subsample, women in Treatment 4 (relative to those in Treatments 1 and 2) had fewer subsequent pregnancies and live births, greater spacing between first and second births; and used food stamps and family aid less. As well, women in Treatment 4 had fewer self-reported alcohol and drug impairments, arrests, convictions and days in jail, and had fewer officially recorded arrests and convictions (primarily accounted for by fewer property crimes, as opposed to personal or other offences). Women who received Treatment 4 had lower rates of identification as perpetrators of child abuse and neglect compared to those in Treatments 1 and 2, an effect found both in the total sample and the higher risk subsample (Olds et al., 1997).

In terms of effects on children's antisocial behaviour, children whose mothers were in Treatment 4 self-reported more frequent stops by the police, but fewer arrests and convictions and parole violations compared to children of Treatments 1 and 2 in the total sample. The effects of Treatment 4 on arrests and convictions and parole violations appeared to be concentrated in the children born to the unmarried, low-socioeconomic women. In the unmarried, low-socioeconomic subsample, children in Treatment 4 had fewer parent-reported arrests and self-reported incidents of running away compared to children in Treatments 1 and 2. Finally, in a substantially smaller subsample of the total sample, official records indicated that Treatment 4 children were less often adjudicated as persons in need of supervision compared to Treatment 1 and 2 children. Many of the differences noted above between Treatment 4 and Treatments 1 and 2 were also found between Treatment 3 and Treatments 1 and 2. For a number of externalizing behaviour dependent variables there were no treatment effects, most notably on teacher-rated acting out in school (Olds et al., 1998).

Preventive experiments that did not reduce conduct problems

During the elementary school years

Much has been written concerning the Cambridge–Somerville Youth Study (McCord, 1978), for a number of reasons. It is one of the earliest controlled prevention experiments. Also, it is the only prevention study in which the participant's criminal behaviour has been assessed well into adulthood. Finally, it is notable in that the intervention was found to have a somewhat negative effect on outcome.

In the mid to late 1930s, 650 boys ranging from ages 5 to 13 were solicited for inclusion in a prevention programme founded on the notion that delinquents lacked close emotional ties. The boys were matched on age, delinquency-proneness, family background and home environments, then assigned according to a coin toss into intervention or control groups. Boys in the intervention group received contact with a social worker for, on average, twice per month for 5.5 years. Social workers arranged tutoring in academic subjects, provided links to medical and psychiatric services, arranged attendance at summer camps, and facilitated involvement in a number of community organizations, including the YMCA and Boy Scouts. A number of the boys were dropped from the treatment group when it was discovered that social worker caseloads were too intense. For these cases, their matched controls were also dropped.

Five hundred and six of the boys were followed up approximately 30 years later when they were, on average, 47-year-old men (McCord, 1978). Rates of juvenile and adult criminal behaviour did not differ between the two groups, and surprisingly, a higher proportion of criminals in the intervention group committed more than one crime compared to criminals in the control group. The intervention group was also found to self-report greater frequencies of alcoholism and stress-related physical disorders, and among those who had died, members of the intervention group had died at a younger age. Later analyses demonstrated that more members of the intervention group could be classified as having an undesirable outcome (convicted for an FBI-indexed crime, received a diagnosis of alcoholism, schizophrenia, or manic-depression, or died prior to age 35) compared to the control group (McCord, 1981).

Additional analyses failed to reveal subgroups within the intervention group that benefited from the intervention. Age at which treatment began, length of treatment, frequency of contact, number of counsellors, degree of closeness of relationship with the counsellor(s), sex of the counsellor(s) or the particular type of assistance provided by the counsellor were tested to see if they were related to desirable/undesirable outcomes (as defined above) (McCord, 1981). Boys who were ages 9 to 11 when treatment began, those visited more frequently (every other week) by a counsellor, those in the programme at least 6 years, and those whose counsellors focused on personal or family problems (as opposed to academics or health) demonstrated greater frequencies of undesirable outcomes relative to controls. These subgroups of intervention boys may have been worse at the start of treatment compared to the other subgroups, thus requiring more attention from counsellors.

McCord has hypothesized that the treatment group as a whole may have done more poorly relative to controls because: (a) counsellors may have imposed their middle-class values on the boys, resulting in difficulties in a lower-class milieu; (b) counsellors may have increased dependency in the boys, not fostering coping abilities; (c) the presence of counsellors may have led to the labelling of the boys as troubled, and them subsequently justifying this label; or (d) the counsellors may have fostered unrealistic expectations of relative successes, leading to disillusionment. Only the final hypothesis received some empirical support in analyses on a reduced sample; treatment group members scored higher on a number of indices of disillusionment with their present life situations (McCord, 1981). In recent analyses, McCord has demonstrated that treated boys who were grouped together in summer camps did worse than treated boys who were not in camp. Furthermore, the frequency of summer camp attendance was associated with poorer outcomes for the treated boys relative to their untreated controls. This suggests that allowing these troubled youth to interact together amplified negative outcomes (Dishion et al., 1999).

During the preschool years

Webster-Stratton (1998) administered parent and teacher training to children in Head Start preschool programmes. Concerning child conduct problem behaviour outcomes, this study can be considered as being partly successful in that modest reductions in child conduct problem behaviour were noted according to one reporting source (observers), but not others (mothers, teachers).

Nine Head Start centres were randomly assigned to either intervention or control groups. Four hundred and twenty-six families completed baseline assessments, 296 in the intervention group and 130 in the control group. Many of the families included in the sample had low incomes. A proportion of the mothers in the sample had their first child during their teen years, had histories of substance abuse and/or depression, had lived at some point in a shelter with their children, had been physically/sexually abused as a child, had engaged in criminal behaviour, or had abused or neglected their own children.

The intervention consisted of an 8 to 9 week programme of parent training in a group format (8 to 16 parents), where parents met weekly for 2 hours to view and discuss videotapes modelling parenting skills. Group discussions were led by a trained family service worker and a parenting clinic staff leader. The emphasis was on problem solving, learning of new skills and support. Intervention integrity was facilitated through the use of treatment manuals, videotaping of parent groups for review by the project director, weekly supervision/feedback of group leaders and comprehensive training procedures.

Additionally, teacher training was implemented, involving teachers viewing the same parenting skill videotapes as shown to parents. The intent was to facilitate teachers' classroom management consistent with the strategies parents were learning. It was hoped that the teachers would support or even encourage the parents' efforts in the classroom setting. Effective classroom behaviour management strategies were also emphasized (e.g. clear rules, positive feedback etc.). The degree to which teachers implemented these behaviours was not assessed systematically.

At the long-term (1 year) follow-up of the sample, there were no differences in mother- or teacher-reported conduct problem behaviour in the intervention children relative to controls. Notably, however, observer-rated total deviance and noncompliance in the home decreased both in the intervention and control groups but somewhat more so in the intervention group. Gains in observer-rated positive affect behaviours, as well as reductions in negative affect behaviours, in the intervention group relative to controls were also found. As well, intervention mothers were observer-rated as being more positive in their parenting (displaying more positive affect, praise and physical positive behaviour), displaying less negative affect valence, being less harsh or critical, and showing more competence in disciplining their children relative to control mothers. Intervention mothers self-reported being less harsh and less likely to use negative verbal discipline techniques, as well as more consistent and more apt to use appropriate limit setting compared to controls.

Why was there a reduction in observer-rated aversive behaviour but not mother- or teacher-rated conduct problem behaviour? It may be that mothers' attitudes concerning their children's behaviour lag behind actual behaviour changes. (An additional follow-up would address this question, as mothers' attitudes would presumably catch up with their children's actual behaviour.) Alternatively, Webster-Stratton suggested that control mothers may have been reluctant to report existing child behaviour problems because of a lack of benefit in doing so, whereas intervention mothers, after participating in group discussions concerning child behaviour problems, may have felt less stigmatized in reporting them. Webster-Stratton suggests that teacher-rated changes in child conduct problem behaviour may not have been found because (a) the teacher-training intervention may not have been long enough to produce reductions in child externalizing behaviour, (b) teachers may have already been maximally promoting child prosocial behaviour by virtue of their training, and/or (c) the base rates of externalizing behaviour in the classroom may have been too low to detect a change. Nevertheless, the observer-rated reductions in conduct problem behaviour in the children of intervention parents, as well as the positive changes in children's moods and mothers' parenting techniques, are promising results arising from this preventive intervention programme.

During infancy

In the Abecedarian project (Clarke & Campbell, 1998), 111 infants were randomly assigned at birth to receive either 5 years of preschool education in a child-care setting, or no treatment. Healthy infants born into conditions of poverty were targeted. The infants were considered to be at risk for suboptimal cognitive development due to a number of socioeconomic and psychological factors, including low parental education levels, low parental IQ, poor maternal social/family support and others (Campbell & Ramey, 1995).

The preschool programme was carried out in a child care centre. The intervention covered four primary domains: cognitive and fine motor development, social and self-help skills, language and gross motor skills. Areas within the child care centre were set up for art, housekeeping, blocks, fine-motor manipulatives, language and literacy. Language instruction was less focused on syntax and more on practical usage. Prephonics training, to prepare children for reading, was also provided.

The intervention and control groups were re-randomized at kindergarten entry for a 3-year school-age intervention, however only the long-term effects of the preschool intervention have been reported. Fifteen participants were lost to attrition during the preschool years (eight in the intervention group, seven in the control group) (Campbell & Ramey, 1995), however some of these individuals were included in the 105 (54 intervention, 51 controls) followed up 13 years later (Clarke & Campbell, 1998).

Analyses on criminality at age 18 failed to reveal significant differences between the intervention and control groups. There were no group differences in the proportion charged with at least one offence, the proportions charged with specific offences (violent, property, drug or other charges), the mean number of total charges, the mean number of specific charges, the mean number of all arrests, or the mean number of specific arrests. This despite the fact that follow-up at age 15 revealed higher IQs, higher reading test scores, fewer students retained in a grade at least once and less assignment to special education classes in the intervention group relative to the control group (Campbell & Ramey, 1995).

During pregnancy

We found no studies initiated during pregnancy which were unsuccessful in reducing disruptive behaviour. In fact, the only two preventive interventions commencing during pregnancy had follow-ups of disruptive behaviour in adolescence and showed positive effects (see Table 16.1). A number of preventive interventions have been initiated with pregnant women, especially adolescent women. Follow-up assessments did not assess their children's disruptive behaviour probably because this was not the area of research of the initiators of the study. These studies could provide ideal samples to trace and further assess the effectiveness of early preventive interventions for disruptive behaviour.

Hypothesized mechanisms: what works and how?

The question of what works is perhaps best answered by looking closely at those preventive experiments that produced positive results. Certainly the two High/Scope studies make a strong case for the long-term efficacy of preschool interventions focusing on cognitive development. Causal modelling in the Perry Preschool Study suggests that the preschool experience directly improved participant's early childhood IQ, which in turn led to increased motivation early in elementary school, leading to completion of a higher level of schooling, ultimately resulting in both fewer lifetime arrests and higher monthly earnings at age 27 (Schweinhart et al., 1993). This is contrasted with the results of the Abecedarian Project which found no differences in crime rates at age 18 between intervention and control groups despite finding IQ differences and less school difficulties at age 15 (Clarke & Campbell, 1998). Clarke & Campbell suggest that the lack of services to parents, and/or differences in the larger social environments in which the studies were carried out, may explain the ineffectiveness of the Abecedarian project in reducing crime vis-à-vis the Perry Preschool Project. It may be that generalization of the learning achieved in preschool to the home environment is necessary to increase school motivation, increase the length of tenure in school and reduce crime. Alternatively, the Abecedarian project may yet show a positive impact on crime rates in the intervention group when assessed later, at a comparable time point to the Perry Preschool Study (i.e. age 27).

The notion that the addition of home visits is important in improving disruptive behaviour outcomes is reinforced by the findings of other studies intervening at or near birth. Studies by Seitz et al. (1985) and Lally et al. (1988) demonstrate that day care coupled with home visits to improve parental skills can lead to reduced disruptive behaviour and delinquency down the road. In fact, it may be a strong emphasis on parent training during the home visit that leads to more positive outcomes. One home visit component not emphasizing parent training failed to demonstrate effects on delinquency or disruptive behaviour (Stone et al., 1988).

Preventive interventions may also reduce disruptive behaviour through their impact on associations with deviant peers. Vitaro and colleagues (Vitaro et al., 1999; Vitaro & Tremblay, 1994) investigated whether the positive effects of the preventive intervention in the Montreal Longitudinal Experimental Study (Tremblay et al., 1995) were mediated in part by a reduction in intervention boys' associations with deviant peers. They found that the combination of parent training and child social skills training reduced the prevalence of conduct disorder in the intervention group at age 13, which was partly mediated by a reduction in disruptive behaviour at post-intervention (age 9), leading to affiliation with less aggressive peers (assessed at ages 10 through 12). The child social skills training component of the preventive intervention in this study was delivered in the context of a peer group with a 3 : 1 ratio of prosocial peers to disruptive boys. Other preventive interventions not necessarily containing this component may still lead to reductions in associations with deviant peers by reducing the likelihood of rejection by conventional peers and increasing access to nondeviant peers. Also, increased parental supervision through parent training may also lead to better regulation of children's friend selection, increasing the likelihood of affiliation with nondeviant peers. It should be noted that grouping together problem children in an intervention may have the reverse effect, i.e. may foster associations with deviant peers, increasing deviant behaviour via modelling and reinforcement, particularly if the number of deviant children exceeds the number of nonproblem children within the group (Dishion & Andrews, 1995; Dishion et al., 1999) (see above).

It appears that, in general, multicomponent interventions lead to positive outcomes (Hawkins et al., 1999; Tremblay et al., 1995). Additionally, intervening for a longer period of time, and at an earlier age, may produce better outcomes on conduct problem behaviours, although this is by no means assured. Some long-term interventions that commenced at birth have failed to demonstrate an effect on conduct-problem behaviours (Stone et al., 1988; Clarke & Campbell, 1998). In general, however, starting younger and intervening longer may be more efficacious (Yoshikawa, 1994).

Ongoing large-scale experiments

There are a number of ongoing, large-scale preventive interventions for conduct disorder presently being undertaken. Two of these programmes will be briefly reviewed here, in order to describe the most recent work in this field. One distinctive preventive intervention study is the Fast Track Project (Conduct Problems Prevention Research Group, 1992). This project combines a universal programme with an indicated intervention directed toward high-risk children. Elementary schools in four cities in the United States deemed at high risk based on crime and poverty were selected, matched within city and randomized to intervention or control groups. Starting in grade 1, a teacher-led classroom curriculum focusing on the development of emotional concepts, social understanding and self-control was administered, lasting for 5 years. Additionally, high-risk children (the top 10% in teacher- and parent-rated aggressive, disruptive and oppositional behaviour) were administered social skills training, tutoring in reading, and classroom friendship enhancement (peer pairing). Their parents were given group training (to foster positive family–school relationships, and teach problem-solving skills, time-out and self-restraint) and home visits (to promote their self-efficacy and life management). It is anticipated that the sample will be followed into early adulthood.

Early results for the universal intervention indicate that the intervention reduced teacher ratings of conduct problems, peer-rated aggression, and led to a more positive classroom environment as rated by observers after the first year of intervention (Coie, personal communication). Results for the high-risk sample show that the intervention reduced parent-reported oppositional aggressive behaviour up to grade 3, and prevented an increase in teacher-rated disruptive behaviour noted in the control group (Coie, personal communication). A strength of this study is the focus on measuring intervening variables in order to model how the intervention may be resulting in decreased aggression. For example, preliminary analyses suggest that a number of child and parent factors mediate (although modestly) the intervention effects on teacher- and parent-rated conduct problems (Coie, personal communication; see also Conduct Problems Prevention Research Group, 1999a, b).

A second recent preventive intervention programme currently being implemented in Ontario, Canada, is the Better Beginnings, Better Futures project (Peters & Russell, 1996). In this project, universal preventive interventions are delivered by social services in high risk communities (i.e. those with high levels of poverty, disorganization), and evaluated by a separate research unit. This project involves the implementation of two types of models to children in different age groups. In the first model, prenatal and infant development programmes are combined with preschool programmes and delivered to children from conception to age 4. In the second model, preschool and primary school programmes are administered to children ages 4 to 8. There are 11 communities participating; eight (including four Native Canadian communities) are implementing prenatal/preschool programmes, while three are implementing preschool/primary programmes. Children will be followed beginning prenatally or at age 4 until age 20. Outcome measures will encompass a wide variety of child, family and community characteristics.

This type of project is notable in that individuals within the communities themselves, in consultation with the government and a research unit, are primarily responsible for the conceptualization and implementation of the preventive intervention. Individuals in the communities are presumably better able to assess and thus address the needs of the community; as a result, participation in the intervention may be greater compared to a programme designed from the top down. One of the primary drawbacks of the project from a design point of view is the lack of random assignment of participants to intervention and control groups. In lieu of this, pre- and postintervention measures will be taken in intervention communities, matched comparison communities, as well as no-treatment control cohorts within the intervention communities.

Design and implementation issues

As can be seen from Table 16.1, the majority of prevention experiments (17 of 20) employed random assignment of participants to intervention and control groups. Random assignment increases the likelihood that observed differences at posttreatment and follow-up can be attributed to the intervention, and not to other variables on which the intervention and control groups may have differed (unintentionally) at the outset. Some investigators incorporated pre-intervention measures with random assignment to ensure that groups are similar on important dimensions (e.g. initial externalizing behaviour, IQ) (Szapocznik et al., 1989; Tremblay et al., 1995) or on the outcome measures themselves (e.g. Webster-Stratton, 1998). Pre-intervention measures can be used as covariates or in the calculation of change scores (when the outcome measure is given pre-intervention) to ensure that the groups are similar before treatment.

In order to fully capitalize on the preventive experiment design, hypotheses concerning the mechanisms mediating the development of conduct disorder should be systematically tested. Mediating variables represent the mechanisms through which an independent variable influences a dependent variable of interest, in this case, conduct disorder (Baron & Kenny, 1986). Early social and familial variables previously shown to predict later conduct disorder can be chosen as intervention targets. For example, a preventive intervention might focus on modifying harsh and inconsistent parenting, which has been shown to predict later conduct disorder (Patterson & Stouthamer-Loeber, 1984; Yoshikawa, 1994). In this case, it is necessary to measure the degree to which the intervention impacts on the proximal target that has a putative mediating role (in our example, the degree to which parents implement newly learned parenting techniques). A significant association between change on a putative mediating variable (e.g. a positive change in parenting style) and positive outcome (a reduction in conduct disorder), as well as a significant reduction in the magnitude of the relationship between the intervention and the distal outcome after accounting for the effects of the mediator, would provide evidence that the intervention was responsible for the behaviour change through its impact on the mediating mechanism. Ultimately, this leads to a refinement of theoretical models of the development of conduct disorder. This level of analysis of outcome is relatively rare in the preventive experiments for disruptive behaviour, with notable exceptions (Coie, personal communication; Schweinhart et al., 1993; Vitaro et al., 1999). Thus, a minimum requirement for future preventive intervention experiments should be the inclusion of an assessment not only of proximal outcomes of interest, but of putative mediating variables of distal effects. If an intervention is carried out and, despite it, intervention children continue to be disruptive, parenting is only slightly improved, and children continue to associate with deviant peers, then perhaps additional intervention is warranted, and indeed necessary. Alternatively, an intervention may have an effect on a hypothesized mediator, with no effect on the distal outcome. On theoretical grounds, results such as these (see, for example, Webster-Stratton, 1998) demand greater refinement of models linking specific mediating variables to distal outcomes.

The effects of moderating variables on intervention outcome are also important to assess. Moderating variables are person and contextual variables that facilitate or protect against the development of a disorder. Moderating variables specify when certain effects will occur or not (i.e. because of adverse circumstances), whereas mediating variables specify how or why such effects occur (Baron & Kenny, 1986). Moderating variables include, for example, socioeconomic status, gender, age and intelligence level. Measuring moderating variables at the outset of a preventive intervention will help to identify specific subgroups that benefit from a particular intervention (e.g. unmarried, low-socioeconomic women in the Elmira Home Visitation Study; Olds et al., 1998).

The notion that moderating variables place certain individuals at higher risk for the development of disruptive behaviour is reflected in the classification of preventive interventions as universal, selective or indicated. Judging by the emphasis on selective and indicated interventions in Table 16.1, the effects of moderating variables have been considered in the planning and implementation of prevention experiments. Low IQ, poverty, teen mothers, alcoholic fathers, low birth weight, and other social stressors have been identified as factors placing offspring at heightened risk for the development of disruptive behaviour (Webster-Stratton, 1990). Subgroups characterized by these qualities have been specifically targeted for intervention.

Other issues in the implementation of preventive interventions deserve attention. Eleven prevention experiments in Table 16.1 included interventions in more than one context (e.g. in the home and at school). Intervening in multiple contexts is likely to have a greater effect than in one context. In 11 of the 20 prevention experiments, the intervention period was one year or greater. Longer interventions would be expected to produce larger effects. Follow-up periods also need to be long enough to assess the impact on disruptive and delinquency in adolescence and early adulthood. A number of prevention experiments have recently extended their follow-up periods into adolescence and early adulthood (Hawkins et al., 1999; Olds et al., 1998; Schweinhart et al., 1993; Schweinhart & Weikart, 1997), greatly adding to our knowledge concerning the long-term impact of preventive interventions for disruptive behaviour. The preventive interventions reviewed in Table 16.1 also incorporate, and find significant effects on, outcome measures in multiple contexts (school, home), from multiple perspectives (parent, teacher, observer, participant), and in multiple areas of functioning (drug/alcohol use, self-esteem, sexuality). As well, the majority of preventive interventions listed in Table 16.1 include some effort to compare follow-up samples to dropouts to ensure that the results of an intervention were not due to differential attrition (Hawkins et al., 1999; Kellam et al., 1994; Webster-Stratton, 1998).

The degree to which a preventive intervention is implemented has been assessed in only a few of the experiments reviewed in Table 16.1. Systematic measurement of the degree to which an intervention is implemented by the deliverers of the intervention (e.g. therapists) (Szapocznik et al., 1989), and the use of intervention manuals to ensure that an intervention is delivered as conceptualized and similarly across participants and over time (Webster-Stratton, 1998), will increase the internal validity of a study. As well, measuring the degree to which participants utilized particular aspects of the prevention programme (e.g. the percentage of parents who attended parenting classes) (Hawkins et al., 1999; Tremblay et al., 1995) is also important. Finally, as mentioned above, assessing the degree to which parents implement the techniques introduced by the prevention researcher in their day-to-day lives is important. None of the prevention experiments reviewed in Table 16.1 have incorporated this degree of implementation assessment.

A number of other design characteristics have yet to be incorporated into experiments designed to prevent disruptive behaviour. Random assignment of intervention personnel to study participants or cohorts ensures that the effects of the intervention are not attributable solely to a specific case worker or a case worker/participant interaction but to the intervention itself. Furthermore, assessment of case worker variables would allow for the specification of case worker qualities that are associated with positive outcome. These more complex design features will likely not be implemented until a consistent positive effect of preventive interventions on disruptive behaviour is demonstrated, and the intervention components that have an impact are identified.

Conclusions

The available evidence to date, as reviewed in this chapter, suggests that conduct disorder can be prevented: some interventions did have substantial positive effects on distal disruptive behaviour outcomes, including externalizing behaviour, aversive behaviour, and delinquency. One must certainly be cognizant, however, of the fact that relatively few long-term preventive intervention studies for conduct disorder have been undertaken. The newest generation of large-scale preventive intervention experiments promises to further clarify the issue, as well as confirm/reveal mediators and moderators of preventive interventions on long-term outcome measures. Finally, there are a number of preventive interventions implemented for the prevention of problems other than disruptive behaviour which could be used to assess their effects on disruptive behaviour, and thus accelerate the accumulation of knowledge on how to prevent conduct disorder.

REFERENCES

Andry, R.G. (1960). *Delinquency and Parental Pathology*. London: Methuen.

Baron, R.M. & Kenny, D.A. (1986). The moderator–mediator variable distinction in social psychological research: Conceptual, strategic, and statistical considerations. *Journal of Personality and Social Psychology*, *51*, 1173–82.

Bierman, K., Miller, C. & Stabb, S.D. (1987). Improving the social behavior and peer acceptance of rejected boys: Effects of social skill training with instructions and prohibitions. *Journal of Consulting and Clinical Psychology*, *55*, 194–200.

Bovet, L. (1951). *Psychiatric Aspects of Juvenile Delinquency*. Geneva: World Health Organization.

Cabot, P.S. de Q. (1940). A long-term study of children: The Cambridge-Somerville Youth Study. *Child Development*, *11*, 143–51.

Campbell, F.A. & Ramey, C.T. (1995). Cognitive and school outcomes for high-risk African–

American students at middle adolescence: Positive effects of early intervention. *American Educational Research Journal, 32,* 743–72.

Carpenter, M. (1851). *Reformatory Schools for the Children of the Perishing and Dangerous Classes and for Juvenile Offenders.* London: The Woburn Press (1968).

Clarke, S.H. & Campbell, F.A. (1998). Can intervention early prevent crime later – The Abecedarian Project compared to other programs. *Early Childhood Research Quarterly, 13,* 319–43.

Cohen, J. (1977). *Statistical Power Analysis for the Behavior Sciences* (Rev. Edn). New York: Academic Press.

Conduct Problems Prevention Research Group (1992). A developmental and clinical model for the prevention of conduct disorder: The FAST Track Program. *Development and Psychopathology, 4,* 509–27.

Conduct Problems Prevention Research Group (1999a). Initial impact of the Fast Track prevention trial for conduct problems: I. The high-risk sample. *Journal of Consulting and Clinical Psychology, 67,* 631–47.

Conduct Problems Prevention Research Group (1999b). Initial impact of the Fast Track prevention trial for conduct problems: II. Classroom effects. *Journal of Consulting and Clinical Psychology, 67,* 648–57.

Dishion, T.J. & Andrews, D.W. (1995). Preventing escalation in problem behaviors with high-risk young adolescents: Immediate and 1-year outcomes. *Journal of Consulting and Clinical Psychology, 63,* 538–48.

Dishion, T.J., McCord, J. & Poulin, F. (1999). When interventions harm: Peer groups and problem behavior. *American Psychologist, 54,* 755–64.

Dolan, L.J., Kellam, S.G., Brown, C.H., et al. (1993). The short-term impact of two classroom based preventive interventions on aggressive and shy behaviors and poor achievement. *Journal of Applied Developmental Psychology, 14,* 317–45.

Earls, F. (1986). Epidemiology of psychiatric disorders in children and adolescents. In G.L. Klerman, M.M. Weissman, P.S. Appelbaum & L.H. Roth (Eds.), *Psychiatry: Social, Epidemiologic, and Legal Psychiatry* (Vol. 5, pp. 123–52). New York: Basic Books.

Farrington, D.P., Ohlin, L.E. & Wilson, J.Q. (1986). *Understanding and Controlling Crime: Towards a New Research Strategy.* New York: Springer-Verlag.

Glueck, S.E. & Glueck, E.T. (1934). *One Thousand Juvenile Delinquents: Their Treatment by Court and Clinic.* Cambridge, MA: Harvard University Press.

Gordon, R. (1983). An operational definition of prevention. *Public Health Reports, 98,* 107–9.

Gordon, R. (1987). An operational classification of disease prevention. In J.A. Steinberg & M.M. Silverman (Eds.), *Preventing Mental Disorders: A Research Perspective* (pp. 20–6). Rockville: MD: Department of Health and Human Services.

Hart, H.H. (1910). *Preventive Treatment of Neglected Children: Correction and Prevention.* New York: Arno Press & The New York Times 1971.

Hawkins, J.D., Catalano, R.F., Kosterman, R., Abbott, R. & Hill, K.G. (1999). Preventing adolescent health-risk behaviors by strengthening protection during childhood. *Archives of Pediatrics and Adolescent Medicine, 153,* 226–34.

Hedges, L.V. & Olkin, I. (1985). *Statistical Methods for Meta-analysis*. New York: Academic Press.

Jenkins, R.L. & Glickman, S. (1947). Patterns of personality organisation among delinquents. *The Nervous Child, 6*, 329–39.

Johnson, D. L. & Walker, T. (1987). Primary prevention of behavior problems in Mexican American children. *American Journal of Community Psychology, 15*, 375–85.

Kellam, S.G., Rebok, G.W., Ialongo, N. & Mayer, L.S. (1994). The course and malleability of aggressive behavior from early first grade into middle school: Results of a developmental epidemiologically-based preventive trial. *Journal of Child Psychology and Psychiatry, 35*, 259–81.

Kolvin, I., Garside, R.F., Nicol, et al. (1986). *Help Starts Here*. New York: Tavistock.

Lally, J.R., Mangione, P.L. & Honig, A.S. (1988). The Syracuse University Family Development Research Program: Long-range impact of an early intervention with low-income children and their families. In D.R. Powell (Ed.), *Advances in Applied Developmental Psychology: Parent Education as Early Childhood Intervention: Emerging Directions in Theory, Research, and Practice* (Vol. 3, pp. 79–104). Norwood, NJ: Ablex Publishing.

Lipton, D., Martinson, R. & Wilks, J. (1975). *The Effectiveness of Correctional Treatment: A Survey of Treatment Evaluation Studies*. New York: Praeger.

Lochman, J.E. (1992). Cognitive–behavioral intervention with aggressive boys: Three-year follow-up and preventive effects. *Journal of Consulting and Clinical Psychology, 60*, 426–32.

Lochman, J.E., Coie, J.D., Underwood, M.K. & Terry, R. (1993). Effectiveness of a social relations intervention program for aggressive and nonaggressive, rejected children. *Journal of Consulting and Clinical Psychology, 60*, 426–32.

McCarton, C.M., Brooks-Gunn, J., Wallace, I.F., et al. (1997). Results at age 8 years of early intervention for low-birth-weight premature infants. The Infant Health and Development Program. *Journal of the American Medical Association, 277*, 126–32.

McCord, J. (1978). A thirty-year follow-up of treatment effects. *American Psychologist, 33*, 284–9.

McCord, J. (1981). Consideration of some effects of a counseling program. In S. E. Martin, L. B. Sechrest & R. Redner (Eds.), *New Directions in the Rehabilitation of Criminal Offenders* (pp. 394–405). Washington, DC: National Academy of Sciences.

McCord, J. (1992). The Cambridge–Somerville Study: A pioneering longitudinal experimental study of delinquency prevention. In J. McCord & R.E. Tremblay (Eds.), *Preventing Antisocial Behavior: Interventions from Birth through Adolescence* (pp. 196–206). New York: Guilford Press.

Mrazek, P.J. & Haggerty, R.J. (Eds.) (1994). *Reducing Risks for Mental Disorders: Frontiers for Preventive Intervention Research*. Washington, DC: National Academy of Sciences.

Olds, D.L., Eckenrode, J., Henderson, C.R., Jr., et al. (1997). Long-term effects of home visitation on maternal life course and child abuse and neglect. *Journal of the American Medical Association, 278*, 637–43.

Olds, D., Henderson, C.R., Jr., Cole, R., et al. (1998). Long-term effects of nurse home visitation on children's criminal and antisocial behavior: 15-year follow-up of a randomized controlled trial. *Journal of the American Medical Association, 280*, 1238–44.

Patterson, G.R. & Stouthamer-Loeber, M. (1984). The correlation of family management practices and delinquency. *Child Development, 55*, 1299–307.

Peters, R.D. & Russell, C.C. (1996). Promoting development and preventing disorder: The Better

Beginnings, Better Futures Project. In R.D. Peters & R.J. McMahon (Eds.), *Preventing Childhood Disorders, Substance Abuse, and Delinquency* (pp. 19–47). Thousand Oaks, CA: Sage.

Pitkanen, L. (1969). A descriptive model of aggression and nonaggression with application to children's behaviour. *Jyvaskyla Studies in Education, Psychology, and Social Research* (No. 19). Jyvaskyla, Finland: University of Jyvaskyla.

Quetelet, A. (1833). *Research on the Propensity for Crime at Different Ages,* 2nd edition. Bruxelles: M. Hayez.

Robins, L.N. (1966). *Deviant Children Grown Up.* Baltimore: Williams & Wilkins.

Robins, L.N. (1992). The role of prevention experiments in discovering causes of children's antisocial behavior. In J. McCord & R.E. Tremblay (Eds.), *Preventing Antisocial Behavior: Interventions from Birth to Adolescence.* New York: Guilford Press.

Rutter, M., Tizard, J. & Whitmore, K. (Eds.). (1981). *Education, Health and Behavior.* Huntington, NY: R.E. Krieger Publishing Company.

Schweinhart, L.L., Barnes, H.V. & Weikart, D.P. (1993). *Significant Benefits. The High/Scope Perry School Study through age 27.* Ypsilanti, MI: High/Scope Press.

Schweinhart, L.L. & Weikart, D.P. (1997). *Lasting Differences: The High/Scope Preschool Curriculum Comparison Study through age 23.* Monographs of the High/Scope Educational Research Foundation, 12. Ypsilanti, MI: High/Scope Press.

Seitz, V., Rosenbaum, L.K. & Apfel, H. (1985). Effects of family support intervention: A ten-year follow-up. *Child Development, 56,* 376–91.

Shaw, C.R. & McKay, H.D. (1942). *Juvenile Delinquency and Urban Areas.* Chicago: University of Chicago Press.

Stone, W.L., Bendell, R.D. & Field, T.M. (1988). The impact of socio-economic status on teenage mothers and children who received early intervention. *Journal of Applied Developmental Psychology, 9,* 391–408.

Strayhorn, J.M. & Weidman, C. (1991). Follow-up one year after parent–child interaction training: Effects on behavior of preschool children. *Journal of the American Academy of Child and Adolescent Psychiatry, 30,* 138–43.

Szapocznik, J., Rio, A., Murray, E., et al. (1989). Structural family versus psychodynamic child therapy for problematic Hispanic boys. *Journal of Consulting and Clinical Psychology, 57,* 571–8.

Tonry, M., Ohlin, L.E., Farrington, D.P., et al. (1991). *Human Development and Criminal Behavior: New Ways of Advancing Knowledge.* New York: Springer-Verlag.

Tremblay, R.E., Kurtz, L., Mâsse, L.C., Vitaro, F. & Pihl, R.O. (1995). A bimodal preventive intervention for disruptive kindergarten boys: Its impact through mid-adolescence. *Journal of Consulting and Clinical Psychology, 63,* 560–8.

Vitaro, F., Brendgen, M., Pagani, L., Tremblay, R.E. & McDuff, P. (1999). Disruptive behavior, peer association, and conduct disorder: Testing the developmental links through early intervention. *Development and Psychopathology, 11,* 287–304.

Vitaro, F. & Tremblay, R.E. (1994). Impact of a prevention program on aggressive children's friendships and social adjustment. *Journal of Abnormal Child Psychology, 22,* 457–75.

Webster-Stratton, C. (1990). Long-term follow-up of families with young conduct problem children: From preschool to grade school. *Journal of Clinical Child Psychology, 19,* 144–9.

Webster-Stratton, C. (1998). Preventing conduct problems in Head Start children: Strengthening parenting competencies. *Journal of Consulting and Clinical Psychology, 66,* 715–30.

Yoshikawa, H. (1994). Prevention as cumulative protection: Effects of early family support and education on chronic delinquency and its risks. *Psychological Bulletin, 115,* 28–54.

17

Economic evaluation and conduct disorders

Martin Knapp

Introduction

Cost and outcomes

Conduct disorder in early childhood can be responsible for scholastic failure, poor peer relations and delinquency in adolescence. It can severely impair individual development and social functioning, and a substantial proportion of children with conduct disorder go on to have psychiatric and other medical problems in adult life, including 'phobia, major depressive disorders, obsessive-compulsive disorder, schizophrenia, panic disorder, manic episodes and somatisation' (Maughan & Rutter, 1998). They also have a higher risk of poor social functioning, alcohol and substance use rates, unemployment, broken marriages, criminality and imprisonment.

Each of these common childhood and adulthood consequences of conduct disorder has a personal and a social cost: there are potential losses (costs) to the person with conduct disorder, to their family and to the wider society. Some of these losses are direct economic costs and some are more indirect. Treatments or other interventions intended to tackle the conditions or disorders underlying these personal and social problems are themselves costly because of the need to devote staff time, office space and other resources to support and care.

Of course, the treatments and other interventions which professional staff provide to children and families would be expected to generate beneficial effects – to reduce the amount of antisocial behaviour, to improve peer relations and personal development, to reduce the likelihood of social and personal problems in adulthood, and so on. Different interventions by health care and other bodies could produce different effects. Economic evaluation is concerned with the relationship between these effects (or outcomes) and the costs of achieving them.

The primary reason for wanting to understand this relationship is because the resources available to meet the needs of children and families are in limited supply relative to the demands made upon them. It is this scarcity which generates the need for economic evaluation. Whenever there is a scarcity of resources or services a choice is needed between alternative uses of them, and the choice or allocation cannot always be left to the free play of market forces. Whether the need for economic evaluation remains latent or is turned into an expressed demand depends a lot on the policy context. Indeed, the policy environments within which child and adolescent mental health problems are identified and treated – and the social, political and economic contexts more generally – have a major bearing on practice (who gets what treatment), its effectiveness and also its cost. This is always the case, but it sometimes takes a change in policy to draw attention to the fact. Recent reforms and other policy initiatives in a number of countries have highlighted how changes in context affect the nature and level of needs, the abilities and willingness of service providers to respond to them, the effectiveness of services in terms of child and family outcomes, and the costs of achieving those outcomes. Two examples – from the US and the UK – illustrate how economic issues have recently moved higher up policy and practice agenda.

Managed care

In the United States the dominant change of recent years has been the growth of 'managed care'. The main reason for that growth was that the costs of mental health care that fell to employers and other payers were increasing more rapidly than these funders found acceptable (Dorwart, 1990; Frank et al., 1991). For example, among the population aged under 18, mental health admissions increased more than fourfold just between 1980 and 1984 (Scherl, 1985). The incentives inherent in many insurance reimbursement arrangements were apparently pushing children into more restrictive settings than were apparently needed (Behar, 1985; Frank & Dewa, 1992; Knitzer, 1982), and there were pressures from third-party payers (employers and government) to reduce length of inpatient stay (Patrick et al., 1993). Finding cost-effective alternatives to inpatient treatment was expected to reduce overall expenditures without damaging outcomes. There were also concerns about the fragmentation of service responses to needs (Bickman et al., 1996; Fairfield et al., 1997).

The total level of health care expenditure on a particular population can be expressed as a simple product of five elements:

Expenditure = number of people with an underlying need for treatment
× proportion referred (expressing an actual demand) for treatment
× proportion receiving treatment

× amount of treatment received

× unit cost of treatment

Managed care can be seen as the set of initiatives designed to put limits on the last three elements in this equation. For example, gatekeeping and screening can restrict the proportion of people getting a service; utilization reviews and other practice guidelines can restrict the amount of care actually received; and contract negotiation might bring down the unit cost of a service. Case management might work across a number of the elements to improve service coordination and improve cost-effectiveness. Evidence from the US, where managed care initiatives have had easily their biggest impacts, remains mixed (Dickey, 1998; Kavanagh, 1997; Wells et al., 1995) but this is hardly surprising given the enormous variations in managed care arrangements across states and between public and private sectors (Unützer & Tischler, 1995). Much of the debate has centred on whether to introduce capitated payments, whether to 'carve out' mental health into separate arrangements, and the need to monitor the activities of private (for-profit) providers. The latter have taken a larger market share of both in-patient and other services (Friedman & Kutash, 1992). Mean length of stay is greater for children than for adults (Padgett et al., 1993) – the fourth element in the equation above – increasing pressure from purchasers to cut costs, and raising questions about supplier-induced demand and quality monitoring.

Managed care raises ethical questions. The clinician has a duty to the individual patient to provide or prescribe the most efficacious treatment, but arguably also a responsibility to funders and/or the community of taxpayers to pursue efficiency in the broader provision of care (Sabin, 1994). The tension between the two is not easily resolved (Almond, 1995; Pomerantz, 1995). Not surprisingly, much of the argument about managed care has revolved around the influence that cost and cost-effectiveness does and should have on who gets what amount of what kind of treatment.

Identifying and meeting needs

The UK has long had a 'managed care' National Health Service, although not often labelled as such (Fairfield et al., 1997). Cost consciousness and certainly expenditure constraints have a longer history. Recent organizational reforms have prompted a closer look at the economics of care and treatment. The introduction of the so-called 'internal market' in the National Health Service in the 1990s made it necessary to be much more explicit about the costs and the expected effects of interventions. Even if contracts between purchasers and providers did not set prices for particular types of intervention, or did not disaggregate child and adolescent from adult services, there was nevertheless a sufficiently major overhaul of the system of health care funding to increase economic awareness among the main internal market 'stakeholders'.

However, there have been specific events which have resulted in conduct disorder, and child and adolescent mental health problems more generally, having a higher public profile than perhaps ever before. Small contributions to this profile-raising have been made by some official reports – such as those from the House of Commons Health Committee (1997), Health Advisory Service (1995) and the Audit Commission (1999) – and also by a number of research studies (see below). However, of more importance has been the growing public concern with juvenile crime, truancy and antisocial behaviour generally. The cost of youth crime in England has been estimated at £1 billion annually (Audit Commission, 1996), and it is not surprising that the 1997 Labour government's stated priorities included improved educational standards, lessening of social exclusion as well as reductions in crime rates.

Achieving these grand policy objectives in relation to young people will be no mean task. The difficulties to be overcome, both nationally and locally, have been set out in the informed and informative reports mentioned earlier. The House of Commons Health Committee (1997) pointed out that mental health had been given prominence in the Conservative government's *Health of the Nation* strategy of 1992, but that children and adolescents were not specifically mentioned in its targets. Two years earlier, the Health Advisory Service (1995) made recommendations for the improvement of child and adolescent mental health, suggesting an agenda which many local purchaser and provider or- ganisations have been keen to follow. The more recent Audit Commission (1999) report painted the most comprehensive picture to date of child and adolescent mental health services in England and Wales, giving it a platform from which to make recommendations, not only for health, social services, education and other services, but particularly for their improved coordination.

Many of the issues identified and addressed by these two UK reports have a distinctly economic flavour, not in the narrow sense of financial constraints or goals – although these are mentioned – but in that they relate to such key considerations as: unmet needs for services; the limited availability of specialist resources; poorly coordinated strategies for commissioning by health, educa- tion and social services agencies; poorly coordinated services on the ground; low effectiveness services in some localities and geographical inequalities more generally; and a lack of data on provision and service organization.

Economics: topic and discipline

These two context-setting discussions – one for the US and the other for the UK – illustrate how economic issues have grown in perceived importance in the child mental health field. More generally, there is an inherent familiarity about economics which follows from regular exposure to the topic through everyday transactions – purchases of goods and services – and through the media coverage of, for example, poverty, unemployment, government expenditure and taxation plans, and markets. In fact, each of these illustrative economic topics has relevance for any discussion of child and adolescent mental health problems, their prevalence and their treatment: poverty is associated with a greater incidence of such childhood problems; unemployment is more common in adulthood among those who experienced childhood disorders; government decisions on spending levels greatly influence how much is available for intervention programmes; and market forces clearly play a role in the allocation of health care services, even in so-called welfare state countries.

Although each of these topics will be touched upon later in this chapter, it is the discipline of economics which is more pertinent to the discussion. The discipline of economics starts with recognition of the basic problem of resource scarcity, emphasizes the need for informed choices as to how those resources are to be deployed, identifies criteria for choice from observations as to how individual people and organizations behave in principle and in practice, and suggests means by which those criteria can be both measured and achieved. Economic evaluation is essentially measurement of the success achieved by an economic system (or component parts thereof) in the pursuit of choice criteria, or more generally in pursuit of personal and societal goals, particularly in circumstances where markets cannot be relied upon to generate efficient allocations of goods and services. Sometimes economic evaluation is referred to by more specific terms, such as cost-effectiveness or cost-benefit analysis, but strictly speaking the terms are not interchangeable.

The main purposes of the chapter are to introduce the different types of economic evaluation and to discuss their respective uses and advantages in the child and adolescent mental health field. The chapter cannot provide a detailed step-by-step guide to conducting your own economic evaluation, but the main practical tasks to be undertaken in an evaluation will certainly be covered. The main aim, however, is to highlight, for those people seeking to use the results of economists' evaluations, the methods that are employed and some of the applications.

In the next section, the discussion concentrates on scarcity in relation to child and adolescent mental health, and its implications. The following sections introduce the three main criteria of both choice and economic evaluation (effectiveness, efficiency and equity), and show how they are linked one with another. The chapter then moves to the principles of the main modes of economic evaluation (cost-benefit analysis and its near relatives) and, finally, some of the core practical tasks to be accomplished.

Needs, services and scarcity

The UK Health Advisory Service (1995) report laid out a disarmingly simple strategic approach which separated four service tiers and the links or filters between them. The first tier comprises services and professionals whose primary activities are not necessarily mental health promotion but who will have an influence on whether the needs of children and adolescents with mental health problems are recognized and whether they receive appropriate attention. Often the best course of action will remain a first-tier responsibility. Primary care doctors, social workers, school health service providers and police officers are among the key professionals in this first tier. Identification of a mental health problem such as a conduct disorder could lead these professionals to refer the child and family on to a second-tier specialist service (or to commission such services within a market-like system). In the second tier are the mental health professionals, educational psychologists and specialist social workers who work with children, adolescents and their families, either peripatetically or at specialist bases such as psychiatric hospitals.

Some young people will need more specialized services by virtue of the rarity and/or complexity or intensity of their needs. These are the third- and fourth-tier services. The third tier comprises multidisciplinary teams working with specific therapeutic approaches (for example to tackle eating disorders, substance abuse, special education or child protection needs), whilst the fourth tier is the set of very specialized interventions and care, such as inpatient facilities, secure units and highly specialized outpatient services for particular disorders.

Using this tiered model of interventions as a template it is clear that current practice, not just in the UK but internationally, does not measure up particularly well. The prevalence of mental health problems in childhood and adolescence has historically been quite seriously under-estimated, and for some disorders may now in fact be growing. In consequence, only a small proportion of those in need of services actually receive them, and many of the proven interventions for meeting identified needs are available in some but not all localities. Only a minority of children with behavioural problems in England

and Wales see a specialist psychiatrist or psychologist (the second to fourth tiers). For example, Cooper & Goodyer (1993) found that none of the girls in their study who had serious depression was in contact with specialist mental health services. The gap between need and treatment – which is perhaps widening – has been evidenced by, for example, Evans & Brown (1993), Light & Bailey (1993), Garralda (1994) and Kurtz et al. (1995). Specialist (fourth-tier) provision was described by the House of Commons Health Committee as 'patchy and inadequate' (1997, p. xliv), reinforcing the HAS view:

[M]ental health services for children and adolescents are, essentially, unplanned and historically determined. Their distribution is patchy and they are very variable in quality and composition. The work they do seems unrelated in strength or diversity to systematically considered local need. (1995, p. 11)

Such features are not peculiar to the UK. Costello et al. (1993) concluded from their review of epidemiological and other studies in the US that:

. . . whereas one child in five has a [formerly-diagnosed] DSM disorder, and perhaps one in 10 has significantly impaired functioning, only one in 20 receives any kind of mental health care, and only one or two in 100 are treated in a speciality mental health setting. . . . Service availability is far lower than need. (1993, p. 1109)

Burns et al. found that only 40% of children aged 9, 11 and 13 with serious emotional disturbances 'had received any kind of mental health care during the three months preceding the . . . interviews' (1995, p. 155), and the problem would certainly seem to be quite widespread internationally (Fergusson et al., 1993; Gureje et al., 1994; Friedman & Kutash, 1992; John et al., 1995).

Establishing the prevalence of conduct disorders and other mental health problems of childhood and adolescence is notoriously difficult (see Dunn, chapter 3, this volume), but there are reasons for believing that prevalence may be increasing, and with it the problem of the comparative scarcity of the resources necessary to meet individual needs. Wilkinson (1994) documents marked increases since the late 1970s in the UK along a number of dimensions of need or social problem: juvenile crime, drug problems, solvent abuse, numbers on local authority child protection registers, young children in care ('looked after'), exclusions from school and suicides among young people. In many parts of the world the prevalence of depression and suicide appear to be on the increase (Diekstra, 1995; Klerman & Weissman, 1989; Ryan et al., 1992; Shaffer, 1988), as is the prevalence of conduct disorder (Robins, 1986).

Cultural, social and economic changes are surely at the root of some of these prevalence increases. The number of children in Britain living in poverty tripled between 1979 and 1995 (Oppenheim & Harker, 1996), and family poverty (or deprivation more generally) is known to be correlated with child and family welfare and the needs for health and social care intervention (Bebbington & Miles, 1989; Routh, 1994; Woodroffe et al., 1993). Farrington & West (1990), among others, have shown the link between childhood poverty and offending in adulthood, and Offord et al. (1992) report how children in low income families are more likely to have one or more psychiatric disorders, including conduct disorder, four years later. (This income effect applied to the preadolescent group but not to adolescents.)

In other words, the international picture is one of marked scarcity of services relative to the identified needs for them. Scarcity is the root of economics, and scarcity is endemic. For example, almost all resources employed in the care and support of children and families are scarce relative to identified prevalence. Relative scarcity could obviously be reduced somewhat by training more child psychiatrists, hiring more social workers, or closing fewer inpatient beds – but to eradicate all need would require an enormous diversion of resources from other uses. Moreover, there are other scarcities, less conventionally defined perhaps, which are not so easily tackled because they are not bought or sold in markets and have no readily identified price or cost. Nevertheless, they exert potentially considerable influences on child and family welfare. These are called 'nonresource inputs' in the conceptual framework set out below (see 'A framework for evaluation'), and include, for example, a child's relations with their parents and siblings, the school environment, community attitudes to antisocial behaviour, and so on.

If scarcity is widespread, is there blame to be apportioned? Are governments not spending enough on child and family services, have insurance companies limited reimbursements too much, or have service purchasers generally put too many limitations on the budgets for child and adolescent mental health? Does responsibility for scarcity lie with primary care doctors who refer too many children to already overstretched specialist services? Are previous cutbacks in preventive services the real cause of today's difficulties? Or is it that schools are excluding too many difficult children, or that social services departments are not adequately tackling the social care needs of children and families within their own resources? Is the basic problem that the general public holds unrealistic expectations of what health care and other services can achieve? It would be possible to line up some support for each of these views, but this would risk diverting attention from the fundamental fact that scarcity will always be with us: the needs and demands for interventions to tackle conduct disorders and other mental health problems of childhood and adolescence will almost always outstrip available supplies.

Criteria for choice and evaluation

Scarcity necessitates choice: how can resources be used to best effect? What criteria might we use in making those decisions? One of the most important will be effectiveness – the abilities of resources to improve the health and welfare of children and families – but increasingly attention is also being paid to the costs of achieving those effects. The generic term for the criterion which combines the effectiveness and resource sides is efficiency. A third criterion of importance is equity, or fairness in the distribution either of access to treatment resources, or of the burden of financing them, or of their effects on health and quality of life.

This chapter focuses on these three criteria. This focus is chosen partly because effectiveness, efficiency and equity are most relevant to economic evaluations, partly because they have intuitive appeal – we are likely to use similar criteria in spending our personal resources – and partly because they also underpin public policy in many countries. (They were reiterated, for example, in the UK government's new 'Best Value' initiative for local government services and in the December 1997 White Paper on the National Health Service.) There will often be tensions between the criteria: maximizing effectiveness may well not represent the most efficient use of resources, whilst efficiency and equity may pull in opposite directions. Additionally, there may be other criteria to consider, notably autonomy, liberty and diversity.

Effectiveness

Effectiveness in the sense of outcome achievement is usually defined in terms of improvements to child and family welfare, health or quality of life. It can also be defined as movement towards an organization's operational or policy objectives (such as to provide services to 10% more children next year or to postpone the need for further intervention in particular families). The demands for effectiveness insights and data are universal: clinicians and other service professionals want to know what effects their interventions exert on symptoms, behaviour and quality of life; governments want to know what returns they are getting from their investment of taxpayers' money; pharmaceutical companies want to be able to demonstrate the beneficial effects of their products; and of course families want to know that the problems faced by their children are being tackled. We shall see in a moment that many of these same constituencies – clinicians, governments, pharmaceutical companies and families – are increasingly likely to be demanding proof of *efficiency* as well as effectiveness.

Effectiveness measurement is complex, for – in addition to the aim of tackling antisocial behaviour itself – the objectives of child and adolescent services include improvements along the somewhat nebulous dimensions of quality of life and family welfare. The familiar reasons for this difficulty will be rehearsed in the final part of the chapter when we look at outcome measurement in economic evaluations. Such difficulties are not unique to child mental health care, but they can mean that many policy and practice decisions are hampered by serious information deficiencies on effectiveness (and hence also on efficiency and some aspects of equity). Consequently, effectiveness discussions in practice settings must often be conducted in terms of 'intermediate' indicators of service volume, quality and patient throughput. The relationships between (say) service quality and symptom reduction may or may not have been established reliably by empirical research.

Economists generally do not employ any particular or different definition of effectiveness from that used by other disciplines. Some economic evaluations do not look at effectiveness at all (as discussed below), but the majority will try to combine some effectiveness measures with resource (cost) indicators. This takes us to the efficiency criterion.

Efficiency

Efficiency combines the resource and effectiveness dimensions. In fact, efficiency has many different meanings, but basically the pursuit of efficiency means either reducing the cost of achieving a given level of effectiveness, or improving the effectiveness achieved from a fixed budget or set of resources. Efficiency has been seen as a controversial criterion in some quarters, but much of this controversy probably stems from the tendency of some policy makers to use the term 'efficiency' as a euphemism for cheapness and to refer to 'efficiency improvements' when they mean cutbacks. Understood properly, the criterion really ought to be quite widely accepted, particularly when used in combination with equity.

In economic evaluations the efficiency criterion underpins cost-benefit, cost-effectiveness and cost-utility analyses, although we shall see later that slightly different concepts of efficiency are being addressed. Governments charged with the responsibility of making the best use of public resources are among the most ardent enthusiasts for efficiency measures, but the constituencies of interest and demand are actually quite wide. For example, health service and other public sector commissioners or purchasers are similarly exercised with the task of allocating the resources under their command so as to have the biggest impact on need, which will mean weighing up the costs and the effects of deploying resources in different ways.

Equity

Equity in the use of or access to resources, or in the distribution of outcomes, can get overlooked when acute scarcity or an urgent need for (constrained) choice or rationing produces a headlong rush for what might look like better 'value for money'. Equity, fairness or justice was of course one of the founding principles of the UK National Health Service 50 years ago and remains an important aim today in many countries. Nevertheless there is no shortage of evidence on the detrimental effects of wide (and widening) income and wealth gaps on the health and quality of life of children and adolescents (Roberts, 1997).

The distinction can be made between horizontal and vertical equity. Horizontal equity is the equal treatment of equals: individuals with the same 'needs' should receive equivalent amounts of care or support, or individuals with the same personal means (for example, in relation to income or wealth) should bear equal burdens of funding. Vertical equity is the differential allocation of treatments or outcomes to individuals with different needs, or a differential burden of payment such as a progressive tax. If the prevalence of conduct disorder is higher in urban than in rural areas (Rutter et al., 1975a, b), resource allocation within a nationally funded health service should, *ceteris paribus*, direct more resources to urban areas. More generally, a public health system like Britain's, for example, should really not be characterized by such wide variations as are currently to be found (Kurtz et al., 1994). Targeting services on needs is the most common example of the pursuit of greater equity, and it is therefore also legitimate to question the efficiency with which equity is pursued, which has been termed 'target efficiency' (Bebbington & Davies, 1983).

A framework for evaluation

The associations between the three allocation criteria of effectiveness, efficiency and equity can be appreciated by employing a simple framework, which also makes plain the links between these criteria and the theoretical and empirical constructs widely used by economists. The framework assists in the interpretation of empirical measures of these and other concepts. This production of welfare approach, as it is known, was developed and employed in the early 1980s in studies of social care for elderly people (Davies & Knapp, 1981; Knapp, 1980), and was also suggested for child social care research (Knapp, 1979). It is summarized in a simple form in Fig. 17.1.

The key elements in the production of welfare framework are:

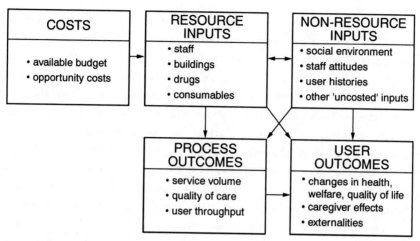

Fig. 17.1. Production of welfare.

Σ The resource inputs to treatment or care, mainly professional and other staff, capital and consumables, and including pharmaceutical products such as methylphenidate (Ritalin).

Σ The costs of those resource inputs expressed in monetary terms or alternatively the budget for a service-providing agency which is used to purchase resource inputs, plus recognition of opportunity costs for all resources whether or not they have a price. Opportunity costs are defined later in the chapter.

Σ The non-resource inputs to the treatment or care process, these being the influences on the achievement of effectiveness which do not have an identifiable price because they are not marketed and do not have an opportunity cost which can sensibly be calculated. They are not outcomes in their own right, nor are they resources to be purchased from existing budgets. Examples are biosocial influences, environmental adversity, cultural expectations, the social milieu of a care setting, the attitudes of the professionals delivering services, and the backgrounds and characteristics of the children and young people being treated (age at onset of the disorder, early behavioural difficulties, gender, attitudes, previous treatment experiences) (see, for example, Maughan & Rutter, 1998).

Σ The outputs or intermediate outcomes, which are the volumes of service output, almost certainly with a quality of care requirement, and perhaps weighted in some way for the characteristics of the children and young people using the service ('casemix'), produced from combinations of the resource and nonresource inputs.

Σ The final outcomes, which are changes over time in the symptoms, welfare and quality of life of children (and their families if relevant to the context), relative to some standard or comparator circumstances. Final outcomes are clearly measures of effectiveness. They can also be defined as reductions in need.

The production of welfare approach assumes that the final outcomes of a mental health care intervention will be influenced ('produced') by the nature of the services provided, the types, levels and mixes of resources employed, the 'social environment' of the care setting and other nonresource factors. This core theme of the production of welfare model is obviously not built up from economic theory as such, but it is a logical corollary of theory and evidence from psychology, child psychiatry and certain other disciplines. However, the formalization of the links between intervention characteristics, resource inputs and child and family outcomes owes much to economic theories of cost and production relations and their empirical investigation. By drawing analogies of this kind it is possible to draw up testable hypotheses and to employ the empirical tools of certain branches of applied economics, including the modes of evaluation discussed in this chapter.

Cost-effectiveness analysis and other evaluations

Market allocations

The simplest model in the most elementary economics textbook assumes that markets work sufficiently well to ensure that society's scarce resources are allocated efficiently. Few markets are as well-behaved as in the elementary textbook, but nevertheless market forces can very often be relied upon to allocate goods and services reasonably well between competing demands. If this is the case, then the need for economic evaluations of the costs and outcomes flowing from alternative uses of scarce resources is lessened some-what. Child and adolescent mental health care services in Britain are purchased and provided within internal or quasi-markets within the state sector (mainly), and these muted market forces have had some influence over allocations (Parry-Jones, 1995; Subotsky, 1992). Market forces play a much larger role in countries like the US, strongly influencing who gets what service and at what cost to different parties (Bickman et al., 1996; Padgett et al., 1993). However, it is difficult to imagine circumstances where techniques such as cost-effectiveness analysis would not be needed to guide the decision making of key actors in any of the world's health care and related systems.

Modes of evaluation

The most commonly discussed and most useful modes of economic evaluation are cost–benefit and cost-effectiveness analyses, but in fact there are quite a few different approaches. These different modes have some common elements, in particular their conceptualization and measurement of costs, but they differ in two main respects: (1) they measure outcomes differently and (2) consequently they address slightly different policy or practice questions.

The underlying aim of each mode of economic evaluation is to examine the efficiency with which resources are being utilized. If the evaluation is comparing two alternative treatments, the question to be addressed is whether one treatment achieves better outcomes for children and families than the other treatment, relative to their respective costs. If the outcomes that follow from the two treatments are known or found to be identical, the economic question would be whether one treatment is less costly than the other. These are efficiency questions and could obviously be employed to compare alternative accommodation settings, family support arrangements or national policies. The various modes of economic evaluation frame these efficiency comparisons in slightly different contexts. Overlaid onto these efficiency analyses are questions of equity in the availability and utilization of resources and in the attainment of health and welfare improvements. Are efficiency improvements achieved at the cost of greater inequity? Do the costs of a new policy fall disproportionately on an already disadvantaged group? Are the beneficial effects of a new treatment made available only to children and families who are perhaps not seen as the greatest priorities for support?

Three evaluative modes will be discussed here: cost–benefit analysis, cost-effectiveness analysis (and its recently distinguished variant cost–consequences analysis) and cost–utility analysis. An excellent, recently updated book by Drummond et al. (1997) gives a more thorough discussion of these modes of economic evaluation, and interested readers are referred there for more advanced discussions of these methods. Introductory accounts in the mental health field are offered by, for example, Kavanagh & Stewart (1995) and Yates (1994).

Cost–benefit analysis

Cost–benefit analysis (CBA) is unique among economic evaluations in that it addresses the extent to which a particular course of action, such as a form of family therapy or an inpatient admission, is socially worthwhile in the broadest sense. A CBA measures all costs and benefits in the same units – usually monetary units – and thus the two sides can be directly compared: if the benefits exceed the costs, the CBA evaluation would recommend undertaking the course of action, and vice versa. The other modes of evaluation cannot provide this degree of guidance. For two or more alternative treatments or interventions, cost-benefit differences can be computed and compared: the intervention which gives the biggest excess of benefits over costs would be deemed to be the most efficient. Note, however, that the most efficient intervention may not actually be chosen: for example, equity, ideology, ethical qualms or political necessity may dominate.

It must be emphasized that a CBA seeks to put monetary values on one or more of the final or intermediate outcomes. It does not simply compare the amount spent with the amount saved as a result of a treatment. This latter would be a cost-offset analysis, which compares two different levels of expenditure. Many evaluators have carried out cost-offset analyses but erroneously given them the CBA label. Without outcome data an evaluation is most certainly not worthless, but its relevance for decision makers is reduced.

There have been a few studies which have looked at how preventive action has been able to cut longer-term expenditure in criminal justice and other areas. Whether these are cost-offset or CBAs is debatable. The best known is the Perry Pre-school or High/Scope programme evaluation. This programme concentrated on children aged 3 or 4 years and achieved, at age 27 and compared to a nonintervention control group, fewer delinquent acts, less use of special education, higher employment and college enrolment rates, higher earnings, lower teenage pregnancy rates, less reliance on social assistance and better peer relationships. The cost-offset compared with the control group was US $15 000 per child at age 19 (Schweinhart & Weikart, 1981), and there was an estimated net benefit of almost $29 000 by age 27 (Barnett, 1985). Over the lifetime of the participants it was suggested that the programme returned to the public $7.16 for every dollar spent.

In another well known evaluation which included an economic component, Seitz et al. (1985) report a cost-offset of $20 000 per family in the Yale Child Study Center Program once children had reached age 13. School performance and attendance were better, and behavioural problems fewer. Again this could perhaps be seen as a CBA, although by no means all of the outcome measures used in the (full) evaluation were expressed in monetary terms. Despite some methodological limitations, both the Perry and Yale evaluations offer good examples of quite wide-ranging assessments of both outcomes and costs.

Generally, it is not hard to see why it is so difficult to conduct proper cost-benefit analyses in a field such as interventions for conduct disorder. The major difficulties arise with attempts to value outcomes in monetary terms. Methodologies for this purpose have been developed by economists – for example, asking various stakeholders how much they are willing to pay for different levels of a particular outcome, and are now being used in some health economics evaluations. However, none has yet been applied in the child or adolescent mental health fields.

Cost-effectiveness and cost–consequences analyses

Cost-effectiveness analysis (CEA) is concerned with ensuring that resources allocated to the treatment of child mental health problems (or one particular diagnosis such as conduct disorder) are used to maximum effect. CEA is usually employed to help decision makers choose between alternative interventions available to or aimed at specific patient groups:

Σ If two care or intervention options are of equal cost, which option provides the greater benefits from a given budget?

Σ If two options have been found to be equally beneficial in terms of child or population impact, which is less costly?

Σ Or if the two options have different costs and effects, which has the better cost-effectiveness ratio?

In the strict application of this evaluation mode, a CEA looks at a single effectiveness dimension and constructs a cost-effectiveness ratio. For example, a research evaluation in the conduct disorder setting might consider measuring changes in antisocial behaviour, and for young offenders one might measure effectiveness in terms of 'offending-free months'. Of two interventions, the one with the lowest cost-effectiveness ratio (lowest cost per unit improvement in outcome) would be the more efficient.

A generalization of CEA to multiple outcomes – which is surely necessary in an area of such symptomatic complexity as conduct disorder – is sometimes called a cost-consequences analysis (Drummond et al., 1997). There is now no single outcome measure to combine with costs in order to compute cost-effectiveness ratios but a set of relevant outcome indicators to be weighed up less formalistically, and compared with costs. What this mode of evaluation lacks in computational simplicity (with direct implications for decision making) it makes up for in its ability to evaluate policies and practices in a way which comes much closer to everyday reality. Findings from such an analysis would need to be reviewed by decision makers, and the different outcomes weighed up. But this is what child mental health care decision makers do every day of the week, so there should really be no hesitation among economists and other researchers about using such a technique.

Siegert & Yates (1980) evaluated three systems for training parents to use social learning techniques with children with behaviour problems. Thirty parents were randomly allocated to individual training at home or in the therapist's office, group training in the therapist's office or a no-training control group. The three interventions were 'equally effective in transmitting social learning principles into improved child-management' (p. 147). The families included in this study were not recruited from mental health or other agencies, their behavioural problems were comparatively mild, and the training techniques studied may now look less interesting than the videotapes developed for parent training by Webster-Stratton (1984), but Siegert & Yates' cost-effectiveness analysis would repay careful reading for its methodology. Unlike Webster-Stratton's otherwise impressive and widely influential work, they formally assessed cost-effectiveness rather than merely asserted it (cf. Webster-Stratton et al., 1988). Comprehensive costs were measured, including those borne by the families themselves, and cost comparisons were made from a variety of perspectives (agency, family, society).

Another example of a cost-effectiveness analysis is offered by Greenwood et al. (1996). They compared four prevention strategies to reduce the risk of eventual trouble with the law: (a) home visits by child care professionals before birth, continuing until age 2, and then day care until age 4; (b) parent training and family therapy with young school-age children; (c) four years of cash and other incentives to graduate; and (d) supervision of young people of high-school age. In each case, the target clients had exhibited antisocial behaviour (or in the first case the families were deemed to be high risk). Each of the four was compared with incarceration for criminal activities (California has harsh repeat-offence sanctions). All but intervention (a) were more cost-effective than incarceration. This study has numerous methodological limitations, an inevitable consequence of the meta-analytic approach which patched together data of varying qualities from a variety of sources, but offers a good jumping-off point for the discussion of preventive measures and their economic consequences.

Cost-utility analysis

The most recently developed mode of economic evaluation is cost-utility analysis (CUA). It is similar to CEA with the important exception that it measures and then values the impact of an intervention not in terms of a single effectiveness indicator such as re-offending or change in a behaviour rating but in terms of a global indicator of a child's health-related quality of life. This global indicator is labelled utility, and aims to summarize more than one effectiveness dimension. Costs are again measured as opportunities forgone, and now represent the costs of achieving the observed changes in quality of life.

The most commonly used measure of 'utility' in the health economics literature is the quality-adjusted life year or QALY, which weights longevity by life quality, and the most familiar measure of health-related quality of life is the EuroQol or EQ-5D (EuroQol Group, 1990). Utility scores are now being developed to convert from Short Form (SF) 36 quality of life measures. Other generic currencies in use today are healthy-year equivalents (HYEs) and disability-adjusted life years (DALYs), although both are used less often than the QALY.

Cost-utility analyses avoid the potential ambiguities with multidimensional outcomes. They can also be seen as an improvement on a single effectiveness measure in what is generally regarded as an inherently multidimensional world. The transparency of the methods used to derive 'utility' scores is a particular strength of the approach. CUAs can be applied to choices across a range of treatments or diagnoses: they can compare one health care area to a quite different area. This has resulted in the construction of 'league tables' of cost per QALY gained. However, there is a danger that QALY or similar measures gloss over the complexities of real-life situations. Where they are most useful is as an adjunct to a CEA or cost-consequences analysis.

CUA was pioneered in the broader health care field in the 1970s and is now quite widely applied there, but there appear to be no examples of its use in child mental health care.

Putting principles into practice

The main modes of economic evaluation have a common aim in their approach to cost measurement, which – if a societal perspective is adopted (which is usually the case; see below) – is to range widely across all direct and indirect costs (Table 17.1). Every resource impact and every opportunity cost is to be included. The types of evaluation obviously differ with respect to their measurement of outcomes. Many problems must be overcome when seeking to turn these economic evaluative principles into practical (and helpful) empirical studies. Three problem areas warrant particular attention: cost measurement, outcome measurement and the duration of an evaluation.

Table 17.1. Economic evaluations – measurement of costs and outcomes

Mode of evaluation	Cost measurement	Outcome measurement
Cost-offset analysis	Comprehensive	No outcomes measured
Cost–effectiveness analysis	Comprehensive	One outcome only
Cost–consequences analysis	Comprehensive	Multiple outcomes measured
Cost–benefit analysis	Comprehensive	Monetary valuation of outcomes
Cost–utility analysis	Comprehensive	Summary utility score of outcomes

Cost measurement

Many research studies on conduct disorder have pointed to the comprehensive nature of children's needs and the consequent (potential) utilization of a range of services with a wide cost base. For example, antisocial behaviour has implications which are not all related to health care, but which impact upon schools, social services agencies, the criminal justice system and elsewhere. Consequently, a well-conducted economic evaluation should normally aim to measure costs and outcomes comprehensively (or to employ partial measures advisedly). Almost any evaluation in the child mental health field would be likely to need to adopt a societal perspective – looking at the widest set of costs and effects – and not the narrower health service or child and family perspectives. For a start, many agencies could be active with young people with conduct disorders, and the consequences of their actions will generally be of quite wide societal concern. Given that inter-agency boundaries are a root cause of some of the operational difficulties in this field, it would generally be misleading to take a narrower view. As the UK House of Commons Health Committee concluded when commenting on school exclusions:

[T]he current arrangements, under which no effective alternative education is arranged for excluded children, are clearly unsatisfactory, and may well contribute not to reducing but to perpetuating patterns of conduct disorder and anti-social behaviour. They also mean that benefits from treatments such as methylphenidate (Ritalin) cannot be fully realised. (1997, p. xliii)

Techniques are needed to record the services used by children and families and to calculate their associated costs. These are separate activities. Numerous pragmatic instruments have been developed to collect service utilization data, one of them by Beecham & Knapp (1992), originally for a particular multiple-casemix group study, but now employed in a large number of studies in the UK and elsewhere. This is the Client Service Receipt Inventory (CSRI).

The second activity is to attach unit costs to services. The economic cost of a resource is the value of the benefits forgone from not using that resource in its highest valued alternative use. This is the economist's concept of 'opportunity cost' (see, for example, Knapp, 1993). Given that all resources are finite in their availability, any health care or other intervention will impose an opportunity cost even when apparently provided free of charge (for example, the use of volunteers is usually not costless). Most resources used directly in the provision of a service (such as psychologist, psychiatrist or social worker time, drugs, equipment and administrative resources) will have market values – they are bought and sold in markets where prices are set by the interplay of the forces of demand and supply, even if imperfectly. In ideal circumstances, these values reflect the opportunity costs of the resource input. In reality, the hourly price of providing specialist family therapy, for example, might not equal the private or social opportunity cost of an hour's use of the therapist's time, but pragmatism dictates that these values are usually the best estimates likely to be reached (see Bickman et al., 1996, ch. 7; Drummond et al., 1997, ch. 4).

Beecham (1995) details a general methodology for costing the service inputs provided by a range of professionals and in a number of accommodation and other congregate settings. Beyond the costing of the 'human resource input' into care, it is also vital to recognize the full range of operating and capital costs associated with service delivery, including those associated with administrative and other overheads. For the UK, there is now an annual publication, *Unit Costs of Health and Social Care*, published by the Personal Social Services Research Unit (PSSRU) which provides up-to-date costings for many health and social welfare services, together with guidelines as to how these are to be employed for different purposes (Netten & Dennett, 1997). For example, in 1996/97 the cost of an inpatient paediatric bed was £237 per day, a child clinical psychiatry team contact with a client cost £51 per hour (and £258 per hour of team working/meeting), a social worker's face-to-face contact with a client cost £78 per hour, and the full package of services used by a child in a local authority community home amounted to £1538 per week. These are all public sector costs. All are, of course, averages.

A number of economic evaluations of child and adolescent mental health services and current or past users are underway at the Institute of Psychiatry/ Maudsley Hospital. One pilot study of ten children referred to the Maudsley Hospital with behavioural problems (diagnosed as conduct disorder) found that the total annual costs attributable to their problems amounted to an average of £15 000 during 1996/97, including allowances and benefits (transfer payments). The breakdown of costs is shown in Table 17.2, and illustrates the range of

Table 17.2. Ten children with conduct disorder: annual costs

National Health Service costs	£2469
Local authority social services	£991
Local authority education services	£4754
Voluntary sector services	£56
(Subtotal: all direct costs)	(£8270)
Lost employment for parents	£3925
Additional housework burden	£538
Extra household repairs	£288
Allowance and benefits	£2261
Total cost (including allowances and benefits) per child	£15 370

Source: Knapp, Scott & Davies (1999).

agencies involved and the consequent need for comprehensive costing if we are to understand the full effects of a mental health problem. The costs in this pilot study also illustrate the potential for wide interpersonal variations in cost. Among the ten children and families, annual costs ranged from £5411 in one case to £40 896 in another. Variations of this magnitude and their implications for research strategy are discussed further below.

Outcome measurement

The measurement of outcomes in conduct disorder, as in other areas of child and adolescent mental health care, social care and education, is quite widely discussed. Most of the discussions point to the difficulty of the task. The reasons for this difficulty are probably familiar but are worth rehearsing because of the strong pressures from various quarters to base expenditure or funding decisions on evidence relating to proven effectiveness:

Σ Changes in child health, behaviour, welfare or quality of life sometimes take years to be achieved. Indeed some policy and practice aims are rightly linked to influencing lifetime behaviour and long-term life chances.

Σ Effectiveness might actually be achieved by slowing down a deteriorative trend or accelerating an upward trend. This makes effectiveness difficult to assess without a comparison group or a set of norms, for there will be ageing and other trending effects (Maughan & Rutter, 1998). This in turn opens up issues concerning study 'design' and the comparability of different settings, user groups and care arrangements.

Σ   Effectiveness is partly subjective (health and social care and education are what economists would call 'experience goods'), and should be based partly on users' and families' own experiences and views. But users may be poorly placed to express their views reliably, because of their behavioural problems, confusion or age, or reluctant to do so because of the compulsory nature of their care. Sometimes families, too, may not make reliable 'raters': they may not be as disinterested as one would like for this kind of task.

Σ   Many interventions have 'multiple clients' (e.g. a child and their family; an offender and the community in which he offends; a disabled teenager and her caregiving network), raising questions as to whose effectiveness should be assessed (or what weights to attach to different perspectives), and indeed whose perspectives on that effectiveness are legitimate or relevant.

Other things being equal, the greater and the more diverse a child's needs, the broader the range of services likely to be utilized and the greater the number of outcome dimensions which an evaluation might be expected to need in order to gauge impact fully. What outcomes are important depends on the objectives that a service or policy is trying to meet. In just the same way as costs should usually be comprehensive, outcome measurement should also be comprehensive in (i) measuring changes in health and welfare status across all relevant domains of the person's life, and (ii) measuring the change in the welfare of all the persons concerned.

Outcome measurement will not be discussed further in this chapter, but it should be emphasized that some distinctive contributions could be made by economics. These include the development of summary unidimensional measures (discussed in the cost-utility section earlier), benefit valuation in monetary terms (with its attendant difficulties, even though new methods are breaking new ground in other fields), and offset measurement (which is quite often undertaken without other outcome assessment, and therefore will usually be inadequate on its own, but which has been most commonly used in child mental health, behaviour and crime prevention evaluations). We would also emphasize, however, that perfectly acceptable (and potentially enormously insightful) economic evaluations can be conducted without resorting to utility, benefit or offset measurement. Cost-effectiveness and cost-consequences approaches have a great deal to offer, building on outcome measures which will be more familiar to noneconomist researchers in this field. It is for this reason that cost-effectiveness and cost-consequences analyses, linked to ongoing clinical trials or other evaluations, are the most likely to be employed over the next few years.

Length of research period

Some of the frequently observed childhood and adulthood implications of conduct disorder were noted at the start of the chapter. These are well-charted waters in child psychiatry and psychology. For example, Zoccolillo et al. (1992) looked at the outcomes of childhood conduct disorder in terms of adulthood social functioning, particularly work, sexual/love relationships, social relationships and criminality; and Maughan & Rutter (1998) discussed continuities and discontinuities between childhood and adulthood along these and other dimensions. There is the related issue that some behavioural, social and economic problems will be transmitted to later generations. There is plenty of evidence of intergenerational transmission of problems, with its own implications for service support networks and public expenditure (Göpfert et al., 1995; Robins & Rutter, 1990).

These potential long-term implications of conduct disorder make it imperative that economic evaluations should endeavour to map the longer-term costs and outcomes of alternative services, treatments or policies. The challenge for a research study is to choose an appropriate length of study: too short a follow-up period will risk missing the full cost and outcome consequences of an intervention, whereas too long a follow-up will risk a large number of dropouts from the study and will also possibly complicate the untangling of causal connections. An important requirement for an economic evaluation is to be clear about causal connections: cost and outcome consequences may be difficult to attribute to a particular intervention or event without very careful research design.

Another requirement is to recognize that more distant, future costs and outcomes might not be valued as highly as costs and outcomes which occur much sooner. This is characteristic of most people's rates of time preference, and an evaluation spanning many years will usually need to discount future or later costs and outcomes back to a present value via an appropriate weighting procedure.

There is a third consideration to bear in mind when looking at a health problem with such potential long-term consequences. This is the problem of different time profiles for costs and outcomes: the full benefits of an intervention in childhood may not be observed for many years, creating a possible disincentive for funders. When resources are particularly tight and when performance is under close scrutiny, it can become increasingly difficult to justify expenditure now on areas which show no or only modest benefits for a few years. Even if there is strong evidence linking treatment expenditure in childhood to favourable outcomes in adulthood – and the evidence in relation to conduct disorder has perhaps not reached such strength just yet – the political imperative of demonstrating 'payback' may just be too pressing to justify the allocation of sufficient resources to the area.

Conclusions

As we have seen, awareness has grown in many quarters of the need for careful evaluation of the economic consequences, both short-term and long-term, of mental health problems in childhood and adolescence, and particularly of conduct disorder. The enormous pressures on health, education and social services resources make it wildly unrealistic to imagine that society could spend its way out of the present problems of under-resourcing and poor coordination. Health insurance companies in countries with predominantly private health care systems are unlikely to be prepared to commit substantial extra funds to tackling conduct disorder, particularly given the often overlapping responsibilities with schools and criminal justice agencies. In countries with public health care systems governments face many competing demands for tax revenue, and increases in the marginal rate of taxation are usually difficult for politicians to sell to the general public. But even if these private or public purchasers were willing to spend more on child and adolescent mental health services they would simultaneously be looking for ways to improve the effectiveness achieved from given levels of resources.

Additional pressures on available treatment and support resources come from the growing prevalence of some childhood needs and evidence of a wide (and perhaps widening) gap between need and the supply of effective treatments or interventions. A number of socioeconomic changes – such as growing rates of divorce and single parenthood, and problems associated with social exclusion – might be partly to blame. There is also the pressure that comes from the higher expectations of public services held by the general public, by service users and their families, and by the professionals who deliver the services.

In consequence there are many expressed demands for economic evaluations across the wide span of public and social policies, including in the areas of health and social care, education, criminal justice, employment and social exclusion. For example, governments and public sector bodies request economic evaluations to inform or reflect upon their strategic policy decisions. Service providers (in all sectors) look for evidence to help them improve the effectiveness and cost-effectiveness of their activities. Service commissioners aim to achieve value for money or 'best value' when purchasing services to meet the needs of their populations.

In stark contrast to the various expressed demands for economic data there have been very few completed studies of treatments, support arrangements or policies (Knapp, 1997; Utting, 1996). Costello et al. (1993) even offer the suggestion that there is an inverse relationship between the cost of a service and the likelihood of it being evaluated: inpatient services have, for example, been particularly neglected. This raises a more specific point about the distribution of costs. For a small number of young people the costs of their disorders and treatment are especially high compared to the average because these individuals account for a markedly disproportionate number of poor outcomes. Economic evaluative research should perhaps give especial attention to these children and families, not to the exclusion of all others but to ensure that the cases which most concern purchasers (funders) and policy makers can begin to be better understood.

Economic evaluations raise no insurmountable technical or practical difficulties, so this cannot be the reason for their relative scarcity in this field. Probably the primary reasons for the shortage of such studies have been a reluctance among other disciplines (until recently) to invite economists to join them and a shortage of economists able and willing to respond. As the few completed studies in this field demonstrate, there are interesting cost consequences of different intervention types. There is, for example, a suggestion from the meta-analyses and reviews of Tremblay & Craig (1995) and Greenwood et al. (1996) that complementary interventions in both the teenage and earlier years could be most effective and cost-effective in tackling criminality. Whether these (tentative) findings would carry over to antisocial behaviour more generally is not altogether clear, and of course there are a host of therapeutic and other interventions for conduct disorder (as discussed in other chapters) which might benefit from economic evaluation. To quote the House of Commons Health Committee again:

The cost of conduct disorders, both in terms of the quality of life of those who have conduct disorder and the people around them, and in terms of the resources necessary to counteract them, is high. It is therefore important that treatment for conduct disorder is both effective and cost-effective. (1997, p. xxiii)

REFERENCES

Almond, R. (1995). Ethical managed care (letter). *Psychiatric Services, 46*, 410.

Audit Commission (1996). *Misspent Youth: Young People and Crime.* London: HMSO.

Audit Commission (1999). *Children in Mind: Child and Adolescent Mental Health Services*. Abingdon: Audit Commission Publications.

Barnett, W.S. (1985). Benefit-cost analysis of the Perry Preschool Program and its policy implications. *Educational Evaluation and Policy Analysis*, 7, 333–42.

Bebbington, A.C. & Davies, B.P. (1983). Equity and efficiency in the allocation of the personal social services. *Journal of Social Policy*, 12, 309–30.

Bebbington, A.C. & Miles, J. (1989). The background of children who enter local authority care. *British Journal of Social Work*, 19, 349–68.

Beecham, J. (1995). Collecting and estimating costs. In M.R.J. Knapp (Ed.), *The Economic Evaluation of Mental Health Care* (pp. 61–82). Aldershot: Arena.

Beecham, J.K. & Knapp, M.R.J. (1992). Costing psychiatric options. In G. Thornicroft, C. Brewin & J. Wing (Eds.). *Measuring Mental Health Needs* (pp. 179–90). Oxford: Oxford University Press.

Behar, L. (1985). Changing patterns of state responsibility: a case study of North Carolina. *Journal of Clinical Child Psychology*, 14, 188–95.

Bickman, L., Guthrie, P.R., Foster, E.M., et al. (1996). *Evaluating Managed Mental Health Services: The Fort Bragg Experiments*. New York: Plenum Press.

Burns, B.J., Costello, E.J., Angold, A., et al. (1995). Children's mental health service use across service sectors. *Health Affairs*, 14, 147–59.

Cooper, P.J. & Goodyer, I. (1993). A community study of depression in adolescent girls. I: estimates of symptom and syndrome prevalence. *British Journal of Psychiatry*, 163, 369–74.

Costello, E.J., Burns, B.J., Angold, A. & Leaf, P.J. (1993). How can epidemiology improve mental health services for children and adolescents? *Journal of American Academy of Child and Adolescent Psychiatry*, 32 1106–14.

Davies, B.P. & Knapp, M.R.J. (1981). *Old People's Homes and the Production of Welfare*. London: Routledge and Kegan Paul.

Dickey, B. (1998). Managed care for mental illness: the Massachusetts experience. *Mental Health Research Review*, 5, 33–7.

Diekstra, R.F.W. (1995). Depression and suicidal behaviours in adolescence: sociocultural and time trends. In M. Rutter (Ed.), *Psychosocial Disturbances in Young People*. Cambridge: Cambridge University Press.

Dorwart, R.A. (1990). Managed mental health care: myths and realities in the 1990s. *Hospital and Community Psychiatry*, 41, 1087–91.

Drummond, M.R., O'Brien, B., Stoddart, G.L. & Torrance, G.W. (1997). *Methods for the Economic Evaluation of Health Care Programmes*, Second edn. Oxford: Oxford Medical Publications.

EuroQol (1990). EuroQol – a new facility for the measurement of health-related quality of life. *Health Policy*, 16, 199–208.

Evans, S. & Brown, R. (1993). Perception of need for child psychiatry services among parents and general practitioners. *Health Trends*, 25, 53–6.

Fairfield, G., Hunter, D.J., Mechanic, D. & Rosleff, F. (1997). Managed care: origins, principles and evolution. *British Medical Journal*, 314, 1823–6.

Farrington, D.P. & West, D.J. (1990). The Cambridge study in delinquent development: a long-term follow-up study of 411 London males. In H.J. Kerner & G. Kaiser (Eds.), *Criminality: Personality, Behaviour and Life History*. Berlin: Springer-Verlag.

Fergusson, D.M., Horwood, L.J. & Lynskey, M.T. (1993). Prevalence and comorbidity of DSM–III–R diagnoses in a birth cohort of 15 year olds. *Journal of the American Academy of Child and Adolescent Psychiatry, 32,* 1127–34.

Frank, R.G. & Dewa, C.S. (1992). Insurance, system structure, and the use of mental health services by children and adolescents. *Clinical Psychology Review, 12,* 829–40.

Frank, R.G., Salkever, D. & Sharfstein, S. (1991). A new look at rising mental health insurance costs. *Health Affairs, 10,* 116–23.

Friedman, R.M. & Kutash, K. (1992). Challenges for child and adolescent mental health. *Health Affairs, 11,* 125–36.

Garralda, M.E. (1994). Primary care psychiatry. In M. Rutter, E. Taylor & L. Hersov (Eds.). *Child and Adolescent Psychiatry: Modern Approaches* (pp. 1055–70). Oxford: Blackwell Scientific Publications.

Göpfert, M., Webster, J. & Seemen, M.V. (1995). *Disturbed Mentally Ill Parents and their Children*. Cambridge: Cambridge University Press.

Greenwood, P.W., Model, K.E., Rydell, C.P. & Chiesa, J. (1996). *Diverting Children from a Life of Crime: Measuring Costs and Benefits*. Santa Monica: RAND.

Gureje, O., Omigbodun, O.O., Gater, R., Acha, R.A. & Ikuesan, B.A. (1994). Psychiatric disorders in a paediatric primary care clinic. *British Journal of Psychiatry, 165,* 530–3.

Health Advisory Service (1995). *Child and Adolescent Mental Health Services: Together We Stand*. London: HMSO.

House of Commons Health Committee (1997). *Child and Adolescent Mental Health Services*. Fourth Report, Session 1996–97, HC 26-I. London: HMSO.

John, L.H., Offord, D.R., Boyle, M.H. & Racine, Y.A. (1995). Factors predicting use of mental health and social services by children 6–16 years old: Findings from the Ontario Child Health Study. *American Journal of Orthopsychiatry, 65,* 76–86.

Kavanagh, S.M. (1997). Purchasers, providers and managed care: developments in the mental health market place. *Current Opinion in Psychiatry, 10,* 153–9.

Kavanagh, S.M. & Stewart, A. (1995). Economic evaluations of mental health care. In M.R.J. Knapp (Ed.), *The Economic Evaluation of Mental Health Care* (pp. 27–60). Aldershot: Arena.

Klerman, G.L. & Weissman, M.M. (1989). Increasing rates of depression. *Journal of the American Medical Association, 261,* 2229–35.

Knapp, M.R.J. (1979). Planning child care from an economics perspective. *Residential and Community Child Care Administration, 1,* 229–48

Knapp, M.R.J. (1980). Production relations for old people's homes. PhD thesis, University of Kent at Canterbury.

Knapp, M.R.J. (1993). Background theory. In A. Netten & J.K. Beecham (Eds.), *Costing Community Care: Theory and Practice*. Aldershot: Ashgate.

Knapp, M.R.J. (1997). Economic evaluations and interventions for children and adolescents with mental health problems. *Journal of Child Psychology and Psychiatry, 38,* 3–25.

Knapp, M.R.J., Scott, S. & Davies, J. (1999). The cost of antisocial behaviour in younger children:

a pilot study of economic and family impact. *Clinical Child Psychology and Psychiatry, 4,* 457–73.

Knitzer, J. (1982). *Unclaimed Children.* Washington, DC: Children's Defense Fund.

Knitzer, J. (1993). Children's mental health policy: challenging the future. *Journal of Emotional and Behavioural Disorder, 1,* 8–16.

Kurtz, Z., Thornes, R. & Wolkind, S. (1994). *Services for the Mental Health of Children and Young People in England: A National Review.* London: South West Thames RHA.

Kurtz, Z., Thornes, R. & Wolkind, S. (1995). *Services for the Mental Health of Children and Young People in England: Assessment of Needs and Unmet Need.* London: South West Thames RHA.

Light, D. & Bailey, V. (1993). Pound foolish. *Health Service Journal,* 11 February, 16–18.

Maughan, B. & Rutter, M. (1998). Continuities and discontinuities in antisocial behaviour from childhood to adult life. In T.H. Ollendick & R.J. Prinz (Eds.), *Advances in Clinical Child Psychology* (pp. 1–47). New York: Plenum Press.

Netten, A. & Dennett, J. (1997). *Unit Costs of Health and Social Care 1997.* Personal Social Services Research Unit, University of Kent at Canterbury.

Offord, D.R., Boyle, M.H., Racine, Y.A., et al. (1992). Outcome, prognosis, and risk in a longitudinal follow-up study. *Journal of the American Academy of Child and Adolescent Psychiatry, 31,* 916–23.

Oppenheim, C. & Harker, L. (1996). *Poverty: The Facts.* London: Child Poverty Action Group.

Padgett, D.K., Patrick, C., Burns, B.J., Schlesinger, H.J. & Cohen, J. (1993). The effect of insurance benefit changes on use of child and adolescent outpatient mental health services. *Medical Care, 31,* 96–110.

Parry-Jones, W.L. (1995). The future of adolescent psychiatry. *British Journal of Psychiatry, 166,* 299–305.

Patrick, C., Padgett, D.K., Burns, B.J., Schlesinger, H.J. & Cohen, J. (1993). Use of inpatient services by a national population: do benefits make a difference? *Journal of the American Academy of Child and Adolescent Psychiatry, 32,* 144–52.

Pomerantz, J.M. (1995). A managed care ethical credo: for clinicians only? *Psychiatric Services, 46,* 329–30.

Roberts, H. (1997). Children, inequalities and health. *British Medical Journal, 314,* 1122–5.

Robins, L.N. (1986). Changes in conduct disorder over time. In D.C. Farran & J.D. McKinney (Eds.), *Risk in Intellectual and Psychosocial Development.* Orlando: FL: Academic Press.

Robins, L.N. & Rutter, M.L. (1990). *Straight and Devious Pathways from Childhood to Adolescence.* Cambridge: Cambridge University Press.

Routh, D.K. (1994). Impact of poverty on children, youth, and families: introduction to the special issue. *Journal of Clinical Child Psychology, 23,* 346–8.

Rutter, M.L., Cox, A., Tupling, C., Berger, M. & Yule, W. (1975a). Attainment and adjustment in two geographical areas. I: The prevalence of psychiatric disorder. *British Journal of Psychiatry, 126,* 35–56.

Rutter, M.L., Yule, B., Quinton, D., Rowlands, O., Yule, W. & Berger, M. (1975b). Attainment and adjustment in two geographical areas. III: Some factors accounting for area differences. *British Journal of Psychiatry, 126,* 520–33.

Ryan, N.D., Williamson, D.E., Iyengar, S., et al. (1992). A secular increase in child and adolescent onset affective disorder. *Journal of the American Academy of Child and Adolescent Psychiatry, 31,* 600–5.

Sabin, J.E. (1994). A credo for ethical managed care in mental health practice. *Hospital and Community Psychiatry, 45,* 859–60.

Scherl, O.J. (1985). Are psychiatric benefits worth the cost? *Journal of the American Medical Association, 253,* 3300–1.

Schweinhart, L.J. & Weikart, D.P. (1981). Perry Preschool effects nine years later: what do they mean? In M. Begab, H.C. Haywood & H.L. Garber (Eds.), *Psychological Influences in Retarded Performance.* Baltimore: University Park.

Seitz, V., Rosenbaum, L. & Apfel, N. (1985). Effects of family support intervention: a ten year follow-up. *Child Development, 56,* 376–91.

Shaffer, D. (1988). The epidemiology of teen suicide: an examination of risk factors. *Journal of Clinical Psychology, 156,* 866–70.

Siegert, F.E. & Yates, B.T. (1980). Behavioral child-management cost-effectiveness: a comparison of individual in-office, individual in-home, and group delivery systems. *Evaluation and the Health Professions, 3,* 123–52.

Subotsky, F. (1992). Psychiatric treatment for children – the organisation of services. *Archives of the Disabled Child, 67,* 971–5.

Tremblay, R.E. & Craig, W.M. (1995). Developmental crime prevention. In M. Tonry & D.P. Farrington (Eds.), *Building a Safer Society.* Chicago: University of Chicago Press.

Unützer, J. & Tischler, G.L. (1995). Differences in managed care (letter). *Psychiatric Services, 46,* 731–2.

Utting, D. (1996). *Reducing Criminality among Young People: A Sample of Relevant Programmes in the UK.* London: Home Office Research and Statistics Directorate.

Webster-Stratton, C. (1984). Randomized trial of two parent-training programs for families with conduct-disordered children. *Journal of Consulting and Clinical Psychology, 52,* 666–78.

Webster-Stratton, C., Kolpacoff, M. & Hollinsworth, T. (1988). Self-administered videotape therapy for families with conduct-problem children: comparison with two cost-effective treatments and a control group. *Journal of Consulting and Clinical Psychology, 56,* 558–66.

Wells, K.B., Astrachan, B.M., Tischler, G.L. & Unützer, J. (1995). Issues and approaches in evaluating managed mental health care. *Milbank Quarterly, 75,* 57–75.

Wilkinson, R. (1994). *Unfair Shares.* Ilford: Barnardo's.

Woodroffe, C., Glickman, M., Barker, M. & Power, C. (1993). *Children, Teenagers and Health: The Key Data.* Buckingham: Open University Press.

Yates, B.T. (1994). Towards the incorporation of costs, cost-effectiveness analysis and cost-benefit analysis into clinical research. *Journal of Consulting and Clinical Psychology, 62,* 729–36.

Zoccolillo, M., Pickles, A., Quinton, D. & Rutter, M. (1992). The outcome of childhood conduct disorder: implications for defining adult personality disorder and conduct disorder. *Psychological Medicine, 22,* 971–86.

18

Antisocial children grown up

Barbara Maughan and Michael Rutter

Introduction

Much adult psychopathology has its roots in childhood difficulties; nowhere is that tendency more apparent than in the antisocial domain. From the time of the first long-term follow-ups (Robins, 1966, 1978) it has been clear that most severely antisocial adults have long histories of disruptive and deviant behaviour reaching back to childhood. Yet these same studies also highlighted an apparent paradox: looking forward from childhood, the picture was a rather different one. Most conduct-disordered children did not grow up to be severely antisocial adults, and for many, discontinuity, rather than continuity, seemed the more usual course.

Identifying the mechanisms that account for these patterns constitutes a central challenge for developmental psychopathology. Which early risks or intervening processes contribute to the long-term persistence of antisocial problems in some individuals, but allow an apparently more benign course in others? Do the majority of antisocial children indeed 'recover' before adulthood, or do they too face continuing vulnerabilities, albeit of a less severe or possibly different kind? And can these varying developmental trajectories help us understand the underlying heterogeneity within the population of antisocial children, and so illuminate classifications of childhood disorders?

Conceptual and methodological issues

Heterogeneity

As other chapters in this volume highlight, childhood behaviour problems are far from homogeneous. At one extreme, the majority of young people are involved in occasional illegal acts; at the other, a minority show long-term,

An earlier version of this chapter (Maughan, B. & Rutter, M. (1998) Continuities and discontinuities in antisocial behavior from childhood to adult life) appeared in T.H. Ollendick & R.J. Prinz (Eds.), *Advances in Clinical Child Psychology*, Volume 20 (pp. 1–47). New York: Plenum Press. We are grateful to the publishers for permission to reproduce this revision.

persistent difficulties that span not only criminality but also severe dysfunction in a range of life domains (Robins et al., 1991). Opinions vary widely, however, on what these variations mean. Some investigators have argued that all manifestations of antisocial behaviour are best viewed in terms of a single underlying syndrome or propensity (Gottfredson & Hirschi, 1990; Jessor & Jessor, 1977), while others have focused on factorially derived dimensions (Frick et al., 1993; Loeber & Schmaling, 1985), and psychiatric classifications involve discrete syndromes. Each of these perspectives is reflected in the long-term follow-up literature. Rather than restrict our focus to diagnostic groupings, we have thus included findings from each of these traditions – along with the extensive literatures on adult outcomes of juvenile offending and delinquency – in the present chapter.

Categories and dimensions

A closely related issue, still unresolved, concerns whether antisocial behaviours are best conceptualized as qualitatively distinct categories or varying admixtures of dimensional traits and risks (Cantwell & Rutter, 1994; Clark et al., 1995; Waldman et al., 1995). Although much existing literature is premised on categorical models, it is far from clear that this is in fact the most appropriate stance. Studies in both medicine and psychology suggest that behaviours can function dimensionally for some purposes, but categorically for others. Clearly categorical outcomes (such as the occurrence of a heart attack) may have their origins in dimensional variables (such as cholesterol levels), and clinically important dimensions can often be identified within qualitatively distinct disease categories. Diagnostic assessments of childhood disorders show considerable overlap with dimensional syndrome scores (Gould et al., 1993; Jensen et al., 1996), and, as we discuss in more detail below, subclinical levels of difficulty frequently show correlates and consequences similar to those of more severe disorder categories. From a methodological perspective, dimensional approaches offer greater power, and categorical models are sensitive to threshold variations (Farrington, 1991). In some instances, however, especially when constellations of factors are examined, categorical models can have considerable force (Magnusson & Bergman, 1990). At this stage, the issue is an empirical one, and longitudinal data offer one important means of testing alternative formulations.

Continuity and change

Several rather different concepts of continuity and change arise in studies of behavioural development (Kagan, 1980; Rutter, 1987). First, there is the question of normative consistency, or the stability of individual differences over time. In relation to antisocial behaviours, such stability is high. Olweus (1979) estimated disattentuated correlations of 0.60 for measures of aggression over 10-year age spans in childhood and early adulthood, with relatively stable individual differences in aggressive tendencies evident from the preschool years. This consistency extends beyond measures of phenotypically similar behaviours; heterotypic continuity (Kagan, 1969) – whereby differing, but conceptually coherent, indicators of antisocial tendencies are related across development – is also strong. Huesmann et al. (1984), for example, reported significant correlations between peer-nominated aggression at age 8 and the number and seriousness of convictions, rates of drunk driving, and harsh physical punishment of children over 20 years later. Rydelius (1988) documented markedly increased risks of violent death amongst previously incarcerated delinquents. Numerous other studies, using a range of different indicators, have reached similar conclusions: individual differences in antisocial and aggressive tendencies are relatively stable across development. Equally important, this is so even over developmental periods when the overall level of antisocial behaviour is rising – as in early adolescence – or falling sharply, as in early adulthood (Farrington, 1990).

These age trends form a second key part of the backdrop to studies of the development of antisocial behaviours. Probably the best-known example here is the age–crime curve. Beginning at the age of criminal responsibility, rates of recorded male crime show a gradual increase over the early teens, a sharp rise in the later teens, then an equally sharp decline in the mid-20s. Studies of offenders reveal a similar pattern. In the UK, for example, under 5% of males are convicted of offences in the early teens and again in the mid-20s, but some 12% of young men are likely to be involved with the criminal justice system in their late teenage years (Farrington, 1992; Home Office, 1995). Self-reports highlight a similar pattern, suggesting that illegal behaviours are so common as to be virtually normative among boys in adolescence (Elliott et al., 1983). Although age trends in disruptive and antisocial disorders have been less systematically documented, they too show a marked adolescent peak. Before age 11, rates of oppositional and conduct disorders occur at around 6% in boys and 2% in girls (Offord et al., 1987). For both sexes, reported rates of oppositional disorders then rise to levels as high as 15–16% among 13 to 16-year-olds, with a sharp decline thereafter (Cohen et al., 1993a). Prevalence curves differ between the sexes in conduct disorder. Rates for boys fall after the early- to midteens, whereas those for girls increase to around age 16, then decline steeply. In early adulthood, some 6% of males and 0.6% of females have been reported as meeting criteria for antisocial personality disorder (Newman et al., 1996); rates fall further in the later adult years (Robins et al., 1991). Drug and alcohol disorders emerge for the first time in the late teens. They too show a marked male preponderance and a decline in prevalence with age across the adult years (Anthony & Helzer, 1991; Helzer et al., 1991).

Individual trajectories will not, of course, necessarily follow this same pattern. Indeed, longitudinal studies of offending (Blumstein et al., 1986; Farrington, 1986a; Nagin et al., 1995) have highlighted the very different implications that emerge from cross-sectional and longitudinal designs. Longitudinal analyses make clear that the adolescent peak in offending is composed of at least two elements: an increase in the prevalence of offenders, along with an adolescent increase in rates of offending among those already involved in crime (Farrington & West, 1993; Nagin et al., 1995). Alongside relatively stable individual differences in antisocial behaviours, the developmental picture also gives clear evidence of important within-individual change.

Reports and reporters

Multiple informants have been seen as essential in assessing child psychopathology, yet epidemiological studies have consistently found that agreement among them is poor (Achenbach et al., 1987). Measurement issues of this kind raise three main types of issue in the context of longitudinal studies. First, different accounts may suggest quite different patterns of stability and change in antisocial behaviours. Self-reports, for example, suggest longer-term persistence in illegal activities and antisocial lifestyles in early adulthood than is reflected in official records (Graham & Bowling, 1995; Nagin et al., 1995), and stability coefficients may differ depending on whether they are based on parent, teacher or self-reports. Second, in longitudinal as in cross-sectional analyses, differing methods of combining reports may give rise to differing conclusions (Canino et al., 1995). Third, attention to measurement error and method factors is crucial in deriving appropriate estimates of effects. In principle, analyses based on observed measures could either over- or underestimate the true extent of continuity. In practice, most empirical demonstrations to date have found higher levels of continuity when measurement error has been taken into account (Fergusson et al., 1995; Zoccolillo et al., 1992). Latent class or latent variable models (Dunn et al., 1993; Waldman et al., 1995) offer important advantages here, though their assumptions may not always mirror the constructs investigators are aiming to test.

One further reporting issue is more specific to longitudinal studies: the reliability of retrospective reports. Although prospective evidence on continuities in antisocial behaviour is expanding rapidly, large-scale retrospective studies of adult samples, such as the Epidemiologic Catchment Area studies (ECA; Robins & Regier, 1991), and the National Comorbidity Study (Kessler et al., 1994) continue to provide key data sources, especially for small or extreme groups. Direct tests of the reliability of retrospective reports of childhood problems remain limited (Maughan & Rutter, 1997). It seems likely that the presence or absence of childhood symptoms can be documented reliably in adulthood using appropriate interviewing styles (Holmshaw & Simonoff, 1996), but accuracy in the timing and dating of symptoms is much more questionable (Angold et al., 1996), especially when recall is for events many years in the past. Retrospective accounts typically involve some 'telescoping', with events brought closer to the present, or systematically moved further into the past, than contemporaneous reports suggest (Menard & Elliott, 1990; Sudman & Bradburn, 1973). Simulations (Guiffra & Risch, 1994) have shown how relatively small tendencies to forget events in the past could mimic true cohort effects, giving rise to spurious conclusions on secular trends. At this stage, retrospective reports continue to provide important sources of data on continuities in conduct problems. Because of these difficulties, however, we have attempted to confirm and complement retrospective accounts with prospective findings wherever possible.

Gender differences

Male gender is perhaps the best established correlate of antisocial behaviour, and many (though not all) measures of antisocial difficulties show a marked male preponderance. In principle, these consistent gender differences could provide a rich source of hypotheses about the etiology and maintenance of conduct problems in both sexes. In practice, with a few notable exceptions, the research literature to date has concentrated almost exclusively on males. The dearth of empirical data is compounded by concerns that current diagnostic criteria fail to detect behaviours relevant in assessing conduct disorder and its sequelae in girls (Zoccolillo, 1993). Loeber & Hay (1994) have charted early stages in the development of gender differences in aggression and conduct problems, and Rutter et al. (1998) have recently summarized evidence on the biological, social and developmental factors that may contribute to evolving differences between the sexes in socially disapproved behaviours. Pajer (1998) provides an overview of existing outcome studies on 'bad girls'. Here, we have noted similarities and differences between the sexes in longer-term continuities so far as current data allow; by comparison with the extensive literatures on childhood–adult continuities in males, however, the database on girls remains extremely limited.

Continuity and change: longitudinal findings

With these issues in mind, we turn to a brief overview of existing longitudinal findings. Many early studies centred on clinical and high-risk samples, or on community samples drawn from severely disadvantaged inner urban areas (Offord & Bennett, 1994). Much of the most detailed and informative evidence still comes from studies of this kind. More recently, however, these sources have been supplemented by large-scale retrospective studies, and by prospective follow-ups of more representative samples. We begin by surveying evidence from 'broad-range' studies, charting adult outcomes for groups assessed at varying points in childhood. To fill in the developmental picture, we then provide a brief summary of continuities over more focused age-periods.

Broad-range childhood–adult studies

Diagnostic criteria for antisocial disorders have been much influenced by Robins's (1966) early findings that the central adult outcome of childhood conduct problems lies in the pattern of severe antisocial difficulties, evident across domains of functioning, typified by antisocial personality disorder (ASPD). Subsequent studies have confirmed this view with striking consistency. In replications of her original child guidance study, Robins (1978) found that the great majority of severely antisocial adults had shown severe behaviour problems in childhood. 'New onset' of antisocial behaviour in adulthood was rare, occurring in only 5–12% of cases. Looking forward from childhood, persistence was much less strong: between 23% and 41% of severely antisocial children went on to become antisocial adults, but the majority, whatever the severity of their initial difficulties, seemed, on these criteria, to have 're-covered'.

Very similar estimates emerged from retrospective reports of childhood conduct problems collected in the ECA studies (Robins et al., 1991). Rates of ASPD rose with the number of childhood symptoms but never went above half, even among those reporting multiple childhood problems. The number of childhood problems functioned dimensionally as a predictor of later disorder, and was a better predictor than any individual type of early behaviour problem. The same pattern of childhood–adult continuities held for both men and women, and across different age cohorts, despite marked secular changes in overall rates of childhood difficulties. Finally, early-onset conduct problems seemed especially ominous in terms of long-term persistence: the average age at onset of the first childhood symptom was 8–9 years, and 80% of future cases reported occurrence of at least one symptom by age 11.

Childhood conduct problems and aggression also show robust links with later offending (Farrington et al., 1990*a*; Hämäläinen & Pulkkinen, 1996; Huesmann et al., 1984; Magnusson, 1988; Moffitt, 1994; Pulkkinen & Pitkanen, 1993; Robins, 1993; Stattin & Magnusson, 1989, 1996). Here, much of the available evidence is prospectively ascertained and based on representative samples. Modest associations with early adult offending have been reported from behavioural observations made as early as age 3 (Caspi et al., 1996), and later in childhood, stronger links are found. Stattin & Magnusson (1989), for example, examined associations between teacher ratings of aggression at ages 10 and 13 and offending up to age 26 in a socially representative Swedish cohort. Among males, the majority of delinquents and recidivist offenders were drawn from early aggressive boys. Aggression predicted to violent crimes, damage to public property, and most strongly to diversified offence patterns, including both acquisitive and other crimes. Among females, aggression also predicted later offending, but only from age 13.

For men, offence histories paint a similar picture. In US samples, between 31% and 71% of juvenile offenders have some subsequent arrests in adult life (Blumstein et al., 1986), and comparable patterns have been documented in European cohorts (Farrington & Wikström, 1994). Individual offenders vary widely in the length and seriousness of their criminal careers. As many as half of the men who come in contact with the criminal justice system do so only once; at the other end of the spectrum, all studies reaching into adulthood have identified small groups of chronic male offenders with extended criminal 'careers' who account for large proportions of recorded crime (Farrington & Wikström, 1994; Wolfgang et al., 1972). Typically, these chronic offenders show an early onset of offending and engage in a diverse range of offences, both violent and nonviolent.

Offence histories have been less widely documented for women, but available evidence suggests that they differ in important ways (Home Office, 1995; Kratzer & Hodgins, 1999; Wikström, 1990). First, recidivist criminality is relatively unusual among women, and the great majority of those who receive official convictions receive only one. Second, ages at offending show a much less marked peak in the teens than for males, and relatively stable (though very low) proportions of women continue to receive first convictions well into their 20s. In one UK birth cohort, for example, the median age for first convictions among women was 22 years, and a quarter of female offenders had their first conviction after age 28 (Home Office, 1995). In a large-scale Swedish cohort (Kratzer & Hodgins, 1999), adult onset cases accounted for the largest proportion of crimes up to age 30.

In addition to these specifically antisocial outcomes, it has long been clear that childhood conduct problems are associated with later risks of much wider kinds (Robins, 1966). Some of these – most notably elevated rates of alcohol and substance use (McCord & McCord, 1960; Robins, 1966; Robins & McEvoy, 1990; Vaillant, 1983) and 'dramatic' personality disorders – fall within a broadly 'externalizing' spectrum of difficulties. In addition, small-scale follow-ups of referred and high-risk samples have pointed to increased risks for a range of other adult disorders (Zoccolillo, 1992). Using ECA data, Robins & Price (1991) confirmed this same picture in community samples, documenting significant relationships between childhood conduct problems (often below current thresholds for disorder) and later phobia, major depressive episode, obsessive-compulsive disorder, schizophrenia, panic disorder, manic episodes and somatization. In general, these risks were dependent on the presence of externalizing disorders in adulthood, though there were also modest direct associations with childhood conduct problems. Some evidence (Quinton et al., 1990; Robins, 1986) suggests that risks of affective disorder are higher for women than for men. In addition, where depressive phenomena are associated with ASPD, they seem almost exclusively of a relatively mild kind, as judged by the type of symptomatology rather than chronicity or degree of social impairment (Rutter et al., 1994).

Finally, other findings suggest that the legacy of childhood conduct problems extends well beyond conventional assessments of psychopathology or crime. Findings from the National Comorbidity Study have underscored the impact of conduct disorder for risks as varied as school dropout (Kessler et al., 1995), teenage parenthood (Kessler et al., 1997) and marital stability (Kessler et al., 1998). Adolescents with conduct problems show accelerated patterns of early adult role transitions, moving into both sexual and cohabiting relationships earlier than their peers (Bardone et al, 1996; Stattin & Magnusson, 1996), and showing persistent problems in intimate and other interpersonal relationships. Health outcomes are poorer among conduct-disordered groups in early adulthood (Bardone et al., 1998), and increased rates of violent death have been reported for both men and women (see Pajer, 1998; Rydelius, 1988; Stattin & Romelsjoe, 1995). Zoccolillo et al. (1992) assessed functioning in work, marriage and social relationships, as well as in offending, in an early adult follow-up of a high-risk sample (children raised in institutional care), together with an inner-city comparison group. In addition to those meeting criteria for ASPD, the great majority of previously conduct-disordered subjects showed poor outcomes in two or more domains of adult functioning. Problems in individual role areas were not uncommon in subjects without childhood conduct problems; the characteristic feature of the outcome for conduct-disordered children, however, lay on the pervasiveness of their difficulties across domains. This pattern has since been replicated in other samples (Maughan et al., 1995; Quinton et al., 1993).

These findings raise central questions about the nature of the long-term risks associated with conduct problems, and the mechanisms by which they are sustained. In particular, they suggest that later outcomes are not confined to severe personality difficulties and criminality, but show effects on interpersonal relationships and social functioning on a much more extensive scale. At this stage, it is unclear how far this wider spectrum of difficulties constitutes an inherent part of the conduct disorder syndrome, or secondary features that arise as a consequence of early impairments. Many of the samples assessed to date have been at high psychosocial risk, or from disadvantaged inner city areas. In more middle class groups, adolescent conduct problems appear to hold few implications for early adult work histories, family relationships or friendship patterns (Jessor et al., 1991). Psychosocial adversities – all too often faced by conduct-disordered young people – may thus play a central role in the persistence of poor functioning.

Assessments over more focused age spans

These findings provide a broad overview of childhood–adult links, but tell us little about developments over the intervening period. As yet, no prospective studies have provided detailed coverage of continuities across the full age span from early childhood to adult life. Follow-up data on representative samples are, however, available over more focused periods. Beginning early in childhood, these show that behavioural precursors of stable antisocial difficulties in late childhood and early adolescence can be reliably detected in the preschool years (White et al., 1990). In epidemiological studies, between 50% and 75% of children who meet criteria for disruptive disorders before adolescence continue to do so in their early teens, and a further proportion go on to show predominantly emotional difficulties (Esser et al., 1990; Graham & Rutter, 1973; Offord et al., 1992; Moffitt et al., 1996; Rutter et al., 1976). These findings may underestimate the extent of continuities (Fergusson et al., 1995). Many childhood onset behaviour problems persist; a minority, however, do appear more transitory.

Prospective studies of epidemiological samples are now beginning to detail developments between the late teens and early 20s. At this stage, continuities in broadly externalizing disorders are most marked among young people who showed severe or aggressive conduct disorder in adolescence (Cohen et al., 1993b; Feehan et al., 1993). New onset of CD/ASPD (cases not showing comparable symptomatology at previous study contacts) seems relatively rare, occurring in only around 10% of cases (Newman et al., 1996). Increased risks for later mood and anxiety disorders have been noted in a number of samples. In the Dunedin Multidisciplinary Health and Development Study, for example, emotional disorders at age 18 were the most common consequences of non-aggressive CD at age 15, and occurred at only slightly lower rates than for groups with internalizing disorders in the mid-teens (Feehan et al., 1993). Increased risks of early adult depressive symptomatology have also been documented in the National Child Development Study (Rutter, 1991; Rutter et al., 1997). Comorbidity with other disorders is associated with increased risks for a range of aspects of later adolescent functioning. Lewinsohn et al. (1995), for example, found that whereas only 5% of adolescents with pure disruptive disorders reported suicide attempts, over one-third with comorbid disorders did so. Bardone et al. (1996) provide some of the few prospective data on early adult outcomes of CD in girls. Adolescent CD exclusively predicted ASPD symptoms and substance dependence; it was also associated with increased risks for anxiety disorders and polydrug use, though not, in this sample, for depression.

Studies using empirically derived syndrome scores, rather than diagnostic categories, have reported similar findings. In a large-scale US study, Achenbach et al. (1995) found that preadult aggressive syndrome scores showed strong predictive links with aggression in early adulthood. Delinquent syndromes also showed clear specificity for males, though a wider range of earlier predictors, including small contributions from both somatic complaints and earlier attention problems, were associated with later delinquency in females. Similar patterns have been reported in Dutch samples (Ferdinand & Verhulst, 1995). In addition, whereas high scores on global measures of externalizing problems in early adulthood were only predicted by previous externalizing scores, early adult internalizing problems were predicted by both prior internalizing and externalizing scores.

Secular change

These findings are drawn from study cohorts spanning a range of historical eras, and, in the case of retrospective studies, for subjects of widely differing ages at the time the data were collected. Effects associated with chronological age will thus inevitably be compounded with either general historical (period) effects, or secular influences specific to individual cohorts (Rutter, 1995). The last 50 years have seen major increases in rates of conduct problems and juvenile offending in most Western societies, along with a narrowing of the sex ratio for many, though not all, types of offence (Smith, 1995). Cohort and cultural differences in rates of antisocial behaviours, and in peak ages of offending, have been documented in both retrospective and prospective studies (Harada, 1995; Robins et al., 1991; Tracey et al., 1990), and a range of social structural factors advanced to explain them. Over such a relatively short period, increases of this magnitude must reflect changes in the environmental risks for antisocial behaviour. Changes in family structure and functioning, increasing mobility and declines in the cohesiveness of local communities, along with changes in the pattern of crime opportunities, seem likely to be among the central factors involved (Smith, 1995).

How far these changes also imply variations in the persistence of antisocial tendencies is unclear. Moffitt (1993), for example, has argued that secular increases in crime largely reflect 'adolescence-limited' behaviours and have few implications for persistent offenders whose criminality extends across the life span. Data from the ECA studies, by contrast, showed that secular changes in rates of childhood conduct problems were associated with parallel increases in adult ASPD (Robins et al., 1991), and that patterns of childhood–adult continuity were similar across all the age cohorts studied. Two different processes may thus be involved here, one influencing the proportions of adolescents expressing relatively time-limited antisocial tendencies, the second affecting expression of an underlying liability to persistent antisocial behaviour of a possibly quite different kind. In addition, secular change in opportunity structures around the transition to adulthood, or the increased availability of alcohol and drugs, may also impact on risks for the persistence of conduct problems from adolescence to adult life. Though relatively little examined as yet, these issues constitute important areas for future study.

Accounting for continuities and discontinuities

As these findings make clear, any comprehensive model of continuities in antisocial behaviour must account for both continuity and change, the stabilization of antisocial tendencies in some individuals, but their more temporary expression in others. A variety of models has been explored to account for these effects. Some have focused on individual susceptibilities, others on variations in age at onset, and yet others on the role of intervening experiences in fostering or inhibiting persistence over time. We begin by examining the role of individually based risks.

Individual susceptibilities

Hyperactivity/impulsivity, low autonomic reactivity, sensation seeking/risk taking, aggressivity, cognitive impairments or executive planning deficits, and problems in social cognition have all been identified as risks for persistent antisocial behaviour (Stoff et al., 1997). It is unclear at this stage how far these reflect different facets of the same risk dimension, or differing routes to long-term impairment. Each is likely to include heritable elements; indeed, twin studies have shown that antisocial behaviour that persists to adulthood includes a clear genetic component, whereas adolescent delinquency seems more strongly environmentally determined (DiLalla & Gottesman, 1989; Lyons et al., 1995; Simonoff et al., reported in Rutter et al., 1997). But heritable factors will, of course, depend crucially on environmental effects for their expression. Although we must await multivariate quantitative genetic studies to identify the behaviours for which genes code, several pointers to the form of the associations are already available. In particular, adoption studies have reported gene–environment interactions for a number of antisocial outcomes (Bohman, 1996; Cadoret et al., 1995; Crowe, 1974). Though neither the genetic nor the environmental influences involved here have been specified in any detail as yet, the pattern of findings points to what has been described as genetic control of sensitivity to the environment (Kendler & Eaves, 1986): the genetic factors contributing to antisocial traits depend heavily for their expression on exposure to adverse environmental circumstances. As we examine evidence of individual risks for persistent antisocial behaviours, we highlight some possible avenues for effects of this kind.

Hyperactivity

Hyperactivity, impulsivity and attentional difficulties have consistently been identified as among the more important markers of poor long-term outcome for conduct problems, at least in males. When the two disorders co-occur in childhood, conduct problems appear to arise as a complication of hyperactivity. Hyperactive symptoms emerge first in comorbid groups (Barkley et al., 1990), and early hyperactivity predicts the development of conduct problems, but the reverse does not apply (Taylor et al., 1996). In addition, behaviour genetic analyses suggest that etiologic factors for 'pure' CD and the comorbid pattern differ in important ways. Comorbid groups include a strong genetic component, while pure CD, especially when defined in terms of adolescents' own accounts, seems largely environmental in origin (Silberg et al., 1996).

Prospective studies have now examined the specific contributions of hyperactivity and conduct problems to later outcomes at a number of stages. Kindergarten measures of restless, impulsive behaviour predict early onset delinquency (Tremblay et al., 1994), and hyperactivity is associated with the persistence of CD across childhood and adolescence (August & Stewart, 1982;

Schachar et al., 1981). Taylor et al. (1996) followed sub-groups of boys from an epidemiological sample over longer age-spans, from early childhood to age 17. Although the threshold for conduct problems used in this study fell below diagnostic criteria for conduct, the findings were striking in pointing to hyper-activity as the main risk for poor later outcome. Defiant and disruptive behaviours, problems in peer relationships and poor social adjustment at age 17 were all most strongly predicted by early hyperactivity; the only outcome specific to conduct problems were behaviour problems in school and aggres-sion. In a similar way, Farrington et al. (1990*a*) found that a composite measure of hyperactivity-impulsivity-inattention, though strongly related to indicators of early conduct problems, independently predicted both early onset and chronicity of offending among males up to age 25.

These findings leave little doubt that hyperactivity constitutes a central marker for the persistence of poor global functioning. Several key questions then arise. First, which aspects of this complex – temperamental impulsivity, motor restlessness or inattentiveness – convey the prime risk? Babinski et al. (1999), analysing these different components separately, found that ratings of childhood hyperactivity/impulsivity and conduct problems each predicted official arrests and self-reports of crime independently and in interaction in males, but that measures of inattentiveness showed no comparable effects. Second, does hyperactivity function predominantly as a dimensional risk factor, a discrete diagnostic category, or as part of a wider constellation of problem behaviours? Genetic analyses (Silberg et al., 1996) suggest that the genetic effect extends beyond the small group of children who show a severe hyperkinetic syndrome. The genetically influenced risk characteristics may thus also operate more widely and depend on co-occurrence with other risks for effects on persistence. Parental emotional disorder, family discord and negative parent–child relationships, especially negative expressed emotion towards the child (Rutter & Quinton, 1984; Rutter et al., 1997; Taylor et al., 1996) are all known to be associated with the persistence of disruptive disorders across childhood and adolescence. Markers of this kind may provide valuable starting points in examining gene–environment interactions that may be specific to the persist-ence of antisocial behaviour across development. Alongside these issues, we need to know more about the role of hyperactivity in girls, and to clarify the basis for the genetic vulnerability.

Neuropsychological deficits, cognitive impairments and school achievements

Neuropsychological deficits offer a second possibility here (see Lynam & Henry, chapter 9, this volume). Depressed IQ scores, most marked on measures of verbal skills, have been widely documented among both juvenile and adult offenders (Hirschi & Hindelag, 1977; Wilson & Herrnstein, 1985), and modest but consistent longitudinal associations have been reported between early childhood verbal skills and criminality in adult life (Stattin & Klackenberg-Larssen, 1993). Tests of executive function have also been found to discriminate between antisocial and nonantisocial adolescents (Moffitt, 1993). These latter deficits seem especially characteristic of comorbid CD/ADHD, but not of conduct disorder alone (Pennington & Ozonoff, 1996).

Poor verbal skills and difficulties in executive planning might contribute in quite direct ways to the onset and persistence of antisocial behaviours. Moffitt (1993), for example, has argued that relatively subtle neuropsychological deficits (whether genetically or environmentally mediated) when they occur in stressed family environments, may initiate a chain of developments that culminate in conduct problems. Early temperamental and communication problems may challenge parenting capacities and possibly also compromise attachment bonds. As the child enters school, so new environmental demands compound the process, and problems in peer relations and learning difficulties are added to an escalating pattern of risk.

Spiralling difficulties of this kind, affecting relationships and social competence in a range of domains, may cumulate across the life-course. During schooling, they are likely to have particular implications for achievement. Criminological theories have posited a particular role for poor school achievement in the genesis of delinquency, running through effects on self-esteem, or reduced attachment to the school system as a support for conventional values (Hawkins & Lishner, 1987). In a recent review of the extensive literature on academic performance and delinquency, Maguin & Loeber (1996) concluded that intelligence and attentional problems were likely to constitute shared causes for both difficulties, but that academic performance made additional contributions to the prediction of delinquency when both SES and prior conduct problems were controlled.

These models suggest rather different predictions for the persistence of antisocial behaviour beyond the end of schooling. On the one hand, since verbal deficits and reading difficulties themselves persist (Maughan et al., 1994; Rodgers, 1986), associated antisocial behaviours might also be expected to show high levels of persistence. On the other, if much of the initial impetus for delinquent activity among low achievers arises from relatively phase-specific stressors in adolescence, links between reading problems and antisocial behaviours might decline in adulthood, as other sources of accomplishment become available. In relation to reading difficulties, the limited prospective evidence available to date favours the second of these accounts. Poor reading males in an inner city sample showed somewhat elevated rates of offending in the teens, but no excess of officially recorded crime or self-reported antisocial behaviours in adulthood (Maughan et al., 1996). These young men left school at a time when opportunities for skilled manual work were relatively plentiful; importantly, social outcomes for women with childhood reading problems were rather less positive (Maughan & Hagell, 1996). Contextual effects of this kind may hold important implications for later outcomes.

Aggressive and other behavioural trajectories

Among specific manifestations of antisocial difficulties, aggression has long been canvassed as a key element in persistence (Stattin & Magnusson, 1989). Individual differences in aggression show considerable stability from early childhood onwards (Olweus, 1979) and Robins (1978) argued that, in the absence of later onset major mental disorders, violent and aggressive patterns do not appear in adults if they have not been evident earlier in life. Violence is a dominant component of antisocial personality disorder in both women and men (Robins et al., 1991), and chronic male offenders show high rates of interpersonal as well as criminal aggression (Farrington & West, 1993). Genetic influences, however, seem less marked for violent than for nonviolent crime, and specific links with aggressive outcomes have proved elusive, reflecting the strong overlaps between aggression and other indices of antisocial behaviour in adult life. In general, early family risks seem similar for both violent and nonviolent crime (Farrington, 1989). Once again, the key may lie in the interplay between individual and environmental characteristics. Henry et al. (1996), for example, found that although violent offending in the late teens showed links with temperamental lack of control in early childhood, effects were most marked in the small group where temperamental difficulties were combined with disrupted parenting. In a similar way, Moffitt et al. (1996) found that elevated serotonin levels were predominantly associated with violent convictions among young men who grew up in incohesive and conflictual families. Langbehn et al. (1998), in an adoption study, explored the effects of adolescent conduct problems and an oppositional behaviour component, argued to reflect temperamental factors, in predicting adult antisocial personality disorder. In males, each showed independent effects. In addition, the oppositional factor was associated with antisocial personality in biological parents, while conduct problems appeared to reflect environmental adversities in the adoptive home. In females, biological background or biological–environmental interactions predicted each of the components.

Behavioural trajectories might offer alternative approaches to examining variations in persistence. Building on factor analytic findings (Loeber & Schmaling, 1985), Loeber (Loeber et al., 1993, 1997; see also Loeber & Coie, chapter 14, this volume) has proposed that there may be different behavioural trajectories associated with progressions in overt, confrontational behaviours; covert, concealing acts; and aspects of antisocial behaviour that reflect conflict with authority. Some individuals will show escalations in all three types of deviance, whereas others may take more 'exclusive' routes. Empirical tests thus far have shown that although boys showing overt, aggressive behaviours often progressed to more covert types of deviance, the reverse pattern was much less common. Hypothesized progressions within each pathway were more evident for boys with persistent difficulties than for 'experimenters', and although ADHD was associated with initiation into all three types of deviance, it showed no additional links with escalating difficulties beyond that point.

To date, these models have only been applied to boys up to the midteens. From the opposite developmental perspective, a number of investigators have explored offence histories of known chronic offenders, in an effort to identify early behavioural trajectories characteristic of long-term persistence in crime. In practice, however, although chronic offenders have long been known to account for disproportionate numbers of serious and violent offences, only a minority are convicted of any serious violent crime (Weitekamp et al., 1995). In the Cambridge Study in Delinquent Development, chronic offenders (all of whom had been convicted of at least nine offences) accounted for exactly equal proportions of both serious and nonserious offences; 'the chronic offenders committed more serious offences in total purely because they committed more offences in total' (Farrington & West, 1993, p. 498).

Chronic offenders may nonetheless show characteristic patterns of escalation in offence seriousness. This possibility raises difficult methodological issues: because later offences are committed at older ages, and older offenders in general commit more serious crimes, it is important to disentangle general age-related changes from those reflecting escalation within individual careers. Strikingly, Weitekamp et al. (1995) found that the mean seriousness of early offences committed by chronic offenders in the Philadelphia cohorts was no higher than that of early offences committed by youth with much shorter criminal careers. In the Cambridge study, Farrington & West (1993) noted an increase in the seriousness of chronic offenders' crimes between the third and tenth offence; after this, seriousness levels began to fall, probably reflecting changes in the types of offences more usual at older ages. The issue is a complex one; to date, however, it has proved difficult to identify characteristic behavioural features of the criminal careers of chronic offenders.

Multiproblem groupings

Hyperactivity, aggression and cognitive deficits frequently overlap. The prime risks for poor adult outcomes might thus emanate from just one of these domains, or might lie in multiproblem subgroups showing all of these difficulties. To test these possibilities, Magnusson & Bergman (1990) advocated a different style of analysis from the usual variable-oriented approach, focusing instead on 'person-oriented' clustering of problems within individuals. Using this strategy, they found strong support for a multiproblem model in a cohort of 13-year-old boys. High scores on aggressiveness, motor restlessness, lack of concentration and low school motivation always occurred in multiproblem groupings; importantly, these groups also showed low autonomic activity. Pervasively poor outcomes in the mid-20s (including psychiatric hospitalization, as well as criminality and alcohol problems) were most strongly concentrated in the multiproblem group. Equally striking, neither poor peer relations nor early adolescent aggression showed any links with adverse later outcomes when it occurred alone. Pulkkinen and colleagues (Hämäläinen & Pulkkinen, 1996; Pulkkinen, 1992), clustering cases in terms of prosociality, aggression and school achievement, confirmed a similar pattern. Constellations of individual susceptibilities, rather than individual risk traits, may thus play a key role in long-term persistence.

Depression, anxiety and shyness/withdrawal

Childhood conduct problems also show frequent overlaps with both anxiety and depression (Hinshaw et al., 1993; Loeber & Keenan, 1994), and, as we have seen, antisocial behaviour is associated with increased risks of affective disorder in adult life. Early links between conduct problems and depression seem likely to reflect correlated or shared risks (Fergusson et al., 1996), and the mixed pattern appears to share more in common with pure conduct than pure emotional difficulties (Steinhausen & Reitzle, 1996). From the limited evidence available to date, comorbid depression appears to have little effect in modifying the course of antisocial behaviour. In follow-ups of child guidance samples, Harrington et al. (1991) and Fombonne et al. (1999) found that antisocial outcomes for groups showing mixed conduct disorder and depressive disorders were closely similar to those with conduct disorder alone, with both groups facing high risks of ASPD, officially recorded crime and alcohol abuse/dependence. In the small sample reported on by Harrington et al. (1991), risks of major depressive disorders were lower than for subjects with a primary diagnosis of depression. In the more extensive series followed by Fombonne et al. (1999), however, the comorbid group showed high rates of depression as well as antisocial outcomes in adult life.

Risks for adult depression might arise in a variety of ways. Continuities from earlier mixed disorders may provide one route, though questionnaire-based data suggest that this is unlikely to be the whole story (Rutter, 1991). Antisocial adolescents showed elevated rates of emotional distress in early adulthood, independent of levels of emotional problems in the teens. Instead, effects may be dependent on later antisocial lifestyles. Robins (1978) was among the first to note that job troubles, poor marital relationships and other concomitants of ongoing antisocial difficulties could function as stressors in adult life. Champion et al. (1995) tested this directly in a 20-year follow-up of community samples. Childhood behavioural deviance showed strong links with severely adverse life events in adulthood, in particular those known from other studies to act as 'provoking agents' for psychiatric disorder (Brown & Harris, 1978). In many instances, these were dependent on features of the young people's behaviour; in addition, early deviance was also associated with increased rates of independent life events, especially those reflecting more chronic psychosocial difficulties and lack of supportive adult relationships. Both directly and indirectly, early behaviour problems appeared to place individuals in adult environments carrying heightened risks for affective disorder.

Links between anxiety and antisocial behaviours have proved more complex (Lahey et al., 1995). The key may lie in the frequent overlap of two related but distinct aspects of anxiety/shyness: behavioural inhibition and social withdrawal. Assessing these separately, Kerr et al. (1997) showed that it is behavioural inhibition that acts as a protective factor, rather than a lack of social connections with delinquent peers. In their study, inhibited-aggressive boys were protected against delinquency, while withdrawn-disruptive boys were at risk for both ongoing antisocial behaviours and depression. The poor outcomes associated with shy/withdrawn and aggressive groups in other studies (Fleming et al., 1982; McCord, 1988; Serbin et al. 1991) may thus largely reflect patterns of this latter kind. Possible biological influences on inhibition and withdrawal are reviewed by Hill, chapter 5, this volume.

Age at onset

A more explicitly developmental approach to conceptualizing variations in persistence has emerged from studies of age at onset. Early onset is among the strongest predictors of continuities in disruptive disorders across childhood

(Loeber, 1982), and early onset delinquency shows similar links with persistence in adult crime (Farrington et al., 1990b). Risks for childhood- and adolescent-onset antisocial behaviours differ in systematic ways, and, as we have seen,
although adult offending shows a clear heritable component, adolescent delinquency is largely attributable to shared environmental effects (DiLalla &
Gottesman, 1989; Lyons et al., 1995).

Building on these observations, a number of investigators have proposed
divisions according to age at onset (DiLalla & Gottesman, 1989; Hinshaw et al.,
1993; Patterson & Yoerger, 1993). The most comprehensive model is Moffitt's
(1993) developmental taxonomy, which divides the overall 'pool' of antisocial
children into two distinct groups: a small, early-onset group showing many of
the risks discussed thus far, and assumed to show strong persistence of antisocial behaviour into adulthood, and a second, adolescent-onset group,
accounting for the short-lived rise in prevalence rates in adolescence. These
'adolescence-limited' delinquents are argued to display a much less pervasive
array of early risks and difficulties; instead, their delinquent behaviours are
largely prompted by status frustration during adolescence, and by social
mimicry of delinquent peers. Importantly, they are also argued to be of
relatively limited duration.

If confirmed, this model could provide a powerful organizing framework.
Initial tests on childhood and adolescent data seem promising (Jeglum
Bartusch et al., 1997), identifying a childhood-onset factor showing the hypothesized links with childhood hyperactivity, poor verbal skills, impulsive
personality traits and increased risks of violent offending, and a separate
adolescent-onset factor, more strongly associated with peer delinquency. Several questions do, however, arise. Firstly, as we have seen, by no means all
childhood-onset conduct problems persist into adolescence (Moffitt et al.,
1996). This suggests that early onset cases include a separate 'childhood-
limited' group, not facing a severe long-term prognosis. It is unclear at this
stage whether this group is characterized by less severe individual vulnerabilities, less serious or persistent environmental risks, or positive protective factors.

Secondly, a main prediction of the model is that adolescence-onset groups
will desist from antisocial behaviour once they gain access to adult statuses and
roles. Nagin et al. (1995) found only mixed support for this proposition in the
Cambridge study males. By age 32, men whose official crime records were
limited to the teens and early 20s had, as expected, made good adjustments in
their working lives and showed little evidence of severe discord in relationships
with their wives. In other respects, however, their adult functioning was by no

means problem-free. Antisocial lifestyles continued, though registered crime did not. In this disadvantaged sample, a variety of factors may have contributed to this pattern. Further tests, in more diverse social groups, are needed to determine the basis for such ongoing difficulties.

Thirdly, we need to know why early onset is associated with long-term risk: does it serve primarily as a marker for other early vulnerabilities; as an index of severity; or does early onset per se affect the likelihood of persistence? The few direct tests of this last possibility have produced inconsistent findings. Nagin & Paternoster (1991), for example, found evidence for 'state dependence' – prior involvement in offending itself influencing the likelihood of future involvement – in self-reports of relatively minor offending in the late teens. Over more extended age ranges, however, Nagin & Farrington (1992) found that associations between age at onset and persistent offending were almost entirely accounted for by time-stable individual differences. And Tolan & Thomas (1995) found a small but significant effect for age at onset on later involvement in offending across adolescence, most marked for persistence in serious crime; age at onset was less influential than psychosocial variables and also of rather less importance for females than for males.

Is early onset also associated with persistence in girls? Retrospective reports of age at onset were very similar – and early – for both males and females who met criteria for ASPD in the ECA samples (Robins et al., 1991), but other findings suggest a more mixed picture. Adolescent, but not childhood, aggression appears to predict offending in girls (Stattin & Magnusson, 1989), and affiliations with deviant peers only become marked for girls in adolescence (Cairns et al., 1988). As we have seen, official offence histories suggest much more diversity in the onset of criminality in women than in men (Home Office, 1995; Kratzer & Hodgins, 1999), and Tolan & Thomas (1995) found age at onset a less important factor in predicting persistence of self-report offending among females in the late teens. Building on these observations, along with evidence of the high rates of family adversities and other risks faced by severely antisocial girls, Silverthorn & Frick (1999) have proposed that the two trajectory model may be less applicable to females, and that age of onset may be a less salient marker of later outcomes than for males; instead, the majority of severely antisocial girls may resemble boys with an early onset of conduct disorder. As yet, this intriguing hypothesis remains to be tested.

Finally, for both males and females, there is the important issue of 'adult' onset. DiLalla & Gottesman (1989) proposed the inclusion of a separate group of 'late bloomers' in their developmental model, and it is clear that using either diagnostic criteria or offence histories, small but nontrivial groups of individuals appear in prevalence estimates for antisocial behaviour and offending for the first time in adult life. Surprisingly little is known about these groups. In some instances, late onset may be more apparent than real. Elander et al. (2000), for example, found evidence of at least minor juvenile delinquency in almost all members of a clinic sample whose first recorded convictions occurred after age 22. Some severe antisocial behaviours are known to develop in the context of major mental disorders, or in response to trauma; new onset of pervasive antisocial behaviour in adulthood may predominantly reflect influences of this kind (Hodgins, 1993). In relation to offending, alcohol and drug-related crime may also play an important part (Kaplan, 1995), and feminist sociologists have argued for some routes into adult crime particular to women, reflecting rational responses to severe environmental pressures or demands (Daly, 1993; Heidensohn, 1994). Comprehensive developmental models need to provide a more systematic picture of these important groups.

Mechanisms for stability and change: person–environment interactions

Identifying the individual vulnerabilities associated with persistence, or sub-groups of conduct-disordered children that follow differing developmental trajectories, constitutes an important first step in understanding continuities over time. On their own, however, these approaches tell us nothing about the mechanisms that contribute to the stabilization of antisocial tendencies in some individuals, but their more time-limited expression in others. Implicitly or explicitly, much early research from a clinical perspective assumed a relatively autonomous unfolding of pathogenic processes. Sociological accounts, by contrast, attributed continuities at the individual level to parallel consistencies in the environment. More recent evidence suggests a more complex pattern, with development reflecting the impact of both organismic and environmental forces, and the expression and maintenance of antisocial tendencies depends crucially on the evolving interplay between individual and environmental effects (Magnusson & Cairns, 1996). In the sections that follow, we outline some of the key processes that seem likely to be involved here.

Social cognitions

A first route for the stabilization of behaviours may run through views of the self and others. Social psychology suggests that most effects of experience operate through cognitive transduction, and that the self is made up of an arrangement of schemas representing past experiences and personal characteristics, as well as future hopes and fears (Markus & Cross, 1990). Aggressive individuals have been found to show characteristic patterns here, believing, for example, that behaving aggressively increases self-esteem and helps avoid a negative image in the eyes of others (Slaby & Guerra, 1988). Among delinquents, Oyserman & Markus (1990) found an imbalance between fears and expectations for the future: although young offenders feared negative outcomes such as being on drugs, many lacked the 'possible selves' that could provide an organizing vision of ways to avoid such adverse outcomes.

Pettit et al. (chapter 11, this volume) discuss the links between biased social cognitions and conduct problems in childhood. As they highlight, attributional biases appear to play some, albeit modest, role in the links between preschool abuse and later risks for conduct problems some 5 years later. The longer-term role of social cognitions remains to be established. Similar cognitive biases to those found in younger age groups have, however, been identified among incarcerated delinquents (Dodge et al., 1990), and among partners in distressed and violent marital relationships (Bradbury et al., 1996; Holtzworth-Munrow & Anglin, 1993). Biased social cognitions, in relation to both the self and others, seem likely to be among the mechanisms that foster persistence in deviant behaviours, or militate against the possibility of change.

Accentuation effects

A second mechanism for the stabilization of behaviour reflects what Elder & Caspi (1990) have described as the 'accentuation principle': new or challenging experiences, though often assumed to prompt change in behavioural development, may in some circumstances function to reinforce existing patterns. Previously vulnerable individuals are most susceptible to the effects of stressors (Rodgers, 1990), and in novel, uncertain or unpredictable situations, individuals must have recourse to their own inner resources in deciding how to act (Caspi & Moffitt, 1993). For antisocial children and adolescents, new environmental demands – whether prompted by developmental transitions or situational stressors – may only go to reinforce deviant tendencies.

Effects of this kind have been noted in a range of domains (Rutter, 1994). The hostile attributions of aggressive boys are most apparent in ambiguous situations, or those lacking familiar cues. In a similar way, the increase in delinquent activities associated with unemployment is most marked for young men with previous histories of delinquency (Farrington et al., 1986), and the rise in norm-breaking shown by early maturing girls (Stattin & Magnusson, 1990) is most apparent for those showing behaviour problems before the main changes of puberty occur (Caspi & Moffitt, 1991). In each case, new, challenging or stressful life experiences have been found to accentuate pre-existing behavioural tendencies.

As these examples suggest, both the biological and the social role changes of adolescence and early adulthood hold the potential for accentuation effects of this kind. It is less clear at this stage how far they carry long-term implications. In relation to early puberty, for example, Stattin & Magnusson (1990) found that by age 15, most differences in deviance between early and later maturing girls had diminished. The most clear consequences for early adult development arose if girls had dropped out of school; then, educational attainments continued to be compromised many years in the future. As in other arenas, the effects of adverse experiences seem likely to be most marked if they close off later opportunities, or trap individuals into adverse circumstances that provide few avenues for escape.

Environmental continuities

If changed environments can contribute to the persistence of antisocial behaviours, continuities in environmental conditions also play a key role. For many antisocial children, adverse environments are likely to persist across development. As we discuss elsewhere in this volume (Maughan, chapter 7) many antisocial children grow up in disadvantaged and disorganized neighbourhoods, antithetical to development at any stage. The same communities that lack adequate supports for early parenting or health care of young children offer limited activities and poor supervision for adolescents, and restricted work opportunities in adult life (Caspi & Moffitt, 1995). To date, research linking macrosocial contextual processes of this kind with more individually oriented measures is still in its infancy (Farrington et al., 1993; Sampson, 1992), and there have been few direct tests of the impact of such broader ecological consistencies on the course of behavioural development. In childhood, much of the effect of neighbourhood disadvantage seems mediated via family risks (Rutter et al., 1975; Sampson, 1992). In adolescence and adulthood, more direct effects may arise. As we have seen, much current evidence on the long-term outcomes of conduct problems derives from disadvantaged samples, likely to have faced ongoing difficulties of this kind. Comparative studies in less distressed groups, along with the integration of community-level indicators in individually oriented analyses, are crucial to clarify the processes involved here.

Selecting and shaping environments

In addition to these broader environmental consistencies, it is now clear that individual actions also play a part in selecting and shaping the environments that individuals experience. Both evocative and active person–environment interactions seem likely to be involved here (Caspi & Moffitt, 1995). Early in childhood, evocative processes may be most salient. Child characteristics are known to elicit differing reactions from caregivers (Bell & Chapman, 1986; Lytton, 1990), and early oppositional behaviours fuel spiralling cycles of coercive interchanges within the family (Patterson, 1982). Later in development, as individuals gain increasing autonomy of action, so options for more direct selection and shaping of environments increase (Scarr, 1992; Scarr & McCartney, 1983).

Behaviour genetic analyses have highlighted the importance of such processes for the persistence of antisocial tendencies (Kendler, 1995). As outlined earlier, genetic and unique environment effects on antisocial behaviour become more salient in adult life. Importantly, however, no new genetic or familial environment risk factors appear to come 'on-line' between adolescence and adulthood (Lyons et al., 1995). Instead, the increased impact of genetic influences later in development arises because they operate at that stage not only to influence behaviour, but also to select individuals into interpersonal and social environments congruent with their dispositions. In some instances, processes of this kind may reflect active selection processes. In others, shaping of environments may arise in less direct but nonetheless powerful ways through the cumulating consequences of early impairments. We focus here on three main routes for effects of this kind: social selection into adolescent peer groups; the implications of conduct problems for transitions to adult roles; and assortative pairing in the selection of life partners.

Peer relations
Deviant peer relationships are among the most powerful correlates of adolescent delinquency (Thornberry & Krohn, 1997; Vitaro et al., chapter 13, this volume). Longer-term effects of adolescent peer relationships have been less widely studied. For some girls, early links with deviant peers appear to constitute a key 'stepping stone' in the progress towards cohabitation with a deviant spouse (Quinton et al., 1993). For males, Warr (1993) has argued that delinquent friendships may be especially 'sticky', and themselves tend to persist over time. Strikingly, evidence from much later in development suggests that continuity in male offending in the 20s and early 30s remains strongly associated with links with deviant peers (Farrington, 1991; Graham & Bowling, 1995). For some individuals, adolescent peer relationships may mark early steps in a chain of developments that contributes, directly or indirectly, to ongoing deviance.

Early adult role transitions

The social role transitions of adolescence and early adulthood provide other routes for shaping environments. Sociological analyses have confirmed that choices made at this period have major implications for subsequent life chances (Hogan & Astone, 1986), and developmental studies suggest that differing transition patterns can also have powerful effects on later psychosocial development. In some circumstances these can be positive, offering breaks from the past and escape from risk trajectories (Elder, 1986). In others, these same role transitions can function to reinforce and amplify earlier difficulties, cutting off opportunities, and trapping individuals in increasingly deviant, unsupportive or stress-prone interpersonal and social worlds (Caspi et al., 1990; Kerner et al., 1995; Rutter et al., 1995).

For many conduct-disordered adolescents, their impulsive behavioural style contributes to a pattern of accelerated early adult role transitions that cut short education, compromise employment options, and precipitate early entry into heterosexual relationships and family formation. In the National Comorbidity Study, for example, early onset conduct disorder was associated with a more than doubled risk of dropout from high school and showed continuing, though less marked, effects on later educational transitions (Kessler et al., 1995). Other studies suggest that these effects are not simply a function of prior associations between conduct problems and poor school achievement. Early exit from schooling is most marked for young people showing both aggressive/antisocial and academic problems, but conduct problems alone also have an effect (Cairns et al., 1989; Maughan et al., 1985).

Not surprisingly, depressed educational qualifications affect entry to the workforce (Sanford et al., 1994). In addition, conduct problems may influence early labour-market involvement more directly through reduced efforts at job search or problems in relationships with colleagues and employers (Caspi et al., 1998). For some young offenders, the stigmatizing effects of arrest and imprisonment will compound these difficulties, further compromising job prospects (Kerner et al., 1995; Sampson & Laub, 1993). Moffitt et al. (1996) found that both early and adolescent onset behaviour problems were associated with increased risks of unemployment in the late teens in males; for girls, however, adolescent conduct disorder appears to have fewer implications for early labour force indicators (Bardone et al., 1996).

Patterns of early partnership and family formation may be more consequential for women. Teenage pregnancy in particular is known to be associated with a plethora of adverse consequences for both mother and child (Furstenberg et al., 1989). In both clinical (Kovacs et al., 1994) and epidemiological samples

(Bardone et al., 1996) conduct-disordered girls have been found at increased risk. These tendencies may be becoming more marked over time. Cohort comparisons (Maughan & Lindelow, 1997) suggest that as secular changes have favoured delayed entry to parenthood, and access to contraception and abortion has become more widespread, so the groups selected into early motherhood have became more behaviourally deviant.

Assorting on deviance

Early and unsupportive marital relationships may also reinforce problems in individual functioning. In the Dunedin study, girls with adolescent conduct disorder were over five times more likely than others to have entered a cohabiting relationship by age 21. Many of these relationships lacked support; by their early 20s, almost half of these girls had already received some form of physical violence from a partner. As yet, relatively little is known of the more proximal processes involved in these effects. Risks of unsupportive partnerships do, however, seem to depend in part on assorting on behavioural deviance. Quinton et al. (1993) found that girls with histories of conduct problems were much more likely than their peers to enter first cohabiting partnerships with deviant men. These relationships reflected the endpoint of a series of prior influences, including adolescent associations with deviant peers, lack of supportive guidance from families, early pregnancy, and the lack of a 'planning' disposition among many of the girls themselves. Similar evidence of assortment on deviance is emerging in other samples (Krueger et al., 1998).

Alcohol and substance use

We cannot conclude this section without noting the strong and mutually reinforcing associations between drug and alcohol problems and antisocial behaviour (see Kaplan, 1995; Tonry & Wilson, 1990, for overviews). It is beyond the scope of this chapter to review the extensive literatures that have examined these associations. For our present purposes, just a few key links can be highlighted. First, childhood conduct problems are strong predictors of alcohol and drug use (Robins & McEvoy, 1990), and deviant adult life-styles further increase the probability of heavy alcohol consumption (Kerner et al., 1997). The complex links between alcohol and aggression have been much debated, and are likely to include pharmacological, psychological and social effects (Fagan, 1990). In the case of drug use, US data suggest that although small groups of heavy polydrug users account for a large proportion of predatory crime, in the majority of cases links are much less apparent (Chaiken & Chaiken, 1990). Possibly as important for the persistence of antisocial behaviour, heavy alcohol use also compromises many other aspects of social functioning; marital relationships and job stability are likely to be especially vulnerable (Sampson & Laub, 1993; Vaillant, 1983). As we discuss in later sections, these often play a key role in desistance from crime. In addition to their direct links with aggressive or criminal acts, alcohol and drug use may thus contribute to the maintenance of antisocial behaviour in more indirect ways, through jeopardizing adult roles and relationships that themselves offer options for change.

Cumulating consequences: indirect chains

Taken together, these findings clearly argue that important routes for continuities in antisocial behaviour run through selection into adverse environments, and the cumulating consequences of early behaviour difficulties (Rutter et al., 1995). Through their characteristic patterns of peer and partnership choices, many conduct-disordered youth will enter their early adult years with limited material resources, restricted labour-force prospects, unsupportive personal relationships and responsibilities for dependents. From a developmental perspective, the key questions concern the extent to which these patterns contribute to the persistence of poor functioning, and the extent to which, if such negative outcomes are avoided, opportunities exist for trajectories to be re-directed over time.

A number of investigators have now shown that processes of this kind do indeed contribute in important ways to the persistence of antisocial behaviour over time. Adverse outcomes at one stage of development elevate risks of persistence at the immediately succeeding stage, acting as 'stepping-stones' into increasingly more deviant pathways. The models advanced – variously described as stepping-stone effects (Farrington, 1986b), processes of cumulative continuity (Caspi & Moffitt, 1995), indirect chain mechanisms (Rutter & Rutter, 1993; Rutter, 1997), or, more specifically in the criminology field, processes of social exclusion and marginalization (Kerner et al., 1995) – all suggest that continuities in antisocial behaviour depend not only on trait persistence, but also crucially on indirect mechanisms of this kind.

Several empirical demonstrations of these effects have now been reported. Fergusson & Horwood (1996), for example, found that affiliation with delinquent peers accounted for a substantial proportion of the continuity between childhood behaviour problems and adolescent offending. Direct behavioural continuities were apparent, but peer-mediated effects accounted for up to half of the associations observed. Caspi et al. (1990), tracing adult outcomes of men with early histories of temper tantrums, reported a similar pattern. Impulsive personality styles persisted to adulthood; in addition, however, progressive deteriorations in occupational status derived in part from indirect effects of truncated educational careers. In a parallel way, Kerner et al. (1995) argued for dynamic processes in the development of criminal careers, whereby the cumulating effects of behaviours, attributions, sanctions and stigma across the life course progressively limit options for escape into nondeviant pathways, and increase risks of persistence in crime. And, as we have seen, similar processes appear to contribute to girls' risks of cohabitation with a deviant spouse (Quinton et al., 1993). Lack of family support in adolescence, lack of a 'planning' disposition in approaching life choices, and association with deviant peers each, in succession, increased girls' risks of achieving deviant partners. Pathways to more distal outcomes depended crucially on these intervening links.

Breaking the chain: turning points in the life course

A key corollary of these models is, of course, that conduct-disordered children who avoid these adverse consequences should show a much reduced likelihood of persistence in deviant behaviours. For those at greatest risk, supportive adult roles or relationships have been argued to function as turning points in the life course, offering opportunities for the redirection of more long-standing deviant trajectories (Caspi & Moffitt, 1993; Pickles & Rutter, 1991; Rutter, 1996; Sampson & Laub, 1993). Three broad categories of experience seem likely to offer the potential for turning points of this kind: those that open up new opportunities; those that result in a radical environmental change (perhaps especially in terms of close relationships); and those that have marked effects on the self-system, or on views and expectations of others (Rutter, 1996).

Testing for change

Many apparent changes in behaviour represent no more than error, or random fluctuations between measurement points (Fergusson et al., 1995; Moffitt et al., 1993). To demonstrate systematic change, several methodological steps are required. First and most basic, longitudinal, repeated measurements on the same individuals are needed both before and after the postulated turning point. Weak measures of behaviour may give rise to artefactual impressions of change. Multiple indicators provide one safeguard here, along with the use of statistical techniques designed to take account of measurement error and persistent unobserved heterogeneity between individuals (Nagin & Paternoster, 1991; Sampson & Laub, 1993; Zoccolillo et al., 1992). Next, as we have seen, there is a need to explore a wide range of later outcomes, to distinguish heterotypic continuity from change (Robins, 1986; Zoccolillo et al., 1992).

Third, equally careful attention is needed in delineating aspects of the experiences postulated to be involved in turning point effects. Marriage per se, for example, may have little effect on desistance from offending (West, 1982). A more specific focus on those aspects of relationships theoretically assumed to be of importance – harmonious, supportive marriages that can foster positive social bonds – has revealed a quite different pattern (Quinton & Rutter, 1988; Sampson & Laub, 1993).

To detect possible turning points, analyses must focus on those segments of a study population for whom new experiences have the opportunity to have effects. In disadvantaged and deviant samples, these may be quite small; few previously deviant individuals may achieve harmonious marriages or strong attachments to work (Quinton & Rutter, 1988). Because of this, conventional tests of the proportion of sample variance explained by such experiences may suggest quite minor effects. Instead, analyses must be designed. to focus on those subgroups in the population where change may be expected (Pickles & Rutter, 1991; Zoccolillo et al., 1992). Finally, causal assumptions will be most convincing if reversal effects are also observed; in the case of marriage, for example, the probability of a causal influence would be strengthened if outcomes improve in the context of a supportive relationship, but deteriorate if that relationship breaks down.

Positive adult experiences

A number of studies, including a range of checks of this kind, have now demonstrated that positive adult experiences can act as turning points out of deviant, antisocial trajectories. For both sexes, supportive marital attachments have proved central here. Especially for men, positive labour force involvement and geographical moves to new living environments also appear to play key roles. Sampson & Laub (1993), for example, found strong effects of positive marital attachment and bonds to the labour force in reducing risks of offending in adult life. The effects were similar for previously incarcerated delinquents and in a control group, and held when the effects of early heavy drinking were controlled. In addition, although the most marked changes were associated with roles and relationships formed in early adulthood, later improvements in job stability or marital attachment were also followed by later decreases in crime.

Farrington & West (1995), using a rather different approach, chose two carefully matched subgroups of offenders, closely similar in the severity of their prior offending, to examine the effects of marriage. In the 5 years following their marriage, married men committed significantly fewer offences than their counterparts who remained single. Equally important, if marriages broke down, offence rates rose, suggesting reversal effects. Laub et al. (1998), also exploring effects of marriage on desistance from offending, used more complex techniques to examine effects of relationships year by year. This more dynamic conceptualization – also controlling for prior characteristics – suggested that apparent 'turning points' may be quite gradual in their effects. Reductions in offending were not simply associated with marriage per se, nor were they immediate. Instead, they became increasingly evident over time, and occurred in the context of relationships that began early, and were characterized by social cohesiveness. Focusing on women, Quinton & Rutter (1988) found that marriage to a nondeviant, supportive partner had marked protective effects against parenting problems in their sample of institutionalized women; and Zoccolillo et al. (1992) found similar positive effects of marriage on continuities between conduct disorder and problems in social functioning in these same samples. Importantly, although women's likelihood of achieving a supportive partner was influenced by dispositional protective factors, the positive effects of a supportive marriage applied even when these were not apparent.

These findings provide strong support for the role of positive adult experiences in influencing antisocial trajectories. As yet, the basis for these influences remains to be clarified: do they emanate primarily, as Sampson & Laub (1993) have argued, from the informal social controls implicit in adult social bonds, or do the changes reflect more intrapersonal processes, arising from enhanced self-esteem or altered social cognitions? Equally important, we know very little at this stage about how far such effects generalize, or persist beyond their immediate context. Farrington & West's (1995) findings that marital separations were followed by somewhat increased levels of offending suggest that effects may be time-limited, and context-dependent. Further tests, exploring persisting effects of positive turning-point experiences across subsequent life transitions, are needed here. In addition, the more extended 'timetable' for the transition to adulthood in recent generations may hold important implications for the ages at which young people gain access to constructive adult involvements (Graham & Bowling, 1995), and so for secular trends in persistence in crime.

Protective factors

To conclude, we turn briefly to the question of individual and social factors that may protect against continuance in deviant behaviour or crime. Here, high-risk designs are needed to identify effects, contrasting the development of individuals at equivalent early risk who do and do not show the posited protective factors. Several demonstrations of this kind have now been undertaken.

As expected from the consistent associations of antisocial behaviours with depressed intellectual skills, IQ shows protective effects against criminality in at-risk groups (Kandel et al., 1988), and interventions designed to improve school motivation are also associated with reductions in delinquency (Yoshikawa, 1994). As we have seen, behavioural inhibition can protect against delinquency in adolescence (Kerr et al., 1997), and prosocial tendencies had important effects in moderating longer-term outcomes of childhood deviance in other samples (Hämäläinen & Pulkkinen, 1996).

In addition, an individual disposition to planfulness (Clausen, 1991) has emerged as of central importance in a number of studies. A planful, considered approach to life choices may be especially important for behaviourally deviant youth, and for those in situations where family or wider social supports for life-planning are restricted. Shanahan et al. (1996), for example, found that planning was of greatest consequence for educational and occupational outcomes in cohorts when institutional structures were less supportive of continuance in education. Champion et al. (1995) showed that planning was associated with reduced risks of exposure to adverse life events, and Quinton & Rutter (1988) and Quinton et al. (1993) found important effects of planning on later life-course developments of institution-reared girls. In this sample, planning seemed of most relevance for partnership choices, reducing the likelihood that girls from high-risk psychosocial backgrounds, or those with histories of conduct disorder, would enter unsupportive partnerships. No comparable effects were evident in a community comparison group. There, family supports, along with fewer deviant peer affiliations, seem likely to have offered alternative supports for partnership choices. Effects of planning were also less marked among institution-reared men (Rutter et al., 1990), reflecting their generally lower risks of gaining a deviant partner.

Finally, researchers have begun to investigate psychophysiological factors that may protect against the persistence of antisocial behaviours. Raine et al. (1995), for example, have reported that antisocial adolescents who desisted from crime in adulthood showed high autonomic arousal in the teens, exceeding levels found in a nondeviant comparison group. These first findings clearly require confirmation; if replicated, however, they may offer important clues to heterogeneity in adolescence and provide additional pointers to groups whose deviant behaviour owes little to psychophysiological predispositions and most to environmental and contextual effects.

Conclusions

Recent years have seen major advances in our understanding of developmental continuities in antisocial behaviour. It is now clear that the long-term risks extend well beyond severely antisocial outcomes; that childhood and adolescent onset behaviour problems may vary in both risks and long-term consequences; and that while progress to adult outcome depends in part on trait persistence, it also turns heavily on intervening developments, each holding the potential to maintain or redirect behavioural trajectories over time. Behaviour genetic analyses have begun to illuminate the interplay between heritable and experiential risks, and longitudinal studies are providing an increasingly detailed picture of the complex forces that shape lives through time.

Alongside these advances, key questions remain to be resolved. We have pointed to a number of these in the course of the discussion, and we note just a few central issues in conclusion here. First, the heterogeneity of antisocial behaviour continues to present major challenges. It now seems clear that long-term persistence is associated with hyperactivity/impulsivity, generally involves early onset, often includes low reactivity to stress, and may be dependent on poor peer relationships. How far these features reflect one or several categories, or are better considered in dimensional terms, remains obscure; answers to these questions will hold important implications for the classification of antisocial disorders.

Second, though many broad-range mechanisms for the maintenance of antisocial behaviour have been described, we still know very little of the more proximal processes involved. Assortment on deviance, for example, might reflect a range of processes: active choice of deviant partners; limitations on the 'field of possibles' from whom conduct-disordered youth can select their mates; or residue effects, whereby antisocial individuals are effectively 'deselected' by more conventional others. Comparable questions arise in almost all the areas we have surveyed. To advance theory, and for the lessons they hold for prevention, these more proximal processes are key targets for future research.

Third, we have drawn attention to the indirect causal connections through which later experiences serve to accentuate or alter earlier behavioural patterns. We have also shown how individual differences contribute in shaping and selecting later environments. But almost nothing is known about the role of individual differences in relation to responsivity to environments in later adolescence or adult life. Does a harmonious marriage, for example, have the same effects in individuals with early-onset antisocial behaviour associated with hyperactivity as in individuals with less marked individual risk characteristics?

Does the shaping and selection of environments primarily affect outcome for those initially at highest risk? To date, these differing issues have in general been examined by separate groupings of investigators, each approaching developmental issues in antisocial behaviour from somewhat different perspectives. The richness of research in the field attests to the value of these different approaches. At the same time, undoubtedly the most major advances of future years can be expected from integrations across domains, and from efforts to bring together, both conceptually and methodologically, the currently separate veins of evidence surveyed here.

REFERENCES

Achenbach, T.M., McConaughy, S.H. & Howell, C.T. (1987). Child/adolescent behavioral and emotional problems: implications of cross-informant correlations for situational specificity. *Psychological Bulletin, 101,* 213–32.

Achenbach, T. M., Howell, C.T., McConaughy, S.H. & Stanger, C. (1995). Six-year predictors of problems in a national sample: III. Transitions to young adult syndromes. *Journal of the American Academy of Child and Adolescent Psychiatry, 34,* 658–69.

Angold, A., Erkanli, A., Costello, E.J. & Rutter, M. (1996). Precision, reliability and accuracy in the dating of symptom onsets in child and adolescent psychopathology. *Journal of Child Psychology and Psychiatry, 37,* 657–64.

Anthony, J.C. & Helzer, J.E. (1991). Syndromes of drug abuse and dependence. In L.N. Robins & D.A. Regier (Eds.), *Psychiatric Disorders in America* (pp. 116–54). New York: The Free Press.

August, G.J. & Stewart, M.A. (1982). Is there a syndrome of pure hyperactivity? *British Journal of Psychiatry, 140,* 305–11.

Babinski, L.M., Hartsough, C.S. & Lambert, N.M. (1999). Childhood conduct problems, hyperactivity-impulsivity, and inattention as predictors of adult criminality. *Journal of Child Psychology and Psychiatry, 40,* 347–55.

Bardone, A.M., Moffitt, T.E., Caspi, A., Dickson, N. & Silva, P.A. (1996). Adult mental health and social outcomes of adolescent girls with depression and conduct disorder. *Development and Psychopathology, 8,* 811–29.

Bardone, A.M., Moffitt, T.E., Caspi, A., Dickson, N. & Silva, P.A. (1998). Adult physical health outcomes of adolescent girls with conduct disorder, depression, and anxiety. *Journal of the American Academy of Child and Adolescent Psychiatry, 37,* 594–601.

Barkley, R.A., Fischer, M., Edelbrock, C.S. & Smallish, L. (1990). The adolescent outcome hyperactive children diagnosed by research criteria: I. An 8-year prospective follow-up. *Journal of the American Academy of Child and Adolescent Psychiatry, 294,* 546–57.

Bell, Q. & Chapman, M. (1986). Child effects in studies using experimental or brief longitudinal approaches to socialization. *Developmental Psychology, 22,* 595–603.

Blumstein, A., Cohen, J., Roth, J.A. & Vishner, C.A. (Eds.) (1986). *Criminal Careers and 'Career Criminals'*. Washington DC: National Academy Press.

Bohman, M. (1996). Predisposition to criminality: Swedish adoption studies in retrospect. In G.R. Bock & J.A. Goode (Eds.), *Genetics of Criminal and Antisocial Behaviour. CIBA Foundation Symposium 194* (pp. 99–194). Chichester: John Wiley & Sons.

Bradbury, T.N., Beach, S.R.H., Fincham, F.D. & Nelson, G.M. (1996). Attributions and behavior in functional and dysfunctional marriages. *Journal of Consulting and Clinical Psychology, 64,* 569–76.

Brown, G.W. & Harris, T.O. (1978). *The Social Origins of Depression: A Study of Psychiatric Disorder in Women*. London: Tavistock.

Cadoret, R. J., Yates, W.R., Troughton, E., Woodworth, G. & Stewart, M.A. (1995). Genetic–environmental interaction in the genesis of aggressivity and conduct disorders. *Archives of General Psychiatry, 52,* 916–24.

Cairns, R.B., Cairns, B.D. & Neckerman, H.J. (1989). Early school dropout: configurations and determinants. *Child Development, 606,* 1437–52.

Cairns, R.B., Cairns, B.D., Neckerman, H.J., Gest, S. & Gariepy, J.-L. (1988). Social networks and aggressive behavior: peer support or peer rejection? *Developmental Psychology, 24,* 815–23.

Canino, G., Bird, H.R., Rubio-Stipec, M. & Bravo, M. (1995). Child psychiatric epidemiology: what we have learned and what we need to learn. *International Journal of Methods in Psychiatric Research, 5,* 79–92.

Cantwell, D.P. &. Rutter, M. (1994). Classification: Conceptual issues and substantive findings. In E. Taylor, L. Hersov & M. Rutter (Eds.), *Child and Adolescent Psychiatry: Modern Approaches* (pp. 3–21). Oxford: Blackwell Scientific Publications.

Caspi, A., Elder, J.G.H. & Herbener, E.S. (1990). Childhood personality and the prediction of life-course patterns. In L. Robins & M. Rutter (Eds.), *Straight and Devious Pathways from Childhood to Adulthood* (pp. 13–55). New York: Cambridge University Press.

Caspi, A. & Moffitt, T.E. (1991). Individual differences are accentuated during periods of social change: the sample case of girls at puberty. *Journal of Personality and Social Psychology, 61,* 157–68.

Caspi, A. & Moffitt, T.E. (1993). When do individual differences matter? A paradoxical theory of personality coherence. *Psychological Inquiry, 4,* 247–71.

Caspi, A. & Moffitt, T.E. (1995). The continuity of maladaptive behaviour: from description to understanding in the study of antisocial behaviour. In D. Cicchetti & D. Cohen (Eds.), *Developmental Psychopathology*, Vol. 2 (pp. 472–511). New York: John Wiley & Sons.

Caspi, A., Moffitt, T.E., Newman, D.L. & Silva, P.A. (1996) Behavioral observations at age 3 predict adult psychiatric disorders: longitudinal evidence from a birth cohort. *Archives of General Psychiatry, 53,* 1033–9.

Caspi, A., Wright, B.R. Moffitt, T.E. & Silva, P. (1998). Early failure in the labor market: childhood and adolescent predictors of unemployment in the transition to adulthood. *American Sociological Review, 63,* 424–51.

Chaiken, J.M. & Chaiken, M.R. (1990). Drugs and predatory crime. In M. Tonry & J.Q. Wilson (Eds.), *Drugs and Crime: Crime and Justice, a Review of Research 13* (pp. 203–40). Chicago: University of Chicago Press.

Champion, L.A., Goodall, G.M. & Rutter, M. (1995). Behaviour problems in childhood and stressors in early adult life: a twenty year follow-up of London school children. *Psychological Medicine, 25,* 231–46.

Clark, L.A., Watson, D. & Reynolds, S. (1995). Diagnosis and classification of psychopathology: challenges to the current system and future directions. *Annual Review of Psychology, 46,* 121–53.

Clausen, J. (1991). Adolescent competence and the shaping of the life course. *American Journal of Sociology, 96,* 805–42.

Cohen, P., Cohen, J., Kasen, S., et al. (1993a). An epidemiological study of disorders in late childhood and adolescence – I. Age- and gender-specific prevalence. *Journal of Child Psychology and Psychiatry, 34,* 851–67.

Cohen, P., Cohen, J. & Brook, J. (1993b). An epidemiological study of disorders in late childhood and adolescence – II. Persistence of disorders. *Journal of Child Psychology and Psychiatry, 34,* 869–77.

Crowe, R.R. (1974). An adoption study of antisocial personality. *Archives of General Psychiatry, 31,* 785–91.

Daly, K. (1993). *Gender Crime and Punishment.* New Haven: Yale University Press.

DiLalla, L.F. & Gottesman, I.I. (1989). Heterogeneity of causes for delinquency and criminality: lifespan perspectives. *Development and Psychopathology, 1,* 339–49.

Dodge, K.A., Price, J.N., Bachorowski, J.A. & Newman, J.P. (1990). Hostile attributional biases in severely aggressive adolescence. *Journal of Abnormal Psychology, 99,* 385–92.

Dunn, G., Everitt, B. & Pickles, A. (1993). *Modelling Covariances and Latent Variables using EQS.* London: Chapman & Hall.

Elander, J., Rutter, M., Simonoff, E. & Pickles, A. (2000). Explanations for apparent late onset criminality in a high-risk sample of children followed-up in adult life. *British Journal of Criminology, 40,* 497–509.

Elder, G.H.J. (1986). Military times and turning points in men's lives. *Developmental Psychology, 22,* 233–45.

Elder, G.H. & Caspi, A. (1990). Studying lives in a changing society: sociological and personalogical explorations. In A.I. Rabin, R.A. Zucker, S. Frank & R.A. Emmons (Eds.), *Studying Persons and Lives* (pp. 201–47). New York: Springer.

Elliott, D.S., Ageton, S.S., Huizinga, D., Knowles, B.A. & Canter, R.J. (1983). *The Prevalence and Incidence of Delinquent Behavior: 1976–1980* (The National Youth Survey Report No. 26). Boulder, CO: Behavioral Research Institute.

Esser, G., Schmidt, M.H. & Woerner, W. (1990). Epidemiology and course of psychiatric disorders in school-age children – results of a longitudinal study. *Journal of Child Psychology and Psychiatry, 31,* 243–63.

Fagan, J. (1990). Intoxication and aggression. In M. Tonry & J.Q. Wilson (Eds.), *Drugs and Crime* (pp. 241–320). Chicago: University of Chicago Press.

Farrington, D.P. (1986a). Age and crime. In M. Tonry & N. Morris (Eds.), *Crime and Justice: an Annual Review of Research,* Vol. 7 (pp. 189–250). Chicago: University of Chicago Press.

Farrington, D.P. (1986b). Stepping stones to adult criminal careers. In D. Olweus, J. Block & M.R. Yarrow (Eds.), *Development of Antisocial and Prosocial Behaviour* (pp. 359–84). New York: Academic Press.

Farrington, D.P. (1989). Early predictors of adolescent aggression and adult violence. *Violence and Victims, 4*, 79–100.

Farrington, D.P. (1990). Age, period, cohort and offending. In D.M. Gottfredson & R.V. Clarke (Eds.), *Policy and Theory in Criminal Justice* (pp. 51–75). Aldershot, UK: Avebury.

Farrington, D.P. (1991). Antisocial personality from childhood to adulthood. *The Psychologist, 4*, 389–94.

Farrington, D.P. (1992). Criminal career research in the United Kingdom. *British Journal of Criminology, 32*, 521–36.

Farrington, D.P., Gallagher, B., Morley, L., St Ledger, R.J. & West, D.J. (1986). Unemployment, school leaving and crime. *British Journal of Criminology, 26*, 335–56.

Farrington, D.P., Loeber, R., Elliott, D.S., et al. (1990*b*). Advancing knowledge about the onset of delinquency and crime. In B.B. Lahey & A.E. Kazdin (Eds.), *Advances in Clinical Child Psychology* (pp. 283–342). New York: Plenum Press.

Farrington, D.P., Loeber, R. & Van Kammen, W.B. (1990*a*). Long-term criminal outcomes of hyperactivity-impulsivity-attention deficit and conduct problems in childhood. In L. N. Robins & M. Rutter (Eds.), *Straight and Devious Pathways from Childhood to Adulthood* (pp. 62–81). New York: Cambridge University Press.

Farrington, D.P., Sampson, R.J. & Wikström, P.-O.H. (Eds.) (1993). *Integrating Individual and Ecological Aspects of Crime*. Stockholm: National Council for Crime Prevention.

Farrington, D.P. & West, D.J. (1993). Criminal, penal and life histories of chronic offenders: risk and protective factors and early identification. *Criminal Behaviour and Mental Health, 3*, 492–523.

Farrington, D.P. & West, D.J. (1995). Effects of marriage, separation, and children on offending by adult males. In Z. Smith Blau (Series Ed.) & J. Hagan (Vol. Ed.), *Current Perspectives on Aging and the Life Cycle: Delinquency and Disrepute in the Life Course* (pp. 249–81). Greenwich: JAI Press.

Farrington, D.P. & Wikström, P-O.H. (1994). Criminal careers in London and Stockholm: a cross-national comparative study. In E.G.M. Weitekamp & H.-J. Kerner (Eds.), *Cross-national Longitudinal Research on Human Development and Criminal Behavior* (pp. 65–89). The Netherlands: Kluwer Academic Publishers.

Feehan, M., McGee, R. & Williams, S.M. (1993). Mental health disorders from age 15 to age 18. *Journal of the American Academy of Child and Adolescent Psychiatry, 32*, 1118–26.

Ferdinand, R.F. & Verhulst, F.C. (1995). Psychopathology from adolescence into young adulthood: an 8-year follow-up study. *American Journal of Psychiatry, 152*, 1586–94.

Fergusson, D.M. & Horwood, L.J. (1996). The role of adolescent peer affiliations in the continuity between childhood behavioral adjustment and juvenile offending. *Journal of Abnormal Child Psychology, 24*, 205–21.

Fergusson, D.M., Horwood, L.J. & Lynskey, M.T. (1995). The stability of disruptive childhood behaviors. *Journal of Abnormal Child Psychology, 23*, 379–96.

Fergusson, D.M., Lynskey, M.T. & Horwood, L.J. (1996). Origins of comorbidity between conduct and affective disorders. *Journal of the American Academy of Child and Adolescent Psychiatry, 35*, 451–60.

Fleming, J.P., Kellam, S.G. & Brown, C.H. (1982). Early predictors of age at first use of alcohol, marijuana, and cigarettes. *Drug and Alcohol Dependence, 9*, 295–303.

Fombonne, E., Cooper, V., Wostear, V., Harrington, R. & Rutter, M. (1999). Adult outcomes of childhood depression – Effects of comorbidity. *Poster presented at the 9th meeting of the International Society for Research in Child and Adolescent Psychiatry (ISRCAP), June 1999, Barcelona, Spain.*

Frick, P.J., Lahey, B.B., Loeber, R., et al. (1993). Oppositional defiant disorder and conduct disorder: a meta-analytic review of factor analyses and cross-validation in a clinic sample. *Clinical Psychology Review, 13,* 319–40.

Furstenberg, F.F., Brooks-Gunn, J. & Chase-Lansdale, L (1989). Teenage pregnancy and child-bearing. *American Psychologist, 44,* 313–20.

Gottfredson, M.R. & Hirschi, T. (1990). *A General Theory of Crime.* Stanford: Stanford University Press.

Gould, M. S., Bird, H. & Jaramillo, B. S. (1993). Correspondence between statistically derived behavior problem syndromes and child psychiatric diagnoses in a community sample. *Journal of Abnormal Child Psychology, 21,* 287–313.

Graham, J. & Bowling, B. (1995). *Young People and Crime.* London: Home Office.

Graham, P. & Rutter, M. (1973). Psychiatric disorder in the young adolescent: a follow-up study. *Proceedings of the Royal Society, 66,* 1226–69.

Guiffra, L.A. & Risch, N (1994). Diminished recall and the cohort effect of major depression: a simulation study. *Psychological Medicine, 24,* 375–83.

Hämäläinen, M. & Pulkkinen, L. (1996). Problem behavior as a precursor of male criminality. *Development and Psychopathology, 8,* 443–55.

Harada, Y. (1995). Adjustment to school, life course transitions and changes in delinquent behavior in Japan. In Z. Smith Blau (Series Ed.) & J. Hagan (Vol. Ed.), *Current Perspectives on Aging and the Life Cycle: Delinquency and Disrepute in the Life Course* (pp. 35–59). Greenwich: JAI Press.

Harrington, R.C., Fudge, H., Rutter, M., Pickles, A. & Hill, J. (1991). Adult outcomes of childhood and adolescent depression: II. Links with antisocial disorders. *Journal of the American Academy of Child and Adolescent Psychiatry, 30,* 434–9.

Hawkins, J.D. & Lishner, D.M. (1987). Schooling and delinquency. In E.H. Johnson (Ed.), *Handbook on Crime and Delinquency Prevention* (pp. 179–221). New York: Greenwood Press.

Heidensohn, F. (1994). Gender and crime. In M. Maguire, R. Morgan & R. Reiner, *The Oxford Handbook of Criminology.* Oxford: Oxford University Press.

Helzer, J.E., Burnham, A. & McEvoy, L.T. (1991). Alcohol abuse and dependence. In L.N. Robins & D.A. Regier (Eds.), *Psychiatric Disorders in America* (pp. 81–115). New York: The Free Press.

Henry, B., Caspi, A., Moffitt, T.E. & Silva, P.A. (1996). Temperamental and familial predictors of violent and non-violent criminal convictions: from age 3 to 18. *Developmental Psychology, 32,* 614–23.

Hinshaw, S.P., Lahey, B.B. & Hart, E.L. (1993). Issues of taxonomy and comorbidity in the development of conduct disorder. *Development and Psychopathology, 5,* 31–49.

Hirschi, T. & Hindelag, M.J. (1977). Intelligence and delinquency: a revisionist review. *American Sociological Review, 42,* 571–87.

Hodgins, S. (Ed.), (1993). *Mental Disorder and Crime.* Newbury Park: Sage.

Hogan, D.P. & Astone, N.M. (1986). The transition to adulthood. *Annual Review of Sociology*, 12, 109–30.

Holmshaw, J. & Simonoff, E. (1996). The validity of a retrospective interview on childhood psychopathology. *International Journal of Methods in Psychiatric Research*, 6, 1–10.

Holtzworth-Munrow, A. & Anglin, K. (1993). Attributing negative intent to wife behavior: the attributions of maritally violent versus nonviolent men. *Journal of Abnormal Psychology*, 102, 206–11.

Home Office, The (1995). *Criminal Careers of those Born between 1953 and 1973*. London: Her Majesty's Stationery Office.

Huesmann, L.R., Eron, L.D., Lefkowitz, M.M. & Walder, L.O. (1984). Stability of aggression over time and generations. *Developmental Psychology*, 20, 1120–34.

Jeglum Bartusch, D.R., Lynam, D.R., Moffitt, T.E. & Silva, P.A. (1997). Is age important? Testing a general versus a developmental theory of antisocial behavior. *Criminology*, 35, 13–47.

Jensen, P.S., Watanabe, H.K., Richters, J.E., et al. (1996). Scales, diagnoses, and child psychopathology: II. Comparing the CBCL and the DISC against external validators. *Journal of Abnormal Child Psychology*, 24, 151–67.

Jessor, R. & Jessor, S.L. (1977). *Problem Behavior and Psychosocial Development: A Longitudinal Study of Youth*. New York: Academic Press.

Jessor, R., Donovan, J.E. & Costa, F.M. (1991). *Beyond Adolescence: Problem Behavior and Young Adult Developments*. Cambridge: Cambridge University Press.

Kagan, J. (1969). The three faces of continuity in human development. In D.A. Goslin (Ed.), *Handbook of Socialization Theory and Research* (pp. 983–1002). Chicago: Rand McNally.

Kagan, J. (1980). Perspectives on continuity. In O. Brim & J. Kagan (Eds.), *Constancy and Change in Human Development* (pp. 26–74). Cambridge: Harvard University Press.

Kandel, D., Mednick, S.A., Kirkegaard-Sorensen, L., et al. (1988). IQ as a protective factor for subjects at high risk for antisocial behavior. *Journal of Consulting and Clinical Psychology*, 56, 224–6.

Kaplan, H.B. (Ed.), (1995). *Drugs, Crime and other Deviant Adaptations*. New York: Plenum Press.

Keenan, K., Loeber, R., Zhang, Q., Stouthamer-Loeber, M. & Van Kammen, W. (1995). The influence of deviant peers on the development of boys' disruptive and delinquent behavior: a temporal analysis. *Development and Psychopathology*, 7, 715–26.

Kendler, K.S. (1995). Genetic epidemiology in psychiatry: taking both genes and environment seriously. *Archives of General Psychiatry*, 52, 895–9.

Kendler, K. & Eaves, L. (1986). Models for the joint effect of genotype and environment on liability to psychiatric illness. *American Journal of Psychiatry*, 143, 279–89.

Kerner, H-J., Weitekamp, E.G.M. & Stelly, W. (1995). From child delinquency to adult criminality. First results of the follow-up of the Tübingen Criminal Behavior Development Study. *Eurocriminology*, 8–9, 127–62.

Kerner, H-J., Weitekamp, E.G.M., Stelly, W. & Thomas, J. (1997). Patterns of criminality and alcohol abuse: results of the Tübingen Criminal Behavior Study. *Criminal Behaviour and Mental Health*, 7, 401–20.

Kerr, M., Tremblay, R.E., Pagani-Kurtz, L. & Vitaro, F. (1997). Boys' behavioral inhibition and the risk of later delinquency. *Archives of General Psychiatry, 54*, 809–16.

Kessler, R.C., Berglund, P.A., Foster, C.L., et al. (1997). Social consequences of psychiatric disorders, II: Teenage parenthood. *American Journal of Psychiatry, 154*, 1405–11.

Kessler, R.C., Foster, L.F., Saunders, W.B. & Stang, P.E. (1995). Social consequences of psychiatric disorders, I: Educational attainment. *American Journal of Psychiatry, 152*, 1026–32.

Kessler, R.C., McGonagle, K.A., Zhao, S., et al. (1994). Lifetime and 12 month prevalence of DSM–III–R psychiatric disorders in the United States. *Archives of General Psychiatry, 51*, 8–19.

Kessler, R.C, Walters E.E. & Forthofer, M.S. (1998). The social consequences of psychiatric disorders, III: Probability of marital stability. *American Journal of Psychiatry, 155*, 1092–6.

Kovacs, M., Krol, R.S.M. & Voti, L. (1994). Early onset psychopathology and the risk for teenage pregnancy among clinically referred girls. *Journal of the American Academy of Child and Adolescent Psychiatry, 33*, 106–13.

Kratzer, L. & Hodgins, S. (1999). A typology of offenders: a test of Moffitt's theory among males and females from childhood to age 30. *Criminal Behaviour and Mental Health, 9*, 57–73.

Krueger, R.F., Moffitt, T.E., Caspi, A., Bleske, A. & Silva, P.A. (1998). Assortative mating for antisocial behavior: developmental and methodological implications. *Behavior Genetics, 28*, 173–86.

Lahey, B.B., McBurnett, K., Loeber, R. & Hart, E.L. (1995). Psychobiology of conduct disorder. In G.P. Sholevar (Ed.) *Conduct Disorders in Children and Adolescents: Assessments and Interventions* (pp. 27–44). Washington, DC: American Psychiatric Press.

Langbehn D.R., Cadoret, R.J., Stewart M.A., Troughton E.P. & Yates W.R. (1998). Distinct contributions of conduct and oppositional defiant symptoms to adult antisocial behaviour: Evidence from an adoption study. *Archives of General Psychiatry, 55*, 821–9.

Laub, J.H., Nagin, D.S. & Sampson, R.J. (1998). Trajectories of change in criminal offending: good marriages and the desistance process. *American Sociological Review, 63*, 225–38.

Lewinsohn, P.M., Rohde, P. & Seeley, J.R. (1995). Adolescent psychopathology: III: The clinical consequences of comorbidity. *Journal of the American Academy of Child and Adolescent Psychiatry, 34*, 510–19.

Loeber, R. (1982). The stability of antisocial and delinquent child behaviour: a review. *Child Development, 53*, 1431–46.

Loeber, R., DeLamatre, M., Keenan, K. & Zhang, Q. (1997). Boys' experimentation and persistence in developmental pathways toward serious delinquency. *Journal of Child and Family Studies, 6*, 321–57.

Loeber, R. & Hay, D. (1994). Developmental approaches to aggression and conduct problems. In M. Rutter & D. Hay (Eds.), *Development through Life: A Handbook for Clinicians* (pp. 488–517). Oxford: Blackwell Scientific Publications.

Loeber, R. & Keenan, K. (1994). Interaction between conduct disorder and its comorbid conditions: effects of age and gender. *Clinical Psychology Review, 14*, 497–523.

Loeber, R. & Schmaling, K. (1985). Empirical evidence for overt and covert patterns of antisocial conduct problems. *Journal of Abnormal Child Psychology, 13*, 337–52.

Loeber, R., Wung, P., Keenan, K., et al. (1993). Developmental pathways in disruptive child behaviours. *Development and Psychopathology, 5*, 101–32.

Lyons, M.J., True, W.R., Eisen, S.A., et al. (1995). Differential heritability of adult and juvenile antisocial traits. *Archives of General Psychiatry, 52*, 906–15.

Lytton, H. (1990). Child and parent effects in boys' conduct disorder: a reinterpretation. *Developmental Psychology, 26*, 683–97.

Magnusson, D. (1988). *Individual Development from an Interactional Perspective: A Longitudinal Study.* Hillsdale, NJ: Lawrence Erlbaum.

Magnusson, D. & Bergman, L.R. (1990). A pattern approach to the study of pathways from childhood to adulthood. In L.N. Robins & M. Rutter (Eds.), *Straight and Devious Pathways from Childhood to Adulthood* (pp. 101–15). Cambridge: Cambridge University Press.

Magnusson, D. & Cairns, R.B. (1996). Developmental science: toward a unified framework. In R.B. Cairns, G.H. Elder & E.J. Costello (Eds.), *Developmental Science* (pp. 7–30). Cambridge: Cambridge University Press.

Maguin, E. & Loeber, R. (1996). Academic performance and delinquency. *Crime and Justice, 20*, 145–264.

Markus, H. & Cross, S. (1990). The interpersonal self. In L. Pervin (Ed.). *Handbook of Personality: Theory and Research* (pp. 576–608). New York: Guilford Press.

Maughan, B. & Hagell, A. (1996). Poor readers in adulthood: psychosocial functioning. *Development and Psychopathology, 8*, 457–76.

Maughan, B., Hagell, A., Rutter, M. & Yule, M. (1994). Poor readers in secondary school. *Reading and Writing: an Interdisciplinary Journal, 6*, 125–50.

Maughan, B., Gray, G., Smith, A. & Rutter, M. (1985). Reading retardation and antisocial behaviour: a follow-up into employment. *Journal of Child Psychology and Psychiatry, 26*, 741–58.

Maughan, B. & Lindelow, M. (1997). Secular change in psychosocial risks: The case of teenage motherhood. *Psychological Medicine, 27*, 1129–44.

Maughan, B. & Rutter, M. (1997). Retrospective reporting of childhood adversity: issues in assessing long-term recall. *Journal of Personality Disorders, 11*, 19–33.

Maughan, B., Pickles, A., Hagell, A., Rutter, M. & Yule, W. (1996). Reading problems and antisocial behavior: Developmental trends in comorbidity. *Journal of Child Psychology and Psychiatry, 37*, 405–18.

Maughan, B., Pickles, A. & Quinton, D. (1995). Parental hostility, childhood behavior and adult social functioning. In J. McCord (Ed.), *Coercion and Punishment in Long Term Perspectives* (pp. 34–58). New York: Cambridge University Press.

McCord, J. (1988). Identifying developmental paradigms leading to alcoholism. *Journal of Studies on Alcohol, 49*, 357–62.

McCord, W. & McCord, J. (1960). *Origins of Alcoholism.* Stanford: Stanford University Press.

Menard, S. & Elliott, S. (1990). Longitudinal and cross-sectional data collection and analysis in the study of crime and delinquency. *Justice Quarterly, 7*, 11–55.

Moffitt, T.E. (1993). Adolescence-limited and life-course-persistent antisocial behaviour: a developmental taxonomy. *Psychological Review, 100*, 674–701.

Moffitt, T.E. (1994). Natural histories of delinquency. In E.G.M. Weitekamp & H.-J. Kerner

(Eds.), *Cross-national Longitudinal Research on Human Development and Criminal Behavior* (pp. 3–61). The Netherlands: Kluwer Academic Publishers.

Moffitt, T.E., Caspi, A., Dickson, N., Silva, P. & Stanton, W. (1996). Childhood-onset versus adolescent-onset antisocial conduct problems in males: natural history from ages 3–18 years. *Development and Psychopathology, 8,* 399–424.

Moffitt, T., Caspi, A., Fawcett, P., et al. (1997). Whole blood serotonin and family background relate to male violence. In A. Raine, D. Farrington, P. Brennan & S.A. Mednick (Eds.), *Biosocial Basis of Science* (pp. 231–349). New York and London: Plenum Press.

Moffitt, T.E., Caspi, A., Harkness, A.R. & Silva, P.A. (1993). The natural history of change in intellectual performance: who changes? How much? Is it meaningful? *Journal of Child Psychology and Psychiatry, 34,* 455–506.

Nagin, D.S. & Farrington, D.P. (1992). The stability of criminal potential from childhood to adulthood. *Criminology, 30,* 235–60.

Nagin, D.S., Farrington, D.P. & Moffitt, T.E. (1995). Life-course trajectories of different types of offenders. *Criminology, 33,* 111–39.

Nagin, D.S. & Paternoster, R. (1991). On the relationship of past and future participation in delinquency. *Criminology, 29,* 163–90.

Newman, D.L., Moffitt, T.E., Caspi, A., Magdol, L. & Silva, P.A. (1996). Psychiatric disorder in a birth cohort of young adults: prevalence, comorbidity, clinical significance, and new case incidence from ages 11 to 21. *Journal of Consulting and Clinical Psychology, 64,* 552–62.

Offord, D.R. & Bennett, K.J. (1994). Conduct disorder: long-term outcomes and intervention effectiveness. *Journal of the American Academy of Child and Adolescent Psychiatry, 33,* 1069–78.

Offord, D.R., Boyle, M.H., Racine, Y.A., et al. (1992). Outcome, prognosis and risk in a longitudinal follow-up study. *Journal of the American Academy of Child and Adolescent Psychiatry, 31,* 916–23.

Offord, D.R., Boyle, M.H., Szatmari, P., et al. (1987). Ontario Child Health Study II. Six-month prevalence of disorder and rates of service utilization. *Archives of General Psychiatry, 44,* 832–6.

Olweus, D. (1979). Stability of aggressive reaction patterns in males: a review. *Psychological Bulletin, 86,* 852–75.

Oyserman, D. & Markus, H.R. (1990). Possible selves and delinquency. *Journal of Personality and Social Psychology, 59,* 112–25.

Pajer, K.A. (1998). What happens to 'bad' girls? A review of the adult outcomes of antisocial adolescent girls. *American Journal of Psychiatry, 7,* 862–70.

Patterson, G.R. (1982). *Coercive Family Interactions.* Eugene, OR: Castalia Press.

Patterson, G.R. & Yoerger, K. (1993). Developmental models for delinquent behavior. In S. Hodgins (Ed.), *Mental Disorder and Crime* (pp. 140–72). Newbury Park: Sage.

Pennington, B.F. & Ozonoff, S. (1996). Executive functions and developmental psychopathology. *Journal of Child Psychology and Psychiatry, 37,* 51–87.

Pickles, A. & Rutter, M. (1991). Statistical and conceptual models of turning points in developmental processes. In D. Magnusson, L.R. Bergman, G. Rudinger & B. Torestad (Eds.), *Problems and Methods in Longitudinal Research: Stability and Change* (pp. 131–65). Cambridge: Cambridge University Press.

Pulkkinen, L. (1992). Life-styles in personality development. Special issue: longitudinal research and personality. *European Journal of Personality, 6*, 139–55.

Pulkkinen, L. & Pitkanen, T. (1993). Continuities in aggressive behavior from childhood to adulthood. *Aggressive Behavior, 19*, 249–63.

Quinton, D., Pickles, A., Maughan, B. & Rutter, M. (1993). Partners, peers and pathways: assortative pairing and continuities in conduct disorder. *Development and Psychopathology, 5*, 763–83.

Quinton, D. & Rutter, M. (1988). *Parenting Breakdown: The Making and Breaking of Intergenerational Links.* Avebury: Gower.

Quinton, D., Rutter, M. & Gulliver, L. (1990). Continuities in psychiatric disorders from childhood to adulthood in the children of psychiatric patients. In L. Robins & M. Rutter (Eds.), *Straight and Devious Pathways from Childhood to Adulthood* (pp. 259–77). Cambridge: Cambridge University Press.

Raine, A., Venables, P.H. & Williams, M.A. (1995). High autonomic arousal and electrodermal orienting – at age 15 years as protective factors against criminal behavior at age 29 years. *American Journal of Psychiatry, 152*, 1595–600.

Robins, L.N. (1966). *Deviant Children Grown Up: A Sociological and Psychiatric Study of Sociopathic Personality.* Baltimore: Williams and Wilkins.

Robins, L.N. (1978). Sturdy childhood predictors of antisocial behaviour: replications from longitudinal studies. *Psychological Medicine, 8*, 611–22.

Robins, L.N. (1986). The consequences of conduct disorder in girls. In D. Olweus, J. Block & M. Radke-Yarrow (Eds.), *Development of Antisocial and Prosocial Behavior: Research, Theories and Issues* (pp. 385–414). New York: Academic Press.

Robins, L.N. (1993). Childhood conduct problems, adult psychopathology and crime. In S. Hodgins (Ed.), *Mental Disorder and Crime* (pp. 173–93). Newbury Park: Sage.

Robins, L.N. & McEvoy, L. (1990). Conduct problems as predictors of substance abuse. In L. Robins & M. Rutter (Eds.), *Straight and Devious Pathways from Childhood to Adulthood* (pp. 182–204). Cambridge: Cambridge University Press.

Robins, L.N. & Price, R.K. (1991). Adult disorders predicted by childhood conduct problems: results from the NIMH Epidemiologic Catchment Area Project. *Psychiatry, 542*, 116–32.

Robins, L.N. & Regier, D. (1991). *Psychiatric Disorders in America.* New York: The Free Press.

Robins, L.N., Tipp, J. & Przybeck, T. (1991). Antisocial personality. In L.N. Robins & D.A. Regier (Eds.), *Psychiatric Disorders in America* (pp. 258–90). New York: The Free Press.

Rodgers, B. (1986). Change in the reading attainment of adults: A longitudinal study. *British Journal of Developmental Psychology, 4*, 1–17.

Rodgers, B. (1990). Influences of early-life and recent factors on affective disorder in women: An exploration of vulnerability models. In L. Robins & M. Rutter (Eds.), *Straight and Devious Pathways from Childhood to Adulthood* (pp. 314–28). Cambridge: Cambridge University Press.

Rutter, M. (1987). Continuities and discontinuities from infancy. In J. Osofsky (Ed.), *Handbook of Infant Development*, 2nd edn (pp. 1256–96). New York: John Wiley & Sons.

Rutter, M. (1991). Childhood experiences and adult psychosocial functioning. In G.R. Bock & J.A.

Whelan (Eds.), *The Childhood Environment and Adult Disease. CIBA Foundation Symposium no. 156* (pp. 189–200). Chichester: John Wiley & Sons.

Rutter, M. (1994). Continuities, transitions and turning points in development. In M. Rutter & D. F. Hay (Eds.), *Development through Life: A Handbook for Clinicians* (pp. 1–26). Oxford: Blackwell Scientific Publications.

Rutter, M. (1995). Causal concepts and their testing. In M. Rutter & D.J. Smith (Eds.), *Psychosocial Disorders in Young People: Time Trends and their Causes* (pp. 7–34). Chichester: John Wiley & Sons.

Rutter, M. (1996). Transitions and turning points in developmental psychopathology: As applied to the age span between childhood and mid-adulthood. *International Journal of Behavioral Development, 19*, 603–26.

Rutter, M. (1997). Antisocial behavior: developmental psychopathology perspectives. In D. Stoff, J. Breiling & J.D. Maser (Eds.), *Handbook of Antisocial Behavior.* New York: John Wiley & Sons.

Rutter, M., Champion, L., Quinton, D., Maughan, B. & Pickles, A. (1995). Understanding individual differences in environmental risk exposure. In P. Moen, G.H.J. Elder & K. Luscher (Eds.), *Examining Lives in Context: Perspectives on the Ecology of Human Development* (pp. 61–93).

Rutter, M., Giller. & Hagell, A. (1998). *Antisocial Behavior by Young People.* New York and Cambridge: Cambridge University Press.

Rutter, M., Harrington, R., Quinton, D. & Pickles, A. (1994). Adult outcome of conduct disorder in childhood: implications for concepts and definitions of patterns of psychopathology. In R.D. Ketterlinus & M. Lamb (Eds.), *Adolescent Problem Behaviors: Issues and Research* (pp. 57–80). Hillsdale, NJ: Lawrence Erlbaum.

Rutter, M., Maughan, B., Meyer, J., et al. (1997). Heterogeneity of antisocial behavior: causes, continuities, and consequences. In R. Dienstbier (Series Ed.) & D.W. Osgood (Vol. Ed.), *Nebraska Symposium on Motivation: Vol. 44. Motivation and delinquency* (pp. 45–119). Lincoln, NE: University of Nebraska Press.

Rutter, M. & Quinton, D. (1984). Parental psychiatric disorder: effects on children. *Psychological Medicine, 14*, 853–80.

Rutter, M., Quinton, D. & Hill, J. (1990). Adult outcome of institution-reared children: males and females compared. In L.N. Robins & M. Rutter (Eds.), *Straight and Devious Pathways to Adulthood* (pp. 135–57). Cambridge: Cambridge University Press.

Rutter, M. & Rutter, M. (1993). *Developing Minds: Challenge and Continuity across the Lifespan.* Harmondsworth, UK & New York: Penguin & Basic Books.

Rutter M., Tizard J., Yule W., Graham P. & Whitmore K. (1976). Research Report: Isle of Wight Studies 1964–1974. *Psychological Medicine, 6*, 313–32.

Rutter, M., Yule, B., Quinton, D., Rowlands, O., Yule, W. & Berger, M. (1975). Attainment and adjustment in two geographical areas: III. Some factors accounting for area differences. *British Journal of Psychiatry, 126*, 520–33.

Rydelius, P.A. (1988). The development of antisocial behaviour and sudden violent death. *Acta Psychiatrica Scandinavica, 77*, 398–403.

Sampson, R.J. (1992). Family management and child development: insights from social disorganization theory. In J. McCord (Ed.), *Facts, Frameworks and Forecasts. Advances in Criminological Theory*, Vol. 3 (pp. 63–93). New Brunswick: Transaction Publishers.

Sampson, R. & Laub, J. (1993). *Crime in the Making: Pathways and Turning Points through Life*. Cambridge: Harvard University Press.

Sanford, M., Offord, D., McLeod, K., Boyle, M., Byrne, C. & Hall, B. (1994). Pathways into the work force: Antecedents of school and work force status. *Journal of the American Academy of Child and Adolescent Psychiatry, 33*, 1036–46.

Scarr, S. (1992). Developmental theories for the 1990s: development and individual differences. *Child Development, 63*, 1–19.

Scarr, S. & McCartney, K. (1983). How people make their own environments: A theory of genotype environment effects. *Child Development, 54*, 424–35.

Schachar, R., Rutter, M. & Smith, A. (1981). The characteristics of situationally and pervasively hyperactive children: Implications for syndrome definition. *Journal of Child Psychology and Psychiatry, 22*, 375–92.

Serbin, L.A., Moskowitz, D.S., Schwartzman, A.E. & Ledingham, J.E. (1991). Aggressive, withdrawn and aggressive/withdrawn children in adolescence: into the next generation. In D.J. Pepler & K.H. Rubin (Eds.), *The Development and Treatment of Childhood Aggression* (pp. 55–70). Hillsdale, NJ: Lawrence Erlbaum.

Shanahan, M.J., Elder, G.H. & Miech, R.A. (1996). History and agency in men's lives: Pathways to achievement in cohort perspective. *Sociology of Education, 70*, 54–67.

Silberg, J., Meyer, J., Pickles, A., et al. (1996). Heterogeneity among juvenile antisocial behaviours: Findings from the Virginia Twin Study of Adolescent Behavioural Development. In G.R. Bock & J.A. Goode (Eds.), *Genetics of Criminal and Antisocial Behaviour. CIBA Foundation Symposium 194* (pp. 76–92). Chichester: John Wiley & Sons.

Silverthorn, P. & Frick, F.J. (1999). Developmental pathways to antisocial behavior: The delayed-onset pathway in girls. *Development and Psychopathology, 11*, 101–26.

Slaby, R.G. & Guerra, N.G. (1988). Cognitive mediators of aggression in adolescent offenders: 1. Assessment. *Developmental Psychology, 24*, 580–8.

Smith, D.J. (1995). Youth crime and conduct disorders: trends, patterns and causal explanations. In M. Rutter & D.J. Smith (Eds.), *Psychosocial Disturbances in Young People: Time Trends and their Cause* (pp. 389–489). Chichester: John Wiley & Sons.

Stattin, H. & Klackenberg-Larssen, I. (1993). Early language and intelligence development and their relationship to future criminal behavior. *Journal of Abnormal Psychology, 102*, 369–78.

Stattin, H. & Magnusson, D. (1989). The role of early aggressive behaviour in the frequency, seriousness, and types of later crime. *Journal of Consulting and Clinical Psychology, 576*, 210–18.

Stattin, H. & Magnusson, D. (1990). *Pubertal Maturation in Female Development*. Hillsdale, NJ: Lawrence Erlbaum.

Stattin, H. & Magnusson, D. (1996) Antisocial development: A holistic approach. *Development and Psychopathology, 8*, 617–45.

Stattin, H. & Romelsjoe, A. (1995) Adult mortality in the light of criminality, substance abuse, and behavioural and family-risk factors in adolescence. *Criminal Behaviour and Mental Health, 4*, 279–311.

Steinhausen, H-C. & Reitzle, M. (1996). The validity of mixed disorders of conduct and emotions in children and adolescents: a research note. *Journal of Child Psychology and Psychiatry, 37,* 339–43.

Stoff, D., Breiling, J. & Maser, J.D. (Eds.) (1997). *Handbook of Antisocial Behavior.* New York: John Wiley & Sons.

Sudman, S. & Bradburn, N.M. (1973). Effects of time and memory factors on response in surveys. *Journal of the American Statistical Association, 63,* 805–15.

Taylor, E., Heptinstall, H., Chadwick, O. & Danckaerts, M. (1996). Hyperactivity and conduct problems as risk factors for adolescent developments. *Journal of the American Academy of Child and Adolescent Psychiatry, 35,* 1213–26.

Thornberry, T.P. & Krohn, M.D. (1997). Peers, drug use and delinquency. In D. Stoff, J. Breiling & J.D. Maser (Eds.), *Handbook of Antisocial Behavior* (pp. 218–33). New York: John Wiley & Sons.

Tolan, P.H. & Thomas, P. (1995). The implications of age of onset for delinquency risk II: Longitudinal data. *Journal of Abnormal Child Psychology, 23,* 157–81.

Tonry, M. & Wilson, J.Q. (Eds.) (1990). *Drugs and Crime: Crime and Justice, a Review of Research, 13.* Chicago: University of Chicago Press.

Tracey, P.E., Wolfgang, M.E. & Figlio, R.M. (1990). *Delinquency Careers in Two Birth Cohorts.* New York: Plenum Press.

Tremblay, R.E., Pihl, R.O., Vitaro, F. & Dobkin, P.L. (1994). Predicting early onset of male antisocial behavior from preschool behavior. *Archives of General Psychiatry, 51,* 732–9.

Vaillant, G.E. (1983). *The Natural History of Alcoholism: Causes, Patterns and Paths to Recovery.* Cambridge: Harvard University Press

Waldman, I.D., Lilienfield, S.O. & Lahey, B.B. (1995). Toward construct validity in the childhood disruptive behavior disorders: classification and diagnosis in DSM–IV and beyond. In T.H. Ollendick & R.J. Prinz (Eds.), *Advances in Clinical Child Psychology,* Vol. 17 (pp. 323–63). New York: Plenum Press.

Warr, M. (1993). Age, peers and delinquency. *Criminology, 31,* 17–40.

Weitekamp, E.G.M., Kerner, H-J, Schubert, A. & Schindler, V. (1995). On the 'dangerousness' of chronic/habitual offenders: a re-analysis of the 1945 Philadelphia Birth Cohort data. *Studies on Crime and Crime Prevention, 4,* 159–75.

West, D. J. (1982). *Delinquency: its Roots, Careers, and Prospects.* London: Heinemann.

White, J., Moffitt, T.E., Earls, F., Robins, L.N. & Silva, P.A. (1990). How early can we tell? Preschool predictors of boys' conduct disorder and delinquency. *Criminology, 28,* 507–33.

Wikström, P.-O.H. (1990). Age and crime in a Stockholm cohort. *Journal of Quantitative Criminology, 6,* 61–84.

Wilson, J.Q. & Herrnstein, R.J. (1985). *Crime and Human Nature.* New York: Simon and Schuster.

Wolfgang, M.E., Figlio, R.M. & Sellin, T. (1972). *Delinquency in a Birth Cohort.* Chicago: University of Chicago Press.

Yoshikawa, H. (1994). Prevention as cumulative protection: effects of early family support and education on chronic delinquency and its risks. *Psychological Bulletin, 115,* 28–54.

Zoccolillo, M. (1992). Co-occurrence of conduct disorder and its adult outcomes with depressive and anxiety disorders: A review. *Journal of the American Academy of Child and Adolescent Psychiatry, 31,* 547–56.

Zoccolillo, M. (1993). Gender and the development of conduct disorder. *Development and Psychopathology, 5,* 65–78.

Zoccolillo, M., Pickles, A., Quinton, D. & Rutter, M. (1992). The outcome of childhood conduct disorder: implications for defining adult personality disorder and conduct disorder. *Psychological Medicine, 22,* 971–86.

19

Conduct disorder: future directions. An afterword

Michael Rutter

Problems involving disruptive behaviour constitute one of the most frequent causes of clinical referral. The preceding chapters of this volume provide a most useful, and interesting, range of perspectives on the issues to be considered with respect to such disorders. In this concluding commentary chapter, some of the key issues that span the different chapters are pulled together. In so doing, research findings are used to draw conclusions on what is known now as well as to highlight research and clinical needs for the future.

Do conduct problems constitute a valid psychiatric disorder?

Over the years, doubts have frequently been raised on this issue (Richters & Cicchetti, 1993). The uncertainties are certainly understandable. The fact that someone behaves in ways that are socially objectionable does not provide a justification for regarding the behaviour as reflecting a mental disorder. What criteria might be used? Possibilities include associated social impairment, accompanying unusual psychological features (such as hyperactivity/inattention or cognitive impairment, or depression) and an adverse outcome in adult life. On all of these criteria, the findings seem to justify a disorder concept (Rutter et al., 1997b, 1998; Maughan & Rutter, chapter 18, this volume). Of course, that is not to argue that any isolated antisocial act justifies the designation of disorder. Obviously, that could not be the case, if only because most people commit such an act at some point during their lifetime (Rutter et al., 1998). However, it is to suggest that the concept of disorder may be justified when disruptive or antisocial behaviour is accompanied by these other validating features.

Costello & Angold (chapter 1, this volume) draw attention to the extent to which the symptoms of conduct disorder, as portrayed in official classifications, focus on illegal acts. They raise legitimate queries as to whether this constitutes an appropriate basis for the definition of a psychiatric disorder. The difficulties that they put forward are most applicable if the concept is restricted to the notion of behaviour that is out of other people's control. In addition, personal social malfunction and individual suffering are frequently present. Moreover, it is important to bear in mind that humans are social animals and it may be expected that mental dysfunction will often be manifest in terms of disrupted social relationships and deviant social behaviour. However imperfectly conceptualized, and however inadequately defined, that is what the diagnostic concepts of oppositional/defiant disorder and conduct disorder imply.

Essence of conduct disorder

If conduct disorder is conceptualized in terms of a disturbance of social functioning, rather than in terms of breaking of the law as such, the question still has to be posed as to what is the essence of the particular type of social malfunction that is diagnosed in this way (Rutter et al., 1998). It cannot be claimed that a very satisfactory answer has been obtained to this question. Does it lie in an unusual level of aggression? That might seem to be relevant to oppositional/defiant behaviour, to physical abuse within the family and to many forms of confrontational or violent crime. It is not quite so obvious, however, that that would account for features such as truanting or shoplifting or running away from home. Alternatively, should it be viewed in terms of unusual risk-taking behaviour? Clearly, that is a very important element in some forms of antisocial act. Moreover, for some individuals, this does indeed seem to constitute an important aspect of the rewards they experience through their antisocial behaviour. Alternatively, does the defining feature lie in a lack of normal responsiveness to social rules and social conventions? Certainly, that does appear to characterize much of what is incorporated in both oppositional/defiant and conduct problems. Is an unawareness or disregard for the feelings and sensitivities of others a crucial feature? That seems to be so in certain forms of psychopathy but it does not seem to be a general feature of most of the commoner forms of antisocial behaviour. In all likelihood, there probably is no one single defining feature but the point of asking these questions is that it does have some relevance to what might constitute some of the key predisposing features. Thus, although undue aggressivity may constitute one feature, attention has shifted to such temperamental characteristics as novelty seeking, risk taking and impulsivity. Clearly, too, hyperactivity constitutes a susceptibility characteristic, although exactly how it operates remains rather uncertain. Molecular genetic studies are primarily focusing on these risk characteristics rather than on antisocial behaviour as such or on the clinical diagnostic categories of oppositional/defiant disorder and conduct disorder. Although the mode of mediation of genetic risk factors is not yet known, it does seem appropriate to place priority on temperamental and personality dimensions of this kind.

One key question with respect to psychosocial factors involved in causal processes concerns their mode of operation. Is it that some children learn to behave in an antisocial way or is it that most young children exhibit antisocial features but most learn to channel their activities in other directions? Probably both play a role. Nevertheless, in the past, the usual assumption has been that the children start prosocial and learn to be antisocial. The findings from some studies that disruptive behaviour tends to be maximal in the preschool years (Nagin & Tremblay, 1999; Tremblay et al., 1999) suggests that there may need to be a shift of emphasis in which the question is posed as to why in some children it continues, rather than why it begins in the first place. It is premature to draw firm conclusions on age trends but it would seem worthwhile to pay attention to family and other psychosocial features that might be operative in that process. Similarly, we need to ask whether the main issue concerns either the learning of antisocial behaviour or a failure to divert or channel it in more constructive directions, or whether instead the issues should be posed in terms of a failure to learn positive social problem-solving strategies. Perhaps, to some extent, people drift into antisocial behaviour, not so much because they have a positive impetus to behave in that way, but rather because they lack any means of dealing with the challenges and frustrations they face in their everyday life. In so far as that may be the case, it is important that intervention strategies focus on positive solutions as well as on the control of negative ones.

Finally, if psychosocial influences have enduring effects that are carried forward in the developmental process, it is necessary to ask how that comes about. In short, what do the experiences do to the organism (Rutter, in press a)? Does the persistence of effects lie in altered styles of cognitive processing, in changed styles of interpersonal interaction, in the setting up of behavioural habits, in alterations in neuroendocrine functioning, or in the effects of stress on brain structure, functioning or development? There is a certain amount of evidence in favour of each of these but the findings are singularly inconclusive. The matter requires much more research attention than it has received up to now.

Criminal responsibility

Legal systems around the world have, over the years, come to appreciate that crimes committed by children need to be viewed in a somewhat different way from those undertaken by adults. There are various reasons why that has come about but, amongst other things, it has been accompanied by the concept of 'criminal responsibility' and by the setting of an age above which young people can be expected to take responsibility for their actions and below which they cannot. Clinicians tend not to use a watershed of this kind but they certainly do recognize that the thought processes underlying an act of violence by a 2-year-old are scarcely likely to be the same as those involved in violent assault by a 20-year-old. Costello & Angold (chapter 1, this volume) discuss some of the issues involved. Key among these is the astonishing range of ages of criminal responsibility that operate across the world. Thus, it is 7 years in Eire and Switzerland and 18 years in Belgium and Luxembourg. Even within a single country, such as the United States of America, there is a wide spread of ages. It might be supposed that it ought to be a simple matter to determine when a child's mental abilities reach a point at which it is appropriate to consider that they have criminal responsibility. However, there are several reasons why that is not the case (Rutter, in press b).

To begin with, there is huge individual variation in children's rates of mental development, just as there are in rates of physical development. Also, children vary in their mental capacities. But what provides an even greater difficulty to any standard assessment of when a child reaches responsibility is the fact that the children's understanding will vary considerably with previous experience, with the ways in which decisions are presented, and by the extent to which decision making involves looking ahead and an appreciation of an interlinked chain of indirect connections (Rutter, in press b; Fraser, in press). Moreover, there is evidence that the children can be helped to gain a greater understanding. In short, this is not a fixed quality. Moreover, it is a dimension rather than something that individuals either have or do not have. Clinicians need to appreciate the complexities involved in assessing children's understanding and the need to help children gain better appreciation of what is involved in their decision making. Of course, a categorical approach needs to be adopted with respect to the legal situation, in just the same sort of way that clinicians have to make a categorical decision as to whether to admit a child to hospital or to provide treatment of a particular kind. Nevertheless, the mental processes that underlie responsibility are dimensional, and not categorical.

Concepts of causation

The issues with respect to possible causal influences on conduct disorder raised directly by Maughan (chapter 7, this volume) pervade a much wider range of chapters. One of the big changes that has taken place over recent times has been the growing awareness of the likely importance of biological risk factors. Simonoff (chapter 8, this volume) provides a balanced overview of genetic factors. Lynam & Henry (chapter 9, this volume) summarize the evidence that impaired verbal and executive planning skills predispose to serious conduct problems, going on to emphasize the uncertainties as to how and why this liability operates. Herbert & Martinez (chapter 4, this volume) outline what is known about biological risk mechanisms, such as those involving neurotransmitters or the neuroendocrine system. They make the important point that a unidirectional causal process cannot be assumed. Thus, for example, experimentally induced changes in testosterone levels have predictable effects on sexuality, dominance and aggression, but, equally, experimentally induced failure in a competitive social situation results in a fall in testosterone levels (Rutter et al., 1998). We need to get away from a dualist view of mind–body relationships. One is not basic to the other; rather, they constitute different facets of the same biological system. When, for whatever reason, someone feels angry or afraid this is shown in both their neuroendocrine function and their cognitive and affective thought processes. One does not cause the other; they are both part of the same emotional response.

Recent findings of associations between temperament (after infancy), obstetric complications, and maternal smoking during the pregnancy (discussed by Hill, chapter 5, this volume) raise further issues. First, the fact that temperament predicts psychopathology (quite substantially) from the age of 3 years onwards, but not in the first couple of years, does not mean that biologically induced temperamental features are not important predisposing factors. We need to get away from the notion that genetic factors have to be evident in early life and become less important as we grow older. Characteristics that are strongly genetically influenced may take time to develop (this is obviously the case with respect to language, for example) and may not even be operative until well after the early years of childhood. This will be the case, for example, with the genes influencing the timing of puberty and, even more strikingly, with those that underlie susceptibility to Alzheimer's disease. The issues with respect to obstetric complications and smoking during pregnancy raise a different consideration and that is whether they index a correlated causal influence or whether they represent the causal mechanism itself. It is well established that social risk factors are quite strongly associated with both obstetric complications and maternal smoking. In addition, maternal smoking is associated with conduct problems. Before assuming that obstetric complications or smoking create a risk because of a biological effect on the foetus, we need to be sure that we have effectively ruled out alternative explanations. In addition, it is highly desirable to be able to test the hypothesized biological mechanism more directly. Research has begun to take on those challenges but it is still too early to be at all sure what conclusions should be drawn.

There has long been a tendency to seek simplification in causal conclusions, with the aim of being able to focus on the one main predisposing factor. The wish to do that is understandable but it carries with it dangers that are important for us to recognize. The fact that genetic influences are implicated in risk for conduct disorder does not, of course, mean that most such difficulties are directly caused by genes. With a few possible very rare exceptions, it is highly questionable whether that is the case. Even when there is a single identifiable genetic factor of an important kind (such as an extra Y chromosome) this does not cause antisocial behaviour in anything approaching a direct fashion (Rutter et al., 1998). It is associated with effects on temperament and these may provide an important predisposing susceptibility but whether or not antisocial behaviour develops will depend on the interplay with other risk factors. That is not to say that it is not useful to identify specific genes that play a role in predisposition; to the contrary, that would be an extremely valuable step forward (see Simonoff, chapter 8, this volume). What we have to appreciate is that all human behaviour is genetically influenced and, with only a few exceptions, it is not useful to seek to subdivide syndromes into those that are genetic and those that are not. Rather, we need to understand which genes and which environmental risk factors are involved in susceptibility and how they operate, and especially how they operate together.

One of the major growth areas in the last 10 or 20 years has been the study of both attachment qualities and cognitive processing as mechanisms that may be involved in the predisposition to antisocial behaviour. Hinde (chapter 2, this volume) provides an interesting account of the possible role of the self-system, arguing that the basic issue may be people's need to act independently from others, while at the same time feeling constrained from doing so. He suggests that a deficiency in an understanding of the self in relation to others may play a role in susceptibility to act in an aggressive manner. Dunn (chapter 3, this volume) notes, too, the need to consider the development of conflict in conjunction with the parallel development of prosocial behaviour. Pettit et al. (chapter 11, this volume) present a thoughtful and balanced review of what is known about cognitive processing, arguing simultaneously that there are very good reasons for supposing that it is intrinsically involved in aggressive behaviour and associated antisocial problems but, equally, the existing empirical findings so far provide only relatively weak evidence on its mediating role in this connection. DeKlyen and Speltz (chapter 12, this volume) provide a broadly comparable account of strengths and limitations in relation to attachment qualities. Loeber and Coie (chapter 14, this volume) make the important observation that we need to be as much concerned as to why antisocial behaviour persists or desists as to why it began in the first place. They summarize what is known about the role of emotional and cognitive processes in such persistence.

Traditionally, psychosocial researchers have mainly focused on family influences as the operative aspects of environmental effects on conduct problems. Kiesner et al. (chapter 10, this volume) give a clear account of how such influences may be conceptualized in terms of a reinforcement model, emphasizing the role of coercive interchanges, and noting that the postulated mechanisms involve the peer group as well as the family. What is particularly important in their account is the recognition that it is not enough to focus on punishments and rewards in relation to acts of disapproved behaviour. Instead, it is crucial to consider how patterns of interpersonal interaction operate to make it more, or less, likely that aggressive behaviour will occur. One of the key features with respect to successfully functioning families in which aggression and disruptive behaviour are uncommon is their skill in using diverting and distracting techniques to cut short possible negative interchanges. Holden (1983) provided a vivid illustration of how this operates with respect to the mothers of toddlers negotiating all that is involved in taking their young child to a supermarket with all the temptations that that provides to pull thing off shelves! A recent study by Gardner et al. (1999) provided a development of the same theme. Monitoring and supervision are important elements in successful parenting. What is striking, however, in observations of well-functioning families is that, in a sense, there does not seem to be anything striking that happens. Why are they so lucky that they do not have the untoward events that so plague other families? That is where the focus on anticipatory skills is so important.

Vitaro et al. (chapter 13, this volume) in their thoughtful account of the role of peer relationships, make the very important point that these need to be considered in two rather different ways. First, there is the evidence that individuals who are socially isolated or who have disrupted peer relationships, or who fail to keep friends, have worse social outcomes, including the increased risk of antisocial behaviour (Parker & Asher, 1987). Also, however, the peer group operates as a social influence in which the mores, ethos and attitudes of the group have important influences on the behaviour of members of that group. Of course, people choose which social groups they enter and it is essential for research to be conducted in ways that can separate the effects of social selection and social influence (Rowe et al., 1994) but the evidence suggests that both operate. One consequence of this recognition of the two different ways in which peer relationships operate is that it would be a mistake to assume that all children with conduct disorder are social failures and have low self-esteem. Undoubtedly, that does apply to many but it does not apply to all.

Another trend in recent years has been the appreciation that the concept of causation can not be restricted to the question of individual differences. Of course, individuals do differ markedly in their liability to engage in antisocial behaviour and it is important to gain an understanding of the facts that underlie this individual variation. However, there are several other rather different issues that similarly require a causal approach. Attention has already been drawn to the need to consider why some individuals persist in their antisocial behaviour whereas others do not. That is important, not only at an individual level, but also at a population level. Thus, across all societies, it is striking that individuals become much less likely to engage in crime during early adult life. They do not necessarily lose the lifestyle characteristics that were associated with their antisocial behaviour but nevertheless they become much less likely to commit crimes. To what extent does this reflect biological changes and to what extent is it a consequence of life circumstances? Certainly, experiences in adult life do make an important impact. For example, several studies have shown that a harmonious marriage to a supportive partner makes it much less likely that individuals will persist in crime (Laub et al., 1998; Sampson & Laub, 1993; Zoccolillo et al., 1992). But are there also biological features within the individual that are influential?

Similarly, we need to ask why it is that crime comes to a peak during the years of adolescence. It is not necessarily the case that any conduct disorder associated with crime peaks at that time; often the conduct disorder has been of much longer standing. The difference is in the tendency for this to be translated into the commission of criminal acts. One might suppose that the key factor would be the surge of testosterone that is such a striking feature of male adolescence. However, although testosterone does have an impact on dominance, its effect on aggression is nowhere near so consistent (Tremblay et al., 1997). Also, however, it is relevant that both self-report and parent-report studies (Moffitt et al., submitted), as well as official crime statistics (Rutter et al., 1998) are consistent in showing that the sex difference in antisocial behaviour is least marked in adolescence.

In that connection, it is important that we gain an understanding of the importance of sex differences in antisocial behaviour. Up until now, the question has usually been posed in terms of either what it is that protects females from antisocial behaviour or in terms of what is special about female crime (on the expectation that it will have its own rather distinctive set of causal influences). Analyses of the data from the Dunedin longitudinal study have shown that a shift in focus is required (Moffit et al., submitted). Several findings were striking. To begin with, the risk factors for antisocial behaviour in males and females were closely comparable; there was no need to invoke any special set of mechanisms that applied only to females.

Second, although antisocial behaviour was indeed generally much more frequent in males than females, confirming the findings from numerous previous studies, the sex difference varied greatly according to life stage and social context. Perhaps most surprising was the finding, but again confirming those from other studies, that domestic violence was equally frequent in males and females. Moreover, this was so whether reliance was placed on reports from the women or from their male partners. Self-reports suggested that most men were inhibited in their use of violence in the family by their adherence both to the cultural convention that you don't hit women or those weaker than yourself, and by the expectation that, if they were violent, they would be quite likely to be reported to the police. Conversely, there is no cultural expectation that women should not hit those who are stronger than they are and their expectation was that, if they were violent, it would be unlikely that they would be reported to the police (an expectation in line with the facts). Whatever the explanation, it is noteworthy that, within the context of the family, the sex difference in violence is lacking, although it does remain the case that, because of their greater strength, violence by the male partner is much more likely to lead to serious injury. It might be supposed that women were simply responding, in self-protection, to male violence, but questioning about who started the violence suggested that explanation is not usually correct.

As already noted, the male preponderance in antisocial behaviour is much more marked in childhood and in adult life than it is in adolescence. One might suppose that this would be the age period in which women were least likely to engage in crime, because all-female groups are much less anti-authority than is the case with all-male groups (Maccoby, 1998). However, the females who engage in crime tend to be part of mixed sex groups, rather than all-female ones. The greatest sex difference applies to life-course-persistent antisocial behaviour, beginning in early childhood and persisting into adult life. Not surprisingly, therefore, the risk factors that were least likely to occur in females were hyperactivity, cognitive deficits and adverse temperamental features. It appears that the focus needs to shift from asking the origins of sex differences in antisocial behaviour more generally to asking why it is that those risk factors that seem to have more in common with the neuropsychiatric problems, all of which are much more common in males, occur less often in females. The investigation of this important topic will require a set of research strategies rather different from those that are ordinarily used to tackle individual differences.

Another topic requiring attention from a causal perspective is the very large increase in the rate of crime over the last half century or so in most industrialized countries (Rutter & Smith, 1995). Given the prevailing assumptions about the increased risks for crime associated with unemployment, with social inequities, and with poverty, it is striking that the major increase in crime occurred during the 1950s and 1970s when social inequalities were narrowing, when affluence was increasing, and when rates of unemployment were unusually low in many countries (including the UK). The findings are a reminder that the risk factors accounting for individual differences in crime may not be the same as those accounting for differences in overall rates of crime over time.

Finally, it is crucial to appreciate that the question of individual predisposition is one thing but whether or not the predisposed individual actually engages in antisocial behaviour is another question. There is a good deal of evidence that situational factors play a substantial role and there are many important prevention strategies that have been devised to build on this body of knowledge (Clarke, 1992, 1995; Rutter et al., 1998).

Heterogeneity

Up to this point in this chapter, reference has mainly been made to the generic concept of antisocial behaviour rather than to the clinical diagnostic categories of oppositional/defiant disorder, conduct disorder, attention deficit with hyperactivity disorder, or antisocial personality disorder. The terminology used has been deliberate because of doubts as to whether the prevailing diagnostic conventions provide the best way of classifying antisocial behaviour. To begin with, it is evident that most antisocial behaviour is most appropriately considered in dimensional terms, rather than present or absent diagnostic categories. That is to say, all individuals have an antisocial propensity to some degree, even though some have it to a much greater extent than others. The evidence available so far does not suggest that the extreme disorders are different in kind from variations along the continuous dimension. It would be premature to rule out that possibility, perhaps particularly with respect to hyperkinetic disorder, but, for the most part, a dimensional concept seems most valid. That does not necessarily mean that it is not useful to have diagnostic categories. After all, categorical decisions do need to be made with respect to who has treatment and to the type of treatment provided. It is just that there is an inevitable degree of arbitrariness on the particular cut-off used to define the diagnostic category.

There is also a considerable question mark hanging over the supposed distinction between oppositional/defiant disorder and conduct disorder. Longitudinal and epidemiological studies suggest that, in many cases, oppositional/defiant behaviour constitutes a milder, earlier onset of a variety of the same liability later shown as conduct disorder (Lahey et al., 1999). Also, many individuals with conduct disorder show oppositional/defiant features in addition. In many cases, it probably makes most sense to view these as variations of the same underlying disorder, with one tending to begin at a much earlier age than the other. Of course, not all children with oppositional/defiant disorder go on to show conduct problems later. The possibility remains that this form of oppositional/defiant disorder when it is confined, or relatively confined, to the early years of childhood, could be somewhat different. The possibility warrants study, but the sharp distinction between these two disorders involving disruptive behaviour is almost certainly unwarranted. In addition, it is relevant that genetic studies have shown that the two share, to a very large extent, the same genetic liability (Eaves et al., in press).

If there is some scepticism about the validity of the present diagnostic conventions, how should heterogeneity be conceptualized and dealt with, because heterogeneity undoubtedly exists? There are two reasonably well-validated differentiations. First, as noted by Angold & Costello (chapter 6, this volume) it is useful to differentiate between life-course-persistent antisocial behaviour and adolescence-limited antisocial behaviour (Moffitt, 1993). The former tends to be evident in early childhood, to be associated with hyperactivity and cognitive differences and, typically, there is more widespread social dysfunction that tends to persist into adult life. Family risk factors, including both parental antisocial behaviour and family discordant disruption, are prominent. By contrast, both the individual and the family risk factors are less strongly evident with respect to adolescence-limited antisocial behaviour. Peer group influences seem to be more important in this group than they are in the life-course-persistent variety, although they play a role in both (Fergusson & Horwood, 1996; Patterson & Yoerger, 1997). The distinction between these two varieties is perhaps not quite as clear-cut as was originally envisaged but the differences are nevertheless marked. It remains uncertain whether they are qualitatively distinct or whether, instead, they represent milder and more severe variants of the same liability.

The second differentiation that seems reasonably well-validated concerns the variety of antisocial behaviour that is accompanied by hyperactivity. As is apparent from what has already been stated, there is uncertainty as to whether this differentiation is largely synonymous with the previous one. This form of antisocial behaviour appears to have a much stronger genetic component and a greater male preponderance (Rutter et al., 1998).

There are other differentiations that warrant further investigation (see Rutter et al., 1998) but these are the two that are most strikingly apparent and which, most obviously, need to be taken into account in all future research. In addition, of course, they have substantial practical clinical implications in terms of their prognostic indications.

Comorbidity

Comorbidity, meaning the concurrent or sequential co-occurrence of supposedly separate psychiatric disorders, is a prominent feature of all epidemiological clinical studies of psychiatric disorders in childhood and adolescence (Angold et al., 1999; Caron & Rutter, 1991; Rutter, 1997). As already noted, the concept raises the prior issue as to whether the disorders that are occurring together are truly separate or whether the co-occurrence is simply a function of the overlapping nature of defining symptomatology or the inadequate conceptualization of the disorders. That is a key question, as we have seen, with respect to oppositional/defiant disorder and conduct disorder. There are, however, three rather separate other forms of apparent comorbidity that require attention. First, there is that between ADHD and ODD/CD. Does the co-occurrence of ADHD and antisocial behaviour define a particular type of disruptive behaviour disorder? If so, within samples where the co-occurrence is evident, the correlates and the genetic liability should be much the same for both sets of symptomatology. Alternatively, are these, indeed, truly separate disorders but in which the occurrence of ADHD in some way predisposes to the development of antisocial behaviour? If so, does that come about because of the cognitive impairments that are associated with ADHD, or does it reflect an increased vulnerability to psychosocial stressors that stems from ADHD, or is it that the negative reactions induced in other people by children's overactive/inattentive behaviour makes them more likely to experience psychosocial stress and adversity? Surprisingly little research so far has seriously attempted to pit these alternative explanatory hypotheses one against the other. There are obvious theoretical implications of whatever answer is obtained but, at least as important, is the fact that an understanding of the mechanisms underlying the comorbidity would have important implications for how one might best plan therapeutic interventions.

Somewhat comparable issues arise with respect to the comorbidity between ODD/CD and drug and alcohol problems. To a considerable extent, it seems reasonable to regard both of these as deriving from the same underlying antisocial predisposition. Neither causes the other but, rather, both stem from similar roots. On the other hand, there is evidence suggesting that that does not constitute the whole story (Rutter et al., 1998). Longitudinal studies show that early manifestations of antisocial behaviour carry with them a much increased likelihood that the person will later show substance misuse or abuse. Does the association mean that the early onset antisocial behaviour is indexing a stronger genetic liability to the composite of antisocial behaviour and substance problems, or does the connection arise in some other way, perhaps because involvement in an antisocial peer group both brings people into contact with others using drugs and also provides a pro-drug culture? Twin studies, particularly if used with longitudinal data, could do much to resolve that issue.

In addition, there is evidence that, in some circumstances, substance misuse also fosters antisocial behaviour (Chaiken & Chaiken, 1991; Collins, 1986). One mechanism may involve the disinhibiting effect associated with the use of alcohol and some other drugs (Ito et al., 1996). This could well predispose to violence (although it is not likely to be of much help if you are a cat burglar!). Also, the purchase of some 'hard' drugs is an expensive matter and people may steal in order to sustain their drug habit. A key point, as with ADHD, is that an understanding of the mechanisms (because there are likely to be several) underlying these patterns of comorbidity may well cast important light on the causal processes involved in conduct disorder.

An apparently somewhat different form of comorbidity is represented by the association between conduct problems and depressive symptomatology (Angold et al., 1999). The empirical research findings seem to suggest that the association works in only one direction. That is, the presence of depressive symptomatology in childhood or adolescence involves no increased risk for antisocial behaviour in later adolescence or early adult life. On the other hand, antisocial behaviour in childhood does involve an increased risk for depressive symptoms in early adult life (Rutter, 1991; Rutter et al., 1997b). Moreover, it seems that this is not simply a function of a pre-existing co-occurrence between antisocial behaviour and depression in childhood. The increased risk is evident from antisocial behaviour in childhood even when that was not accompanied by identifiable emotional disturbance at the time. The possible mechanisms involved in this association have been little investigated up to now. It is quite possible that the answer lies in the tendency for antisocial individuals to act in ways that generate interpersonal stresses and create disadvantageous psycho-social situations – a tendency first well demonstrated by Robins (1966) and confirmed in longitudinal studies undertaken since that time (Champion et al., 1995). However, although it seems highly probable that that constitutes part of the explanation, the necessary studies have not been undertaken to determine whether that provides a sufficient explanation.

Moderating effects and resilience

One of the striking features of all studies of psychosocial stress and adversity is the wide diversity in people's responses (Rutter, in press a). That is so even with the most severe and most prolonged of negative experiences. Our understanding of the mechanisms involved remains quite limited. Still, partial answers are available. To some extent, the explanation lies in the importance of combinations of adverse experiences. On the whole, isolated psychosocial adversities have limited effects; the main psychopathological damage comes about from combinations of risk factors. In part, too, it is likely that prior adversities may render individuals more vulnerable to later stresses. Conversely, successfully overcoming challenges and life problems can be strengthening. Probably, too, it matters how people think about their experiences. It may well be helpful to be able to put even severely negative experiences into a balanced perspective that avoids the development of feelings of personal impotence or failure. It is protective for people to develop a sense of their own self-efficacy (Bandura, 1995, 1997). In addition, too, there is growing evidence of the importance of genetic moderation of environmental effects. That is to say, some genetic factors operate through their role in making people more vulnerable to environmental stress and adversity (Rutter et al., 1997a, 1998). Genetic factors may also be important in their role in making it more likely that people will act in ways that make it more likely that they will experience negative interactions with others or which put them in disadvantageous social situations (Rutter et al., 1995). A key priority is research designed to understand the processes involved in nature–nurture interplay (Rutter et al., 1997a). Genetic factors often operate indirectly through their role in influencing (through gene–environment correlations) people's exposure to risk environments as well as their susceptibility to such environments (through gene–environment interactions), and their skills in coping with the challenges involved (through effects on personality features). As Maughan (chapter 7, this volume) emphasizes, we need to think about causal mechanisms in terms of the dynamic interplay among multiple factors as they operate over time, and not in terms of a fixed effect that determines liability in a direct manner at a single point in time.

Evolutionary considerations

It has become fashionable to seek to view different forms of behaviour in relation to evolutionary considerations (see Ketelaar & Ellis, 2000). This gives rise to questions as to why behaviour that is so obviously maladaptive persists, just as it has also raised questions about why behaviour that is so obviously advantageous (as in the case of high IQ) continues to show a strong genetic influence on individual differences despite evolutionary pressures that might have been expected to eliminate them (Bock & Goode, 2000). In that connection, it is important to bear in mind several key considerations. To begin with, the issue is not the adaptive function of particular behaviours in modern day society but rather the role that they might have followed millions of years ago. Inevitably, that involves a good deal of speculation and supposition that is difficult to test. Second, the question is not whether a behaviour is adaptive with respect to either individual functioning or successful societal functioning, but rather its role in relation to reproductive success. Clearly, antisocial behaviour is disadvantageous in many ways for the individual, and for society, but it is not quite so obvious that it impairs reproductive success. Accordingly, there is no reason to suppose that it will have been subject to strong evolutionary pressures. In that connection, it may be relevant that numerous studies have shown the extent to which both antisocial males and females have a much increased tendency to have children early and, probably, thereby, produce more children (Rutter et al., 1998). Although that carries with it substantial disadvantages in present-day society, it might well have had advantages in a hunter-gatherer society. Third, evolution operates on traits that are under strong genetic influence. Certainly, there are important and substantial genetic influences on antisocial behaviour (see Simonoff, chapter 8, this volume) but they are far from overwhelming. In so far as antisocial behaviour is influenced by environmental features, it will not follow the expectation of evolutionary change. Fourth, research findings make clear that evolutionary forces foster variation as well as universal species-typical characteristics; also effects need to be considered with respect to the implications of varying environmental circumstances (Bock & Goode, 2000). There can be no doubting the importance of evolution but it is not obvious that reference to evolutionary features helps an understanding of antisocial behaviour.

Prevention and intervention

In their different ways, both Maughan & Rutter (chapter 18, this volume) and Knapp (chapter 17, this volume) bring out the high personal and societal costs of conduct disorder. Not only is there a substantial tendency for persistence into adult life, but this is associated with sequelae such as failures in parenting, unemployment, breakdowns in relationships, depressive symptomatology, an increased risk of suicide and the range of problems associated with substance abuse. In addition, of course, there are the costs to society associated with the crimes committed by the individual with conduct problems. The successful prevention of conduct disorder, or of its consequences, would have substantial social and economic benefits.

LeMarquand et al. (chapter 16, this volume) provide an admirable summary of the different approaches that have been followed, together with the evidence on their benefits. The research findings give rise to an attitude of cautious optimism. Although antisocial behaviour constitutes one of society's more intractable problems, there are things that can be done.

Kazdin (chapter 15, this volume) provides a comparable service with respect to therapeutic interventions. He notes the lack of evidence for traditional counselling or relationship approaches but points to the modest efficacy of four, somewhat related, modes of intervention; parent management training (PMT), cognitive problem-solving skills training (PSST), functional family therapy (FFT) and multisystemic therapy (MST). Each focuses on interpersonal interactions and on means of coping with real life challenges and problems, but does so with somewhat different emphases and therapeutic techniques.

In pointing to the demonstrated benefits of these forms of intervention, he also draws attention to some of the key challenges that remain. Even the very best of studies have been troubled by rather high dropout rates from treatment. Not only are the interventions quite demanding of what they ask of families but many of the parents do not view the needs in the same way as do the therapists (or for that matter the law enforcers). Provided that there is a high degree of cooperation from the family as a whole, quite a lot can be done to help young people troubled with antisocial behaviour. The difficulty is in knowing how to get that high degree of commitment and to maintain it over time. In addition, Kazdin notes the marked individual differences in response. In some cases there are clear and lasting benefits whereas in others the changes are modest in the extreme, and in some instances things actually get worse. The Patterson group (Patterson & Chamberlain, 1994; Stoolmiller et al., 1993) have paid particular attention to the need to understand better what underlies these individual differences, because such an understanding seems needed if we are to improve our methods of intervention. That constitutes one key priority. A somewhat related question is the need to determine which elements in the therapeutic programme bring the benefits. For very good reasons, most of the successful interventions are multifaceted (because the problems being dealt with involve many elements and the difficulties experienced by the young people extend, of course, to many social settings). Nevertheless, if we are to improve our methods of treatment in the future, we do need to learn more about the mechanisms involved in successful treatments. That requires the research to be planned in such a way as to measure the different postulated therapeutic mediating variables and to analyse the factors involved with individual differences in change within the treated group (see Forgatch & De Garmo, 1999). Kazdin also notes that we know rather more about the effects of treatment on targeted specific behaviours than we do about the effects on positive social functioning and on a reduction in overall social impairment.

Conclusions

In the past, many clinicians have groaned with each referral of a new child with a conduct problem, feeling that little could be done to help, that they had a rather limited understanding of the meaning and origins of such behaviour, and that it was most uncertain whether psychiatrists had anything very useful to offer for disorders of this kind. The chapters in this volume indicate the extent to which the field has moved ahead in a positive direction. A neat package of answers is not yet available but not only has a greatly increased level of understanding been provided but there are excellent leads available on both how research might take things further and on how clinical practice might be improved.

REFERENCES

Angold, A., Costello, E. & Erkanli, A. (1999). Comorbidity. *Journal of Child Psychology and Psychiatry*, 40, 55–87.

Bandura, A. (Ed.) (1995). *Self-efficacy in Changing Societies*. Cambridge: Cambridge University Press.

Bandura, A. (1997). *Self-efficacy: The Exercise of Control*. New York: Freeman.

Bock, G. & Goode, J. (2000). *The Nature of Intelligence*. Novartis Foundation Symposium 233. Chichester: John Wiley & Sons.

Caron, C. & Rutter, M. (1991). Comorbidity in child psychopathology: concepts, issues and research strategies. *Journal of Child Psychology and Psychiatry, 32,* 1063–80.

Chaiken, J. & Chaiken, M. (1991). Drugs and predatory crime. In M. Tonry & J. Wilson (Eds.), *Drugs and Crime* (pp. 203–40). Chicago: University of Chicago Press.

Champion, L.A., Goodall, G. & Rutter, M. (1995). Behavioural problems in childhood and stressors in early adult life. I: A 20-year follow-up of London school children. *Psychological Medicine, 25,* 231–46.

Clarke, R.V. (1992). *Situational Crime Prevention: Successful Case Studies.* Albany, NY: Harrow and Heston.

Clarke, R.V. (1995). Situational crime prevention. In M. Tonry & D.P. Farrington (Eds.), *Crime and Justice,* Vol. 19 (pp. 91–149). Chicago: University of Chicago Press.

Collins, J. J. (1986). The relationship of problem drinking to individual offending sequences. In A. Blumstein, J. Cohen, J.A. Roth & C.A. Visher (Eds.), *Criminal Careers and Career Criminals* (pp. 89–120). Washington, DC: National Academy Press.

Eaves, L., Maes, H., Rutter, M. & Silberg, J. (in press). Genetic and environmental causes of covariation in interview assessments of disruptive behavior in child and adolescent twins. *Behavior Genetics.*

Fergusson, D.M. & Horwood, L.J. (1996). The role of adolescent peer affiliations in the continuity between childhood behavioral adjustment and juvenile offending. *Journal of Abnormal Child Psychology, 24,* 205–21.

Forgatch, M.S. & DeGarmo, D.S. (1999). Parenting through change: An effective prevention program for single mothers. *Journal of Consulting and Clinical Psychology, 67,* 711–24.

Fraser, I.W. (in press). Decision making and assessment of competence in individuals with a learning disability. *Appendix to Guidelines for Researchers and Ethics Committees on Psychiatric Research Involving Human Participants.* London: Royal College of Psychiatrists.

Gardner, F.E.M., Sonuga-Barke, E.J.S. & Sayal, K. (1999). Parents anticipating misbehaviour: An observational study of strategies parents use to prevent conflict with behaviour problem children. *Journal of Child Psychology and Psychiatry, 40,* 1185–96.

Holden, G.W. (1983). Avoiding conflict: Mothers as tacticians in the supermarket. *Child Development, 54,* 233–40.

Ito, T., Miller, N. & Pollock, V.E. (1996). Alcohol and aggression: A meta-analysis on the moderating effects of inhibitory cues, triggering events, and self-focused attention. *Psychological Bulletin, 120,* 60–82.

Ketelaar, T. & Ellis, B.J. (2000). Are evolutionary explanations falsifiable? Evolutionary psychology and the Lakotosian philosophy of science. *Psychological Inquiry, 11,* 1–21, 56–68 (& commentary 22–55).

Lahey, B.B., Waldman, I.D. & McBurnett, K. (1999). The development of antisocial behavior: An integrative causal model. *Journal of Child Psychology and Psychiatry, 40,* 669–82.

Laub, J.H., Nagin, D.S. & Sampson, R.J. (1998). Trajectories of change in criminal offending: Good marriages and the desistance process. *American Sociological Review, 63,* 225–38.

Maccoby, E.E. (1998). *The Two Sexes: Growing Up Apart, Coming Together.* Cambridge, MA: Belknap.

Moffitt, T.M. (1993). Adolescence-limited and life-course-persistent antisocial behavior: A developmental taxonomy. *Psychological Review, 100*, 674–701.

Moffitt, T., Caspi, A., Rutter, M. & Silva, P. (submitted). Sorting out sex differences in antisocial behavior: Findings from the first two decades of the Dunedin longitudinal study.

Nagin, D. & Tremblay, R.E. (1999). Trajectories of boys' physical aggression, opposition, and hyperactivity on the path to physically violent and nonviolent juvenile delinquency. *Child Development, 70*, 1181–96.

Parker, J.G. & Asher, S.R. (1987). Peer relations and later personal adjustment: Are low-accepted children at risk? *Psychological Bulletin, 102*, 357–89.

Patterson, G.R. & Chamberlain, P. (1994). A functional analysis of resistance during parent training therapy. *Clinical Psychology and Scientific Practice, 1*, 53–70.

Patterson, G.R. & Yoerger, K. (1997). A developmental model for late-onset delinquency. In R. Dienstbier & D.W. Osgood (Eds.), *The Nebraska Symposium on Motivation. Vol. 44: Motivation and Delinquency* (pp. 119–77). Lincoln: University of Nebraska Press.

Richters, J.E. & Cicchetti, D. (1993). Mark Twain meets DSM–III–R: Conduct disorder, development, and the concept of harmful dysfunction. *Development and Psychopathology, 5*, 5–29.

Robins, L. (1966). *Deviant Children Growing Up*. Baltimore: Williams & Wilkins.

Rowe, D.C., Woulbroun, E.J. & Gulley, B.L. (1994). Peers and friends as nonshared environmental influences. In E.M. Hetherington, D. Reiss & R. Plomin (Eds.), *Separate Social Worlds of Siblings: Impact of Nonshared Environment on Development* (pp.159–73). Hillsdale, NJ: Lawrence Erlbaum Associates.

Rutter, M. (1991). Childhood experience and adult psychosocial functioning. In G.R. Bock & J. Whelan (Eds.), *The Childhood Environment and Adult Disease*, CIBA Foundation Symposium 156 (pp. 189–200). Chichester: John Wiley & Sons.

Rutter, M. (1997). Comorbidity: Concepts, claims and choices. *Criminal Behaviour and Mental Health, 7*, 265–85.

Rutter, M. (in press *a*). Psychosocial influences: Critiques, findings and research needs. *Development and Psychopathology*.

Rutter, M. (in press *b*). Children's level of understanding of medical decisions. In *Guidelines for Researchers and Ethics Committees on Psychiatric Research Involving Human Participants*. London: Royal College of Psychiatrists.

Rutter, M. & Smith, D.J. (Eds.) (1995). *Psychosocial Disorders in Young People: Time Trends and their Causes*. Chichester: John Wiley & Sons.

Rutter, M., Champion, L., Quinton, D., Maughan, B. & Pickles, A. (1995). Understanding individual differences in environmental risk exposure. In P. Moen, G.H. Elder, Jr. & K. Luscher (Eds.), *Examining Lives in Context: Perspectives on the Ecology of Human Development* (pp. 61–93). Washington, DC: American Psychological Association.

Rutter, M., Dunn, J., Plomin, R., Simonoff, E., Pickles, A., Maughan, B., Ormel, J., Meyer, J. & Eaves, L. (1997*a*). Integrating nature and nurture: Implications of person–environment correlations and interactions for developmental psychology. *Development and Psychopathology, 9*, 335–64.

Rutter, M., Giller, H. & Hagell, A. (1998). *Antisocial Behavior by Young People*. New York: Cambridge University Press.

Rutter, M., Maughan, B., Meyer, J., et al. (1997b). Heterogeneity of antisocial behavior: Causes, continuities and consequences. In R. Dienstbier & D.W. Osgood (Eds.), *Nebraska Symposium on Motivation. Vol. 44: Motivation and Delinquency* (pp. 45–118). Lincoln, NE: University of Nebraska Press.

Sampson, R.J. & Laub, J.H (1993). *Crime in the Making: Pathways and Turning Points through Life*. Cambridge, MA: Harvard University Press.

Stoolmiller, M., Duncan, T., Bank, L. & Patterson, G.R. (1993). Some problems and solutions in the study of change: Significant patterns in client resistance. *Journal of Consulting and Clinical Psychology, 61*, 920–8.

Tremblay, R.E., Schall, B., Boulerice, B. & Perusse, D. (1997). Male physical aggression, social dominance and testosterone levels at puberty: A developmental perspective. In A. Raine, P. Brennan, D.P. Farrington & S.A. Mednick (Eds.), *Biosocial Bases of Violence* (pp. 271–92). New York: Plenum Press.

Tremblay, R.E., Japel, C., Pérusse, D., et al. (1999). The search for the age of 'onset' of physical aggression: Rousseau and Bandura revisited. *Criminal Behaviour and Mental Health, 9*, 8–23.

Zoccolillo, M., Pickles, A., Quinton, D. & Rutter, M. (1992). The outcome of childhood conduct disorder: Implications for defining adult personality disorder and conduct disorder. *Psychological Medicine, 22*, 971–86.

Index

Note: page numbers in bold indicate figures; those in italic, tables.

Lightning Source UK Ltd.
Milton Keynes UK
UKOW020851090413

208924UK00002B/4/A